# Burt and Eklund's Dentistry, Dental Practice, and the Community

# Burt and Eklund's Dentistry, Dental Practice, and the Community

SEVENTH EDITION

**Ana Karina Mascarenhas, BDS, MPH, DrPH, FDS RCPS (Glasgow)**

Past President
American Association of Public Health Dentistry
Fort Lauderdale, Florida

**Christopher Okunseri, BDS, MSc, MLS, DDPH RCSE (England), FFD RCSI (Ireland)**

Marquette University School of Dentistry
Milwaukee, Wisconsin

**Bruce A. Dye, DDS, MPH**

National Institute of Dental and Craniofacial Research
National Institutes of Health
Bethesda, Maryland

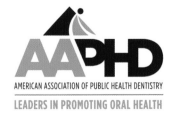

ELSEVIER

AMERICAN ASSOCIATION OF PUBLIC HEALTH DENTISTRY
LEADERS IN PROMOTING ORAL HEALTH

# ELSEVIER

Elsevier
3251 Riverport Lane
St. Louis, Missouri 63043

BURT AND EKLUND'S DENTISTRY, DENTAL PRACTICE, AND THE COMMUNITY,
SEVENTH EDITION
ISBN: 978-0-323-55484-8

Previous editions copyrighted 2005, 1999, 1992, 1983, 1969, and 1964.

**Library of Congress Control Number: 2019955907**

*Content Strategist:* Joslyn A. Dumas/Alexandra Mortimer
*Content Development Specialist:* Joanie Milnes
*Publishing Services Manager:* Deepthi Unni
*Project Manager:* Radjan Lourde Selvanadin
*Design Direction:* Brian Salisbury

Printed in China

Last digit is the print number: 9  8  7  6  5  4  3  2  1

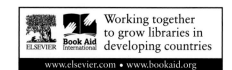

*To Brian Burt*
*Teacher, Mentor, and Friend*
*And To Our Families*

# Preface to the Seventh Edition

The preface to the sixth edition noted "Change is the only true constant in our uncertain world." The world described by Brian and Steve came to pass with substantial social and political change that has impacted our profession and the populations we care for, not only in the US but across our world. A world that constantly continues to shrink not in time and space, but in impacts of our actions and the reach of connectivity and technology.

As in the sixth edition, the purpose of this book is to prepare the next generation of Dental Public Health specialists by presenting concepts against the backdrop of social events: economic, technological, and demographic trends, as well as the distribution of the oral diseases that dental professionals treat and prevent. While substantial changes and rewriting were done, a reasonable amount of work from the sixth edition and Brian and Steve's words have been retained, hence the naming of this new edition as Burt and Eklund's Dentistry, Dental Practice, and the Community. Another purpose and guiding principle for this new seventh edition is the recognition that the practice of Dental Public Health is not undertaken by specialists alone, but is advanced by the efforts of a wide range of oral health professionals and like-minded individuals. Consequently, it is our hope this edition can serve this diverse *community* of dental public health practitioners well.

The lineage of this book can be traced from the landmark work of Pelton and Wisan's *Dentistry in Public Health*, first published in 1949, up to the sixth edition in 2005 by Brian Burt and Stephen Eklund. We carry on the tradition in this seventh edition, which has 28 chapters in four parts. There has been substantial reorganization and several new chapters included. Part I, Dentistry and the Community looks at the dental profession, the public they serve, social determinants of health, access to care, and deals with ethics. Part II Dental Care Delivery deals with the everchanging delivery and financing of dental care, the emerging dental workforce, infection control and mercury safety, reading the literature, and evidence-based dentistry. Part III Methods and Measurement of Oral Diseases and Conditions, besides the traditional nitty-gritty of oral epidemiology, to the various indexes used to measure oral disease, and the distribution of these diseases in the population and associated risk factors, now includes a new robust chapter on applications of biostatistics in dental public health. Part IV Health Promotion and Prevention of Oral Disease addresses oral health promotion, oral health literacy, and the prevention of oral diseases and conditions.

We have continued the style used in the sixth edition, such as the use of the term *dental professionals*, to include dental hygienists, dental therapists, and dentists as colleagues working together. The goal for all working together in dental public health is to improve the oral health of the communities we work in. As our world becomes more connected and the knowledge base expands, we learn from the global experiences of others. An example of recognizing the importance of this is the inclusion of a chapter on dentistry in Canada, which was not part of the sixth edition, but was present in the fourth edition. Other, smaller examples of the global knowledge gained in dental public health populates many of the chapters in this new edition.

We owe a debt of gratitude to the many chapter authors and the Elsevier team who have made this seventh edition a reality for the next generation of our specialty of Dental Public Health. We pay special tribute to Dr. Howard L. Bailit for his many contributions to dental public health and his last chapter in this seventh edition. The final responsibility however for this book lies with us, and with us alone.

As we pass into the third decade of this twenty-first century in an ever-changing world both socially and politically, as health professionals, we dental public health professionals and oral health professionals must provide leadership, adapt, and innovate. We hope that this book will encourage and engage readers to innovate and lead.

**Ana Karina Mascarenhas, BDS, MPH, DrPH,
FDS RCPS (Glasgow)
Bruce A. Dye, DDS, MPH
Christopher Okunseri, BDS, MSc, MLS,
DDPH RCSE (England), FFD RCSI (Ireland)**

# Foreword

I am indebted to be the Executive Editor for the Seventh Edition of Burt and Eklund's Dentistry, Dental Practice, and the Community as this brings my life full circle. In my dental school in Goa, India, the Third Edition co-authored by Striffler, Young, and Burt was a required textbook. This book then led me to apply to the University of Michigan to study with Brian Burt. Since then, there has been no looking back. And so, it is with a heavy heart that during the writing of this book both men who played a large part in my life, my father Rico and Brian passed. It is only fitting that this book is dedicated to them. Much love and respect for the long-standing support to my loved ones, both personal and professional in India and the US.

**– Ana Karina**

As I reflect back upon the early years of my career in public health, Brian's presence was instrumental in reminding me of the importance of the foundational sciences in public health – epidemiology and biostatistics in transforming data to information that could guide change. It has been a great honor to participate in the development of this new edition. Many thanks to my family and colleagues for their support and encouragement throughout.

**– Bruce**

My services as a co-editor of this book would not have been possible without the support of my family. To my amazing wife Elaye, thank you for your patience and unwavering support through long hours of review and editing. My children, Tesse and Tenny, thank you for bringing such joy and wonder into my life and for motivating me to seek excellence in all I do.

**– Chris**

# Contents

[†]Deceased

# List of Contributors

Jasim M. Albandar, DDS, DMD, PhD
Temple University
Philadelphia, Pennsylvania

David Albert, DDS, MPH
Columbia University
New York, New York

Kathryn A. Atchison, DDS, MPH
UCLA School of Dentistry and Fielding
  School of Public Health
Los Angeles, California

Amir Azarpazhooh, DDS, MSc, PhD, FRCD(C)
University of Toronto
Toronto, Ontario

Victor M. Badner, DMD, MPH
Jacobi Medical Center
New York, New York

Howard L. Bailit, DMD, PhD†
University of Connecticut
Storrs, Connecticut

Jagan Kumar Baskaradoss, BDS, MPH, MJDF
RCS (ENG)
Kuwait University
Kuwait City, Kuwait

Pradeep Bhagavatula, BDS, MPH, MS
Marquette University School of Dentistry
Milwaukee, Wisconsin

Vinodh Bhoopathi, BDS, MPH, DScD
Temple University Kornberg School of Dentistry
Philadelphia, Pennsylvania

Derek R. Blanchette, MS, PStat
University of Iowa
Iowa City, Iowa

Wenche S. Borgnakke, DDS, MPH, PhD
University of Michigan
Ann Arbor, Michigan

Brian Burt, BDS, MPH, PhD†

Benjamin W. Chaffee, DDS, MPH, PhD
University of California San Francisco
San Francisco, California

Matt Crespin, MPH, RDH
Children's Health Alliance of Wisconsin /
  Children's Wisconsin
Milwaukee, Wisconsin

Eve Cuny, MS
University of the Pacific Arthur A. Dugoni School
  of Dentistry, San Francisco
San Francisco, California

Peter Damiano, DDS, MPH
University of Iowa
Iowa City, Iowa

Deborah V. Dawson, PhD, ScM
University of Iowa
Iowa City, Iowa

Bruce A. Dye, DDS, MPH
National Institutes of Health
Bethesda, Maryland

Paul I. Eke, PhD, MPH, PhD
Centers for Disease Control
Atlanta, Georgia

Kathy Eklund, RDH, MPH
The Forsyth Institute
Cambridge, Massachusetts
Regis College
Weston, Massachusetts

Julie Farmer, RDH, MSc
University of Toronto
Toronto, Ontario, Canada

---

†Deceased

**Jay W. Friedman, DDS, MPH**
Los Angeles, California

**Noha Gomaa, BDS, MSc, PhD**
University of Toronto
Toronto, Ontario, Canada

**Michelle M. Henshaw, DDS, MPH**
Boston University
Boston, Massachusetts

**Hiroko Iida, DDS, MPH**
Health Efficient
Albany, New York

**Marita Rohr Inglehart, Dipl Psych, Dr phil, Dr phil habil**
The University of Michigan
Ann Arbor, Michigan

**Amid I. Ismail, BDS, MPH, MBA, DrPH**
Temple University
Philadelphia, Pennsylvania

**Richie Kohli, BDS, MS**
Oregon Health & Science University
Portland, Oregon

**Elizabeth Krall Kaye, PhD, MPH**
Boston University
Boston, Massachusetts

**Jayanth Kumar, DDS, MPH**
California Department of Public Health
Sacramento, California

**Steven M. Levy, DDS, MPH**
University of Iowa
Iowa City, Iowa

**Teresa A. Marshall, PhD, RD/LD**
University of Iowa
Iowa City, Iowa

**Ana Karina Mascarenhas, BDS, MPH, DrPH, FDS RCPS (Glasgow)**
American Association of Public Health Dentistry
Fort Lauderdale, Florida

**Hannah Maxey, PhD, MPH, RDH**
Indiana University School of Medicine
Bloomington, Indiana

**Colman McGrath, BA, BDentSc, DDPHRCS, MSc, FDSRCS, FFDRCSI, MEd, PhD, FPH, FICD**
The University of Hong Kong
Hong Kong SAR, China

**Susan McKernan, DMD, MS, PhD**
University of Iowa
Iowa City, Iowa

**Michelle McQuistan, DDS, MS**
East Carolina University, School of Dental Medicine
Greenville, North Carolina

**Marisol Tellez Merchan, BDS, MPH, PhD**
Temple University
Philadelphia, Pennsylvania

**Elizabeth Mertz, PhD, MA**
University of California
San Francisco, California

**Peter Milgrom, DDS**
University of Washington
Seattle, Washington

**Jean Moore, DrPH, FAAN**
State University of New York
Albany, New York

**Mark E. Moss, DDS, PhD**
East Carolina University
Greenville, North Carolina

**Christopher Okunseri, BDS, MSc, MLS, DDPH RCSE (England), FFD RCSI (Ireland)**
Marquette University School of Dentistry
Milwaukee, Wisconsin

**Bruce L. Pihlstrom, DDS, MS**
University of Minnesota
Minneapolis, Minnesota

**Carlos Quiñonez, DMD, MSc, PhD, FRCD(C)**
University of Toronto
Toronto, Ontario, Canada

**Julie Reynolds, DDS, MS**
University of Iowa
Iowa City, Iowa

**Georgia G. Rogers, DMD, MPH**
Aberdeen Proving Ground Dental Clinic
    Command
Edgewood, Maryland

**Eli Schwarz, DDS, MPH, PhD, FHKAM, FHKCDS, FACD, FRACDS**
Oregon Health & Science University
Portland, Oregon

**Thayer Scott, BS, MPH**
Boston University Henry M. Goldman School of Dental Medicine
Boston, Massachusetts

**Karl Self, MBA, DDS**
University of Minnesota, School of Dentistry
Minneapolis, Minnesota

**Jayapriyaa R. Shanmugham, BDS, MPH, DrPH**
Boston University
Boston, Massachusetts

**Sonica Singhal, BDS, MPH, PhD, FRCD(C)**
University of Toronto
Toronto, Ontario, Canada

**Vladimir W. Spolsky, DMD, MPH**
UCLA School of Dentistry
Los Angeles, California

**Scott L. Tomar, DMD, MPH, DrPH**
University of Florida
Gainesville, Florida

**John J. Warren, DDS, MS**
University of Iowa
Iowa City, Iowa

**Darien Weatherspoon, DDS, MPH**
National Institutes of Health
Bethesda, Maryland

**Jane A. Weintraub, DDS, MPH**
University of North Carolina at Chapel Hill
    Adams School of Dentistry
Chapel Hill, North Carolina

**Athanasios I. Zavras, DMD, DDS, MS, DrMedSc**
Boston University Henry M. Goldman School of Dental Medicine
Boston, Massachusetts

**Domenick T. Zero, DDS, MS**
Indiana University
Bloomington, Indiana

# PART I

# Dentistry and the Community

# 1

# The Practice of Dentistry and Dental Public Health

BRIAN BURT, BDS, MPH, PHD[†]

ANA KARINA MASCARENHAS, BDS, MPH, DrPH, FDS RCPS

## CHAPTER OUTLINE

Dental practice has existed in some form since the dawn of time, but it is only sometime in the last century that its practitioners in most nations have achieved the status of a profession. Webster's dictionary defines a *profession* as "a calling requiring specialized knowledge and often long and intensive academic preparation" and "the whole body of persons engaged in a calling." The definition of *professionalism* is "the conduct, aims, or qualities that characterize or mark a profession or professional person." These dictionary definitions, however, do not fully capture the essence of a profession or of professionalism: Commitment to patient welfare, ethics, and other professional ideals are not included. Nor are all aspects of professionalism necessarily high minded or noble. Admission to some professional groups can be based on self-perpetuation rather than public good.[43]

Three models of professionalism have been described,[26] none of which by itself fully characterizes dentistry, although collectively they may do so. The first is the *commercial model*, in which dental care is viewed as a commodity sold by the practitioner. The services are thus not based primarily on the client's needs but on what the client is able or willing to buy. This rather crass view is distasteful to many, although there are aspects of it in dental practice. The second is the *guild model*, in which dental care is seen as a privilege with the professional dominant in practitioner–patient relations. Here the professional is the repository of all knowledge and wisdom, the patient is a passive recipient, and the practitioner has an ethical trust to provide the best-quality care. This model has probably been dominant in the United States, although it is slowly merging with the third model, the *interactive model*, in which dental care is considered a partnership of equals. In this model,

practitioner and patient jointly determine care provided through a combination of professional expertise and patient values.

What are the criteria that characterize a profession, and how can a profession be distinguished from, say, a trade union? The first is the criterion given in the dictionary definition—a substantial body of knowledge, a corollary of which is the obligation to keep that knowledge up to date through continuing education. The second is self-regulation, a tradition whereby society delegates to professional groups the legal responsibility for determining who shall join them in serving the public and for disciplining those members who do not meet the profession's requirements. A third and perhaps the main distinguishing criterion of a profession is a code of ethics, guidelines for professional conduct that are rooted in a moral imperative rather than in law or regulation (see Chapter 4). A profession sets its own code of ethics and its own procedures for dealing with infringements. Taking the various criteria mentioned, one can distinguish a profession by the features listed in Box 1.1.

A health profession can then be defined by paraphrasing Webster's definition given earlier: a calling in the health sciences requiring specialized knowledge and one that meets the other criteria listed. Dentistry meets all the requirements of a profession.

Public health is one of those aspects of life that most people take for granted or more likely don't think about at all. We take for granted that we can drink a glass of water without thinking about cholera, choose a restaurant without concern about rats in the kitchen, and buy a can of vegetables without worrying about botulism. The source of the occasional outbreak of food poisoning is rapidly identified by the authorities, and thoughts of scarlet fever, typhoid, and poliomyelitis simply never enter our heads. To many of the younger generations, dental caries is almost as distant as these infectious diseases of the past. But this happy state of affairs has not just happened; rather, it is the endpoint of years of public health research and practice.

The low profile of public health has both good and bad aspects. Although it is good that mostly invisible basics like drains, sewage treatment, fluoridated drinking water, food quality and safety, and immunizations against infectious diseases are part of the accepted institutions of modern life, it is not good that most people have so little grasp of how public health functions. It is not good because, without a constituency to press for it, funding and legislation for public health can be eroded—with subsequent threats to health and the quality of life. In contrast, everyone is acutely conscious of access (or lack of it) to personal health services, and that subject is a constant political issue. The development of the public health

---

**• BOX 1.1　Characteristics of a Profession**

- A body of knowledge exists that is constantly being expanded, updated, and archived in a literature record. The purpose is constant improvement of the quality of the profession's service to individuals and to the public.
- Academic preparation is required, carried out in specialized institutions.
- The profession and its members accept a lifelong commitment to continuing education.
- Society awards the profession the privilege of self-regulation, which means determining the requirements for entering and remaining in the profession and dealing with those members who do not meet the requirements.
- Its members subscribe to a code of ethics drawn up by the profession itself.
- The members form organized societies to enhance the development of the group and its societal mission and to serve its individual members.

---

infrastructure has taken a long time and has required some painful lessons in lifting our quality of life to its present level.

The purpose of this chapter is to examine the development, structure, and practice of dentistry and dental public health in the United States and to develop the theme that dental public health and private dental practice need to work together for the good of the community's oral health. The chapter also discusses an essential element of dental public health, the collection and use of data in dental public health.

## Development of the Dental Profession

Dental diseases have afflicted the human race since the dawn of recorded history.[24,40] Dentistry, however, has existed as a vocation only in recent years, historically speaking, and it was not until modern times that any sort of scientific basis was developed for the care of oral diseases. One landmark event was the 1728 publication of Pierre Fauchard's *Le Chirurgien Dentiste, ou Traité des Dents*, a two-volume book of more than 800 pages. Fauchard, a Frenchman, is seen as a seminal figure in the evolution of the dental profession. His work was the first complete treatise on dentistry published in the Western world, and it remained an authoritative document for more than 100 years. Despite his lack of formal training, Fauchard was clearly a first-class empiricist with keen powers of observation.

Aspiring dentists of the time served as apprentices. It is worth noting that even the formal education of G.V. Black, one of the profession's most notable 19th-century pioneers, did not exceed 20 months. His introduction to dentistry consisted of "a few weeks" with one Dr. Speers, who was not considered a particularly good dentist and whose dental library consisted of one book.[9] Fortunately, Dr. Black was a true professional and followed the precept that "a professional person has no choice other than to be a continuous student."

The first American dental school was the Baltimore College of Dental Surgery, later part of the University of Maryland, established in 1840. The course was 16 weeks in length after a year or more of apprenticeship. The initial enrollment was five, of whom two graduated. At about the same time, the first national professional dental journal appeared, the *American Journal of Dental Science*, and the first national dental organization, the American Society of Dental Surgeons, was established. The genesis of the dental profession in the United States can thus be dated fairly precisely to the 1840 period. The path of professional progress was not entirely smooth, however, as the emergence of

dentistry as a fledgling profession was followed by a scramble to open proprietary dental schools. In the best American traditions of free enterprise and entrepreneurship, most of these places were run strictly for profit and turned out thousands of graduates whose professional abilities covered the spectrum from respectable to dreadful.

These events led to dentistry's development in the United States as a profession separate from medicine, a position that has been maintained to the present day. This separate development occurred more by chance than by deliberate policy, as the Baltimore dental school was originally intended to be established within the medical school. It was not, but only because of lack of space and internal friction among medical school faculty. The separation of dentistry from medicine was standard in the English-speaking world, Scandinavia, and some other European countries, but in central and southern Europe, by contrast, there was a division between stomatologists (physicians with specialty training in clinical dentistry) and dentists, who in this context were considered second-level providers. This division of labor is thought not to have benefited oral health in most of the countries concerned[14] and was abandoned in most of them as the European community moves toward standardization of professional training. On the other hand, it is debatable whether American dentistry benefited from its evolution on a branch that grew out of the main medical trunk, rather than being more closely allied to medicine during its formative years. By the early 21st century, there were signs that dentistry might be evolving into something closer to the medical model.

The era of modern dentistry could be said to date from the closing of the last proprietary school in 1929, which came shortly after the landmark Gies report on dental education. Gies collected information from the dental schools of the time and concluded that the dental profession would only progress when dental education became university based and subject to the maintenance of high standards through accreditation. The 1930s and 1940s were a hard time for dental education and dental practice. The teaching of basic science was often perfunctory, and the emphasis in the clinical sciences was almost entirely on restorative dentistry and prosthetics. Subjects such as radiology, oral diagnosis, endodontics, periodontics, and pediatric dentistry were neglected in many dental schools, and full-time faculty were the exception rather than the rule. There were few educational programs for the preparation of specialists, and those that did exist varied in quality and length.[23] One of the few bright spots during this difficult period was the beginning of the first controlled water fluoridation projects in 1945 (see Chapter 25).

With a rapidly expanding postwar economy and population, added to accelerating technologic growth and a spirit of optimism, dentistry entered what some saw as a golden age during the 1950s. New dental materials expanded treatment horizons, and the arrival of the high-speed air-turbine engine in 1957 revolutionized dental practice. Dental research grew rapidly, stimulated by the establishment of the National Institute of Dental Research (now the National Institute of Dental and Craniofacial Research) in 1948, and the publication of *The Survey of Dentistry* in 1961[18] led to improvements in education and practice. Stagnating dental schools were revitalized with the passage of the Health Professions Educational Assistance Act in 1963. This act authorized federal funds for construction and student aid. Later renewals in 1971 and 1976 included per capita funding to support the basic instructional program. In the 15 years from 1963 to 1978, the addition of federal monies to state, local, and private sources spurred the reconstruction of the entire physical plant of dental education.[16] New schools were built too; the number of dental schools had increased from 39 in 1930 to 59 in 1980.[3]

The 1960s and 1970s saw the emergence of comprehensive care, expansion, and growth of the dental team to include dental hygienists and dental assistants, the beginnings of prepaid dental insurance, and the development of a community outlook in dentistry. Growth in the number of dentists and in dental business was sharp—in retrospect perhaps too sharp. The economic downturn following the Vietnam War (1964–1975), added to the decline in dental caries among children (see Chapter 14), led to a growing perception of an oversupply of dentists despite increasing public utilization of services (see Chapters 5 and 8), and continued growth of dental insurance (see Chapter 7). During the 1980s, enrollment in dental schools dropped substantially from its peak during 1977 to 1979 and rose only a little from these levels through the mid-1990s (see Chapter 8). In response, seven dental schools closed during this period (Emory, Fairleigh Dickinson, Georgetown, Loyola of Chicago, Northwestern, Oral Roberts, and Washington University). Applications to dental schools picked up again in the late 1990s, and new dental schools opened in Arizona, Florida, and Nevada, and class sizes grew. By 2019, there were 66 accredited dental schools in the United States.[12]

Today, the major oral diseases continue to be better controlled than ever, and dental practice continues to evolve, adapting to internal and external forces. Research continues to expand our understanding of many oral and craniofacial diseases, including oral-systemic connections, genetics, genomics and bacterial susceptibility, social determinants, and equity. Other features that will shape dental practice are the changing demographic profile (see Chapters 2 and 5), disease patterns (see Chapters 14–19), financing of dental care (see Chapter 7), the dental workforce (see Chapter 8) student indebtedness, interprofessional collaboration, and new restorative materials and technologies.

## What Is Public Health?

*Health* is an elusive concept to define. The often-quoted World Health Organization (WHO) definition[44] states that "health comprises complete physical, mental, and social well-being and is not merely the absence of disease." Noble indeed, but too idealistic to be of much practical value. A sociologist's more pragmatic definition is that health is "a state of optimum capacity for the performance of valued tasks."[27] This is a more useful definition in that it presents health as a means to an end: that of maximizing the quality of life rather than as an end in itself.

*Public health*, too, does not lend itself to easy definition. Among the many definitions, Winslow's is the most widely accepted and quoted as "the science and art of preventing disease, prolonging life, and promoting physical health and efficiency through organized community efforts."[42] A more useful definition of the public health mission, which accepts health as a means rather than an end, is "fulfilling society's interest in assuring conditions in which people can be healthy."[19] That seems to encompass everything from maintaining the stratospheric ozone layer to picking up the garbage to providing recreational facilities, decent housing, or dental care where needed. This definition might have been ahead of its time in stressing the public responsibility for a healthy physical and social environment, while still leaving some room for personal choices ("…in which people *can* be healthy").

The landmark 1988 report of the Institute of Medicine (IOM), from which the last definition came, went on to describe the functions of public health agencies as the following:

- *Assessment.* The regular collection and dissemination of data on health status, community health needs, and epidemiologic issues.
- *Policy development.* Promotion of the use of the base of scientific knowledge in decision making on policy matters affecting the public's health.
- *Assurance.* The provision of services necessary to achieve mutually agreed-upon goals, either directly, by encouraging other entities to supply them, or by regulation.[19]

These three domains have become the foundation for evaluating many aspects of the public health mission. The IOM's follow-up report and assessment in 2002 incorporated the broader, more inclusive view of public health that emerged with the new century. This view states that, although governmental agencies remain the backbone of the public health system, they cannot and should not do the job alone.[20] The IOM report goes beyond the traditional view of individual responsibility for health and bases its recommendations on the concept of *population health*, defined as "the health of a population as measured by health status indicators and as influenced by social, economic, and physical environments, personal health practices, individual capacity and coping skills, human biology, early childhood development and health services."[20]

The essence of understanding population health is grasping that people's health is a function of more than just biology and other individual clinical factors. People influence and are influenced by the values and beliefs of the broader community in which they live and work. To illustrate, exhorting a person to stop smoking is likely to be fruitless if everyone in that individual's world smokes and smoking is an important part of the person's social interactions. Similarly, attempts to persuade a person to eat more vegetables will fail when the social environment calls for a diet of deep-fried foods or when needed items are not available or local food stores do not stock them.

All of this means that in the promotion of public health, governmental public health agencies need to coordinate with community-based organizations, the healthcare delivery system, academia, business, and the media if good population health is to be achieved. A shift of the mindset more toward population health and away from purely individual health could help. The United States is easily the world leader in healthcare expenditures, but its rankings on general population health status measures are low. A shift in where we invest our healthcare resources would help redress that imbalance, which the more recent 2012 IOM report *For the Public's Health: Investing in a Healthier Future* affirmed[21]—though this is not easy in a society in which individualism is dominant.

The core of public health practice is shown in Box 1.2, which presents a succinct definition of the mission and essential services that only public health can provide. This statement, developed by the American Public Health Association in 1994, has since received virtually universal acceptance including by the Centers for Disease Control and Prevention (CDC).

## Identifying a Public Health Problem

Ask people on the street whether they consider human immunodeficiency virus (HIV) or West Nile virus a public health problem, and most will give a resoundingly affirmative reply. What about deaths from traffic accidents? There will be more equivocation,

**Vision:** Healthy people in healthy communities
**Mission:** Promote physical and mental health and prevent disease, injury, and disability

**What Public Health Does: the *Purpose* of Public Health**
- Prevents epidemics and the spread of disease
- Protects against environmental hazards
- Prevents injuries
- Promotes and encourages healthy behaviors and mental health
- Responds to disasters and assists communities in recovery
- Assures the quality and accessibility of health services

**How Public Health Serves: The *Practice* of Public Health –
10 Essential Public Health Services**
1. Monitors health status to identify and solve community problems
2. Diagnoses and investigates health problems and health hazards in the community
3. Informs, educates, and empowers people about health issues
4. Mobilizes community partnerships and action to identify and solve health problems
5. Develops policies and plans that support individual and community health efforts
6. Enforces laws and regulations that protect health and ensure safety
7. Links people to needed personal health services and ensures the provision of healthcare when otherwise unavailable
8. Ensures a competent public and personal healthcare workforce
9. Evaluates effectiveness, accessibility, and quality of personal and population-based health services
10. Researches for new insights and innovative solutions to health problems

health agency for attention, virtually by definition it is a public health problem. If a president, governor, or mayor defines a public health problem by decree, then a public health problem it is, regardless of whether public health professionals agree. These latter two types of decisions, legislative mandate and executive order, can have the advantage of ensuring immediate action and the potential disadvantage of disturbing the orderly process of program planning and operation.

Today, we define a public health problem as an issue that meets the following criteria:
- A condition or situation is a widespread actual or potential cause of morbidity or mortality.
- There is a perception on the part of the public, government, or public health authorities that the condition is a public health problem.

To use cigarette smoking as an illustration, the first condition has been satisfied based on the first report of the Surgeon General of the United States in 1964,[35] and there is no question that the second condition has also been met. These criteria have also been met for the HIV epidemic.[34] Allocation of public resources to deal with a recognized problem is a logical consequence, although not a criterion for problem recognition. In the case of cigarette smoking, there has been considerable action through widespread public education campaigns, advertising bans, efforts to block the sale of cigarettes to minors, and legislation to protect the public and employees from exposure to smoking. On the other hand, the public is divided about condom distribution and needle-exchange programs intended to inhibit the spread of HIV infection.[25]

even though the number of deaths from road accidents in 2016 was almost 10 times higher than that from HIV-related disease.[47] Substance abuse similarly is seen by most as a major social and public health problem, but fewer would view infant mortality as such a problem, even though the United States had only the 56th lowest infant mortality rate globally in 2017.[11] So given that handling a public health problem demands some allocation of resources and some opportunity costs, how is a public health problem determined?

Over the years some criteria have emerged for its definition. As early as 1944, for example, Blackerby listed them as the following: (1) a condition or situation that is a widespread cause of morbidity or mortality, (2) there is a body of knowledge that could be applied to relieve the situation, and (3) this body of knowledge is not being applied.[8] However, these criteria seem unduly restrictive. For example, the Black Death in the 14th century killed off one-third of the population of Europe in 3 years. There is no question that it was a public health problem, even though there was no body of knowledge on how to deal with it. Subsequent epidemics of typhoid, cholera, yellow fever, and other infectious diseases were also public health problems before there were effective means to deal with them, and the same can be said for some viral infections such as the avian flu and Zika today.

Additional criteria can broaden the scope of what constitutes a public health problem. Public perception is one, as in the example of the HIV epidemic. If enough of the public perceive a public health problem, then the mandate exists to allocate resources to deal with it. HIV is in that category. Besides public perception, governmental perception goes far toward defining a public health problem. When a government assigns a problem to its public

## Dental Public Health

Dental public health is one of the nine board-certified specialties of dentistry in the United States and was certified in 1950. The American Board of Dental Public Health adapted Winslow's definition to develop one that was subsequently approved by the American Association of Public Health Dentistry, the Oral Health section of the American Public Health Association, and the American Dental Association (ADA).

That definition—still used today, although there have been attempts to change it to be more contemporary—is:

*Dental public health is the science and art of preventing and controlling dental diseases and promoting dental health through organized community efforts. It is that form of dental practice which serves the community as a patient rather than the individual. It is concerned with the dental education of the public, with applied dental research, and with the administration of group dental care programs as well as the prevention and control of dental diseases on a community basis.[41]*

Implicit in this definition is the requirement that the specialist have broad knowledge and skills in program administration, research methods, the prevention and control of oral diseases, and the methods of financing and providing dental care services. Box 1.3 is the dental corollary of the essential public health functions summarized in Box 1.2, a concise listing of the essential functions of dental public health (sometimes referred to as *core functions*) as adopted by the Association of State and Territorial Dental Directors (ASTDD).

**I. Assessment**

1. Assess oral health status and implement an oral health surveillance system
2. Analyze determinants of oral health and respond to health hazards in the community
3. Assess public perceptions about oral health issues and educate/empower them to achieve and maintain optimal oral health

**II. Policy Development**

4. Mobilize community partners to leverage resources and advocate for/act on oral health issues
5. Develop and implement policies and systematic plans that support state and community oral health efforts

**III. Assurance**

6. Review, educate about and enforce laws and regulations that promote oral health and ensure safe oral health practices
7. Reduce barriers to care and assure utilization of personal and population-based oral health services
8. Assure an adequate and competent public and private oral health workforce
9. Evaluate effectiveness, accessibility and quality of personal and population-based oral health promotion activities and oral health services
10. Conduct and review research for new insights and innovative solutions to oral health problems

1. Manage oral health programs for population health
2. Demonstrate ethical decision-making in the practice of dental public health
3. Evaluate systems of care that impact oral health
4. Design surveillance systems to measure oral health status and its determinants
5. Communicate on oral and public health issues
6. Lead collaborations on oral and public health issues
7. Advocate for public health policy, legislation, and regulations to protect and promote the public's oral health, and overall health
8. Critically appraise evidence to address oral health issues for individuals and populations
9. Conduct research to address oral and public health problems
10. Integrate the social determinants of health into dental public health practice

Dentists and dental hygienists enter the dental public health field when they are employed in the administration of public health programs (which can include health promotion, community prevention, and provision of dental care to specified groups), become faculty members in departments dealing with community-oriented dental practice, or become researchers in epidemiology, prevention, or provision of health services. Some researchers in the behavioral sciences related to dental health can also be considered public health personnel. Dentists become recognized specialists when, in addition to being employed full time in the fields mentioned, they achieve diplomate status with the American Board of Dental Public Health. Specialty certification first requires satisfaction of the educational requirements of the Council on Dental Education and Licensure of the ADA (i.e., at least 2 years of accredited advanced graduate education in the specialty addressing the 10 dental public health competencies in Box 1.4 plus fulfillment of a work experience requirement and then completion of the specialty board examinations).

Although there are fewer than 200 board-certified specialists in dental public health, the specialty's influence on the oral health of the public is greater than those numbers would suggest.[2] Dental public health professionals are employed by federal, state, and local health departments; conduct research in universities and government agencies; and are administrators in the insurance industry, professional organizations, and various foundations. Dental public health practice gets away from the relative isolation of the dental office, as its programs require cooperative effort with other professionals such as physicians, nurses, engineers, social workers, nutritionists, and other public health professionals. Among the rewards is the ability to bring about improvement of the oral health status of whole populations rather than of single patients. Public health dentists serving in the Indian Health Service of the U.S. Public Health Service, for example, have demonstrated over the last generation their ability to upgrade dental care for several million Native Americans from a bare emergency service to comprehensive care for many, carried out in excellent clinical facilities. Similarly, a dental public health professional who institutes water fluoridation in a community has done more for its oral health than could be achieved in a lifetime of private dental practice.

Achievements of dental public health professionals include conducting the epidemiologic studies that established the basis for community water fluoridation, carrying out clinical trials to demonstrate the effectiveness of fluoride toothpastes and other products, and implementing the associated caries-control programs in a wide variety of settings, which have been fundamental to the decline in caries among children.[2] Oral epidemiologists have also charted the natural progression of periodontal diseases,[6] access to dental care, and the dental workforce. Administrators in dental public health pioneered the concept of providing regular dental care in a logical, sequential way for large population groups,[15,17,39] and they demonstrated the increased productivity that efficient use of the dental team brings to patient care.[22,28] Dental hygienists engaged in dental public health have played all the roles above alongside dentists.

To round out this discussion of what dental public health is, it might be useful to state what it is not. It is not just "dentistry for the poor," although provision of care to persons who do not fit the private practice mode is part of it. It is not just "Medicaid dentistry," although improving that creaky and inefficient program should be of concern to all health professionals. Similarly, dental public health is not "socialized dentistry," health maintenance organizations and preferred provider organizations, or expansion of functions of the dental team. And dental public health is not just the provider of last resort. Its function goes well beyond filling the healthcare gaps for those whom the private sector cannot or will not treat.

## Differences Between Personal and Community Healthcare

In addition to the similarities between private and public health practice, there also are some notable differences. It is fair to say that most practitioners do not understand the goals of public health.

That is unfortunate, because both privately and publicly employed dental professionals are working toward the same end: the oral health of the public. At the philosophic level, one major difference between personal care and public health is that the goals of public health are socially determined, whereas the priorities of private care are only coincidentally related to social goals. Another way of looking at this distinction is to say that private care seeks to maximize the chance that the best outcome will occur, often unlimited by resource restraints. Public health, on the other hand, seeks to minimize the chance that the worst outcome will occur.[29]

The private practitioner works more or less alone. Decisions the dentist makes are in the context of his or her training, the legal framework for dental practice, and the dentist–patient relationship. Despite insurance carriers, quality assurance programs, and governmental requirements, the private practitioner is still a relatively independent healthcare provider. By contrast, the public health professional is a salaried employee who is accountable to both an immediate supervisor and to the taxpayers, represented in such forms as a board of health, a community advisory board, and a governing body. Rarely is a major decision in public health made on one's own.

The public health professional often works in communities with special characteristics of culture, language, socioeconomic status, and values. Public health workers often must care for those outside the mainstream, where those characteristics just mentioned make some groups of people more difficult and often more expensive to reach. The challenge in dental public health practice is that patients in these groups often do not share middle-class values with regard to brushing their teeth, keeping appointments, or making regular dental visits, but they still need care if the professional trust of working for the oral health of the public is to be preserved.

## Collection and Use of Data in Dental Public Health

Information on health conditions is fundamental to public health practice, including dental public health practice, and the necessary data can be collected in different ways. Data on vital statistics, plus information on certain infections that could become epidemics, are gathered by a process known as *surveillance.* Surveillance in public health is the ongoing systematic collection, analysis, and interpretation of outcome-specific data for planning, implementation, and evaluation of public health practice.[33] It is an ongoing data collection system that uses methods that are quick, simple, and practical and are designed to put as little burden as possible on the busy health professionals who do the reporting. As a result, the data are usually not as accurate as those collected under a strict protocol in research projects, but they are seen as accurate enough for disease monitoring.

This is a key concept in public health: Data for planning and evaluation, although they must be valid, do not need to be as precise as data in clinical trials. Some data are always better than no data, and the collection of data for public health purposes needs a collection protocol that emphasizes practicality and reliability rather than total precision. One must remember that the main purpose of surveillance is to detect changes in trends or distribution of disease so that investigative or control measures can be initiated if needed. Surveillance is a finger on the pulse of the public's health.

In the United States, surveillance activities at the state and local level are coordinated by the Epidemiology Program Office at the Centers for Disease Control and Prevention (CDC) in Atlanta. Guidelines are available for evaluating surveillance systems.[38] Perhaps the best known of these surveillance systems is the Surveillance, Epidemiology, and End Results (SEER) program for cancer reporting. SEER is the source of virtually all cancer data in the United States (see Chapter 16), including oral cancer.

Data sources for surveillance activities include:
- Vital statistics (e.g., births, deaths)
- Information on reportable diseases (e.g., plague, cholera, yellow fever, and others designated by states)
- Registries (e.g., congenital defects, cancer)
- Administrative data collection systems (e.g., hospital discharge data)

Information is mostly collected by *passive surveillance,* which means that although physicians and hospitals are required to notify appropriate authorities whenever reportable conditions are encountered, the authorities themselves do not actively solicit such data. Some errors of omission undoubtedly occur as a result. On some occasions, health department staff go into the field to collect data, often on a specific disease, for a limited time. The staff people call physicians and hospitals by arrangement to obtain data on new cases and to get demographic and other relevant data. This process is known as *active surveillance* and is similar to investigating an outbreak of an infectious disease.

Until recently, the absence of a surveillance system for oral conditions (other than oral cancer, which is included in cancer registries, and cleft lip and palate, for which some states have registries) hampered the development of targeted approaches to improve oral health. Surveillance in dental public health had been largely restricted to surveys in which samples of a defined population are examined clinically or assessed by questionnaire. Surveys, which have a lot in common with active surveillance, range in scope from large national surveys conducted by federal agencies (see Chapters 12, 14–19), to statewide surveys,[30] to local community surveys conducted by a state or local public health agency.[32] Important though they are, surveys involving clinical examinations can be too expensive and logistically demanding for most state or local agencies. National surveys, conducted by the National Center for Health Statistics and in the past by the National Institute of Dental (and Craniofacial) Research, provide excellent clinical data for the whole nation, but state-level data cannot be pulled out because the sampling system is not so designed. A sampling system that permits extraction of state-level data is possible but would be too expensive for the budget of the National Center for Health Statistics. National data do not work well as a basis for local planning for the reasons given in Box 1.5, and the future of extensive clinical examinations in national surveys continues to be uncertain because of time and cost. More reliance on true surveillance systems, in which useful data can be collected fairly inexpensively, is needed.

A new approach came with the establishment in the mid-1990s of the National Oral Health Surveillance System (NOHSS), a joint venture of the CDC and ASTDD.[37] States wanting to collect their own survey data can now turn to the CDC for help with financing and expertise. The result is that within a fairly short period, a number of states have collected valuable data for planning and evaluation that they otherwise would not have obtained.

The main focus of the NOHSS is on data for a set of eight oral health indicators. In adults these are dental visits, teeth cleaning (professional), complete tooth loss, and loss of six or more teeth. In children these are caries experience, untreated caries, sealants, and fluoridation. The data themselves are state specific and mostly come from several state-based surveys, of which the most used are the Behavioral Risk Factor Surveillance System (BRFSS) for the adult indicators.[36] In these telephone surveys, the core questionnaire developed by the CDC can be adapted by a state health agency for its local needs. Use of chewing tobacco is one example of a topic about which some states want information when the

National surveys that include clinical dental examinations, such as those conducted by the National Center for Health Statistics, provide a superb data set on oral conditions. The data are collected by trained examiners, and the representative sampling ensures that the data are generalizable to the national population. National surveys are not true surveillance, however, and reliance on them as a type of surveillance brings its problems. These can be listed as follows:

- Reliance on primary data collection comes from the underlying view that only trained dental professionals can record oral disease. Experience with the use of death certificates, which are completed by all sorts of untrained persons following standard protocols, is just one example which implies that the traditional attitude has become a dinosaur.
- The protocol for national surveys was developed primarily to record dental caries. However, caries continues to decline, and other conditions are becoming of more concern. In addition, the recording of past disease (restorations and extracted teeth), rather than just present disease, does not fit the philosophy of surveillance and may even be invalid.
- Examination protocols record data at the surface level (caries) and at up to six sites per tooth (periodontitis). However, oral health objectives are stated with the individual person as the unit of measurement, so all that time and effort is probably not well spent.
- There is no good surveillance tool to measure periodontal diseases. Despite all the detailed indexes of periodontal diseases (see Chapter 15), we cannot yet identify a person with active progressing disease.
- Visual-tactile clinical examinations in national surveys consume a lot of resources—they are expensive.
- Public participation in surveys of representative samples of population is diminishing. This problem is severe enough in some instances to introduce response bias—the people who do participate are different in some way from those who do not. This weakens the generalizability of the results, one of the chief reasons for conducting such surveys.
- The sheer logistics of national surveys means that data are nearly always reported late, sometimes years late. More timely data are needed for public health authorities to plan and evaluate programs.

From Beltrán-Aguilar ED, Malvitz DM, Lockwood SA, et al. Oral health surveillance: past, present, and future challenges. *J Public Health Dent*. 2003;63:141–149.

arise from the collected information. For new data collection (step 4 in the seven-step program), a basic screening survey and a training program to use it effectively have been developed by the ASTDD.[5] Again, the principle behind the basic screening survey is to permit limited but valid clinical data to be collected as efficiently and unobtrusively as possible.

WHO has also developed and systematized basic methods of data collection for surveillance of oral conditions in all parts of the world into an approach known as Pathfinder.[45] Although not all details of these methods have received universal acceptance, WHO has succeeded very well in promoting the collection and use of data in parts of the world where previously there was no information at all on oral conditions. The simplicity of the protocol for sampling and data collection permits it to be used by dental personnel with no previous training in survey methods. The country-specific data collected by Pathfinder and other survey methods are maintained in WHO's Global Oral Data Bank.[46]

By whatever method they are collected, dental data are used to identify needs and to plan programs to meet those needs. Functioning programs then need to be evaluated. The results of evaluation can lead to plan modifications, and so the cycle continues. This ongoing process is known as the planning cycle and is illustrated in simplified form in Figure 1.1.

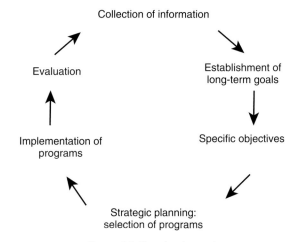

• **Figure 1.1** The planning cycle.

Data from surveys or surveillance are part of the foundation on which public policy at federal, state, and local levels is built. Some federal funding programs for dental public health, such as the Maternal and Child Health block grants, require that needs assessment and planning data be submitted each year with a state's application for funds. Agencies and foundations that fund research use oral survey data to help establish their research priorities, dental schools use them when establishing curricula, state agencies can use them in regulating the activities of dentists and hygienists, and dental insurance companies consult them when establishing benefit packages.

Simply put, dental public health is concern for and activity directed toward the improvement and protection of the oral health of the whole population. Narrowing the role of dental public health only to groups defined as high risk or underserved would exclude such basic activities as the efforts to control tobacco exposure, infection control in dental practice, water fluoridation, dental workforce, access to care, and health disparities.[13] Because organized dentistry also espouses the goal of optimum oral health for all, public and private sectors need to understand each other and work cooperatively if this worthy goal is to be achieved.

habit is known to be a problem, whereas other states do not. The BRFSS telephone surveys began in the early 1980s, and by 1994 all states and territories were participating. These two surveys are the basis for current data on four of the oral health indicators: dental visits, teeth cleaning, complete tooth loss, and fluoridation status.[38] Having both statewide clinical data and BRFSS data gives a state an excellent view of conditions when preparing an oral health plan.

National surveys that include a clinical dental examination of the participants usually involve performance of a lengthy and detailed clinical examination, a type of examination that states could not handle because of the cost—time is money in dental public health as it is anywhere else. Hence, this increased activity in collecting state-level oral health data has been stimulated by the development of quick and simple data collection protocols—again we see the underlying principle of making surveillance as practical as possible, even at the expense of precision.

The first major step toward practical oral health surveillance came in the mid-1990s, when the ASTDD developed a seven-step model for state and local agencies for collecting dental data by choosing from a variety of approaches to best suit local needs.[31] This model includes the planning process, identification of partner organizations, determination of whether new data collection (clinical examinations, telephone surveys, questionnaires) is needed or whether existing data will do, and prioritization of the issues that

# References

1. Altman D, Mascarenhas AK. New competencies for the 21st century dental public health specialist. *J Pub Health Dent.* 2016;76: S18–S28.
2. American Association of Public Health Dentistry, American Board of Dental Public Health. Dental public health: the past, present, and future. *J Am Dent Assoc.* 1988;117:171–176.
3. American Dental Association. Summary of the 1979–1980 annual report on dental education. *J Am Dent Assoc.* 1980;100:926–930.
4. Association of State and Territorial Dental Directors. *Guidelines for State and Territorial Oral Health Programs: Part II. Revised* January 2018. Available from: https://www.astdd.org/state-guidelines.
5. Association of State and Territorial Dental Directors. *ASTDD Basic Screening Surveys.* Available from: https://www.astdd.org/basic-screening-survey-tool.
6. Beck JD, Sharp T, Koch GG, et al. A study of attachment loss patterns in survivor teeth at 18 months, 36 months, and 5 years in community-dwelling older adults. *J Periodont Res.* 1997;32:497–505.
7. Beltrán-Aguilar ED, Malvitz DM, Lockwood SA, et al. Oral health surveillance: past, present, and future challenges. *J Public Health Dent.* 2003;63:141–149.
8. Blackerby Jr PE. Treatment in public health dentistry. In: Pelton WJ, Wisan JM, eds. *Dentistry in Public Health.* Philadelphia, PA: Saunders; 1949:187–221.
9. Burgess K, Ruesch JD, Mikkelsen MC, et al. ADA members weigh in on critical issues. *J Am Dent Assoc.* 2003;134:103–107.
10. Centers for Disease Control and Prevention. *The Public Health System & the 10 Essential Public Health Services.* Available from: https://www.cdc.gov/publichealthgateway/publichealthservices/essentialhealthservices.html.
11. Central Intelligence Agency. *Infant Mortality Rate—The World Factbook.* Available from: https://www.cia.gov/library/publications/the-world-factbook/rankorder/2091rank.html.
12. Commission on Dental Accreditation. *Search for Dental Programs.* Available from: https://www.ada.org/en/coda/find-a-program/search-dental-programs.
13. Corbin SB, Mecklenburg RE. Report on the future of dental public health. *J Public Health Dent.* 1994;54:80–91.
14. Ennis J. *The Story of the Fédération Dentaire Internationale.* London: The Federation; 1967.
15. Freire PS. Planning and conducting an incremental care program. *J Am Dent Assoc.* 1964;68:199–205.
16. Galagan DJ. Back from the brink: how and why U.S. dental schools were rebuilt. *Dent Surv.* 1978;54:14–18.
17. Galagan DJ, Law FE, Waterman GE, et al. Dental health status of children 5 years after completing school care programs. *Public Health Rep.* 1964;79:445–454.
18. Hollinshead BS. *The Survey of Dentistry: The Final Report.* Washington, DC: American Council on Education; 1961.
19. Institute of Medicine. *The Future of Public Health.* Washington, DC: National Academy Press; 1988.
20. Institute of Medicine. *The Future of the Public's Health in the 21st Century.* Washington, DC: National Academies Press; 2003. https://doi.org/10.17226/10548.
21. Institute of Medicine. *For the Public's Health: Investing in a Healthier Future.* Washington, DC: National Academies Press; 2012. https://doi.org/10.17226/13268.
22. Lotzkar SJ, Johnson DW, Thompson MB. Experimental program in expanded functions for dental assistants. Phase 3: experiment with dental teams. *J Am Dent Assoc.* 1971;82:1067–1081.
23. Mann WR. Dental education. In: Hollinshead BS, ed. *The Survey of Dentistry; the Final Report.* Washington, DC: American Council on Education; 1961:239–422.
24. Moore WJ, Corbett ME. The distribution of dental caries in ancient British populations. II. Iron Age, Romano-British and mediaeval periods. *Caries Res.* 1973;7:139–153.
25. Moss AR. Epidemiology and the politics of needle exchange. *Am J Public Health.* 2000;90:1385–1387.
26. Ozar DT. Three models of professionalism and professional obligation in dentistry. *J Am Dent Assoc.* 1985;110:173–177.
27. Parsons T. Definitions of health and illness in light of American values and social structures. In: Jaco EG, ed. *Patients, Physicians, and Illness.* Glencoe IL: Free Press; 1958:165–187.
28. Pelton WJ, McNeal DR, Goggins JK. Student dental health program of the University of Alabama in Birmingham: VI. Chair time expended for the delivery of services. *Ala J Med Sci.* 1971;8:373–377.
29. Pickett G, Hanlon JJ. *Public Health: Administration and Practice.* 9th ed. Times Mirror/Mosby: St. Louis, MO; 1990.
30. Rozier RG, Dudney GG, Spratt CJ. *The 1986–87 North Carolina School Oral Health Survey.* Raleigh, NC: North Carolina Department of Environment, Health, and Natural Resources; 1991.
31. Siegal MD, Kuthy RA. *Assessing Oral Health Needs; ASTDD Seven-Step Model.* Association of State and Territorial Dental Directors: Jefferson City, MO; 1995.
32. Siegal MD, Martin B, Kuthy RA. Usefulness of a local oral health survey in program development. *J Public Health Dent.* 1988;48:121–124.
33. Thacker SB, Berkelman RL. Public health surveillance in the United States. *Epidemiol Rev.* 1988;10:164–190.
34. US Department of Health & Human Services. *U.S. Statistics. Fast Facts.* Available from: https://www.hiv.gov/hiv-basics/overview/data-and-trends/statistics.
35. US Public Health Service. Smoking and Health. Report of the Advisory Committee to the Surgeon General of the Public Health Service. *PHS Publication No. 1103.* Washington, DC: Government Printing Office; 1964.
36. US Public Health Service, Centers for Disease Control and Prevention. *Behavioral Risk Factor Surveillance System.* Available from: http://www.cdc.gov/brfss/index.html.
37. US Public Health Service, Centers for Disease Control and Prevention. *National Oral Health Surveillance System (NOHSS).* Available from: http://www.cdc.gov/oralhealthdata/overview/nohss.html.
38. US Public Health Service, Centers for Disease Control and Prevention. *Updated Guidelines for Evaluating Public Health Surveillance Systems.* Available from: http://www.cdc.gov/mmwr/preview/mmwrhtml/rr5013a1.htm.
39. Waterman GE. The Richmond-Woonsocket studies on dental care services for school children. *J Am Dent Assoc.* 1956;52:676–684.
40. Weinberger BH. *An Introduction to the History of Dentistry, With Medical and Dental Chronology and Bibliographic Data.* St. Louis, MO: Mosby; 1948.
41. Weintraub JA, Rozier RG. Updated competencies for the dental public health specialist: using the past and present to frame the future. *J Pub Health Dent.* 2016;76:S4–S10.
42. Winslow CEA. The untilled fields of public health. *Mod Med.* 1920;2:183–191.
43. Wolfenden CB. What makes a profession? *Br Dent J.* 1975;139: 61–65.
44. World Health Organization. *Constitution of the World Health Organization.* Geneva: WHO; 1946:3.
45. World Health Organization. *Oral Health Surveys; Basic Methods.* 4th ed Geneva: WHO; 1997.
46. World Health Organization. *WHO Oral Health Country/Area Profile Programme.* Available from: https://www.who.int/oral_health/databases/malmo/en.
47. Xu JQ, Murphy SL, Kochanek KD, et al. Deaths: final data for 2016. *Natl Vital Stat Rep.* 2018;67(5):1–76. Available from: https://www.cdc.gov/nchs/data/nvsr/nvsr67/nvsr67_05.pdf.

# 2

# Social Determinants of Health and Oral Health Disparities and Inequities

JANE A. WEINTRAUB, DDS, MPH

MICHELLE M. HENSHAW, DDS, MPH

This chapter starts with describing a few key concepts: health and healthcare disparities, health equity, equality, social determinants of health, and upstream approaches.

## Health and Healthcare Disparities and Inequities

### Health Disparities

Population-specific differences are found across many diseases and healthcare services including oral health. They are important because they are associated with worse health outcomes and generally affect disadvantaged groups. From a population perspective, the factors that contribute to health disparities, such as poorer access to healthcare and poorer health and life expectancy among racial and ethnic minorities, take on particular significance as about 40% of Americans identify as belonging to one of these groups,[48] and this percentage is projected to increase over the next few decades.[9] At individual and population levels, oral health has a great impact on quality of life and well-being. Poor oral health, oral pain, dysfunction, and poor

appearance—whether from tooth loss, craniofacial anomalies, oral cancer, or lack of dental care—can be detrimental to social and emotional well-being and ability to work and learn.[38]

At the turn of the century, *Oral Health in America: A Report of the Surgeon General* brought focus and attention to the "profound and consequential **oral health disparities** within the United States (U.S.) population."[47] This situation is particularly disconcerting in oral health, where many conditions and risk factors are largely preventable. There are several definitions of health disparities and inequities; the scope of the definitions and the goals for overcoming them have expanded over time. In 2002, The Institute of Medicine (IOM; now called the National Academies of Sciences, Engineering, and Medicine) released a landmark report, *Unequal Treatment: Confronting Racial and Ethnic Disparities in Health Care*. The authors defined healthcare disparities narrowly "as racial or ethnic differences in the quality of healthcare that are not due to access-related factors or clinical needs, preferences, and appropriateness of intervention."[20] They raised controversial issues and provided some evidence of bias, prejudice, and stereotyping at the provider, patient, institutional, and health system levels as contributing to differential quality of care.

Almost a decade later, the U.S. Department of Health and Human Services' 2011 report *HHS Action Plan to Reduce Racial and Ethnic Health Disparities* defined health disparities more broadly than the IOM but still limited the focus to differences in racial and ethnic minority groups.[46] Their definition included concepts covered in the IOM definition, such as access to care, preventive care, and preventable hospitalizations, and included additional constructs, such as poorer overall health and more severe forms of serious illness, and identified that these differences are influenced by a diverse set of factors. For example, many American adults have limited English proficiency that exacerbates their inability to navigate the healthcare system and adhere to treatment recommendations.[11]

### National Healthy People Initiative

The National Healthy People Initiative establishes science-based measurable objectives to improve the health of the nation. In Healthy People 2020, the definition of health disparities was broadened even more to include populations beyond racial and ethnic minority groups:

*"... a particular type of health difference that is closely linked with social, economic, and/or environmental disadvantage. Health disparities adversely affect groups of people who have systematically experienced greater obstacles to health based on their racial or ethnic group; religion; socioeconomic status; gender; age; mental health; cognitive, sensory, or physical disability; sexual orientation or gender identity; geographic location; or other characteristics historically linked to discrimination or exclusion."* [41]

Healthy People 10-year goals to address health disparities have also evolved. In Healthy People 2000, the national goal was to reduce health disparities, Healthy People 2010 was to eliminate health disparities, and Healthy People 2020, *"to achieve health equity, eliminate disparities, and improve the health of all groups."* [41]

Although there is not a Healthy People 2020 goal focused specifically on oral health disparities, there are 17 oral health objectives. Progress toward reducing oral health disparities is assessed. [43] Another source of information on health disparities is the Agency for Healthcare Research and Quality (AHRQ)'s annual *National Healthcare Quality and Disparities Report*. This report is based on 250 measures of quality and disparities in care by different racial and socioeconomic groups and trends over time. From 2000 to 2014–15, most measures of disparities continued to show worse care for poor and underinsured populations. [2]

## Health Equity and Equality

Outside of the U.S., the term **health inequalities** has been used more commonly than health disparities. It often refers to health differences among different social class or socioeconomic groups instead of the initial focus on race and ethnicity in the U.S. [8] The two classic Whitehall studies of civil servants in England who all had access to the same healthcare through the National Health Service demonstrated gradients in health and longevity, such as coronary heart disease mortality according to occupation and social class hierarchy in populations where participants were employed and living above the poverty line. [25,26] In contrast to inequalities, which just looks at absolute differences in health outcomes, **health inequities** are health differences among social groups that are avoidable, unnecessary, and unjust. [49,54] Thus, inequities are different from inequalities because they involve the consideration of social justice and fairness.

For example, differences between men and women in the incidence of Sjögren's syndrome are inequalities but not avoidable and inequitable. Differences in incidence of anterior tooth fractures between hockey and non-hockey players would not be considered unfair and unjust. Higher rates of tooth extractions versus endodontic treatment for toothaches among low-income compared to high-income adults would be a health inequity.

The difference between the concepts of equality and equity has been illustrated in a popularized cartoon by artist Angus Maguire, shown in Figure 2.1. [21] Three people of different heights—an adult, a school-age child, and a pre-school child—are trying to look over a fence to watch a baseball game. In the first panel, they are each given one equal-size crate, representing provision of equal resources to stand on, but it does not help them equally, because the shortest person still cannot see over the fence and the taller

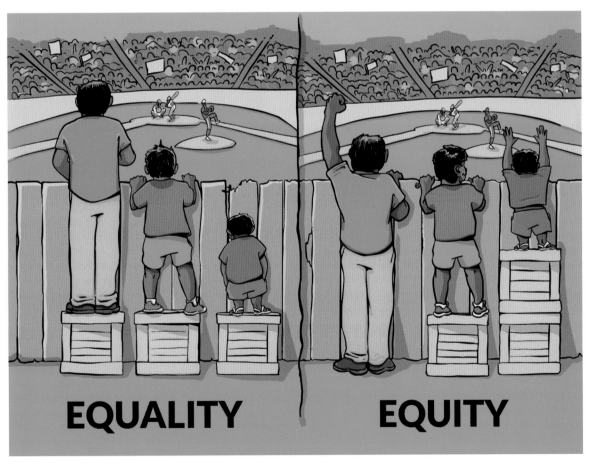

EQUALITY          EQUITY

• **Figure 2.1** Equality Versus Equity. Interaction Institute for Social Change. (Artist: Angus Maguire. interactioninstitute.org and madewithangus.com.) [21]

person does not need the crate. This equal distribution of resources would work if they were the same height, but the short person is at a disadvantage and needs more help. In the second panel, to make the situation equitable, the three boxes are redistributed based on need, so they can stand and all watch the game over the fence—equal outcomes are achieved. Other graphics have emerged that have adapted and modified the original cartoon a step further. Some label the first box "equality" and the second one "justice" or "fairness." Others have added a third image that replaces the wooden fence with a see-through wire fence, and others have removed the fence entirely. These modifications represent system-level changes that reduce or remove the barrier. Some images give each person more boxes to stand on, but the artist argues that would represent adding more resources instead of redistributing existing resources.[14] As applied to oral health, "a short child might need a step stool to reach the sink to brush her teeth, a resource not needed by someone taller, but both should have a tooth brushing opportunity."[16]

Life expectancy is an example of health inequities between and within countries. For example, globally, Japan has the longest life expectancy of 83.7 years, whereas Sierra Leone has the shortest life expectancy, 50.1 years.[51] Where you live within a country also matters to your health. In the U.S., an extensive analysis has shown a 20.1-year gap in geographic inequalities in life expectancy among U.S. counties between those with the lowest (in parts of North and South Dakota, some with Native American reservations) and highest (in Colorado) life expectancies.[10]

An example of geographic oral health inequities are apparent in the prevalence of third graders with untreated caries by state. A PEW 2008 analysis of 28 states revealed a prevalence of 13.2% among children in Iowa and 44% in Nevada, a gap of 30.8%.[33] In an analysis of children's oral health using the 2007 National Survey of Children's Health, state-level variation explained differences in whether a child had a preventive dental visit or fair/poor oral health beyond other child, family, and community factors.[13]

## Social Determinants of Health

To understand the root causes of oral health disparities and inequities, it is necessary to recognize the role of the **social determinants of health**. The World Health Organization (WHO)'s definition of the social determinants of health is "...*the conditions in which people are born, grow, work, live and age, and the wider set of forces and systems shaping the conditions of daily life. These forces and systems include economic policies and systems, development agendas, social norms, social policies and political systems.*"[53] In the geographic oral health disparities example discussed previously, where you live determines your access to healthy food, a safe place to exercise, dental care, and fluoridated water. Some neighborhoods are food deserts that lack fresh fruits and vegetables but have available tobacco products, alcohol, illicit drugs, fast food, and cheap cariogenic snacks. These are some examples of how social determinants of health can influence oral health and contribute to oral health disparities and inequities. However, our understanding of the social determinants of health has expanded as research has begun to explain the underlying biologic pathways of how social determinants such as poverty and living in unsafe neighborhoods impact health.

The Healthy People 2020 objectives address this range of social, economic, and environmental factors that influence health status and serve as the guideposts to measure progress on

addressing health disparities and inequities.[42] Improving social determinants will involve non-health sectors such as education, housing, transportation, and the environment. This intersectoral concept to improve health dates to the WHO Declaration of Alma-Ata in 1978. This declaration called on all countries to work "*to protect and promote the health of all people of the world*" requiring the actions of social and economic sectors in addition to the health sector.[50] It was reaffirmed in 2011 at the World Conference on Social Determinants of Health in Rio de Janeiro as the *Rio Political Declaration on Social Determinants of Health*.[52] To advance these collaborative, intersectoral initiatives, the American Public Health Association with other organizations created the guide *Health in All Policies: A Guide for State and Local Government*.[36] Water fluoridation is an example of successful intersectoral collaboration that brings together boards of health, water treatment operators, dental public health professionals, practicing dentists, pediatricians and other healthcare professionals, community advocates, and political systems to improve oral health. The use of seat belts and child car seats to reduce oral and craniofacial injuries among other types of trauma is another example of intersectoral collaboration.

The "cliff analogy," initially developed by Jones, shown in Figure 2.2, serves to illustrate social determinants of health and of equity and allows us to see how intersectoral initiatives are necessary. Jones and colleagues describe disparities arising from differences in quality of care, access to care, and exposures and opportunities. The illustration depicts different dimensions of interventions to address disparities by: (1) providing health services, (2) addressing the social determinants of health, and (3) addressing the social determinants of equity. To keep people from "falling off the cliff of good health," four interventions are shown, "*including acute care and tertiary prevention (the ambulance at the bottom of the cliff), secondary prevention (the safety net half-way down the cliff face), primary prevention (the fence at the top edge of the cliff), and addressing the social determinants of health (moving the population away from the edge of the cliff).*"[22]

## Upstream Determinants

An important component of social determinants of health are the **upstream determinants**, features of the environment and society that influence individual behavior and disease. The metaphor "upstream" comes from Zola in an article by McKinlay.[27,36] Here is a brief version of his parable:

*I am standing by a swiftly flowing river and hear a man drowning, crying for help. I jump in, pull him out, and provide artificial respiration. As he starts to breathe, there is another cry for help. I go back in the river again and rescue him. Then there is another cry for help. Again, I go into the river, pull him out, help him breathe. This sequence goes on and on. "You know, I am so busy jumping in, pulling them to shore, applying artificial respiration, that I have no time to see who the hell is upstream pushing them all in."*

When allocating resources or developing interventions to eliminate oral health disparities and inequities, addressing the underlying higher order upstream factors, such as poverty and safe, affordable housing, are more likely to be effective than if we continue to focus on treating disease after it occurs.[16] Importantly, many of the upstream factors have an impact on many diseases in addition to oral health and contribute to a multitude of health disparities. So this approach, although complex, is likely to be the most effective way to decrease health disparities and inequity overall.

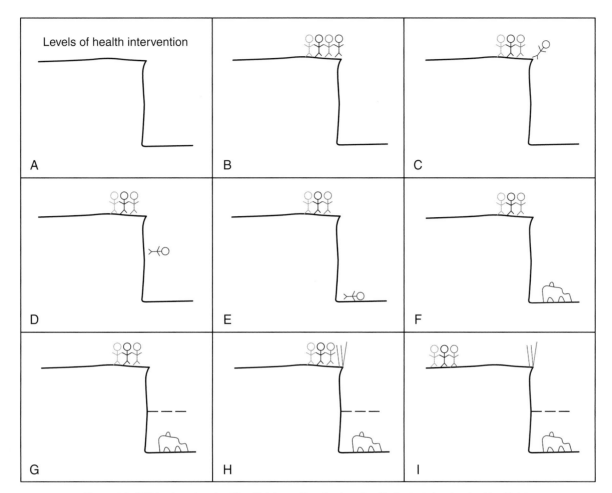

• **Figure 2.2** Cliff Analogy: Levels of health intervention. As described in the text, four levels of health intervention are illustrated, including acute care and tertiary prevention (F-the ambulance at the bottom of the cliff), secondary prevention (G-the safety net halfway down the cliff face), primary prevention (H-the fence at the top edge of the cliff), and addressing the social determinants of health (I-moving the population away from the edge of the cliff).[22]

## Conceptual Models, Frameworks, and Measurements for Understanding Health Disparities and Inequities

The National Institute of Dental and Craniofacial Research (NIDCR) has a long history of supporting oral health disparities research, and one of the four goals in its 2014–19 strategic plan is to: "*Apply rigorous, multidisciplinary research approaches to overcome disparities and inequalities in dental, oral, and craniofacial health.*"[32] The results of this research and studies funded by other organizations have provided a better understanding of the complex interplay of the social determinants of health and their relationship to oral health disparities.[1,7]

Adler and Stewart[1] have described different phases of health disparity research over time. Historically, research focused on the association between poverty and health, and assessing the ramifications of this important relationship continues. Factors that result from differing socioeconomic positions were added to analyses, including psychosocial factors such as stress, lifestyle, social capital, and neighborhood cohesion. Life course analyses started to show disparities across the lifespan and the influence of early childhood experiences and parental socioeconomic status (SES) on health status later in life.

The MacArthur Research Network on SES and Health was established to address the question, "*How does socioeconomic status get under the skin?*" A model was developed showing possible pathways between SES and health. Environmental hazards and exposures such as from hazardous waste and air and water pollution were more likely to be found in low SES communities. SES gradients are also found in unhealthy behaviors, including smoking, lack of exercise and poor diet, and related diseases and conditions such as obesity, type 2 diabetes, hypertension, and oral diseases. The body's response to chronic levels of stress and allostatic load has led to ongoing studies of the biologic mechanisms between SES, aging, and health. For example, chronic stress can disrupt immune systems, trigger inflammatory mediators, shorten telomeres, or in childhood, alter neural development.[8]

### Multilevel Conceptual Models

In addition to research turning inward to the cellular level, it also turned outward to examine neighborhood and community influences. The results were used to develop multilevel conceptual models that incorporate different levels of influence that encompass individual genetic and other biologic factors; individual and family behaviors; extent of health literacy; community, workplace, environmental, and political-social influences over time; and the interaction between these factors. Examples of the models are those developed by Fisher-Owens and colleagues shown in Figure 2.3[12,23,31] to explain factors associated with dental caries in children and another by Lee and Divaris in Figure 2.4.[24] The Fisher-Owens model in Figure 2.3 starts with the traditional intersecting triad associated with dental caries; the teeth, the microflora, and the child's diet. This intraoral focus is expanded to include child, family, community, and environmental factors that change over time. The Lee and Divaris model also includes these multilevels, applied to many oral conditions. They specify additional macro-level political, economic, and social factors and add a place for relevant mediators and pathways. The ultimate goal of these models is to translate what we learn from health disparity research into programs, practices, and policies that improve oral health.

## Measurements

Many different measurements have been used to increase our understanding of disparities and inequalities.[3] Some are measures of absolute disparity. For example, a **rate difference** is the simple arithmetic difference between two groups, usually between the less advantaged and the more advantaged groups. The **slope index of inequality (SII)** is the absolute difference in health status between the bottom and top of the social group distribution. Some are measures of relative disparity. For example, a **rate ratio** measures the relative difference in the rates of the best and worst group, whereas the **relative index of inequality (RII)** measures the proportionate rather than the absolute increase or decrease in health between the highest and lowest group. Health differences across groups with different amounts of social resources may be linear and exhibit a dose-response effect or a threshold effect. For example, if there are linear differences in tooth loss by level of education, then we would compare low versus high income groups. However, if differences level off after a certain amount of education, a threshold effect may be acting.[5]

While overall improvements in oral health may occur in a population, inequalities across income groups may remain or the gap may widen. For example, among adolescents in Brazil, there was a large decline in D(decayed), M(missing), and F(filled) T(teeth)

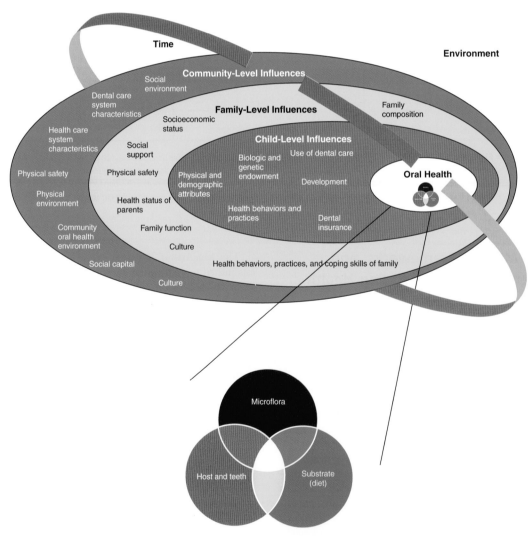

• **Figure 2.3** Child, family, and community influences on oral health outcomes of children.[12] The triad was adapted from Keyes P.H.[23] and the concentric oval design was adapted from the National Committee on Vital and Health Statistics.[31]

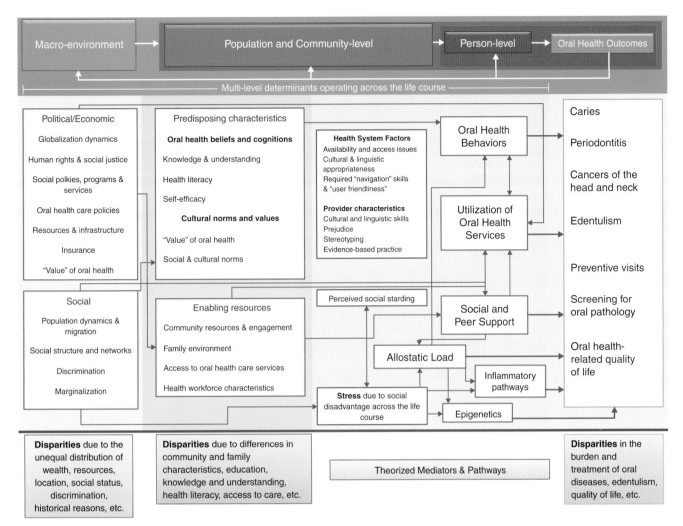

**Figure 2.4** Proposed framework to conceptualize and act on eliminating the sources of oral health disparities. The illustration outlines how hierarchically nested political, social, environmental, population, behavioral, and biologic factors interact with one another to generate health disparities. A feedback loop of oral health outcomes on these factors is also depicted.[24]

between 2003 and 2010. However, when viewed in the context of family income, although adolescents in each income group had lower DMFT scores, differences increased across socioeconomic groups. The SII for DMFT increased from 0.54 to 2.01, from about a difference of half a DMF tooth to two teeth between the lowest and highest social classes. Similarly, the RII increased from 1.09 to 1.50.[35] Because DMFT is cumulative, it may be harder to overcome differences already accrued over the life course. Disparities in both health and healthcare need to be considered.

The **Gini coefficient** (or Gini index) is used to measure inequality in income or wealth distribution of a population.[4] If everyone had the same income, representing equality, the Gini coefficient would equal zero. If one person had all the income and everyone else had none, then it would equal 1 (or 100%). Moeller and Quiñonez[29] used the Gini coefficient to compare 11 Canadian metropolitan areas. They found that areas with greater income inequality were more likely to report their oral health as poor/fair compared to good/very good/excellent and were more likely to have not visited a dentist in the past year or for more than three years.

## Examples of Oral Health Disparities and Inequities

### Oral Health Status

Progress toward the established national health objectives is tracked as part of Healthy People 2020. The clinical oral health status information is largely based on the National Health and Nutrition Examination Survey (NHANES), with 1999–2004 as the baseline and 2013–14 as the most recent data available. Baseline data, the 2020 target, and the most recent national data are documented online, and for many objectives, data are presented by groups such as age, sex, education, family income (percent of poverty threshold), race and ethnicity, and health insurance status. Some oral health conditions are also reported for adults by marital status, veteran status, disability status, country of birth (U.S. or outside U.S.), and obesity status (obese or not).[44]

In the following examples, NHANES data and the Healthy People 2020 objectives are used to illustrate some profound oral health status disparities and inequities for untreated dental caries, tooth loss, and periodontitis. Disparities are apparent by poverty status (below the 100% poverty threshold compared to the highest group reported), race and ethnicity (Mexican American, black or African American only [not Hispanic or Latino] and white only [not Hispanic or Latino]), and for adults, by education (less than, equivalent, or more than high school education). The unequal burden of disease is evident across the lifespan.

For children age 6 to 9 years, the Healthy People 2020 target is 49% for the proportion with dental caries experience. But in 2013–14, 66% of children living below the poverty threshold were affected, twice that compared to the 32% of children affected who live at or above the 500% threshold, a proportion lower than the target. The majority of Mexican American children in this age group (72%) had dental caries experience compared to 42% of white children.[41]

Among adults, the Healthy People 2020 target was to reduce the proportion of adults age 35 to 44 years with untreated dental decay from 27.8% to 25%. However, the recent national average of 31.3% indicated that proportion with untreated caries increased. More than half of those with less than a high school education (52.6%) had untreated caries, a proportion more than twice that of the population with more than a high school education (22%). Similarly, 56% living below the poverty level were affected compared to 13% at or above the 500% threshold. Mexican American and black or African American adults in this age range were more likely than white adults to have untreated caries.[41]

One of the tooth loss objectives is to reduce the proportion of adults age 45 to 64 years who have ever had a permanent tooth extracted because of dental caries or periodontal disease from 76.4% to 68.8%. This target was already met for the populations in this age range who have more than a high school education, are at or above the 500% poverty threshold, or are white. Other groups were much worse than the target, with 91% of those with less than high school education, 92% of those below the poverty threshold, and 88% of black or African Americans having lost at least one permanent tooth due to oral disease.[41]

This pattern is the same for the proportion of adults age 45 to 74 with moderate or severe periodontitis. The Healthy People 2020 objective is to reduce the proportion from 47.5% to 40.8%. The same socioeconomic and racial groups had already met the target. However, about 60% or more of the population groups with lower education, living in poverty, or Mexican American, black, or African American were afflicted with moderate or severe periodontitis.[41]

When assessing oral health disparities, differences in oral health quality of life (OHQOL) are important considerations as are differences in oral health status. Similar to what is seen in clinical oral health measures, there are OHQOL disparities by both ethnicity and poverty status. Using multivariate analysis of NHANES data from 2005 to 2008, Huang and Park found that older adults (age 65+) living in poverty reported significantly worse OHQOL compared to those not living in poverty. Hispanic older adults reported significantly worse OHQOL compared to non-Hispanic whites. However, reported OHQOL was similar for black and white older adults.[17]

## Dental Care Utilization

Healthy People 2020 objectives include both health status measures and indicators of access to care. For example, Healthy People Objective 7, *"increase the proportion of people aged ≥2 years who used the oral health care system in the last 12 months,"* is one of 12 Healthy People 2020 Leading Health Indicators (LHI) and provides an example of an oral health disparity. The LHIs are *"high priority health issues that serve as measurements of the Nation's health."*

Unlike the other examples of oral health disparities, instead of reducing the prevalence of disease, this objective is to increase the proportion from 44.5% to 49% of children, adolescents, and adults who used the oral health system in the past year. The data source is the 2014 Medical Expenditure Panel Survey (MEPS). Among adults age 25 years and older, the proportion with a dental visit in the past 12 months for those with at least some college education was more than three times that of the population with less than a high school education—57.9% and 17.7% respectively. For the age range 2 years and above, the proportion with a dental visit with family incomes 400% or more of the poverty threshold was twice that of those living below the threshold—57.2% compared to 28.7%. Among those under age 65 years with health insurance, 46.1% had a prior year dental visit compared to only 16.1% of those uninsured.[45]

Disparities and inequities in dental use within racial and ethnic groups also exist by poverty level. According to National Health Interview Survey data, among adults age 18 to 64 years in 2015, the proportion with a dental visit in the past year for Hispanic or Latino adults living below the poverty level was 40.8%, and it was much higher (74.8%) for those living at 400% or more of the poverty threshold. These proportions for non-Hispanic or Latino black or African American adults were 44.8% and 75.8% respectively and 46.9% and 80.1% for non-Hispanic or Latino whites. Thus, within each group the dental utilization gap was 31% to 34%.[30]

Similar patterns are evident for medical care. In 2014 and 2015, 10.2% of children and adolescents age 6 to 17 years had not had a healthcare visit to an office or clinic in the past 12 months. This proportion varied by factors such as race/ethnicity (white only 9.7%, black or African American 11.6%, Hispanic or Latino 14.2%, American Indian or Alaska Natives 20.0%), poverty status (12.3% if living <100% poverty level and 6.3% if 400% or above), and dramatically, by insurance status, 8.9% if insured publicly or privately and 31.6% if uninsured.[30]

These trends may continue because financial gaps between low- and high-income households are widening, and the proportion of American adults living in middle-income households is shrinking.[34]

## Emergency Department Use

Low-income, uninsured individuals who often lack employer-sponsored dental insurance and are ineligible for Medicaid dental coverage are more likely to forego regular preventive dental care.[55] Moreover, when they have emergent dental care needs, they are more likely to go to the emergency department (ED) seeking care,[55] in part because for these populations the emergency department is perceived as the only available setting for management of acute dental problems.[39]

Although there are no national data available on ED usage for nontraumatic tooth pain, several studies have found disparities in ED use. In a study conducted using data from the National Hospital Ambulatory Medical Care Survey,[37] the proportion of ED visits due to nontraumatic tooth pain among those who arrived by ambulance was highest among public insurance enrollees (1.9%) and Hispanics (2.3%). In the multivariable analysis, patients with public insurance had four times higher odds of visiting the ED due to nontraumatic tooth pain than people with private insurance.

Similarly, a study of Nevada ED nontraumatic dental visits noted that uninsured patients (OR = 2.75) and Medicaid recipients (OR = 2.16) were two times more likely to seek emergency department treatment than were those with private dental insurance.[55] This study also found that black patients were more likely than white patients to seek emergency department treatment (OR = 1.13). In Oregon, ED visitors with no insurance, Medicaid, or Medicare had, respectively, 5.2, 4.0, and 1.9 times increased odds that their ED visit was associated with a nontraumatic dental problem, compared with those who were commercially insured.[39]

It is clear from these studies that populations who have the highest rates of dental disease are also most likely to seek treatment for dental conditions at EDs. Unfortunately, EDs often treat the symptoms of dental conditions with antibiotics and pain medications while leaving the underlying disease untreated, resulting in costly yet ineffective visits. Increasing access to dental care for those who have the highest levels of disease by expansion of quality, comprehensive dental insurance for adults is one way to reduce the incidence of costly ED visits and to potentially redirect those funds toward getting the population the dental care they need.

## Health Policies and Guidelines Addressing Oral Health Disparities and Inequities

In the United States, several federal agencies and national initiatives have developed policies, guidelines, and strategic plans to address oral health disparities. Some have already been mentioned—the Surgeon General's report,[47] Healthy People 2020,[45] and the NIDCR Strategic Plan, 2014–2019.[32] Another is the U.S. Department of Health and Human Services (DHHS) Oral Health Strategic Framework, 2014–2017,[40] with the vision to eliminate oral health disparities. The five goals in the framework are to: (1) integrate oral health and primary health care, (2) prevent disease and promote oral health, (3) increase access to oral health care and eliminate disparities, (4) increase the dissemination of oral health information and improve health literacy, and (5) advance oral health in public policy and research.

The strategies listed for advancing these goals build on recommendations from two 2011 IOM reports, *Advancing Oral Health in America*[18] and *Improving Access to Oral Health Care for Vulnerable and Underserved Populations.*[19]

The DHHS strategies for goal 3 are:

3-A. Expand the number of health-care settings that provide oral health care, including diagnostic, preventive, and restorative services in federally qualified health centers, school-based health centers, Ryan White HIV/AIDS-funded programs, and IHS-funded health programs.

3-B. Strengthen the oral health workforce, expand capabilities of existing providers, and promote models that incorporate other clinicians.

3-C. Improve the knowledge, skills, and abilities of providers to serve diverse patient populations.

3-D. Promote health professionals' training in cultural competency.

3-E. Assist individuals and families in obtaining oral health services and connecting with a dental home.

3-F. Align dental homes and oral health services for children.

3-G. Create local, regional, and statewide partnerships that bridge the aging population and oral health systems.

3-H. Support the collection of sex- and racial/ethnic-stratified data pertaining to oral health.[40]

Additional policies that help reduce oral health disparities are covered in other chapters that focus on financing and delivery of oral health prevention and treatment (e.g., Medicaid, community health centers, school-based sealant programs, water fluoridation, workforce policies). Oral health and access to dental care are influenced by many individual and external factors, including insurance coverage, availability of providers who accept that insurance and speak the same language, out-of-pocket affordability, transportation, employment issues such as ability to take time off from work, availability of healthcare systems and practices that address health and oral health literacy needs, cultural norms, and perceived need for care and others. With so many social determinants of health, it is necessary to think broadly to create new policies that will address all social determinants at all levels of influence from the individual to the macro enviroment.[16] The successful implementation of these policies will require working collaboratively with other health professionals, community-based and faith-based organizations such as substance abuse treatment centers, and government agencies such as public housing authorities and Women, Infants, and Children (WIC).

There are now several models of the integration of oral health and primary care that provide additional access for preventive oral health services in nontraditional locations to alleviate disparities. Examples include medical providers in pediatric offices and nurses in schools applying fluoride varnish to children enrolled in Medicaid and where scope of practice allows, colocation of dental hygienists providing preventive services to pregnant women as part of prenatal care during obstetric visits and dental hygienists employed by health centers to provide periodontal care for patients with diabetes and cardiovascular disease.[6]

As indicated in the multidimensional conceptual models, untangling why there are differences is an important aspect of health disparity research so that appropriate interventions can be developed. A complex mix of material (e.g., income), psychosocial (e.g., stress, discrimination, social support), behavioral (e.g., smoking, oral hygiene), biologic (e.g., genetics, in utero effects) and many other factors contribute to health disparities across the lifespan, with different exposures, risks, and resources at different times and in different places.[5] Interventions that address inequalities in oral disease such as health promotion and prevention strategies may differ from those addressing differences in access to care and treatment.[28]

We end this chapter with a quote from the poet Dr. Maya Angelou.

*"I think we can move beyond disparity—because I look at the world, at everything, as if it is a half-filled glass. I think the word disparity puts the weight on the already encumbered. I think if I look at it as "equity," I have a different image...more emphasis on opportunity, on seeking, with more resolve, more hope."*[15]

## References

1. Adler NE, Stewart J. Health disparities across the lifespan: meaning, methods, and mechanisms. *Ann N Y Acad Sci.* 2010;1186:5–23.
2. Agency for Healthcare Research and Quality. *National Healthcare Quality and Disparities Report.* Available from: https://www.ahrq.gov/research/findings/nhqrdr/nhqdr16/summary.html#Key; 2016.
3. Agency for Healthcare Research and Quality. *Measures of Absolute and Relative Health Disparity.* Rockville, MD. Available from: http://www.ahrq.gov/research/findings/final-reports/iomqrdrreport/futureqrdrtab4-2.html.

4. Alleyne GA, Castillo-Salgado C, Schneider MC, et al. Overview of social inequalities in health in the region of the Americas, using various methodological approaches. *Pan Am J Public Health*. 2002;12(6):388–397.

5. Arcaya MC, Arcaya AL, Subramanian SV. Inequalities in health: definitions, concepts and theories. *Global Health Action*. 2015;8(1). 27106.

6. Atchison KA, Rozier RG, Weintraub JA. Integrating Oral health, primary care, and health literacy: considerations for health professional practice, education and policy. In: *Commissioned by the Roundtable on Health Literacy, Health and Medicine Division, the National Academies of Sciences, Engineering, and Medicine*; 2017. http://nationalacademies.org/hmd/~/media/Files/Activity%20Files/PublicHealth/HealthLiteracy/Commissioned%20Papers%20-Updated%202017/Atchison%20K%20et%20al%202017%20Integrating%20oral%20health%20primary%20care%20and%20health%20literacy.pdf.

7. Bharmal N, Derose KP, Felician M, et al. *Understanding the Upstream Social Determinants of Health. Working Paper*. RAND Health; May 2015. Available from: https://www.rand.org/content/dam/rand/pubs/working_papers/WR1000/WR1096/RAND_WR1096.pdf.

8. Braveman P. Health difference, disparity, inequality or inequity—what difference does it make what we call it? In: Buchbiner M, Rivkin-Fish M, Walker RL, eds. *Understanding Health Inequalities and Justice*. Chapel Hill, NC: University of North Carolina Press; 2016.

9. Colby SL, Ortman JM. Projections of the size and composition of the U.S. population: 2014 to 2060. In: *U.S. Department of Commerce, Economics and Statistics Administration, U.S. Census Bureau*: 2015. Available from: https://census.gov/content/dam/Census/library/publications/2015/demo/p25-1143.pdf.

10. Dwyer-Lindgren L, Bertozzi-Villa A, Stubbs RW, et al. Inequalities in life expectancy among U.S. counties, 1980 to 2014: Temporal trends and key drivers. *JAMA Intern Med*. 2017;177(7):1003–1011.

11. Ending racial and ethnic health disparities in the USA. *Lancet*. 2011;377(9775):1379.

12. Fisher-Owens SA, Gansky SA, Platt LJ, et al. Influences on children's oral health: a conceptual model. *Pediatrics*. 2007;120(3):e510–e520.

13. Fisher-Owens SA, Soobader MJ, Gansky SA, et al. Geography matters: state-level variation in children's oral health care access and oral health status. *Public Health*. 2016;134:54–63.

14. Froehle C. *The Evolution of an Accidental Meme*. Available from: https://medium.com/@CRA1G/the-evolution-of-an-accidental-meme-ddc4e139e0e4.

15. Garnett C. Angelou brings art to science summit. Health disparities gets intramural research component. *NIH Record*. 2009. Vol LXI, No. 1, January 9. Available from: https://nihrecord.nih.gov/sites/recordNIH/files/pdf/2009/NIH-Record-2009-01-09.pdf.

16. Henshaw MM, Garcia RI, Weintraub JA. Oral health disparities across the lifespan. *Dent Clin North Am*. 2018;62(2):177–193.

17. Huang DL, Park M. Socioeconomic and racial/ethnic oral health disparities among U.S. older adults: oral health quality of life and dentition. *J Public Health Dent*. 2015;75(2):85–92.

18. Institute of Medicine. *Advancing Oral Health in America*. Washington, DC: National Academies Press; 2011.

19. Institute of Medicine. *Improving Access to Oral Health Care for Vulnerable and Underserved Populations*. Washington, DC: National Academies Press; 2011.

20. Institute of Medicine. *Unequal Treatment: Confronting Racial and Ethnic Disparities in Health Care*. Washington DC: National Academies Press; 2002.

21. Interaction Institute for Social Change. *Illustrating equality vs equity. Artist: Angus Maguire*. January 13. Available from: http://interactioninstitute.org/illustrating-equality-vs-equity; 2016.

22. Jones CP, Jones CY, Perry GS, et al. Addressing the social determinants of children's health: a cliff analogy. *J Health Care Poor Underserved*. 2009;20:4A, Figure 1 (1a-1i). © 2009 Meharry Medical College. Reprinted with permission of Johns Hopkins University Press.

23. Keyes PH. Recent advances in dental caries research bacteriology. Bacteriological findings and biological implications. *Int Dent J*. 1962;12:443–464.

24. Lee JY, Divaris K. The ethical imperative of addressing oral health disparities: a unifying framework. *J Dental Res*. 2014;93(3):224–230.

25. Marmot MG, Rose G, Shipley M, et al. Employment grade and coronary heart disease in British civil servants. *J Epidemiol Community Health*. 1978;32(4):244–249.

26. Marmot MG, Smith GD, Stansfeld S, et al. Health inequalities among British civil servants: the Whitehall II study. *Lancet*. 1991;337(8754):1387–1393.

27. McKinlay J. A case for refocusing upstream: the political economy of illness. In: Gartley J, ed. *Patients, Physicians and Illness: A Sourcebook in Behavioral Science and Health*. New York, NY: Free Press; 1979:9–25.

28. Mejia G, Jamieson LM, Ha D, et al. Greater inequalities in dental treatment than in disease experience. *J Dental Res*. 2014;93(10):966–971.

29. Moeller J, Quiñonez C. The association between income inequality and oral health in Canada: a cross-sectional study. *Int J Health Serv*. 2016;46(4):790–809.

30. National Center for Health Statistics. *Health, United States, 2016: With Chartbook on Long-Term Trends in Health*. Hyattsville: MD; 2017.

31. National Committee on Vital and Health Statistics. *Shaping a Health Statistics Vision for the 21st Century*. Washington, DC: Department of Health and Human Services Data Council, Centers for Disease Control and Prevention, National Center for Health Statistics; 2002:viii.

32. National Institutes of Health. *National Institute of Dental and Craniofacial Research. NIDCR Strategic Plan*. 2014. Bethesda, MD; 2014-2019. Available from: https://www.nidcr.nih.gov/research/ResearchPriorities/StrategicPlan.

33. PEW Center on the States. *The Cost of Delay: State Dental Policies Fail One in Five Children*. February 2010. Available from: http://www.pewtrusts.org/~/media/legacy/uploadedfiles/costofdelaywebpdf.pdf

34. Pew Research Center. *The American Middle Class Is Losing Ground*. December 9, 2015. Available from: http://www.pewsocialtrends.org/2015/12/09/the-american-middle-class-is-losing-ground

35. Roncalli AG, Sheiham A, Tsakos G, et al. Socially unequal improvements in dental caries levels in Brazilian adolescents between 2003 and 2010. *Community Dent Oral Epidemiol*. 2015;43(4):317–324.

36. Rudolph L, Caplan J, Ben-Moshe K, et al. *Health in All Policies: A Guide for State and Local Governments*. Washington, DC and Oakland, CA: American Public Health Association and Public Health Institute; 2013. Available from: https://www.apha.org/~/media/files/pdf/factsheets/health_inall_policies_guide_169pages.ashx.

37. Shenkin JD, Warren J, Spanbauer C, et al. Hospital emergency department visits by ambulance for nontraumatic tooth pain in the USA. *Clin Cosmet Investig Dent*. 2018;10:159–163.

38. Sischo L, Broder HL. Oral health-related quality of life: what, why, how, and future implications. *J Dental Res*. 2011;90(11):1264–1270.

39. Sun BC, Chi DL, Schwarz E, et al. Emergency department visits for nontraumatic dental problems: a mixed-methods study. *Am J Public Health*. 2015;105(5):947–955.

40. U.S. Department of Health and Human Services Oral Health Coordinating Committee. U.S. Department of Health and Human Services Oral Health Strategic Framework, 2014–2017. *Public Health Rep*. 2016;131(2):242–257.

41. U.S. Department of Health and Human Services. *Healthy People 2020*. Washington, DC. Available from: https://www.healthypeople.gov/2020/about/foundation-health-measures/Disparities.

42. U.S. Department of Health and Human Services. *Healthy People 2020*. Washington, DC. Available from: https://www.healthypeople.gov/2020/about/foundation-health-measures/Determinants-of-Health.

43. U.S. Department of Health and Human Services. *Healthy People 2020.* Washington, DC. Available from: https://www.healthypeople.gov/2020/topics-objectives/topic/oral-health/objectives.

44. U.S. Department of Health and Human Services. *Healthy People 2020.* Washington, DC. Available from: https://www.healthypeople.gov/2020/data-search/Search-the-Data#topic-area=3511.

45. U.S. Department of Health and Human Services. *Healthy People 2020.* Washington, DC. Available from: https://www.healthypeople.gov.

46. U.S. Department of Health and Human Services. *HHS Action Plan to Reduce Racial and Ethnic Health Disparities.* Washington, DC; 2011. Available from: https://minorityhealth.hhs.gov/npa/files/Plans/HHS/HHS_Plan_complete.pdf.

47. U.S. Department of Health and Human Services. Oral Health in America. *A Report of the Surgeon General.* Rockville, MD: U.S. Department of Health and Human Services, National Institute of Dental and Craniofacial Research. In: *National Institutes of Health*; 2000.

48. U.S. health care: plumbing the depths of disparities. *Lancet.* 2016;387 (10031):1879.

49. Whitehead M. The concepts and principles of equity and health. *Int J Health Serv.* 1992;22(3):429–445.

50. World Health Organization. *Declaration of Alma-Ata. September 6–12. Adopted at the International Conference on Primary Health Care. USSR: Alma-Ata; 1978.* Available from: http://www.who.int/publications/almaata_declaration_en.pdf.

51. World Health Organization. *Life expectancy increased by 5 years since 2000, but health inequalities persist*, news release, May 19, 2016. Available from: http://www.who.int/mediacentre/news/releases/2016/health-inequalities-persist/en.

52. World Health Organization. *Rio Political Declaration on Social Determinants of Health. October 19–21. Adopted at the World Conference on Social Determinants of Health.* Rio de Janeiro: Brazil; 2011. Available from: http://www.who.int/sdhconference/declaration/Rio_political_declaration.pdf.

53. World Health Organization. *Social Determinants of Health.* Available from: http://www.who.int/social_determinants/en.

54. World Health Organization. Commission on Social Determinants of Health. *A Conceptual Framework for Action on the Social Determinants of Health;* April 2007. Available from: http://www.who.int/social_determinants/resources/csdh_framework_action_05_07.pdf?ua=1.

55. Zhou E, Kim P, Shen JJ, et al. Preventable emergency department visits for nontraumatic dental conditions: trends and disparities in Nevada, 2009–2015. *Am J Public Health.* 2018;108(3):369–371.

# 3

# Access to Dental Care

SUSAN MCKERNAN, DMD, MS, PhD

JULIE REYNOLDS, DDS, MS

MICHELLE MCQUISTAN, DDS, MS

## CHAPTER OUTLINE

The Institute of Medicine (IOM) has defined *access* as a broad concept that encompasses "the timely use of personal health services to achieve the best possible health outcomes."[30] Current estimates are that one-third of Americans lack access to dental care, which primarily includes economically disadvantaged populations who lack private dental insurance along with underserved racial and ethnic minorities, institutionalized populations, elderly adults with physical limitations, people with disabilities, and people living in dental health professional shortage areas.[22]

## Conceptualizing Dental Access

Access to dental care is frequently equated with utilization of services. However, utilization is just one aspect of access (Box 3.1). Aday and Andersen drew a distinction between realized access (i.e., utilization) and potential access or the potential for entry to the healthcare delivery system.[1]

## Need for Dental Care

Potential access includes availability of health resources along with characteristics of the population at risk, such as perceived need for care and demand for services. As it relates to access, need often motivates an individual to seek care. If access were equitable, this motivation alone would determine utilization of services, but barriers or mediators often affect who seeks and receives needed dental care.

## Barriers to Dental Care

The IOM has described three sources of barriers to access: structural, financial, and personal (Table 3.1). These categories can be broken down further into descriptive dimensions of access. Originally described by Penchansky and Thomas, these dimensions describe access as the *fit* between consumers and the healthcare system.[53]

The five original dimensions of access *(accessibility, availability, accommodation, affordability, and acceptability),* along with a sixth more recently introduced dimension *(awareness),*[55] provide a useful framework for operationalizing access (see Table 3.1). Access to dental care is facilitated by several interrelated elements: physical *accessibility* of dental providers, *availability* of sufficient providers to meet demand, *accommodations* that meet patients' needs with respect to scheduling, *affordability* of care that includes the ability to pay, culturally appropriate care *(acceptability),* and *awareness* or education about available services. By targeting specific dimensions of access, public health stakeholders can more effectively perform core functions of public health, including monitoring the impact of existing programs, investigating sources of health disparities, and designing policies that target access barriers.

## Utilization of Dental Care

In 1993, the IOM identified 15 key indicators of access to monitor national objectives for healthcare. Annual utilization of dental services was selected as an indicator of progress toward "reducing morbidity and pain through providing timely and appropriate treatment."[30] This indicator includes "all visits made to a dentist, or to a technician or hygienist under a dentist's supervision, for regular, specialized, or emergency dental care."[30]

**• BOX 3.1   Conceptualizing Access to Dental Care**

| Dental Need | |
|---|---|
| Perceived need | Demand for care |

⇩

| Barriers or Mediators | | |
|---|---|---|
| Structural | Financial | Personal/Cultural |

⇩

| Utilization of Dental Care | | | | |
|---|---|---|---|---|
| Provider type | Setting | Purpose | Continuity of care | Quality of care |

⇩

| Oral Health Status | | |
|---|---|---|
| Morbidity | Mortality | Quality of life |

**• TABLE 3.1   Barriers and Dimensions of Access**

| Barriers | Dimension | Description and Examples |
|---|---|---|
| Structural | Accessibility | Location of supply resources with respect to consumer distribution, affecting travel times and costs |
| | Availability | Adequacy of the supply of services and resources with respect to demand |
| | Accommodation | Ability to accept clients in a timely manner, including hours of operation, walk-in facilities, wait times |
| Financial | Affordability | Financial costs of services and ability to pay; includes type of insurance coverage and covered benefits and provider acceptance of insurance plans |
| Personal/cultural | Acceptability | Consumer perceptions about personal and practice characteristics of providers; can include age, sex and ethnicity of the provider, and type or neighborhood of facility |
| | Awareness | Effective communication about services or programs and use of that information to make health decisions; includes aspects of health literacy such as adherence to treatment recommendations |

Medical Expenditure Panel Survey data show that 43% of community-dwelling Americans had a dental visit in 2015.[42] Dental utilization among children and elderly adults showed an increase from 1996 to 2015; the percent of the population with a dental visit increased from 42% to 48% among children and 40% to 47% in older adults (Figure 3.1). Adult dental utilization declined slightly over the 20-year period, from 44% to 39.5%.

When barriers exist, use of dental services is a concern. Thus, characterizing the properties of dental utilization can reveal whether access was sufficient. Various properties of utilization[30] to be considered include:

- *Care setting.* For example, was an individual seen in an emergency department? A private dental office? School-based dental clinic?
- *Provider type.* Who provided dental care? An emergency department physician? A dentist? A dental hygienist working under public health supervision?
- *Purpose of encounter.* Was the patient seen for a dental emergency? Routine dental care?
- *Continuity of care.* Will the patient receive needed follow-up services? A permanent restoration placed after temporization?
- *Quality of care.* Was care provided in a timely manner? Patient centered? Effective?

**• Figure 3.1** Proportion of U.S. population with a dental visit in the year by age group (1996-2015).[42]

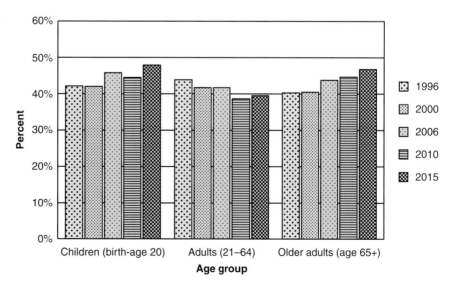

As an example, someone who lacks access to routine dental care may go to an emergency department for treatment of a painful abscessed tooth. Although this represents utilization, it is typically considered an indicator of poor access to dental care. Data from the National Hospital Ambulatory Medical Care Survey (NHAMCS) show that the use of emergency departments for nontraumatic dental conditions was 1.7% in 2007 and that rates had increased by 4% annually since 1997.[52] Patients seen in emergency departments for nontraumatic dental conditions are rarely treated by a dentist and typically only receive palliative treatment for their condition. In addition, reliance on emergency departments as a safety net for dental care is not a cost-effective use of resources.

## Oral Health Status

Health outcomes are the ultimate measure of whether access has been achieved.[30] On a population level, oral health status includes oral disease morbidity, mortality, and oral health–related quality of life. While the widespread burden of oral disease and impacts on quality of life are well known, it is less well known that oral disease can be a cause of death.[57] Thus, the mortality component of oral health status cannot be overlooked.

If differences in oral health status are related to avoidable barriers to care, these are considered to be health disparities (see Chapter 2). Health disparities, or inequities, are of particular concern because "they systematically put groups of people who are already socially disadvantaged (for example, by virtue of being poor, female, and/or members of a disenfranchised racial, ethnic or religious group) at further disadvantage with respect to their health."[11]

## Dimensions of Access to Dental Care

The complex interrelation of dental need, barriers, utilization, and effects on health status all contribute to access. Dimensions of access as they relate to dental care are described subsequently.

## Affordability

Findings from the 2014 National Health Interview Survey (NHIS) show that cost is a greater barrier to dental care than to other types of healthcare services, such as medical care or prescription drugs.[63] Differences in financial barriers to dental versus medical care are driven by the fact that many more people have health insurance for medical care than dental insurance. In 2015, 71% of community-dwelling Americans had dental insurance[42] compared to 91% with health insurance.[5]

In addition to overall coverage, financial barriers to medical versus dental care are affected by differences in the structure of medical and dental insurance plans. Dental insurance plans typically have more cost-sharing mechanisms in place compared to medical care, including higher rates of coinsurance and annual maximum benefit limits. As a result of these differences in coverage and benefit structures for medical and dental insurance, Americans pay a higher share of dental care out of pocket than medical care. In 2017, 41% of total dental spending in the U.S. was paid out of pocket compared to 10% of total health spending.[16]

### Children

Improvements in children's utilization of dental care over the past 20 years have primarily been driven by increases in public insurance enrollment. The proportion of U.S. children under age 19 enrolled in Medicaid or Children's Health Insurance Program (CHIP) increased from 20% to 37% between 1996 and 2015.[42] Because state Medicaid programs are required to provide comprehensive dental coverage for all Medicaid- and CHIP-enrolled children, increases in enrollment translate to increases in dental coverage for this age group.

### Adults

Adults are more likely to report financial barriers to care compared to children or older adults. Findings from the 2014 NHIS show that 13% of nonelderly adults reported unmet dental needs because of cost.[63] Unlike the trends seen in children, enrollment in public insurance among adults has not increased in recent years. The proportion of nonelderly adults with public dental insurance increased from 7% to 13% between 1996 and 2015.[42]

Also in contrast to coverage for children, state Medicaid programs are not required to provide dental coverage for adults. Therefore, dental benefits for Medicaid-enrolled adults vary considerably by state. In 2016, only 15 states provided comprehensive dental coverage to Medicaid-enrolled adults.[28] Thirteen states provided emergency-only coverage, and four provided no dental coverage at all. This variation in dental benefits for low-income adults is a major contributing factor to financial barriers among this age group.

### Older Adults

Adults age 65 and older experience a unique set of issues affecting dental care affordability. This age group has the lowest proportion who are dentally insured compared to children and nonelderly adults. In 2015, only 38% of adults age 65 and older had any form of dental insurance.[42] This is primarily because the Medicare program does not provide coverage for dental care except in cases of medical necessity. Additionally, although low-income older adults may also be eligible for Medicaid, the state-by-state variation in Medicaid dental coverage presents similar financial barriers for all adults. However, older adults are less likely than nonelderly adults to report financial barriers to dental care; 7% of older adults compared to 13% in adults age 19 to 64 reported financial barriers to dental care in 2014.[63] Increasing cost barriers for older adults are likely, as older adults are retaining their teeth longer, thus creating more need for dental care into older age.

## Accessibility and Availability

Accessibility and availability are conceptually related: These dimensions of dental care access are generated by an adequate supply of dental services, which are suitably located relevant to local demand. As these dimensions are influenced by the relative geographical distribution of supply and demand, accessibility and availability can together be considered to comprise spatial accessibility.[24] Spatial barriers to dental care include transportation distance along with other transportation-related factors that disproportionately affect residents of rural and frontier areas and low-income populations. Rural populations have fewer dentists per population and face greater travel distances to access dental care.[59] Low-income populations can also face spatial barriers to dental care in areas where few local dentists are available that accept public dental insurance and where public transportation is lacking.

Supply and demand for dental care are largely sensitive to market forces, including general economic trends, but the profession of dentistry also maintains fairly tight control of workforce supply and scopes of practice (Table 3.2). Between 2008 and 2016, 10 new dental schools opened in the U.S., raising the total number of

| ● TABLE 3.2 | Overview of Factors Affecting Supply and Demand for Dental Care | |
|---|---|---|
| **Supply** | **Demand** | |
| ● **Educational programs and graduating class sizes.** Recent increases in number of dental schools and class size contribute to increased workforce. | ● **Cultural norms.** Perceived need varies by geographical location, generational differences, cultural background, and socioeconomic status. | |
| ● **Composition of dental workforce.** Size, geographical distribution, and age and sex composition contribute to availability and accessibility. | ● **Disease prevalence.** This is influenced by access to prevention, including community water fluoridation and treatment. | |
| ● **Occupational regulation.** State-regulated licensing of members of the oral health team can restrict or expand local availability of dental care. | ● **Dental insurance.** Private dental insurance, along with federal and state programs, reduce financial barriers to care. | |
| ● **Dental office productivity.** Hours worked and patients seen per day can affect overall workforce productivity. | ● **Overall economy.** Dental utilization is highly correlated with disposable income and employment status of the population. | |
| ● **Oral health safety net.** Availability of community health centers, public health supervision of dental hygienists, and school-based services add points of accessibility to the dental system. | ● **Population size and age distribution.** The includes an increasing population and an aging baby boom generation. | |

dental schools operating in the U.S. to 66, plus 10 in Canada.[3] In 2016, there were 207,900 dental hygienists employed in the U.S.; this figure is projected to increase 20% by 2026.[13] Trends in dental workforce supply are discussed in detail in Chapter 8.

Occupational regulation over scopes of practice for members of the oral health team, including dental hygienists, therapists, and assistants, also affects the availability of dental care. In states with restrictive scopes of practice, points of care may be limited to clinics where a supervising dentist is present. With more permissive state practice acts, dental hygienists and dental therapists can work in public health settings, under general supervision, or independent of a supervising dentist.

Demand for dental services fluctuates with cultural norms, disease prevalence, and generational differences. The cohort of Americans born during the post–World War II baby boom began to retire in 2011. By 2030, over 20% of Americans are projected to be aged 65 and older, compared with 13% in 2010.[19] This cohort has benefited from water fluoridation and topical fluoride agents that were not available for previous generations. Additionally, this generation was the first to grow up with dental insurance.[34] As a result, baby boomers have lower prevalence of edentulism than previous generations. As Americans retain their teeth longer, demand for care will keep pace or continue to increase. Need for dental care will also be affected as this cohort shifts from community-dwelling to institutional settings, with elderly adults who are unable to care for their own dentitions having to rely on nursing staff and a flexible dental workforce to obtain care.

## Acceptability

Acceptability refers to patient preferences for certain provider characteristics, including the desire to seek treatment from a same-sex provider due to religious beliefs or personal preference and provider ability to address patients' cultural and social concerns. Acceptability influences dental care access in that individuals who are unable to find a dental provider who is acceptable to them may not use services or continue with follow-up treatment.

Studies have shown that some individuals prefer to seek care from providers who look like them and share similar cultural backgrounds.[7,36] Racial concordance between patient and provider can also lead to greater satisfaction with care.[10] When traditional Western views of individualism and medicine conflict with other cultural values, certain racial/ethnic minority groups may feel unsatisfied with their dental care[58] or feel as though they have been treated disrespectfully.[9]

Acceptability of care is also particularly important with regard to patients' gender identity. In a survey of transgender individuals, nearly 40% of respondents reported a fear of being mistreated in a dental office.[27] This is a realistic concern, given that 33% of respondents who completed the 2015 U.S. Transgender Survey reported negative experiences when seeking healthcare.[32] These experiences ranged from verbal harassment and physical assault to being refused treatment by a healthcare provider or receiving care from providers who did not understand how to appropriately treat patients who identify as being transgender. This can lead to access challenges; 23% of respondents had not sought healthcare because they feared discrimination or mistreatment.[32]

## Accommodation

Accommodation of unique patient needs and preferences increase the likelihood that patients will seek care, thereby reducing access barriers. Examples of accommodations include providing interpretation services, providing space for family members to attend a dental appointment to facilitate shared decision making, and scheduling accommodations such as same-day appointments or extended clinic hours. In primary medical care, same-day access and extended clinic hours have been associated with reduced emergency department visits and less unmet need for care.[41,67] Although these topics are less studied in dental care settings, one study reported reduced barriers to care for dental patients and caregivers attending an adolescent evening clinic.[20]

Individuals with intellectual or physical disabilities may require unique accommodations as well, including appropriate communication, wheelchair access, and scheduling appointment time and duration based on patient needs.[37] Parents of children with special healthcare needs have identified challenges accessing dental care due to the need for dentists to provide special accommodations to deliver dental treatment to the children, along with dentists' inability or unwillingness to accommodate behavior problems.[48,60]

## Awareness

Awareness relates to patient knowledge that dental services or programs exist and provider awareness of local context and population-related factors.[55] Without an awareness about where to go to seek services, one cannot access dental care. For example, patients may not be aware of where they can seek affordable dental care besides private practices or emergency departments. Awareness is related to health literacy, which is defined as "the degree to which individuals have the capacity to obtain, process, and understand basic information and services needed to make appropriate health decisions."[31] Health literacy relies on patients' understanding of when to seek care and how to make a dental appointment. Studies have found that people with low health literacy are less likely to seek preventive medical services[56] and are more likely to report difficulty in finding a medical provider and not having a usual source of care compared to individuals with adequate health literacy.[38] In contrast, studies examining the associations between oral health literacy and attendance at dental appointments have shown conflicting findings.[6,14,29,33,39,40] (See Chapter 22: Health Literacy for more details.)

## Strategies to Improve Access to Dental Care

Recognizing that a large proportion of the population is not served by the existing dental delivery system, strategies to improve access primarily aim to reduce barriers to care noted in Table 3.1. Discussed below are several relevant strategies that have proved successful. Additionally, emphasizing primary prevention of oral disease can help reduce overall need and thus improve access to dental care for the individual and those with high need.

### Address Cost-Related Barriers

Efforts to improve access to dental care must address cost-related factors, from the perspective of both patients and providers, as these are the most important barriers to care. A key strategy to improve dental care affordability for patients is to expand dental coverage for low-income and elderly Americans. Currently, dental coverage in public insurance programs deteriorates over the lifespan; it is mandatory for children, optional for adults, and nearly nonexistent for elderly adults. Recent research and advocacy efforts have targeted these disparities. It has been estimated that introducing comprehensive dental benefits for Medicaid-enrolled adults in states not currently providing it would cost approximately $1.5 billion and would increase state Medicaid spending by only 0.4% to 2.1% depending on the state.[66]

Cost-related strategies to improve access also include incentivizing providers to participate in public dental insurance programs. The level of reimbursement for dental services has consistently been shown to be the most important factor driving dentist participation in Medicaid. Nationally, Medicaid fee-for-service reimbursement for dental care averages less than 50% of what commercial dental plans typically pay, and Medicaid reimbursement rates have declined in most states since the early 2000s.[47] The impact of Medicaid reimbursement on dentist participation influences patients' ability to access care.[17] Therefore, this is a topic that requires attention if access to dental care for low-income Americans is to be improved.

### Strengthen the Oral Health Safety Net

The oral health safety net is intended to provide care to those not able to access the private practice delivery system. The dental safety net includes federally qualified health centers (FQHCs), other community health centers, dental schools, dental hygiene programs, school-based clinics, and mobile dental programs.[22] FQHCs make up the largest portion of the dental safety net by far. Among the 1367 FQHCs nationwide, more than one-quarter do not provide dental services.[26] FQHCs provided dental care to approximately 6.4 million patients in 2016—approximately 23% of all FQHC patients.[25]

Although an impressive number, this system cannot serve the 70 million individuals enrolled in Medicaid alone, further demonstrating that the current capacity of the whole safety net is not sufficient to meet the oral health needs of vulnerable populations. Therefore, efforts to improve access for low-income and other vulnerable populations requires change in both the public and private dental delivery systems. The proportion of FQHCs with an oral health program increased over 20% in 20 years; in 2017, 71% of FQHCs had an oral health program,[26] and concurrently the number of dental visits at FQHCs increased by 74%.[62] These trends in public safety net expansion should continue, along with efforts to engage the private dental delivery system to provide care to underserved populations.

Although volunteer dentistry can be considered a component of the dental safety net, it cannot be relied on as a predictable and sustainable source of access to care for vulnerable populations. Volunteer dentistry includes care provided in a dental office free of charge, donation of dental supplies, and volunteer events such as Missions of Mercy and Give Kids a Smile. Since the goal of the dental community should be to connect individuals with a dental home, one-off volunteer events and services present ethical concerns related to patient follow-up and the ability to meet standards of care.[54] Therefore, sustainable solutions to increase safety net capacity are encouraged; these should focus on solutions that provide patients with ongoing access to needed care rather than expansion of short-term charitable events and services.

### Engage Private Practitioners and Organized Dentistry

The existing safety net is inadequate to meet the oral health needs of currently disenfranchised populations. If dental benefits are expanded to cover elderly and low-income adults, increasing dentist participation in public programs will be critical. Collaboration with private practitioners is required to achieve equitable access to dental care. Given the overall declining trends in the number of total dental visits nationwide, along with reductions in dentist busyness, dentists and dental hygienists in private practice represent untapped workforce capacity.[61] However, the dentist workforce faces imposing financial constrictions related to increases in educational debt without concurrent increases in income.[46] Higher Medicaid reimbursement rates have been shown to be associated with increased dentist participation.[47] Financial encouragement to participate in public dental programs is likely required to see large scale change in dentists' behaviors.

Engaging these providers by setting common goals—even if these goals are motivated by different aims—is a requisite for creating a more efficient, equitable dental system. In order to make broad changes, collaboration with stakeholders at an organizational level offers the potential for higher level impact. Professional organizations acting in partnership can generate consensus among members and direct high-level efforts toward change.

### Optimize the Use of Allied Dental Workforce and Other Healthcare Providers

Another method for increasing dental safety net capacity is to offer oral health services outside of the dental office. Such approaches include expanding the settings in which dental hygienists can provide preventive services, including in medical settings and other outreach settings under public health supervision. Additional approaches include use of the nondental health workforce to provide screenings, referrals, and preventive services.

As of 2018, 42 states allow dental hygienists to provide preventive services, typically only in public health settings without the direct supervision of a dentist.[4] Broadening the utilization of dental hygienists under public health supervision may improve the reach of the dental clinic, especially in areas where spatial barriers to care limit access. In 2015, the Colorado Medical-Dental Integration Project began integrating dental hygienists into primary medical care settings and school-based health centers. In these settings, hygienists provide preventive dental services and coordinate care with the medical team and community dentists.[21]

Advocates for state legislation permitting dental therapists to treat patients under general supervision of dentists argue that these mid-level providers can also improve the reach of the traditional dental practice to rural and low-income populations. In Alaska's remote tribal communities, dental health aide therapists (DHATs) provide preventive and restorative care, including extractions, to populations that were previously served by dentists who visited communities only on an annual basis.[18] From 2005 to 2015, the presence of DHATs in these communities was associated with positive trends in dental utilization, with increasing use of preventive dental services and decreases in the proportion of individuals receiving extractions.

Other alternative workforce designs are being explored to complement the existing dental safety net. Teledentistry can allow dentists in cooperation with dental hygienists or specialists to provide services at a distance: live video, stored health information that can be reviewed by a dentist at distance, and mobile health devices offer dentists a mechanism to provide virtual services to patients living in remote areas, nursing homes, or other populations that cannot be physically present at a dental practice.

One application of teledentistry is the virtual dental home, a workforce innovation demonstration project in California.[23] In the virtual dental home, teledentistry links dental hygienists and dental assistants to a remote dentist who leads a community-based team to provide oral health education, preventive services, and interim therapeutic restorations (ITR) until patients can be seen by a dentist for definitive care.

## Increase Workforce Diversity and Cultural Competency

Although the U.S. population has become increasingly diverse, the field of dentistry has been slow to follow, especially with respect to underrepresented minority populations, including blacks, Hispanics or Latinos, Pacific Islanders, and American Indians or Alaska Natives (AI/AN). From 1977 to 2017, the proportion of graduating dental students who were black, Hispanic, or AI/AN increased from 6% to 13%.[45] However, the proportion of Asian dental school graduates saw a much greater increase during this time period, from 3% to 23%. Consequently, although blacks compose approximately 19% of the U.S. population, they only represent 3% of the dentist workforce.[44] Similarly, the percentage of Hispanic dentists (2.8%) and American Indian or Alaska Native (0.2%) dentists is significantly less than the general population (22% and 1.4%, respectively).[44] Since dentists from underrepresented backgrounds are more likely to treat underserved populations,[44,51] increasing racial and ethnic diversity within the dental profession has the potential to reduce barriers, especially within the dimensions of accessibility and acceptability (see Table 3.1).[61]

One way to increase the diversity of the dental workforce is through pipeline programs such as the Summer Health Professions Education Program, formerly the Summer Medical and Dental Education Program, funded through the Robert Wood Johnson Foundation.[64] Additionally, numerous dental schools have pipeline programs funded at their own institutions. These programs have been successful in increasing the number of underrepresented minority students enrolling in dental school.[12,35,43]

Beyond increasing workforce diversity, it is imperative that all members of the dental team are able to provide acceptable, culturally competent care. This involves providing care "to patients with diverse values, beliefs, and behaviors" and "tailoring delivery to meet patients' social, cultural, and linguistic needs."[8] Culturally competent healthcare addresses the social and cultural factors that impact patients' health beliefs and behaviors, and it encourages active patient participation. Furthermore, it reduces barriers between the patient and the healthcare team by considering differing perspectives on "health, medical care, and expectations about diagnosis and treatment."[8] Skills that are learned through cultural competency training can be applied to any population, including those with varying religious beliefs, racial and ethnic backgrounds, sexual orientation, gender identity, and other identifying characteristics.

Numerous guidelines, training opportunities, and resources are available to members of the dental team to assist with treating diverse patients and addressing health literacy. Examples include the AHRQ Health Literacy Universal Precautions Toolkit,[2] the CDC Clear Communication Index,[15] and Think Cultural Health.[50] In 2000, the U.S. Department of Health and Human Services Office of Minority Health developed the National Standards for Culturally and Linguistically Appropriate Services in Health and Health Care ("National CLAS Standards") to "improve health care quality and advance health equity by establishing a framework for organizations to serve the nation's increasingly diverse communities."[49] These 15 standards are updated periodically and provide suggestions to help organizations and providers consider the cultural beliefs of their patients, provide care in patients' preferred languages, and address patients' health literacy levels and communication needs.

## Conclusions

Access to dental care is a complex phenomenon; several conceptual frameworks have attempted to describe these complexities. Although "access" is often used to mean "utilization of dental services," it can also refer to the potential for utilization of services to occur. Barriers to care may prevent utilization and can be categorized as structural, financial, or personal.[31] When these barriers systematically affect disadvantaged populations, health disparities arise.

Limited resources restrict access to dental care for many Americans. The private dental delivery system employs over 90% of active dental professionals and serves approximately two-thirds of the U.S. population.[65] The oral health safety net exists to address demand among vulnerable populations, but access to the safety net is limited. It is the role of dental public health to prioritize available resources in a way that reduces oral health disparities among populations not readily served by the existing delivery system. Where existing policies and practices create health inequity, the public health professional is called upon to advocate for systematic changes to improve access to dental care through research, policy, and practice.

## References

1. Aday LA, Andersen RM. Equity of access to medical care: a conceptual and empirical overview. *Med Care*. 1981;19(12):4–27.
2. *AHRQ Health Literacy Universal Precautions Toolkit*. Rockville, MD: Agency for Healthcare Research and Quality. Available from:

http://www.ahrq.gov/professionals/quality-patient-safety/quality-resources/tools/literacy-toolkit/index.html.

3. ADEA. *Snapshot of Dental Education, 2016–2017.* Washington, DC: American Dental Education Association; 2016. Available from: http://www.adea.org/snapshot/.

4. American Dental Hygienists' Association. *Direct Access States;* 2019. http://www.adha.org/resources-docs/7524_Current_Direct_Access_Map.pdf.

5. Barnett JC, Berchick ER. *Health Insurance Coverage in the United States: 2016.* Washington, DC: U.S. Government Printing Office; 2017. Available from: https://www.census.gov/content/dam/Census/library/publications/2017/demo/p60-260.pdf.

6. Baskaradoss JK. The association between oral health literacy and missed dental appointments. *J Am Dent Assoc.* 2016;147(11): 867–874.

7. Bender DJ. Patient preference for a racially or gender-concordant student dentist. *J Dent Educ.* 2007;71(6):726–745.

8. Betancourt JR, Green AR, Carrillo JE. *Cultural Competence in Health Care: Emerging Frameworks and Practical Approaches.* New York, NY: The Commonwealth Fund; 2002.

9. Blanchard J, Lurie N. R-E-S-P-E-C-T: patient reports of disrespect in the health care setting and its impact on care. *J Fam Pract.* 2004;53(9):721–730.

10. Blanchard J, Nayar S, Lurie N. Patient-provider and patient-staff racial concordance and perceptions of mistreatment in the health care setting. *J Gen Intern Med.* 2007;22(8):1184–1189.

11. Braveman P, Gruskin S. Defining equity in health. *J Epidemiol Community Health.* 2003;57:254–258.

12. Brunson WD, Jackson DL, Sinkford JC, et al. Components of effective outreach and recruitment programs for underrepresented minority and low-income dental students. *J Dent Educ.* 2010;74(10 suppl):S74–S86.

13. Bureau of Labor Statistics (BLS), U.S. Department of Labor. *Occupational Outlook Handbook, Dental Hygienists.* Available from: https://www.bls.gov/ooh/healthcare/dental-hygienists.htm.

14. Burgette JM, Lee JY, Baker AD, et al. Is dental utilization associated with oral health literacy? *J Dent Res.* 2016;95(2):160–166.

15. Centers for Disease Control and Prevention. *The CDC Clear Communication Index.* Available from: https://www.cdc.gov/ccindex/.

16. Centers for Medicare and Medicaid Services. *National Health Expenditures 2017 Highlights.* Available from: https://www.cms.gov/Research-Statistics-Data-and-Systems/Statistics-Trends-and-Reports/NationalHealthExpendData/downloads/highlights.pdf.

17. Chalmers NI, Compton RD. Children's access to dental care affected by reimbursement rates, dentist density, and dentist participation in Medicaid. *Am J Public Health.* 2017;107(10):1612–1614.

18. Chi DL, Lenaker D, Mancl L, et al. Dental therapists linked to improved dental outcomes for Alaska Native communities in the Yukon-Kuskokwim Delta. *J Public Health Dent.* 2018;78(2):175–182.

19. Colby SL, Ortman JM. The baby boom cohort in the United States: 2012 to 2060. Population estimates and projections. *Current Population Reports.* P25-1141. U.S. Census Bureau; U.S. Department of Commerce Economics and Statistics Administration. Available from: https://www.census.gov/prod/2014pubs/p25-1141.pdf.

20. Cully JL, Doyle M, Thikkurissy S. Impact of an alternative hours dental clinic for adolescents. *Pediatr Dent.* 2018;40(4):288–290.

21. Delta Dental of Colorado Foundation. *Year One Highlights.* Available from: Colorado Medical-Dental Integration Project; September 2015. http://medicaldentalintegration.org/co-mdi-overview/.

22. Edelstein B. The dental safety net, its workforce, and policy recommendations for its enhancement. *J Pub Health Dent.* 2010;70(s1):S32–S39.

23. Glassman P, Harrington M, Namakian M, et al. The virtual dental home: bringing oral health to vulnerable and underserved populations. *J Cal Dent Assoc.* 2012;40(7):569–577.

24. Guagliardo MF. Spatial accessibility of primary care: concepts, methods and challenges. *Int J Health Geogr.* 2004;3(1):3.

25. Health Resources and Services Administration. *2016 National Health Center Data.* Available from: https://bphc.hrsa.gov/uds/datacenter.aspx.

26. *Healthy People 2020.* [Internet]. Washington, DC: U.S. Department of Health and Human Services: Office of Disease Prevention and Health Promotion. Available from: https://www.healthypeople.gov/2020/topics-objectives/topic/oral-health; 2020.

27. Heima M, Heaton LJ, Ng HH, et al. Dental fear among transgender individuals—a cross-sectional survey. *Spec Care Dentist.* 2017;37(5):212–222.

28. Hinton E, Paradise J. Access to dental care in Medicaid: spotlight on nonelderly adults. *Kaiser Family Foundation Issue Brief.* Available from: http://files.kff.org/attachment/issue-brief-access-to-dental-care-in-medicaid-spotlight-on-nonelderly-adults; 2016.

29. Holtzman JS, Atchison KA, Gironda MW, et al. The association between oral health literacy and failed appointments in adults attending a university-based general dental clinic. *Community Dent Oral Epidemiol.* 2014;42(3):263–270.

30. Institute of Medicine (IOM). Access to health care in America. Millman M, editor. *Access to Health Care in America.* Washington, DC: National Academies Press; 1993. 2, A model for monitoring access. 3, Using indicators to monitor national objectives for health care. https://www.ncbi.nlm.nih.gov/books/NBK235882/

31. Institute of Medicine. *Health Literacy: A Prescription to End Confusion.* Washington, DC: National Academy Press; 2004.

32. James SE, Herman JL, Rankin S, et al. *Executive Summary of the Report of the 2015 U.S. Transgender Survey.* Washington, DC: National Center for Transgender Equality; 2016.

33. Jones M, Lee JY, Rozier RG. Oral health literacy among adult patients seeking dental care. *J Am Dent Assoc.* 2007;138(9):1199–1208.

34. Kiyak HA, Reichmuth M. Barriers to and enablers of older adults' use of dental services. *J Dent Ed.* 2005;69(9):975–986.

35. Lacy ES, McCann AL, Miller BH, et al. Achieving student diversity in dental schools: a model that works. *J Dent Educ.* 2012;76(5):523–533.

36. Laveist TA, Nuru-Jeter A. Is doctor-patient race concordance associated with greater satisfaction with care? *J Health Soc Behav.* 2002;43(3):296–306.

37. Lawton L. Providing dental care for special patients. Tips for the general dentist. *J Am Dent Assoc.* 2002;133(2):1666–1670.

38. Levy H, Janke A. Health literacy and access to care. *J Health Commun.* 2016;21(Suppl 1):43–50.

39. Macek MD, Atchison KA, Chen H, et al. Oral health conceptual knowledge and its relationships with oral health outcomes: findings from a multi-site health literacy study. *Community Dent Oral Epidemiol.* 2017;45(4):323–329.

40. Macek MD, Atchison KA, Watson MR, et al. Assessing health literacy and oral health: preliminary results of a multi-site investigation. *J Public Health Dent.* 2016;76(4):303–313.

41. O'Malley A. After-hours access to primary care practices linked with lower emergency department use and less unmet medical need. *Health Aff.* 2013;32(1):175–183.

42. Manski RJ, Rohde F. *Dental services: use, expenses, source of payment, coverage and procedure type, 1996–2015: Research Findings No. 38.* Agency for Healthcare Research and Quality: Rockville, MD; 2017. Available from: https://meps.ahrq.gov/data_files/publications/rf38/rf38.pdf.

43. McClain MA, Jones FR, McClain CR, et al. Increasing dental student diversity through the UNLV Dental Prospects Program. *J Dent Educ.* 2013;77(5):548–553.

44. Mertz EA, Wides CD, Kottek AM, et al. Underrepresented minority dentists: quantifying their number and characterizing the communities they serve. *Health Affairs.* 2016;35(12):2190–2199.

45. *Minority Graduates of U.S. Dental Schools, 1977 to 2017.* Table. American Dental Education Association; 2018. Available from: http://www.adea.org/data/students/.

46. Nasseh K, Vujicic M. The relationship between education debt and career choices in professional programs. The case of dentistry. *J Am Dent Assoc.* 2017;148(11):825–833.

47. Nasseh K, Vujicic M, Yarbrough C. *A Ten-Year, State-By-State, Analysis of Medicaid Fee-for-Service Reimbursement Rates for Dental Care Services.* American Dental Association: Health Policy Institute

Research Brief; 2014. Available from: http://www.aapd.org/assets/1/7/PolicyCenter-TenYearAnalysisOct2014.pdf.

48. Nelson LP, Getzin A, Graham D, et al. Unmet dental needs and barriers to care for children with significant special health care needs. *Pediatr Dent.* 2011;33(1):29–36.

49. Office of Minority Health. *The National CLAS Standards.* Washington, DC: US Department of Health and Human Services Office of Minority Health; 2016. Available from: https://minorityhealth.hhs.gov/omh/browse.aspx?lvl=2&lvlid=53.

50. Office of Minority Health. *Think Cultural Health.* US Department of Health and Human Services. Available from: https://thinkculturalhealth.hhs.gov/.

51. Okunseri C, Bajorunaite R, Abena A, et al. Racial/ethnic disparities in the acceptance of Medicaid patients in dental practices. *J Public Health Dent.* 2008;68(3):149–153.

52. Okunseri C, Okunseri E, Thorpe JM, et al. Patient characteristics and trends in nontraumatic dental condition visits to emergency departments in the United States. *Clin Cosmet Investig Dent.* 2012;4:1–7.

53. Penchansky R, Thomas JW. The concept of access. *Med Care.* 1981;19(2):127–140.

54. Raimann TE, Reynolds E, Ishkanian E, et al. *The Ethics of Temporary Charitable Events.* American Dental Association White Paper; 2015. Available from: https://www.ada.org/~/media/ADA/About%20the%20ADA/Files/ADA-Charitable-Event-White-Paper.pdf?la=en.

55. Saurman E. Improving access: modifying Penchansky and Thomas's theory of access. *J Health Serv Res & Pol.* 2016;21(1):36–39.

56. Scott TL, Gazmararian JA, Williams MV, et al. Health literacy and preventive health care use among Medicare enrollees in a managed care organization. *Med Care.* 2002;40(5):395–404.

57. Shah AC, Leong KK, Lee MK, et al. Outcomes attributed to periapical abscess from 2000 to 2008: A longitudinal trend analysis. *J Endod.* 2013;39(9):1104–1110.

58. Shelley D, Russell S, Parikh NS, et al. Ethnic disparities in self-reported oral health status and access to care among older adults in NYC. *J Urban Health.* 2011;88(4):651–662.

59. Skillman SM, Doescher MP, Mouradian WE, et al. The challenge of delivering oral health services in rural America. *J Public Health Dent.* 2010;70(S1):S49–S57.

60. Stein LI, Polido JC, Najera SO, et al. Oral care experiences and challenges in children with autism spectrum disorders. *Pediatr Dent.* 2012;34(5):387–391.

61. US Department of Health and Human Services. *Oral Health in America. A Report of the Surgeon General–Executive Summary.* Rockville, MD: US Department of Health and Human Services, National Institute of Dental and Craniofacial Research. In: *National Institutes of Health;* 2000.

62. Vujicic M. Where have all the dental care visits gone? *J Am Dent Assoc.* 2015;146(6):412–414.

63. Vujicic M, Buchmueller T, Klein R. Dental care presents the highest level of financial barriers, compared to other types of health care services. *Health Aff.* 2016;35(12):2176–2182.

64. Washington DC: *State Health Professions Education Program.* SHPEP; 2018. Available from: http://www.shpep.org/about/.

65. Wendling WR. Private sector approaches to workforce enhancement. *J Public Health Dent.* 2010;70(s1):S24–S31.

66. Yarbrough C, Vujicic M, Nasseh K. *Estimating the cost of introducing a Medicaid adult dental benefit in 22 states.* American Dental Association: Health Policy Institute Research Brief; 2016. Available from: http://www.ada.org/~/media/ADA/Science%20and%20Research/HPI/Files/HPIBrief_0316_1.ashx.

67. Yoon J, Cordasco KM, Chow A, et al. The relationship between same-day access and continuity in primary care and emergency department visits. *PLoS One.* 2015;10(9). e0135274.

# 4

# Ethics and Dental Public Health

KATHRYN A. ATCHISON, DDS, MPH

JAY W. FRIEDMAN, DDS, MPH

## CHAPTER OUTLINE

Framework for Ethical Standards

Individual Versus Social Responsibility

Individualism in the United States

Right to Healthcare

Professional Ethics and Self-Regulation
    Ethical Standards in Patient Care
    Ethical Standards in Research

Dentistry's Ethical Challenge: Access to Care for Everyone

As noted in Chapter 1, professionalism brings with it the responsibility to adhere to the highest ethical standards. Public trust is a profession's greatest asset, and that trust assumes the dental profession's adherence to ethical practices and the responsibility to follow through with corrective action if there has been a breach. Whether one is in clinical practice treating individual patients or working in public health agencies, even the most conscientious practitioner will find that ethical dilemmas arise frequently. For example, how does a practitioner respond to a patient who wants all her amalgam restorations removed because she believes they are the cause of her chronic fatigue? How does a practitioner respond to a colleague whose practice philosophy is the extraction of a tooth and replacement with an implant rather than endodontically treating teeth? What is the practitioner's role in helping a community fully understand the benefits and risks of water fluoridation so that the community can come to an informed decision via the voting process? A profession's code of ethics provides guidelines for the practitioner to follow.

This chapter discusses aspects of professional ethics relevant to dental care and dental public health. We discuss the framework for ethical codes, the social and cultural background against which U.S. ethical standards have evolved, ethics in patient and population care and research, and the role of the professional associations in defining ethical codes.

## Framework for Ethical Standards

Ethics, a branch of philosophy, is the study of what is right and good with respect to the conduct of an individual or a group.[25] Perhaps our understanding of ethics can be helped by first defining what ethics is not. Ethics is not a set of rules or restrictions, it is not religion, and it is not the law.[25] It is essentially a guide to moral conduct. Much of the ethics literature asks questions about issues that are too complex for simple answers. The literature helps to guide us toward an understanding of what is right and wrong in our behavior. This lack of a "formula" to solve problems can be frustrating, because ethical decisions vary over time and between cultures that historically have different moral standards. Nonetheless, some basic guides are common to all cultures.

Hippocrates' dictum, "First, do no harm," has been around since 400 BCE. Today there are six basic principles (Box 4.1) that are widely accepted as guidelines for decision-making in biomedical ethical dilemmas and that apply to all healthcare professionals, including dentists, dental hygienists, physicians, and nurses. For professional organizations, these principals can take the following forms:

*Aspirational*: A broadly worded statement of ideals, lacking precise definitions of right or wrong behavior

*Educational*: Combines principles with explicit guidelines that can assist professionals in their decision-making during challenging situations

*Regulatory*: Includes a detailed set of rules to govern professional conduct and serve as a basis for adjudicating grievances

Professions adopt ethical codes of conduct to guide their members and to protect the public from charlatans and negligent practitioners including those who present unscientific bias. A patient's trust comes in part from the expectation that the professional's behavior is governed by norms prescribed by the group.[9] The public expects that ethical standards are enforced by the profession, a requirement that comes with the privilege of self-regulation.

As stated earlier, ethical standards are shaped in part by cultural forces, so it is important to examine briefly some of the social and cultural forces that underlie ethical expectations in the United States.

## Individual Versus Social Responsibility

Who is responsible for health? Is health each individual's responsibility, or does society bear some responsibility? Clearly, the answer can only be "both."

It is well understood today that individual lifestyle choices are a major factor affecting our health. The public is well advised: Don't

---

**• BOX 4.1   Summary of Ethical Guidelines for Biomedical Decision Making[2]**

1. *Respect for autonomy* directs the practitioner to respect patients and their points of view and to provide sufficient information for patients or the community to make their decision.
2. *Nonmaleficence* obliges the practitioner to do no harm and to act in the best interests of the patient.
3. *Beneficence* encourages the practitioner to prevent harm, promote good for others, and provide information for the patient to balance the benefits against risks and cost.

4. *Justice* argues for the fair distribution of scarce healthcare benefits and risks associated with interventions in the community.
5. *Veracity* underscores the informed consent process and places expectations on the practitioner to provide sufficient information to the patient or community in plain language that can be understood by the recipient.
6. *Right to dignity* argues that all parties—patients, their families, and health care providers—have a right to respect during the healthcare interaction, and good communication is foremost in achieving a successful interaction and healthcare decision.

---

smoke, drink in moderation, eat a varied diet with lots of fresh fruit and vegetables, get enough sleep, exercise regularly, fasten the car's seatbelt, maintain friendships and social contacts. But what about those individuals who are unfortunate enough to have genetic predispositions to disease or are mentally or physically disadvantaged? What about those who live in rundown neighborhoods where food choices are limited and there is little opportunity to practice a healthy lifestyle? Many people become addicted to cigarettes, alcohol, and drugs even though the danger is well understood. These problems are compounded by the individual's inability to pay for necessary healthcare. What are the professions' ethical obligations in these and related instances?

If we believed that health is solely an individual responsibility, we would shrug our shoulders, say "bad luck," and be thankful that these bad things weren't happening to us. But to lesser or greater degree, most nations accept some measure of public responsibility by means of public health and social support systems for their less fortunate populations. Most European countries, along with Canada, Australia, and New Zealand, have comprehensive national healthcare systems that cost less per capita (compared to the United States) with comparable or better overall indicators of population health, such as longevity.

Although the United States has strengthened its national healthcare coverage, opposition is strong, with arguments about whether such programs should exist at all. Thus, the extent of and eligibility criteria for public financing of health and welfare—and the right balance between public and personal financing for them—continues to be vigorously debated. Since American attitudes toward publicly financed social systems are not as positive as those in other developed countries, it is worth looking at how American cultural attitudes toward individualism and social responsibility have evolved.

## Individualism in the United States

Americans cherish their individual rights and freedoms; individualism is a powerful cultural force in the United States, more so than in many other countries.[7] Many of the early immigrants to America left rigid social, religious, or political systems with little opportunity to advance. They sought a new life where they and their children could prosper in an environment that was free of the constraints they had left behind and where hard work would create its own opportunities and yield its own rewards. An abundance of natural resources and a seemingly limitless frontier gave rise to the attitude that in America people could mold their own destinies largely by their own efforts. The American Dream continues to attract immigrants today.

Social welfare programs grew slowly in the United States. It was not until 1935, in the middle of the Great Depression, that the Social Security Act was passed. Many people lost everything during the Great Depression through no fault of their own, and the response of the federal government was a series of emergency relief measures aimed at providing jobs through the Work Projects Administration (WPA), thus avoiding total societal collapse.

Social Security has not only survived but has become institutionalized as a major entitlement that figures prominently in the current political debate. World War II (1939–45) provided the industrial expansion that brought the country out of the Depression. It also gave rise to the health insurance industry. With increasing recognition of the extent, persistence, and consequences of poverty, the 88th and 89th Congresses (1964–65) passed a series of legislative measures intended to improve social equity, the main ones being Medicare and Medicaid (see Chapter 7), the Voting Rights Act, the Economic Opportunity Act, the Model Cities Program, and the Elementary and Secondary Education Act. The trend toward social programs was slowed, and in some cases reversed, by the more conservative mood that set in during the 1980s.

## Right to Healthcare

American attitudes, historically shaped by individualism, are evolving slowly in recognition that good health contributes to a competent workforce. Further, a growing segment of the U.S. population believes that some level of access to healthcare is a right rather than a privilege.[6] The "right to healthcare" is often misunderstood. Although medical care has been overvalued to some extent as a determinant of health,[6,11,13] most individuals at some time in their lives have a need for it, sometimes an urgent need.

The demand for healthcare exceeds its "supply." Healthcare has always been rationed in one way or another. Traditional rationing is accomplished by fee for service, meaning that those who can afford to purchase it get it; those who lack the money go without. The rationing is simple enough, but it confers an untold cost in wasted human resources through illness, disability, and death. This system of unfettered individual responsibility for one's health was challenged in the 1960s when financing of healthcare was extended to millions of poorer citizens through Medicaid and to the elderly through Medicare. It was extended further when the Children's Health Insurance Program (CHIP) was signed into law in 1997, followed by the Patient Protection and Affordable Care Act of 2010 (see Chapter 7).

As expenditures for both public and private medical care increased exponentially, controlling cost became a high priority.

After the enactment of the Health Maintenance Organization Act, "managed care" grew rapidly as a means to control the cost of health care (see Chapter 7).[19] While reducing the rate of increase in medical expenditures, managed care introduced another form of rationing—the restriction of services and choice of doctor. This interjected additional ethical challenges to the practitioner.

## Professional Ethics and Self-Regulation

The American Dental Association (ADA) maintains a code of ethics, which is reviewed and amended periodically by the association's Council on Ethics, Bylaws and Judicial Affairs. The current version of the code of ethics can be found on the ADA's website.[4] It addresses the following: principles of ethics, code of professional conduct, and advisory opinions. This code is classified as *aspirational* by the ADA.

The Principles of Ethics section provides examples applicable to select behaviors and situations primarily concerned with the care of patients and the handling of a dental practice (e.g. referrals, criticism of colleagues, advertising, and specialty practice). The code is influenced by judicial outcomes, which presumably represent social values, as evidenced by growth in the legal advisory opinions in the code. As an example, the 1982 statement on patient selection stated the following:

> *While dentists, in serving the public, may exercise reasonable discretion in selecting patients for their practices, dentists shall not refuse to accept patients into their practice or deny dental service to patients because of the patient's race, creed, color, sex or national origin.*[2]

An advisory opinion was added in 1988 to include treating infected patients:

> *A dentist has the general obligation to provide care to those in need. A decision not to provide treatment to an individual because the individual has AIDS or is HIV seropositive, based solely on that fact, is unethical. Decisions with regard to the type of dental treatment provided or referrals made or suggested, in such instances, should be made on the same basis as they are made with other patients, that is, whether the individual dentist believes he or she has need of another's skills, knowledge, equipment or experience and whether the dentist believes, after consultation with the patient's physician if appropriate, the patient's health status would be significantly compromised by the provision of dental treatment.*[3]

The advisory opinion, maintained in the 2003 version of the code, is an example of an issue that causes misgivings among some practitioners who do not feel it unethical to turn away a patient who has tested positive for human immunodeficiency virus on the grounds that the health of the dentist and staff would be unduly at risk if treatment were offered. Of note, not only is such behavior unethical, it is also illegal, as was substantiated by the courts in finding that while using universal precautions, there was no evidence that treating an HIV-positive patient presented a direct threat of infection.[26] By the new century, however, the issue had advanced to the point where the code includes sharing the bloodborne status of the healthcare team in Section 2.E:

> *All dentists, regardless of their blood borne pathogen status, have an ethical obligation to immediately inform any patient who may have been exposed to blood or other potentially infectious material in the dental office of the need for post-exposure evaluation and follow-up and to immediately refer the patient to a qualified health care practitioner who can provide post-exposure services. …The dentist's ethical obligation in the event of an exposure incident extends to providing information concerning the dentist's own bloodborne pathogen status to the evaluating health care practitioner, if the dentist is the source individual, and to submitting to testing that will assist in the evaluation of the patient. If a staff member or other third person is the source individual, the dentist should encourage that person to cooperate as needed for the patient's evaluation.*[4]

Section 3 of the ADA code, Principle of Beneficence, states that the dentist has an obligation to put the patient's welfare first:

> *This principle expresses the concept that professionals have a duty to act for the benefit of others. Under this principle, the dentist's primary obligation is service to the patient and the public-at-large. … The same ethical considerations apply whether the dentist engages in fee-for-service, managed care or some other practice arrangement. Dentists may choose to enter into contracts governing the provision of care to a group of patients; however, contract obligations do not excuse dentists from their ethical duty to put the patient's welfare first.*

Not all aspects of practice are covered by the ADA Code of Ethics. For example, the obligation to keep current through continuing education and reading the literature, a prime ethical responsibility,[21] is nonetheless given only cursory mention in the ADA code Section 2 Principle of Nonmaleficence, 2.A Education:

> *The privilege of dentists to be accorded professional status rests primarily in the knowledge, skill and experience with which they serve their patients and society. All dentists, therefore, have the obligation of keeping their knowledge and skill current.*

The states have assumed the role of requiring continuing education in order to apply for dental relicensure, emphasizing the overlap between ethical and legal responsibilities.

The ADA Code of Ethics places little emphasis on the role of the dentist in the community. Section 3.A of the code simply states:

> *Since dentists have an obligation to use their skills, knowledge, and experience for the improvement of the dental health of the public and are encouraged to be leaders in their community, dentists in such service shall conduct themselves in such a manner as to maintain or elevate the esteem of the profession.*[4]

Some dentists working for a fluoridation campaign in the community, for example, have felt that an appearance on local television might be construed as personal advertising, which violates the spirit of the ADA Code of Ethics, even if such an appearance would help the campaign. This unduly cautious interpretation contrasts with those who feel that the statement in the code was never intended to preclude such obviously public-spirited activity. Some would like to see Section 3.A of the code strengthened to encourage dentists to work cooperatively with public health authorities for the benefit of the whole community.

The code of ethics adopted by the American Dental Hygienists' Association (ADHA) is generally similar to the ADA code.[5] The ADHA considers that all people should have access to healthcare and to oral healthcare and that people are responsible for their own health and entitled to make choices regarding their health. No such statement about access to healthcare can be found in the ADA code. The ADHA also describes standards of professional responsibility that include serving the clients without discrimination and serving as advocates for the welfare of their clients.

A national survey of ADHA members in the late 1980s disclosed that the three most frequent ethical issues faced by hygienists were: (1) observation of a dentist's behavior in conflict with standard infection control procedures; (2) failure of the dentist to refer patients to specialists, such as periodontists; and (3) nondiagnosis of oral disease by the dentist.[12] Although 86% of those hygienists responding said that they had some instruction in ethical theory, only 51% reported that they had received instruction in how to cope with these ethical challenges encountered in their employment. A survey of the factors influencing dental hygienists with 5 or more years of practice to remain in private practice reinforced the importance of ethical concerns over the quality of care experienced in practice.[8] Three of the top five issues related to retention in private practice, after salary and working conditions, were the quality of the dentist's work, the maintaining of current infection control standards in the practice, and being given adequate time to provide high-quality and complete patient treatment. The ADHA code contains some statements about dental hygiene practice that reflects a stronger community outlook than is found in the ADA code.

*The Principles of the Ethical Practice of Public Health* provides guidance for dental professionals performing community engagement.[22] Rather than focusing on the practice of a professional serving the individual patient, the code (Box 4.2) emphasizes the type of tools that a professional employs when serving the community. These include promotion of population health, such as implementation of community-based fluoride in areas with insufficient naturally occurring fluoride and the corollary prevention of disease. Professionals may advocate the collection and use of epidemiologic data or the use of surveillance data to better understand the challenges and needs of the community.

Specific principles describe the need to respect the interdependence, cultural diversity, and the variety of socioeconomic conditions of the people who make up the community. The principles challenge professionals working within the community to simultaneously recognize and balance the health of the community and its individual residents; to provide opportunities for

public input before developing policies, practices, priorities, and programs; and to gain the community's approval before implementing programs.

The emphasis on community is a keystone of public health, as recognized also in the ethical code of the American Association of Public Health Dentistry.[1] It is not intended to be at odds with the individualist tradition described earlier but recognizes a different lens within which practice takes place.

## Ethical Standards in Patient Care

The world was shocked by the atrocities committed by Nazi Germany on prisoners in concentration camps during World War II in the name of medical experimentation. In a reaction against these appalling crimes, the World Medical Association—a group of national medical associations rather like the Fédération Dentaire Internationale (FDI) adopted the Declaration of Geneva in 1948.[30]

Society bestows self-governance upon the dental profession in recognition that the profession conducts itself in a fair and honorable manner in its contacts with patients. As discussed in Chapter 1, this is one of the cornerstones of professionalism. The ADA states that "the ADA Code is, in effect, a written expression of the obligations arising from the implied contract between the dental profession and society."[4]

Because the professional has knowledge that the patient does not have, the professional can evaluate likely treatment outcomes better than the patient can. The professional therefore is obligated to minimize the effects of *paternalism* by providing sufficient information, in language the patient can understand, to allow the patient to make truly informed decisions.[21]

This is easier said than done:

*Although intellectually patients—including doctors when they become patients—know that doctors are not infallible, emotionally we want to believe that they are, that they know what they are doing and are capable of doing it. The most skeptical of us longs to leave such skepticism in the waiting room.*[10]

The 1998 *Consumer Bill of Rights and Responsibilities,* also known as the Patient's Bill of Rights, was adopted to increase

---

**• BOX 4.2    Principles of the Ethical Practice of Public Health[22]**

The code of ethics adopted by the Public Health Leadership Society presents the key principles of an ethical practice of public health followed by a statement describing the values and beliefs inherent to a public health perspective.

1. Public health should address principally the fundamental causes of disease and requirements for health, aiming to prevent adverse health outcomes.
2. Public health should achieve community health in a way that respects the rights of individuals in the community.
3. Public health policies, programs, and priorities should be developed and evaluated through processes that ensure an opportunity for input from community members.
4. Public health should advocate and work for the empowerment of disenfranchised community members, aiming to ensure that the basic resources and conditions necessary for health are accessible to all.
5. Public health should seek the information needed to implement effective policies and programs that protect and promote health.
6. Public health institutions should provide communities with the information that is needed for decisions on policies or programs and should obtain the community's consent for their implementation.
7. Public health institutions should act in a timely manner on the information they have within the resources and the mandate given to them by the public.
8. Public health programs and policies should incorporate a variety of approaches that anticipate and respect diverse values, beliefs, and cultures in the community.
9. Public health programs and policies should be implemented in a manner that most enhances the physical and social environment.
10. Public health institutions should protect the confidentiality of information that can bring harm to an individual or community if made public. Exceptions must be justified on the basis of the high likelihood of significant harm to the individual or others.
11. Public health institutions should ensure the professional competence of their employees.
12. Public health institutions and their employees should engage in collaborations and affiliations in ways that build the public's trust and the institution's effectiveness.

patients' confidence that the U.S. healthcare system was fair and responsive to patients' needs, that a strong relationship between the patient and the doctor was important, and that patients needed to assume an active role in getting or staying healthy.[28] This advisory opinion recognized the ethical challenges brought by the unequal knowledge between the patient and professional and sought to define patients' rights and professionals' responsibilities.

The unbalanced knowledge between doctor and patient can easily lead the professional to take a paternalistic role, no matter how reluctantly, and it can sharpen the conflict between professional and proprietary values that frequently arises in dental practice.[18] Some have argued that dentistry needs well-defined standards of care to fall back on in such circumstances,[10] but the profession has never been comfortable about defining such *educational* standards because of its reluctance to infringe upon professional judgment.

Nonetheless, the ADA began developing standards with its Dental Practice Parameters, adopted by the House of Delegates in 1994–1995, which described clinical aspects of diagnosis and treatment. The standards are presented as voluntary aids to the dentists' clinical decision-making.[24] These parameters have been followed by "evidence-based" clinical recommendations, now termed "evidence-based dentistry" (see Chapter 11). Dentists are obligated to understand what constitutes scientific evidence (see Chapter 10) and to keep current with evidence-based dentistry through continuing education. Maintaining professional competence is a prime ethical responsibility.[21]

## Ethical Standards in Research

Much research involves experimental studies using humans and human tissues, as well as animals, and there are strict codes or regulations to protect them from abuse. The first detailed codes were developed in the shadow of World War II. The revulsion that followed the disclosure of Nazi "experiments" gave rise to patients' rights and resulted in the 1947 Nuremberg Code,[17] which required that subjects be able to exercise choice, have the legal and intellectual capacity to give consent, and be able to understand to what they are consenting.[16]

Since then, the Nuremberg Code has served as the basis for the extensive legal regulations many countries have developed to govern the participation of humans in research. In addition to drafting the Declaration of Geneva, which was aimed at patient care, the World Medical Association has further refined the rights of human participants in research through the Declaration of Helsinki in 1964, its subsequent amendments,[31] and a host of national and professional codes since then. The Declaration of Helsinki states definitively: "While the primary purpose of medical research is to generate new knowledge, this goal can never take precedence over the rights and interests of individual research subjects."

Legal requirements aside, researchers always have the ethical obligation to treat all human research volunteers with respect and dignity. The treatment of animals in research has also become more regulated to ensure humane treatment of the animals, although there is still cause for caution and concern.

In the United States, formulation of codes of ethics in research considers both the World Medical Association code and the *Belmont Report.*[27] The *Belmont Report* identified the basic ethical principles for the conduct of biomedical and behavioral research involving human subjects: respect for persons' autonomy, beneficence, and justice. It also developed guidelines to ensure that such research is conducted properly.

The International Association for Dental Research (IADR) is the umbrella organization for dental research activities around the world. The IADR adopted the principles for a code of ethics in 1994.[14,23] Given the range of laws for each country, their healthcare systems, and cultural norms among those involved in research, the IADR Ethics Committee presented specific principles that would have wide recognition.

Each of the five regions (usually groups of countries) is encouraged to use the IADR's comprehensive report on ethics[14] to develop their own codes. The IADR's 1994 statement of research principles, shown in Box 4.3, is clearly aspirational in nature. In addition to the principles, the code of ethics provides statements referring members to the Declaration of Helsinki for ethical principles related to research with human subjects and with animals.

The trend in guidelines for ethical conduct within the United States is toward ever-expanding regulations governing research with human subjects, especially documentation of informed consent. Every institution in which research involving human subjects takes place is required to have an institutional review board whose task is to review all proposals before the research actually starts to ensure that regulations for the protection of human subjects have been followed.

Punishment for not complying with these regulations can be strict—several major research universities have had all research funding cut off until alleged transgressions against human subjects have been corrected. Complying with the institutional review board requirements should be viewed not as a burden but as an obligation to the subjects who have generously given their time and personal contribution to expanding our scientific knowledge.

In addition to physical abuse, fabrication and falsification of data and plagiarism must be guarded against.[29] *Fabrication* involves the manufacturing of research data out of thin air. *Falsification* includes the manipulation of the research materials, equipment, or processes or selectively including or omitting data or results so that the

---

**• BOX 4.3** **Statement of Principles Within the Code of Ethics for the International Association for Dental Research (IADR) Intended to Guide Members in Their Research and Scholarly Activities[14]**

All members of the IADR shall:
1. Act with honor and in accordance with the highest standards of professional integrity;
2. Conduct work with objectivity;
3. Communicate in an honest and responsible manner;
4. Show consideration and respect for all components of and individuals associated with the research process;

5. Cultivate an environment whereby differences in perspective, experience and culture are recognized and valued;
6. Maintain appropriate standards of accuracy, reliability, credit, candor and confidentiality in all research and scholarship activities;
7. Use all resources prudently, taking into account appropriate laws and regulations.

ultimate research findings do not accurately represent the research record. *Plagiarism* is the taking of another individual's words, results, ideas, or work without giving appropriate credit to the author. Plagiarism has always been around, but the Internet has raised it to unprecedented heights. It seems that people who would never lift a paragraph from a book or journal without attribution have no such qualms about lifting Internet material without attribution, even though the principles are the same.

## Dentistry's Ethical Challenge: Access to Care for Everyone

In 2007, a 12-year-old boy, Deamonte Driver, died from an infection that spread from an abscessed tooth to his brain before his family could find a dentist who would accept him as a Medicaid patient. His tragic death, widely reported in the news, outraged the public and led to nationwide discussion over access to dental care for the disadvantaged population and the ethical responsibility of the dental profession to provide it.[20]

Access to dental care is a function of geography and financial resources. Most dentists practice in affluent cities and suburbs where there are sufficient patients with the means to afford their services. But in the "inner cities" and in many rural areas, access to care is limited by a shortage of dentists. There are over 5800 dental health professional shortage areas[15] in the United States, defined as 1 dentist or less per 5000 people. It would take approximately 10,000 additional dentists to meet this minimal level of access.

As discussed in Chapter 2, some 12% of Americans (39 million) exist below the federal poverty line, and millions of others live on the fringe of poverty. Eighteen percent or 58 million people are eligible for Medicaid. Yet adults who have Medicaid, which does not cover dental care in many states, are almost five times as likely to have poor oral health as adults with private health insurance. A survey of the population showed that high cost was the main reason that poor adults do not visit a dentist when they have an oral health problem. Not only is dental care financially out of reach for the poor, many practitioners prefer not to treat such patients. Intertwined with the world of poverty are the homeless, the unemployed and unemployable, and the homebound and chronically ill—all of whom suffer dental neglect. Then there is a virtual army of working poor, usually uninsured and in minimum-wage positions, who simply cannot afford the high cost of dental care.

As a consequence, the need for dental public health services is self-evident, but there are still formidable practical obstacles to making them available. Public services in the United States, in contrast to their counterparts in most developed nations, are chronically underfunded. This is partly an offshoot of the individualist culture described earlier, which leads to public services being held in low esteem. Even when resources are adequate, treatment for these special groups is usually less efficient than it is for patients in private practice. Their oral health needs are often greater, appointments are missed for lack of transportation or assistance of caregivers, and the mentally or physically disabled require special management skills and take more time to treat.

There are no simple answers to the problem of ensuring access to dental care. However, the problems are compounded without adequate funding of public health agencies. A nationwide health center infrastructure, known as Federally Qualified Health Centers (FQHCs), was developed as a means to increase access to comprehensive primary health, mental health, and substance abuse services for vulnerable populations, but many FQHCs do not yet offer dental care. Adequate funding and an increase in the supply of dentists, dental hygienists, dental assistants, and dental therapists are essential if the underserved population is ever to have access to not only emergency care but also primary preventive services to achieve and maintain optimum oral health.

The ultimate ethical challenge to everyone in dentistry is achieving the noble goal of adequate oral health for all. Finding the appropriate mix of public and private services that serves the entire population is needed for this to occur.

## References

1. American Association of Public Health Dentistry. *Code of Ethics and Standards of Professional Conduct.* Interim policy adopted October 16, 1997. Available from: http://www.aaphd.org/index. php?option=com_content&view=article&id=120:aaphd-code-of-ethics-and-standards-of-professional-conduct&catid=19:site-content.
2. American Dental Association, Council on Ethics, Bylaws, and Judicial Affairs. American Dental Association principles of ethics and code of professional conduct. *J Am Dent Assoc.* 1982;105: 493–495.
3. American Dental Association, Council on Ethics, Bylaws, and Judicial Affairs. American Dental Association principles of ethics and code of professional conduct. *J Am Dent Assoc.* 1988;117: 657–661.
4. American Dental Association, Council on Ethics, Bylaws, and Judicial Affairs. *Principles of Ethics and Code of Professional Conduct.* Available from: https://www.ada.org/en/about-the-ada/principles-of-ethics-code-of-professional-conduct; 2018.
5. American Dental Hygienists' Association. *Code of Ethics for Dental Hygienists.* Adopted June 13, 2016. Available from: http://www.adha. org/sites/default/files/7611_Bylaws_and_Code_of_Ethics_0.pdf.
6. Banta D. What is health care? In: Jonas S, ed. *Health Care Delivery in the United States.* 1st ed. New York, NY: Springer; 1977:12–39.
7. Billington RA. Frontiers. In: Woodward CV, ed. *The Comparative Approach to American History.* New York, NY: Basic Books; 1968: 75–90.
8. Calley KH, Bowen DM, Darby ML, et al. Factors influencing dental hygiene retention in private practice. *J Dent Hyg.* 1996;70(4): 151–160.
9. Frankel MS. Developing ethical standards for responsible research. *J Dent Res.* 1996;75:832–835.
10. Friedman JW, Atchison KA. The standard of care: an ethical responsibility of public health dentistry. *J Public Health Dent.* 1993;53: 165–169.
11. Fuchs V. *Who Shall Live? Health, Economics, and Social Choice.* New York, NY: Basic Books; 1974.
12. Gaston MA, Brown DM, Waring MB. Survey of ethical issues in dental hygiene. *J Dent Hyg.* 1990;64:216–223.
13. Illich I. *Medical Nemesis: The Expropriation of Health.* New York, NY: Bantam Books; 1976.
14. International Association for Dental Research. *Code of Ethics.* Adopted May 2009. Available from: http://www.iadr.org/IADR/ About-Us/Who-We-Are/Code-of-Ethics.
15. The Kaiser Family Foundation State Health Facts. *Dental Care Health Professional Shortage Areas (HPSAs).* Data source: Bureau of Health Workforce, Health Resources and Services Administration (HRSA), U.S. Department of Health & Human Services, Designated Health Professional Shortage Areas Statistics: Designated HPSA Quarterly Summary, as of December 31, 2016. Available from: https://www.kff.org/other/state-indicator/dental-care-health-professional-shortage-areas-hpsas/?currentTimeframe=0&sortModel=%7B% 22colId%22:%22Location%22,%22sort%22:%22asc%22%7D.

16. McCarthy CR. Legal and regulatory considerations concerning research involving human subjects. *J Dent Res.* 1980;59(Spec Issue C): 1228–1234.

17. Mitscherlich A, Mielke F. *Doctors of Infamy: The Story of the Nazi Medical Crimes.* Schuman: New York, NY; 1949.

18. Nash DA. A tension between two cultures. Dentistry as a profession and dentistry as a proprietary. *J Dent Educ.* 1994;58:301–306.

19. National Council on Disability. Appendix B. A brief history of managed care. Available from: https://www.ncd.gov/policy/appendix-b-brief-history-managed-care.

20. Otto M. For want of a dentist. *Washington Post*, February. 2007;28. Available from: http://www.washingtonpost.com/wp-dyn/content/article/2007/02/27/AR2007022702116.html.

21. Ozar DT. A framework for studying professional ethics. *J Am Coll Dent.* 1991;58:4,6–9.

22. Public Health Leadership Society. *Principles of the Ethical Practice of Public Health. Ver. 2.2.* Available from: https://www.apha.org/-/media/files/pdf/membergroups/ethics/ethics_brochure.ashx; 2002.

23. Shah RM. Introduction: proceedings of a symposium, Ethics in Dental Research. *J Dent Res.* 1994;74:1757–1758.

24. Shugars DA, Bader JD. Practice parameters in dentistry: where do we stand? *J Am Dent Assoc.* 1995;126:1134–1143.

25. Snyder JE, Gauthier CC. *Evidence-Based Medical Ethics: Cases for Practice-Based Learning.* Totowa, NJ: Humana Press; 2008.

26. Turner R. Bragdon v. Abbott—First circuit rules on direct threat defense to ADA claim. In: *University of Houston Law Center.* 1999. 4/13/. Available from: https://www.law.uh.edu/healthlaw/perspectives/Disabilities/990413Bragdon.html.

27. U.S. Department of Health, Education, and Welfare, National Commission for the Protection of Human Subjects of Biomedical and Behavioral Research. *The Belmont Report.* Available from: https://www.hhs.gov/ohrp/regulations-and-policy/belmont-report/index.html; April 18, 1979.

28. U.S. Department of Health and Human Services, Agency for Healthcare Research and Quality, Presidents' Advisory Commission on Consumer Protection and Quality in the Health Care Industry. *Consumer Bill of Rights and Responsibilities.* Available from: https://archive.ahrq.gov/hcqual/final/append_a.html.

29. U.S. Department of Health and Human Services, Office of Research Integrity. *Definition of Research Misconduct.* Available from: https://ori.hhs.gov/definition-misconduct.

30. World Medical Association. *Declaration of Geneva.* Adopted 1948, with amendments in 2017. Available from: https://www.wma.net/policies-post/wma-declaration-of-geneva/.

31. World Medical Association. *WMA Declaration of Helsinki – Ethical Principles for Medical Research Involving Human Subjects.* Adopted 1964, with amendments in 2013. Available from: https://www.wma.net/policies-post/wma-declaration-of-helsinki-ethical-principles-for-medical-research-involving-human-subjects/.

# PART II

# Dental Care Delivery

# 5

# Delivery of Oral Health Care in the United States

**HOWARD L. BAILIT, DMD, PhD**[†]

**PETER MILGROM, DDS**

## CHAPTER OUTLINE

Dentistry in the United States separated from the profession of medicine in 1840, and until recently, private dental care delivery has largely been by independent dentist-owner in solo offices. From the 1970s into the second millennium, there were small numbers of practitioners sharing space but rarely sharing revenue. This practice form was maintained by custom and curtailed by practice laws that prohibited corporate ownership. More recently, the practice of dentistry has evolved and corporate ownership has increased. The private dental practice is organized to provide comprehensive dental care to individuals who can afford and seek care in their offices and clinics. Most people receive dental care in the private dental practice and a small number of special patients who are institutionalized—such as prisoners, armed forces, and low-income groups—receive care within the public health care delivery system. The voluntary sector is made up of largely not-for-profit health facilities that are small in number and are neither publicly nor privately owned, such as many community hospitals.

[†]Deceased

The public dental care delivery systems are focused on the treatment and prevention of dental diseases at the community level. The systems are the primary responsibility of the public health workforce and are mostly operated by local, state, and federal governments. Some examples of community level interventions include public water fluoridation and the use of mass media to effect behavior change that will lead to the prevention of common dental diseases.

## Private Dental Care Delivery System

About 95% of all dentists provide care in privately owned dental practices. As of 2018, more than 65% of private dentists were in groups of two or more in a practice setting. For dentists who graduated in the last 10 years, only 15% are in solo practices.[27] Large group practices that employ 500 or more people are growing faster than small groups.[35] In the next decade, these large groups will almost dominate the private dental practice in many states and urban communities. Satellite offices of groups and some solo practices are likely to continue in rural areas of the country. Some particularly affluent communities will continue to have small numbers of private solo practices.

Longer-term group practices are likely to consolidate at the local market level as large practices and have the capital to buy or merge with smaller practices. Larger groups are better positioned to negotiate with private insurers and government over reimbursement rates, with their suppliers for the price of equipment and supplies, and to accept the financial risk associated with capitation payment systems (versus the traditional fee-for-service payment system). Federal tax law changes in 2018 will contribute to changes in the form of practice entities as practices seek to take advantage of changes in the way costs are expensed and profits taxed.

### Corporate Practice

Most group practices are dentist owned and operated, but a growing percentage is corporate owned.[6] Until recently, most state dental practice acts required practice owners to be licensed dentists. Now some 12 states (e.g., Texas, California, Florida) allow corporations to own practices, and the number is growing.

Corporations are investor owned, private, or publicly traded businesses. To get around legal restrictions that have remained, dental service organizations (DSOs) have formed and exist in almost every state.[25]

DSOs own the clinical facilities and equipment, employ the administrative and clinical staff, and manage the practice. The DSO hires a local dentist who is ostensibly the office owner. In fact, the employed dentists only own the patient records and serve at the pleasure of the corporation. This complicated legal arrangement will not be needed as more states change dental practice acts and allow corporations to own dental offices. In 2016, about 8% of dentists worked in DSOs, but this varied widely among states.[3] In the Northeast, less than 5% of dentists worked for these organizations, whereas in Texas and Arizona around 20% of dentists were employed.

## Specialty Practice

About 20% of dentists are specialists. Table 5.1 lists the dental specialties, describes the types of services they deliver, and notes the approximate number of dentists and their primary delivery sites. There are nine specialties of dentistry recognized by the American Dental Association (ADA): dental public health, endodontics, oral and maxillofacial pathology, oral and maxillofacial radiology, oral and maxillofacial surgery, orthodontics, pediatric dentistry, periodontics, and prosthodontics.[34] Since 2017, the approval system changed due to the demand for the recognition of new specialties. It is now the responsibility of the newly formed National Commission on Recognition of Dental Specialties and National Certifying Boards for Dental Specialists. Other specialist groups have put forward applications to be recognized, but approval remains difficult because of the competing interests of the established specialties.

## Organization, Revenue, and Expenses of Typical Practices

### Solo Practice

Most solo practices are small, with two or three employees, including full- or part-time dental assistants and administrators and a part-time dental hygienist. About 75% of solo general practitioners (GPs) employ a hygienist for an average of 22 hours per week.[7] The primary reason they do not have a larger employed staff is the lack of patient demand and also preferred dentist lifestyle issues (e.g., hours worked per day and week). The average owner solo GP works 33 hours per week, sees about 1350 patients per year, and averages 2.5 visits per patient per year. In a 33-hour week, this comes to about seven patients per day. The number of patients treated annually is very sensitive to changes in demand. After the 2007 economic recession, dentists averaged 1000 patients per year. In periods of high demand, solo owner GPs may see between 1500 and 1600 patients per year.[23]

Solo dentists and small groups typically operate on a fee-for-service basis. That is, each sets its unique price for each service and is paid per service or at a discount if the dentist is affiliated with a preferred provider organization (PPO) organized by an insurer or dental services intermediary company. The primary fee-for-service payers are insurers who pay a portion of charges and patients who

| • TABLE 5.1 | Description of the Dental Specialties and Estimates of the Number of Specialists in the United States in 2018 | | |
|---|---|---|---|
| Specialty | Description | Number of Dentists | Delivery Setting |
| Dental public health | Concerned with preventing and controlling dental diseases and promoting dental health through organized community efforts | 753 | Public health departments |
| Endodontics | Concerned with the morphology, physiology, pathology, and treatment of the dental pulp and periradicular tissue | 5469 | Private practices |
| Oral and maxillofacial pathology | Deals with the nature, identification, and management of diseases affecting the oral and maxillofacial regions | 351 | Dental schools Hospitals |
| Oral and maxillofacial radiology | Concerned with the production and interpretation of images and data produced by all modalities of radiant energy that are used for the diagnosis and management of diseases and disorders and conditions of the oral and maxillofacial region | 117 | Dental schools Hospitals |
| Oral and maxillofacial surgery | The diagnosis, surgical and adjunctive treatment of diseases, injuries, and defects involving both the functional and aesthetic aspects of the hard and soft tissues of the oral and maxillofacial region | 7756 | Private practices Hospitals |
| Orthodontics | Focuses on the diagnosis, prevention, interception, and correction of malocclusion | 7163 | Private practices |
| Pediatric dentistry | Provides both primary and comprehensive preventive and therapeutic oral health care for infants and children | 6150 | Private practices Hospitals |
| Periodontics | Encompasses the prevention, diagnosis, and treatment of diseases of the supporting and surrounding tissues of the teeth or their substitutes | 5524 | Private practices |
| Prosthodontics | Involved in the diagnosis, treatment planning, rehabilitation, and maintenance of the oral function, comfort, appearance, and health of patients with clinical conditions associated with missing or deficient teeth and/or oral and maxillofacial tissues | 3531 | Private practices |

| TABLE 5.2 | Median GP Owner Practice Gross Billings and Expenses Excluding Owner Wages, 2016 and Estimated Percentage by Category | |
| --- | --- | --- |
| Median Gross Billings | | $600,000 |
| Median Gross Expenses | | $350,000 |
| Expense Categories | | % Expenses |
| Staff (wages/benefits) | | 27.7 |
| Taxes | | 5.6 |
| Rent | | 5.6 |
| Supplies | | 12.1 |
| Laboratory | | 5.6 |
| Communications | | 0.8 |
| Maintenance | | 0.5 |
| Fees and Services | | 1.2 |
| Depreciation | | 1.8 |
| Travel and Meetings | | 2.1 |
| Utilities | | 0.5 |
| Profit Sharing Plan | | 2.9 |
| Other | | 33.6 |

pay all remaining charges out of pocket. Most solo dentists and small groups do not have the economic resources to accept capitation payment, where they take the financial risk.

Table 5.2 shows the median annual gross billings and expenses per GP owner practice (solo and group) for 2016 and the percent of expenses by category reported in the 2017 ADA Survey of Dental Practice[4] and estimated from practice consultants in 2016.[17] The exact proportions of expenses vary by market. About 28% of expenses are for practice staff excluding the dentist(s). If dentist wages and benefits are included, they are responsible for 25% of total expenses. Thus, the major expenses of dental practice are related to facilities, staff, technology and supplies, etc. This means that just reducing payments to dentists by 20% to 30% will have a

limited overall impact on expenses, unless other practice-related expenses are addressed.

In terms of revenues, the median gross annual gross billings of the typical private practice were reported to be about $600,000 with median expenses at about 58%. Owner GP dentists (solo and group) self-reported average earnings of $180,000 per year in 2016, reflecting the great variation among practices in patient mix, hours worked per week, practice efficiencies, and the particular market. Note also that these data are provided in voluntary surveys collected by the ADA and are not validated. For all dentists combined, median earnings in 2017 were $158,120 according to the U.S. Department of Labor.[14]

Figure 5.1 shows GP and specialist dentist self-reported average income trends from years 1981 to 2016.[1] Again, these are unvalidated data provided in voluntary surveys. Adjusted for inflation, dentist incomes have clearly plummeted. Nonowner dentist incomes were substantially less than for owners (data not shown).

Another chapter in this book addresses quality assurance (QA) programs in private practices. There are no organized internal or external formal QA systems in most practices, except if they are integrated into large medical organizations. Compliance with evidenced-based guidelines is part of internal dental management control programs. In terms of external control systems, the dental clinical operations are reviewed by the Joint Commission on the Accreditation of Health Organizations.

## Group Practices

In 2018, most large group practices were made up of two to five dentists and employed many personnel and saw large numbers of patients. Large groups having 20 or more dentists at the same site are unusual.[23] All the dentists in the group models are employed by the group owners, corporations, or dentists. Much like solo dentists, almost all large groups receive fee-for-service payment from insurers and patients, and the employed dentists are paid a base salary with a productivity bonus.[16]

The exception to this is a few large groups that are part of health maintenance organizations (HMOs) that provide both medical and dental care. These HMOs often contract directly with employers or state or municipal unions under capitation contracts and provide fee-for-service care to insured and noninsured patients. That is, the HMO is at financial risk for providing care for a fixed capitation amount per enrollee and delivering the care. In this

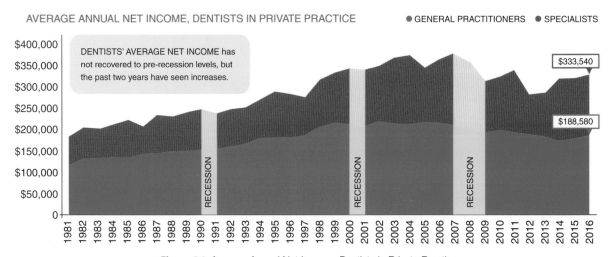

• **Figure 5.1** Average Annual Net Income, Dentists in Private Practice.

model, dentists and physicians are paid on the basis of relative value units (RVUs) per unit time and compliance with explicit evidence-based guidelines. RVUs encourage productivity but not for specific services. The evidence-based guidelines come from many sources but mainly the American Dental Association.

HMOs all accept capitation payment and appear to have a competitive price advantage in the marketplace.[23] Their premiums are lower than for noncapitated groups or insurance plans. HealthPartners, a large medical and dental HMO centered in Minneapolis, Minnesota, and the surrounding areas, serving more than 1.8 million medical and dental health plan members nationwide appears to have a price advantage compared to competing traditional private insurance plans.[23]

Some possible reasons for this advantage are that all patients are put into caries risk groups that determine what services they receive and how often they are scheduled for visits. The best estimate is that 60% of patients are low risk in the average practice. These patients do not need to be seen every 6 months or even yearly. Also, they do not benefit from many preventive services given to higher risk patients. In addition, the groups are staffed to meet demand, and if there is less demand, the dental workforce is reduced. Unused capacity is less of a problem in large group practices than in solo and small group practices. Capitated groups appear to use more allied dental health personnel per dentist, especially dental hygienists, and delegate more duties to them. Finally, the dental plan can be embedded into the medical plan, reducing administrative costs.

One indication of this delivery model's efficiency is that the average HealthPartners GP manages 2100 patients per year versus 1350 for solo dental GPs.[23] It is difficult to estimate the cost advantage of such models, but they are probably substantial. Group practices integrated with medical plans should gain market share and eventually dominate the dental care delivery system in one state or region. Unlike medicine, which is highly concentrated around hospital systems and their associated medical practices at the state level, few large dental groups have substantial negotiating leverage with payers and suppliers. This is likely to change in the future.

## Medical Practices

Most states allow physicians to bill Medicaid or private insurance for providing screening and preventive dental services to children below age 5. This practice is rapidly becoming part of the clinical routines of pediatric and family medicine practitioners.[31] The rationale is that physicians see young children more than dentists do. This makes preventive services available to many more young children and helps with the early identification of problems that need to be treated by dentists. The American Academy of Pediatrics is in full support of this practice. Operationally, the biggest problems are finding a dentist who would accept Medicaid-enrolled patients and having caretakers make and keep appointments with dentists.

Because few physicians graduate from medical schools with any knowledge of the oral cavity, the medical specialty organizations have established web-based courses to assist physicians and their staff to become familiar with screening for oral disease and applying preventive dental services.[32] In addition, more medical schools and residency programs are now covering basic information on oral diseases as part of their core curriculum. Furthermore, the nurses and nurse assistants employed in practices deliver the screening and preventive dental services. In some areas of the country (e.g.,

Colorado) medical practices employ dental hygienists to provide these services.[22] So far this activity has been limited to young children, but there is no clinical reason for not providing these services to children and adults of all ages. However, the future of these activities in medical practices remains unclear. As noted earlier, about 50% to 60% of dental visits consist of diagnostic and preventive services only. A related activity is for large integrated medical care organizations to contract with or purchase large dental group practices in their area. This will help them sell medical care, reduce the cost of dental care, and become a new profit center. Some large HMOs are already doing this including HealthPartners in Minnesota and Kaiser Permanente Northwest in Oregon and Washington.[8]

## Public Delivery System

There is a small publicly owned or not-for-profit system for providing dental care. Most relevant to this chapter is federally qualified health centers (FQHCs). These are developed and operationally subsidized by the federal government and by federal regulation, and 51% of their boards must be active patients. FQHCs focus on providing medical and dental care to low-income and migrant populations who do not have the resources to pay for care in the private system.

In 2016, the program served more than 24 million patients nationally, including 1 in 7 Medicaid beneficiaries. Nationally, there are about 1300 FQHC clinics and approximately 850 of them provide dental care to patients.[9] The dental facilities usually consist of two or three operatories and one full-time dentist with clinical support staff. There are exceptions, and a few FQHCs employ 20 or more dentists working out of multiple FQHC-owned practices. However, for the most part they are small operations and generate perhaps 10% of total FQHC revenues. Because they are so small, they do not receive much senior management attention, and the employed dentists are not part of the senior management team.

FQHCs generally are paid per visit rather than fee for service and are reimbursed at a higher rate for Medicaid patients than private dental offices. They also receive an annual grant from the Health Resources and Services Administration under Section 330 of the Public Health Service Act to cover the costs of indigent non-Medicaid patients who cannot pay out of pocket, even on a sliding scale. FQHC dental clinics see somewhere between 4 and 5 million patients each year and employ or contract with about 4500 dentists. Although FQHC dental clinics are slowly expanding, it is unlikely they will become a dominant force in the dental care delivery system. Even for Medicaid patients, they only treat 30% of those receiving any care. The great majority of Medicaid patients obtain care in the private dental care delivery system.

A second group of public dental care facilities are in county health departments, prisons, Indian reservations, armed forces, Veterans Administration, and similar government-owned organizations. These clinics together serve no more than 200,000 dental patients, as their workforce is small. Control of many of the clinics serving American Indians and Native Alaskans has evolved, and many tribal organizations now operate their own clinical services and employ dentists. Regardless, the majority of dentists are employed to provide care and are usually paid a salary and sometimes receive a productivity bonus. Some will be part of the small U.S. Public Health Service Commissioned Corps, a nonmilitary

| • TABLE 5.3 | Estimate of the Number of Dentists Employed by Government Organizations in 2018 | |
|---|---|---|
| **Agency** | **Number of Dentists** | |
| Department of Defense | 2900 | |
| Veterans Administration | 600 | |
| Public Health Service | 215 | |
| Bureau of Prisons | 170[a] | |
| Indian Health Service | 1050 | |
| Federally Qualified Health Centers | 4474 | |

[a]A small percentage of dentists working in the Bureau of Prisons are part of the Public Health Service Commissioned Corps.

uniformed federal service. A small but unknown number of private dentists have full- or part-time contracts with these organizations. In most cases the programs are funded by the sponsoring government or tribal organization, and when possible, the Medicaid program is billed. Table 5.3 provides data from the U.S. Public Health Service.

In the past it was difficult to recruit dentists to work in publicly owned dental systems because of relatively low incomes compared to private practitioners and in some cases difficult working conditions. This is no longer true. Most clinics have many applicants because of the growing number of dentists and because the federal government provides loan forgiveness toward a percentage of the student's federal educational loans for up to 4 years. This loan forgiveness is not considered a wage and therefore the funds are not taxed. Recruitment and retention of dentists in rural areas remains a problem for tribal organizations and other government-related entities. Turnover is also a concern.

## Hospital Dentistry

This system is mainly within the purview of community hospitals. There are approximately 4800 community hospitals (voluntary, public, and private) and about 20% have dental departments with full-time clinical chiefs and few full- and part-time dentists. These hospital clinics are mainly seen in large urban hospitals. The primary objective of these programs is to provide dental care to hospital inpatients who are undergoing medical treatment that is related to oral health. For example, head and neck cancer patients need to have their teeth in good health before undergoing surgery and radiation treatment. Hospital dental programs also care for patients referred to hospitals for technology or expertise that is not available in community-based practices. This includes some types of radiologic examinations, oral pathology, and medicine.

Many of these hospital dental programs also operate dental residency programs for general practice dentistry (GPR), oral and maxillofacial surgery, and pediatric dentistry. They manage a significant number of patients under sedation or general anesthesia, which takes place in both in- and outpatient hospital operating rooms. They also serve the needs of community-based patients from a wide range of socioeconomic classes. Hospital dental residents are eligible for support from the graduate medical education (GME) program for medical residents. Funded by Medicare, GME

funds are used to cover the direct and indirect cost of residency programs. The direct support goes for resident stipends and some program faculty.

For most of the hospitals without dental programs, patients who seek care in emergency rooms (ER) for dental pain and infection (80% pulpal and periapical abscess) are treated symptomatically and referred to local community practices and clinics.[2] The percentage of referred patients who obtain comprehensive dental care is not known, but it is likely small. Most ER dental patients are adults and have no insurance or only Medicaid and are from low-income families.[33] In one study, the encounters resulted in opioid (56%) and antibiotic (56%) prescriptions and generated $402 (95% confidence interval [CI] = $396, $408) in hospital costs per visit.[33]

The cost of ER dental visits is much higher than office visits, so some experts argue that substantial funds could be saved by having dental care for low-income adults more fully covered by the Medicaid program. This position is supported by the fact that ER use increases when adult Medicaid dental coverage is stopped.[36] Nevertheless, the number of people seeking dental ER care is about 48.8 per 1000 population and a significant percentage of Medicaid patients continue to seek ER dental care even when covered by Medicaid.[8] Hospitals without dental departments usually allow oral and maxillofacial surgeons and pediatric dentists to treat their patients who need sedation or general anesthesia in their in- and outpatient operating rooms.

## Dental Practice in Dental Educational Institutions

Overall, the dental educational institution clinics provide care to about 1,176,000 patients per year with most of them from low-income households. While significant, it is quite a small part of the dental delivery capacity in the United States. There are approximately 21,237 junior and senior dental students, residents, and full-time clinical faculty working in dental schools and hospital dental programs who treat patients. The total number exceeds the number of dentists who are employed by FQHCs. Dental schools and hospitals, unlike FQHCs, receive no state or federal subsidies for treating low-income patients. State schools receive a relatively modest state educational subsidy that accounts for 20% or less of their total budgets. Two states, North Carolina and New York, increased Medicaid reimbursement levels for clinical care in medical and dental education programs.

It is estimated that dental students provided services to about 518,000 patients in school clinics and another 168,000 patients in community clinics for a total of close to 687,000 patients in 2013 and 2014.[10] Most patients come from lower income families who are attracted to dental schools because student fees are 50% to 60% lower than average market fees in private practices. Nevertheless, many of the institutional clinics have financial problems operating standalone programs in the current financial environment and in the future may need to colocate with FQHCs or other not-for-profit community providers. In 2010 and 2011, there were 365 advanced education in general dentistry (AEGD)/GPR and 1066 specialty graduate students in dental schools. Another 3100 residents were based in hospitals, for a total of 4541 dentists.[10] As an upper boundary estimate, in 2012 and 2013 dental residents provided treatment to 489,500 patients from lower income households annually. The fees charged for dental procedures performed in resident specialty clinics are 70% to 80% of market fees and are often beyond the financial capacity of most low-income patients.

In total there are about 3706 full-time clinical faculty in U.S. dental schools, excluding dentists in administration. However, clinical faculty members spend most of their time supervising the care provided by students and postgraduate students and provide small amounts of care directly. In schools with faculty practice, the faculty spend 4 to 8 hours per week providing care to patients. Patients treated in dental school faculty practices are usually charged market level fees and, as such, mainly come from middle- and high-income families.

## Future Dental Care Practice in the United States

Dental practice is transforming as medicine did 20 years ago. The changes in medical practice are therefore instructive. Only 18% of physicians are in solo practice, and the fastest model of group medical practice is seen in groups with 100 or more physicians.[26] Many of these medical groups are part of integrated medical systems built around hospitals that are horizontally (multiple area hospitals linked together by mergers, purchases, and contracts) and vertically integrated (hospital systems with medical practices, rehabilitation centers, and long-term care programs). In many predominantly urban states, three or four of these large integrated medical systems have 85% market share.[26] This level of concentration was intended to improve system efficiency to reduce costs, improve the quality of care, and increase negotiating leverage with payers and suppliers. There is little evidence that integration has had a notable impact on costs and quality. In fact, greater consolidation has increased costs.[13] There is strong evidence that consolidation has increased their negotiating leverage with payers.[13]

In response to this challenge, the large national insurers have tried to consolidate within regions and states. They have been partially successful, but they still do not have the market share of strong state or region-based payers, and federal government regulators have turned down several attempts by national companies to purchase or merge with other national insurers. However, in the current political environment in the United States, regulators may permit more mergers and takeovers.

At the same time, many integrated medical systems are becoming insurers as well as deliverers of care.[19] These are large multibillion dollar systems, and as they mature administratively and economically they have the capacity to serve as both insurers and deliverers of care. In this respect they are in direct competition with insurers for health insurance contracts with local employers and public payers. Because of this competition, some large insurers are being bought by other health companies (e.g., CVS purchase of Aetna to explore different delivery models).

## The Changing Marketplace

What changes are occurring in dental practice? The number of dentists per 100,000 people is growing 2.5 times as fast as the increase in population.[5] This is mainly the result of the 10 new dental schools that have opened since 1990 and the increase in class size in established schools. Moreover, in a relatively short period the average age of retirement went from 64 to 69 years, further increasing the supply of dentists.[5] Already about 35% of solo GPs claim that they are not busy enough.[38] These data suggest much greater competition in the future.

The increased competition means that group practices in dentistry—corporate or dentist owned—will consolidate and become much larger organizations at state and regional levels. This will increase their negotiating leverage with national and state insurers. Because of the growing surplus of dentists and because most dental groups are not consolidated in local markets, regional insurers have reduced the fees paid per service from 20% to 10% in many states. This is likely to continue without consolidation.

So far, most large medical systems have not offered dental insurance to employers or developed the capacity to deliver dental care to them. There are some exceptions, and a few large HMOs do include dentistry as another medical service with employed dentists. A good indication of this trend is seen in Medicare Advantage plans. Some 40% of Medicare eligibles now receive their medical care from Medicare Advantage HMOs and PPOs, and about 65% of the plans now include a "bare bones" dental insurance.[29] The dental care insurance is funded by the money the HMOs/PPOs receive from the Medicare system to provide medical care to their members. This business decision is an effort to attract more members. If members want higher quality dental plans, they are available to those willing to pay higher out-of-pocket premiums. This trend will probably continue, as the population wants dental coverage, and medical systems that offer it will become more competitive.

Also, the cost of dental insurance is decidedly lower when it is embedded in a medical insurance plan. The savings appear to come from reduced administrative costs. There are substantial profits possible from efficiently run dental delivery systems. For all these reasons, many large integrated medical systems are likely to offer dental coverage to employers and develop the capacity to own and operate dental group practices. This is going to have a profound impact on the careers of dentists. Similar to physicians, they will be employed and function as another medical department in the system. In this environment, dentists and physicians will work closely together, ending the clinical isolation between the practice of dentistry and medicine.

Following the same path as medical organizations, some large dental group practices that dominate local markets are beginning to offer insurance plans to private and public payers under fixed price capitated plans. They have the economic capacity to take and manage the financial risk. This is especially important as increasingly states require their Medicaid members to receive care in capitated programs. In response to this challenge, some dental insurers are buying large dental group practices or starting dental practices.[18] Whether these insurers will be able to manage and grow these practices remains to be seen. In the long term, standalone dental insurers may not be able to survive from the competition of large medical and dental provider organizations to offer dental insurance to employers and other purchasers of dental insurance.

When local markets are dominated by large group dental practices, these organizations will have the economic and political strength to change dental practice acts to meet the needs of their business model. Current state practice acts are designed to support and protect the solo practice model from competition. The practice act changes are likely to expand the role of other dental team members where dental hygienists and therapists provide most primary dental care. These may also provide many specialty services. Dentists will have a major role supervising these dental team members, but most of their time will be spent managing patients with more complex medical and dental conditions. Practice act change will also continue to eliminate barriers to nondentist ownership and operation of dental practices, as has happened in medicine.

Further, we can expect that practice acts will be changed to allow foreign-trained dentists to practice without having a U.S.

dental degree. Foreign graduates will have to pass an examination and complete a Commission on Dental Accreditation (CODA)–approved residency program to be eligible to take state licensing examinations. This general model already exists for foreign-trained physicians, and a substantial percentage of currently practicing physicians do not have U.S. medical degrees.[15]

## The Impact of Changing Dental Caries Risk on Practice Models

The current model for both solo and group practices is to have central facilities where dentists and support staff provide a full range of services to patients. These practices are expensive to operate largely because of all the capital needed to cover the costs of facilities, equipment, supplies, and highly skilled dentists. This model made sense when most patients required extensive treatment. It makes less sense now when most patients are healthy.

In some states, where large dental group practices provide care mainly to Medicaid patients under fixed-price capitation plans, they are starting to use the hub and spoke system.[12] This is an effort to still make an acceptable profit under low Medicaid reimbursement rates. In this model, most basic screening and primary and secondary preventive dental services are provided in community-based satellite practices staffed mainly by dental hygienists. In public schools, factories, worksites, nursing homes, and related community sites, patients are screened and provided primary and secondary preventive dental services. These satellite operations use portable equipment and a minimum of technology and expensive space. Often they are linked to central hub dental practices through telehealth, so they have immediate access to dentists if needed. As such, they are typically less expensive to operate than conventional practices, because they require far less capital to start and operate. The substitution of dentists by dental hygienists is also a factor.

Patients needing more extensive care by a dentist are referred to the central hub practices. This referral process is difficult to operate, and some patients do not follow up and seek care in the hub practices. The number of satellite practices needed per hub practice is not known at this time, but it is likely at least 6 to 10. This model will become even more effective when most caries in the enamel are treated by remineralization and the use of silver diamine fluoride to stop the carious process. This model recognizes that most patients need relatively little care.

Currently, for a middle-class population with private insurance, some 65% to 85% only receive diagnostic and preventive services per visit, and this percentage is increasing 1% per year.[21] In the average practice it is estimated that 50% to 60% of patients are at low risk for dental caries and can receive most of their care in satellite practices. Data on the distribution of dental caries risk levels come from multiple sources, including the National Health and Nutrition Examination Survey[11] and several studies of the caries risk levels in low-income children[28] (as well as from private general dentist practices[20]).

The measurement of dental caries risk level is based on the use of commercially available survey instruments. Those based on in-mouth examinations by dentists appear to be superior. Several dental insurance plans now require dentists to send them caries risk level data on their insured patients. Low caries risk also determines the frequency of visits and the preventive services that they receive. As expected, these patients do not need to be seen every 6 months. Visits every 12 to 18 months should be adequate for most low-risk

patients. Further, current ADA and American Academy of Pediatric Dentistry evidence-based guidelines indicate that preventive services such as fluoride varnish and dental sealants are not needed in most low caries risk patients.[30,37] These guidelines are likely to change further as national authorities have begun to question the validity of existing studies supporting widespread use of dental sealants.[24]

A second major advantage of the public health/community delivery model is that it is more effective than the traditional model in reducing social barriers to care. The latter includes education, transportation, and language.

It is not surprising that even with financial access to care through public insurance, many low-income families still do not use dental care at the rate of higher income families. The community dental clinic sites in schools have continuous access to children and do not have to depend on caregivers to seek dental care in traditional practices.

If more states move to managed care and require Medicaid patients to receive care in capitated group dental practices as expected, more of these group practices will move to community-based care using the hub and spoke model. Even privately insured employer groups may move to this delivery model to increase access to care and at the same time lower the cost of dental insurance. Oregon has had several years of experience with this delivery model, and the largest group practice, Advantage Dental Services, provides care in many schools and other community sites. This trend is also seen in some FQHC dental programs. For example, in Connecticut, they deliver care in more than 300 public schools to low-income children using the hub and spoke delivery model.

## Reasons for the Ongoing Change in Dental Practice

Even though the changes in the dental delivery system are of importance, relatively little research has investigated the reasons for this transformation. It is known that student educational debt is a factor. Graduates with greater debt do not have the resources to start or purchase their own practices. In an effort to pay back their debt, they seek employment in group practices as employees. Many other factors are in play, and these are discussed based on the literature and common sense but nonetheless are speculative.

Group practices are likely to have a competitive advantage over solo practices in efficient practice operations. They are much better positioned to manage complex technologies such as advanced information systems and to employ and manage a large staff of clinical and administrative support staff. Further, as they grow in size, large groups have better access to capital to adapt to a changing delivery system and to negotiate more favorable rates with payers and suppliers. With larger size, groups can also take the financial risk of capitation plans and sell directly to employers, reducing their dependence on traditional standalone dental insurers and increasing their profitability. Another factor is the large number of female graduates who do not want the responsibility of owning and operating solo practices and prefer working for group practices. This is not just an economic issue but also one of preferred life style. Working as an employee removes the problems and headaches of operating practices and offers more benefits and time for family. There may be many other factors driving the change from solo to group practice, and thus more research is needed.

## Implications for Patients

In 25 years the dental delivery system will be dominated by large group practices, and some of these practices will be part of integrated medical systems. Low caries risk patients (50%–60% of all patients) will receive screening and primary and secondary preventive services in community-based satellite offices that are part of the group. Most low risk patients will be scheduled for visits every 12 to 18 months with midlevel dental providers. Patients at high dental caries risks and those who have other problems will be treated in hub practices/clinics by midlevel staff who will provide most of the routine general and specialty services under the direct and indirect supervision of dentists. Only those patients with complex medical, dental, and behavioral problems will see the dentist more frequently. These complex patients will be treated by physicians and dentists who work together on the underlying systemic diseases.

The quality of care should improve for two reasons. First, quality will improve because the performance of employed dentists will be monitored frequently to ensure it complies with internal evidenced-based guidelines and other clinical and administrative procedures. Additionally, groups will be reaccredited every few years by an external accreditation agency such as the Joint Commission for the Accreditation of Health Care Organizations (JCAHO) and the results will be public.

In the long term, the costs of dental services faced by patients should be relatively lower. Initially, the savings from this new delivery model will be used by large dental groups to increase their profits. In competitive markets these savings will eventually be passed on to payers and patients.

## Implications for Dentists

In the future, most dentists will be employed in group practices and will not have an equity interest in practices. They will spend almost all their time caring for patients rather than in administration. The business functions will be carried out by professional managers. Dentists will have to learn to work in large organizations and to take direction from practice clinical and administrative leaders. Some dentists will rise in their groups and assume larger clinical and administrative roles. Average dentist incomes may be relatively lower, because they will not have a large financial investment in their own practices to recover, but their incomes will still be relatively high and commensurate with other highly educated professionals. They will likely receive better fringe benefits such as healthcare, pensions, and paid vacations. Once established in the practices, they will not have to worry about having enough patients.

Change in dental practice will be uneven and take time, and progress will be characterized by both successes and failures. This has been the path in medicine and still many issues are not resolved. Both patients and dentists will need to accommodate the necessary adjustments over time. Adaptation to change is one of the great strengths of American business culture.

## References

1. American Dental Association. Health Policy Institute. *Dentist Earnings and Busyness in the U.S.* Available from: https://perma.cc/P733-VUAV

2. American Dental Association. Health Policy Institute. *Emergency Department Visits for Dental Conditions—a Snapshot.* Infographics. 2017. Available from: https://perma.cc/4A79-QFN3.

3. American Dental Association. Health Policy Institute. *How Big Are Dental Service Organizations?* Available from: https://perma.cc/6WMM-NZPG

4. American Dental Association. Health Policy Institute. *Income, Gross Billings, and Expenses. Selected 2016 Results from the Survey of Dental Practice.* Chicago, IL: American Dental Association; 2017.

5. American Dental Association. Health Policy Institute. Munson B, Vujicic M. Supply of full-time equivalent dentists in the U.S. expected to increase steadily. Health Policy Institute Research Brief. American Dental Association. July 2018. Available from: https://perma.cc/TYU7-6RXG.

6. Deleted in review.

7. American Dental Association, Health Policy Institute. Table 10: percentage of dentists employing dental hygienists, 1960–2009. In: *Survey of Dental Practice.* Chicago, IL: American Dental Association; 2011.

8. Baicker K, Allen HL, Wright BJ, et al. The effect of Medicaid on dental care of poor adults: evidence from the Oregon Health Insurance Experiment. *Health Serv Res.* 2017;9(17):2147–2164.

9. Bailit H, Devitto J, Myne-Joslin R, et al. Federally qualified health centers dental clinics: financial information. *J Public Health Dent.* 2013;73(3):224–230.

10. Bailit HL. Are dental schools part of the safety net? *J Dent Educ.* 2017;81(8 Suppl):eS88–96.

11. Bailit H, Lim S, Ismail A. The oral health of upper income Americans. *J Public Health Dent.* 2016;76(3):192–197.

12. Bailit HL, Plunkett M, Schwarz E. The Oregon dental market: a case study. *J Am Coll Dent.* 2016;83(2):14–23.

13. Baker L, Bundorf M, Kessler D. Vertical integration: hospital ownership of physician practices is associated with higher prices and spending. *Health Aff.* 2014;33(5):756–763.

14. Bureau of Labor Statistics, U.S. Department of Labor. *Occupational Outlook Handbook, Dentists.* Available from: https://www.bls.gov/ooh/healthcare/dentists.htm.

15. Carroll A. Why America needs foreign medical graduates. *The New York Times.* October, 2017;6.

16. Conrad DA, Milgrom P, Shirtcliff RM, et al. Pay-for-performance incentive program in a large dental group practice. *J Am Dent Assoc.* 2018;149(5):348–352.

17. Dental Practice Overhead Survey. Somerset CPAs and Advisors. Available from: https://perma.cc/LE3C-Z3HK.

18. *Denta Quest finalizes acquisition of Advantage Dental, creating partnership to enhance oral health across the U.S. DentaQuest News and Updates*; 2017.

19. Dignity seeking license to take full risk for care. *Modern Healthcare*; 2015. 28 Feb.

20. Deleted in review.

21. Eklund SA, Bailit HL. Estimating the number of dentists needed in 2040. *J Dent Educ.* 2017;81(8):eS146–eS152.

22. Gauger TL, Prosser LA, Fontana M, et al. Integrative and collaborative care models between pediatric oral health and primary care providers: a scoping review of the literature. *J Public Health Dent.* 2018;78(3):246–256.

23. Gesko DS, Bailit HL. Dental group practice and the need for dentists. *J Dent Educ.* 2017;81(8):eS120–eS125.

24. Kumar SV, Bangar S, Neumann A, et al. Assessing the validity of existing dental sealant quality measures. *J Am Dent Assoc.* 2018;149:756–764.e1.

25. Langelier M, Wang S, Surdu S, et al. *Trends in the Development of the Dental Service Organization Model: Implications for the Oral Health Workforce and Access to Services.* Rensselaer, NY: Oral Health Workforce Research Center, Center for Health Workforce Studies, School of Public Health, SUNY Albany; 2017.

26. Muhlestein D, Smith N. Physician consolidation: rapid movement from small to large group practices, 2013 to 2015. *Health Aff (Millwood).* 2016;35(9):1638–1643.

27. Nasseh K, Vujicic M. The relationship between education debt and career choices in professional programs. The case of dentistry. *J Am Dent Assoc.* 2017;148(11):825–833.

28. Nelson S, Mandelaris J, Ferretti G, et al. School screening and parent reminders in increasing dental care for children in need: a retrospective study. *J Public Health Dent.* 2012;72(1):45–52.

29. Pope C. Supplemental benefits under Medicare Advantage. *Health Affairs Blog.* Jan. 21, 2016. Available from: https://www.manhattan-institute.org/html/supplemental-benefits-under-medicare-advantage-10157.html.

30. Council on Scientific Affairs. Professionally applied topical fluoride: evidenced-based clinical recommendations. *J Am Dent Assoc.* 2006;137(8):1151–1159.

31. Silk H. The future of oral health care provided by physicians and allied professionals. *J Dent Educ.* 2017;81(8):eS171–eS179.

32. Silk H, Sachs Leicher E, Alvarado V, et al. A multi-state initiative to implement pediatric oral health in primary care practice and clinical education. *J Public Health Dent.* 2018;78(1):25–31.

33. Sun BC, Chi DL, Schwarz E, et al. Emergency department visits for nontraumatic dental problems: a mixed-methods study. *Am J Public Health.* 2015;105(5):947–955.

34. Thierer TE, Meyerowitz C. Trends in general and specialty advanced dental education and practice. 2005-06 to 2015-16 and beyond. *J Den Educ.* 2017;81(8):eS162–eS170.

35. Wall T, Guay A. *Very Large Dental Practices Seeing Significant Growth in Market Share.* Health Policy Institute, American Dental Association: Research Brief; 2015. Available from: https://perma.cc/ZEQ5-QTUK.

36. Wides C, Alam S, Mertz E. Shaking up the dental safety-net: elimination of optional adult dental benefits in California. *J Health Care Poor Underserved.* 2014;25(1):151–164.

37. Wright JT, Crall JJ, Fontana M, et al. Evidence-based clinical practice guideline for the use of pit-and-fissure sealants. A report of the American Dental Association and the American Academy of Pediatric Dentistry. *J Am Dent Assoc.* 2016;147(8):672–682. e12.

38. Yarborough C. *State of the Dental Market: Slide 20, Percent of Dentists Not busy Enough.* 2014. Arizona: Presentation at Institute of Oral Health Meeting; October 2015.

# 6

# Oral Health and Oral Health Care in Canada

CARLOS QUIÑONEZ, DMD, MSc, PhD, FRCD(C)

JULIE FARMER, RDH, MSc

NOHA GOMAA, BDS, MSc, PhD

SONICA SINGHAL, BDS, MPH, PhD, FRCD(C)

## CHAPTER OUTLINE

## Introduction

Canada and the United States are natural foils to each other. While they share significant political and sociocultural similarities—they are both neoliberal welfare states, meaning they privilege economic freedoms and use private markets to distribute social goods—they also differ substantially in relation to their approaches to healthcare. Such differences are a common policy trope that views the Canadian approach to organizing, financing, and delivering health care—or how care is governed and managed, paid for, and provided—as superior.

For example, it is regularly reported that, due to Canada's national and universal (meaning it covers the whole population) system of health insurance (termed "Medicare"), Canada provides much better access to healthcare compared to the United

States.[12,23,32] Yes, Canadians do not have the affordability challenges that Americans can experience when accessing healthcare, but can the same thing be said about oral healthcare?

What is often surprising to health policy actors north and south of the border (and internationally as well) is that Canada's approach to oral healthcare is actually equivalent to the American approach, albeit with much less complexity. It is a fact that oral healthcare is not included in Canada's national system of health insurance (Medicare). Canadians face many of the same financial barriers to accessing oral healthcare that Americans do.[23,38] It is also a fact that on a per capita basis, the United States pays for more public (or government-funded) oral healthcare than Canada.[38] Further, the United States has a much more robust public option (publicly funded and supported clinics) than Canada.[38] Given this, our traditional policy tropes around the Canadian approach to healthcare may, at best, not be as accurate as we think and, at worst, may be uncritical and damaging to policy clarity around what oral healthcare means in each country.

This chapter will detail how Canada organizes, finances, and delivers oral healthcare, with the ultimate aim of comparing both nations. Such a comparison is beneficial for understanding the dynamics of oral healthcare in each country. Thus, describing the Canadian approach in the context of an American textbook on dental public health can provide a window into potential solutions to the challenges that face each country in terms of population oral health and oral healthcare.

## The Organization, Financing, and Delivery of Oral Healthcare in Canada

### The Organization of Oral Healthcare

In terms of governance, whereas the United States is a federal republic, Canada is a confederation. Broadly speaking, the difference relates to whether membership in the nation state is voluntary. In a federation, it is not, in a confederation, it is. And whereas the United States has member "states," Canada has member "provinces" and "territories." For Canada, this means that powers are divided between a federal government, 10 provincial governments, and three territorial governments. The provinces/territories have the primary governance authority over healthcare, and each has its own universal health insurance plan that operates under standards established by federal legislation, or the Canada Health Act. The Canada Health Act mandates the public financing of hospital and physician care across the country and only includes oral healthcare by noting that the provinces/territories must fund "surgical-dental services" delivered in hospital (essentially boiling down to major and/or catastrophic oral and maxillofacial surgery care). Importantly, given decades of health and social services restructuring in Canada, municipalities now have decision-making powers over healthcare programming as well.[25]

Through other federal legislation and regulations, specifically related to social services, the federal government also provides funding support to the provinces/territories for the different types of services (including some healthcare) that the provinces/territories provide to socially and economically marginalized groups (e.g., low-income families). Unlike the Canada Health Act, however, such legislation and regulations are largely unspecific in terms of what the provinces/territories must do, meaning there is no specificity as to whether oral healthcare must be provided to the specific populations that the provinces/territories target in their social services legislation. That said, at the provincial/territorial level, different forms of social services legislation do include—although not always—requirements to provide oral healthcare for targeted (socially and economically marginalized) groups.[33]

Thus, for oral healthcare, the governance structure described earlier results in a patchwork of programs and services. For example, apart from providing funding for surgical-dental services delivered in hospital at the provincial/territorial level, the federal government also finances oral healthcare for specific groups, including state-recognized Indigenous groups and the country's armed forces. In turn, within their jurisdiction, the provinces/territories finance surgical-dental services delivered in hospital, along with targeted care for groups like low-income children, social assistance recipients, those with developmental disabilities, and those with craniofacial disorders. And through cost-sharing agreements with the provinces, municipalities finance care for low-income children, social assistance recipients, and sometimes independently for groups such as low-income seniors.[33]

Due to this governance and jurisdictional structure, some say that there are actually 14 health systems in Canada: 10 provincial, three territorial, and one federal.[25,33] The same could be said for oral healthcare, but in fact it is more accurate to say that there are two systems, the public oral healthcare system and the private oral healthcare system. As described earlier, the public system varies across municipal, provincial/territorial, and federal jurisdictions. The private system is ubiquitous, with little variation across the country. Based on this fact, some will argue that it is even more accurate to describe oral healthcare in Canada as one system, a private oral healthcare system.[25] This private system ensconces and dwarfs the public system, meaning that the public system functions within and in the context of the private system, namely through public payment in the form of fee-for-service delivery in private dental clinics.[25,38] This will become more apparent when we discuss how oral healthcare is financed and delivered in Canada.

In summary, many describe Canada's healthcare system as "socialized medicine." Formally, this means that healthcare is universal (it covers everyone) and that it is both publicly financed and delivered. Yet, although it is universal, Canadian Medicare is actually more accurately described as "public payment, private delivery."[21] What is more, Canadian Medicare only really publicly finances hospital and physician services (excluding many other services, like oral healthcare) and allows hospitals and physicians to be independent, private entities, meaning care is privately delivered even though most or even all of the funding comes from public sources.

## The Financing of Oral Healthcare

In comparison to Organisation for Economic Co-Operation and Development (OECD) nations, Canada, like the United States, ranks low in the public financing of oral healthcare (Table 6.1). Out of all oral healthcare spending in Canada, only about 5% is paid for by governments.[38] Oral healthcare in Canada is almost wholly privately financed and paid for on a fee-for-service basis, with approximately 59% of the population paying for care through private insurance (of which greater than 90% is employment-based insurance or group plans vs. individually purchased plans) and 41% through out-of-pocket payments.[9,30] Again, of the 5% of the public financing that remains, almost all is targeted to socially marginalized groups (as described earlier) and delivered in the private sector through public forms of third-party financing (public insurance paying on a fee-for-service basis).

A defining feature of the financing of oral healthcare in Canada (as in the United States) is the role of employment-based insurance. Employers offer "nonwage benefits" to employees (income that is not part of a person's wage) partly in the form of health and dental benefits. The employee generally pays a monthly premium that is matched by the employer (an amount that the employee and employer must pay for the insurance policy). These benefits have historically made up the majority of nonwage benefit packages in Canada, are meant to improve the employer/employee contract, and are incentivized by favorable tax treatment by federal and provincial governments.[7,17]

Cost sharing is also the norm in Canada, meaning that those who are insured often pay a deductible (a specified amount that the insured must pay before accessing the benefits) and/or a copayment (a partial amount of the covered service). And finally, over time, on a relative basis, it appears that Canadians made more and more private investments in oral healthcare while Canadian governments have made less and less of a public investment in oral healthcare (Figure 6.1).

## The Delivery of Oral Healthcare

A variety of oral healthcare providers exist to support the delivery of oral healthcare in Canada, and they are governed through provincial/territorial health professional legislation (Table 6.2). These are the regulated oral healthcare professions, or dentistry, dental hygiene, dental therapy, and denturism. There are other oral healthcare providers who work in a supporting role to dentists, including dental assistants and dental technologists. In some provinces/territories, dental regulators are separate from dental associations; in others they are not. Regulators govern oral healthcare professionals with the aim of protecting the public and acting in the public interest. Associations represent oral healthcare professionals and represent their interests. This is akin to the notion and role of state dental boards and state dental associations in the United States.

Dentistry, dental hygiene, and dental assisting make up the largest share of oral health human resources in Canada, whereas other groups, such as denturists and dental therapists, only make up a very small proportion.[30,33] Available estimates demonstrate that as of 2015, there were 21,880 dentists (88% general dentists, 12% specialists) in Canada (Table 6.2). Again, the delivery of oral healthcare in Canada occurs almost exclusively in private settings or through independent, sole-proprietorship, fee-for-service

**• TABLE 6.1** **Oral Healthcare Spending and Financial Barriers to Care in Select OECD Nations[32,38]**

| | Per Capita Dental Expenditure ($2011 PPP) | Percentage of Spending From Private Sources | Dental Spending as a Percentage of Total Health Spending | Skipped Dental Care or Dental Checkups Because of the Cost |
|---|---|---|---|---|
| Australia | 223 | 77.6 | 5.9 | 21.0 |
| Canada | 313 | 94.7 | 6.9 | 28.0 |
| France | 176 | 66.1 | 4.3 | 23.0 |
| Germany | 278 | 36.1 | 6.2 | 14.0 |
| Netherlands | 214 | 72.6 | 4.2 | 10.6 |
| New Zealand | 107 | 63.5 | 3.4 | 22.0 |
| Norway | 274 | 63.5 | 3.4 | 20.0 |
| Sweden | 248 | 65.1 | 6.3 | 19.0 |
| Switzerland | 338 | 93.6 | 6.0 | 21.0 |
| United Kingdom | NA | NA | NA | 11.0 |
| United States | 348 | 90.3 | 4.1 | 32.5 |
| OECD average | 186 | 68.5 | 5.2 | NA |

*OECD,* Organisation for Economic Co-operation and Development; *PPP,* purchasing power parity; *NA,* comparable data is unavailable.

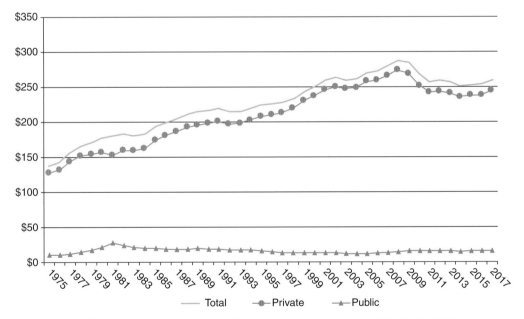

**• Figure 6.1** Total, private, and public per capita dental expenditure, Canada, 1975–2017 In 2002 dollars. (Source: Original analysis of the National Health Expenditure Database, Canadian Institute for Health Information. Thank you to Mr. Mark Gera for his research assistance in producing this data.)

practices, most often made up of dentists, dental hygienists, and dental assistants. Partnerships and group practices do exist, but they are the minority. There is also some corporate ownership of dental practices, but currently this too is minor, as compared to the United States, where this sector of the dental care market is well established and growing. To a much lesser extent, oral healthcare is provided in hospitals (surgical-dental services delivered in hospital as per the Canada Health Act) and in public clinics run by governments or the not-for-profit sector.

Finally, given historical and recent American debates over oral health human resources and service delivery models, of interest are dental therapy and alternative models of care in Canada. Canada is a historical bastion of dental therapy in North America, with successful programs existing in two provinces and in federal jurisdictions from the mid-1970s through to the mid-1990s.[13,18,20] Although due to largely unsupported concerns held by dentists and dental associations (concerns similar to those in the United States over safety and effectiveness) and the pressure that

**• TABLE 6.2** Oral Healthcare Providers in Canada

| | Number | Delivery Settings |
|---|---|---|
| General dentists | 19,181 | Private practices, public clinics, hospitals |
| Dental public health specialists | 43 | Governments, professional regulators, professional associations, public clinics |
| Endodontists | 311 | Private practices, hospitals |
| Oral and maxillofacial pathologists | 46 | Private practices, hospitals |
| Oral and maxillofacial radiologists | 25 | Private practices, hospitals |
| Oral and maxillofacial surgeons | 444 | Private practices, hospitals |
| Orthodontists | 841 | Private practices, hospitals |
| Pediatric dentists | 312 | Private practices, hospitals |
| Periodontists | 418 | Private practices, hospitals |
| Prosthodontists | 226 | Private practices, hospitals |
| Dentist anesthesiologists | 33 | Private practices, hospitals |
| Dental hygienists | 29,246 | Private practices, hospitals, public clinics |
| Dental therapists | 300 | Private practices, public clinics |
| Dental assistants | 29,000 | Private practices, hospitals, public clinics |
| Dental technologists | 2,000 | Private practices, hospitals, public clinics |
| Denturists | 2,393 | Private practices, public clinics |

Notes: Numbers are estimated. Estimates for general dentists and specialists are for 2015. Dentist anesthesiologists are only recognized as a specialty in Canada's most populated province, Ontario. Denturist, dental hygienist, dental therapist, dental assistant, and dental technologist estimates are for 2018. Thank you to the Canadian Dental Association and Denturist Association of Canada for providing this data.

dentists and dental associations were able to bring to bear on governments to not support the dental therapy model, there has been a significant decline in dental therapy in Canada over time.[13,18] Other than dental therapy, Canada has also never really supported any robust alternative models of care. Canada is different from the United States here in that it does not have any dental management or service organizations or anything of that sort (e.g., preferred provider networks), nor does it have any form of robust public delivery. In this regard, from the American perspective, the Canadian dental care market is quite simple in its organization, financing, and delivery.

## Oral Healthcare and Canadian Medicare

Given the general confusion among American and international researchers and policy actors about oral healthcare's positioning within Canada's national system of health insurance, understanding the factors that contributed to the exclusion of oral healthcare from Canadian Medicare deserves some attention. In general terms, from the mid-1800s onward and most importantly after World War II, like the United States and other OECD nations, Canada began to develop its welfare state, or the idea that government should play a role in helping to determine the health and well-being of citizens. Through a series of legislative and policy instruments, Canadian governments (particularly the federal government) shaped social and health policy to eventually support things like public education, unemployment benefits, income support programs, old age security, and universal healthcare (or universal access to hospital and physician care).[22]

The key period for oral healthcare occurred in the 1960s, as the federal government began to formally explore a national system of health insurance,[21] including the place of oral healthcare within it.[25] Governments were faced with scarcity, and oral healthcare presented a significant economic concern, because the experience of the United Kingdom—who did include oral healthcare within its national system of health insurance—demonstrated how expensive it could be. Epidemiologically, dental caries in the population (particularly among children) was in significant decline with improvements in the oral health status of the population due to improved social, economic, and living conditions; the introduction of community water fluoridation (CWF); and broad societal changes in oral health–related behaviors linked to the rise of the cultural importance of teeth in social life.

Thus, with alternatives like CWF, the large-scale coverage of oral health was not seen as necessary. The dental profession also played an important role by strongly promoting CWF and health education and by noting the significance of individual responsibility in terms of oral health. It is important to note that things like universal healthcare and other welfare state programs and policies are meant to stress and support the idea of social responsibility. Yet, as in any liberal democracy, these two ideas are juxtaposed and create an inherent tension that drives social and health policy. The American two-party system, or schism between Republicans and Democrats, specifically cuts along this line.

The same is true in Canada as a policy context, and governments tend to speak about issues in this way. Thus, given the economic and epidemiological realities of the time, oral healthcare was ultimately positioned as an individual responsibility and not included in Canadian Medicare. What is more, the Canadian electorate also perceived oral health and oral healthcare in these terms, especially at a time when an increasing number of them were being insured through the introduction of employment-based benefits. Simply put, Canadian society did not see the same immediate need to include oral healthcare in Canadian Medicare as it did hospital and physician care.

However, the landscape has now changed. Employment-based insurance is not as robust as it used to be, with less of it being offered to new employees due to changes in the labor market.[27,29] An aging population has put into focus the plight of seniors who no longer get to keep their employment-based insurance upon retirement, as was the case for many in the past, while being challenged by increasing oral healthcare needs as they age.[10] Incomes have stagnated, and more middle-class families are experiencing cost barriers to care.[27,29] Dental caries remains a public health challenge, given significant and often severe inequalities in oral health and access to oral healthcare.[3,9] The construct and ethos of oral health is now linked to systemic health for the average Canadian as more research supports the important and sometimes serious links between the two. Poor access to oral healthcare is having impacts on Canadian Medicare through increasing visits to physicians and hospital emergency departments for toothaches.[11,26,27,34]

All of this is pushing governments and civil society toward a renewed focus on oral health and oral healthcare policy. What the future may hold is unknown, but as in the United States, people are now wondering whether it is time to consider universal oral healthcare or a more nuanced and/or complex oral healthcare system in order to more appropriately meet the needs of the most vulnerable and to better meet the changing and emerging needs of all society.

## The Epidemiology of Oral Health and Oral Healthcare in Canada

### Clinical and Self-Reported Oral Health Outcomes

Unlike in the United States with its National Health and Nutrition Examination Survey (NHANES), Canada does not regularly gather clinical data on the oral health status of its population. The last time this was done was through the Canadian Health Measures Survey (CHMS) 2007/09[9] and before that, through the Nutrition Canada National Survey (NCNS) 1970/72.[2] Nevertheless, on the whole, Canadian and American populations are similar enough that differences in oral health status and their trends are arguably not substantially different. For example, in the mid- to late 2000s, the mean decayed, missing, and filled teeth (DMFT) among 12-year-olds in Canada and the United States were reported as 1.0 and 1.2, respectively,[5,9] placing them in the middle of the pack when compared to other OECD nations in the same period: Germany (0.7), Denmark (0.8), Belgium (1.0), Australia (1.1), France (1.6), and Greece (2.1).[38]

In terms of trends, there has been an epidemiological transition in oral disease in both Canada and the United States. For example, since the early 1970s and into the first decade of the 2000s, the prevalence of caries (DMFT >0) has significantly reduced among Canadian and American children, from 74.3% and 54.8% to 23.6% and 21.1%, respectively.[2,4,5,6,9] The mean DMFT among Canadian and American children has also fallen, from 2.5 and 1.7 in the 1970s respectively to 0.5 in both countries in the 2000s.[2,4,5,6,9] Over the same period, the prevalence of caries

(DMFT >0) among Canadian and American adults has remained relatively stable, from 95.2% and 98.7% in the 1970s to 95.9% and 91.6% in the 2000s respectively, while the mean DMFT has also fallen from 18.0 and 16.9 in the 1970s to 10.7 and 10.3 in the 2000s, respectively.[2,4,5,6,9] Finally, the prevalence of edentulism among Canadian and American adults has also fallen, from 23.6% and 14.7% in the 1970s to 6.4% and 3.8% in the 2000s.[2,4,5,6,9]

Significant inequalities in oral health outcomes exist across social groups in both countries as well (comparisons with the United States will be made later in this chapter). For now it is important to note that in Canada, oral health outcomes tend to be worse in populations that experience social and/or economic marginalization, whether by income, dental insurance status, education, place of birth, and/or Indigenous status (Table 6.3).

In terms of periodontal conditions, although time trend information is not available in Canada, similar inequalities in the population are seen, meaning periodontal conditions are worse by income, dental insurance status, education, place of birth, Indigenous status, and/or smoking status.[9] Interestingly, compared to the United States, Canadian estimates for periodontitis among adults are surprisingly low (i.e., in the 2000s, 9.2% vs. 5.7% had a loss of clinical attachment of 5 mm, respectively), yet this may have to do with the way periodontitis was measured in the CHMS; it was not a full periodontal exam and only included measurements on World Health Organization indicator teeth.[2,4,5,6,9] As for self-reported outcomes, although most Canadians rate their oral health as good to excellent and do not report pain and/or other negative oral health–related quality-of-life outcomes, similar inequalities to clinical oral health outcomes exist (see Table 6.3).

## The Utilization of and Access to Oral Healthcare

The majority of Canadians access and use oral healthcare on a yearly basis. Children visit the dentist most often, and there are variations in use and access based on age, gender, income, dental insurance status, and/or Indigenous status (see Table 6.3). In general terms, utilization trends are similar in both countries, although Canadian adults appear to visit the dentist more often than American adults (i.e., in the 2000s, 71.6% vs. 59.9% visited a dentist in the past year, respectively). Also, affordability is a significant issue given that Canada and the United States have similar oral healthcare systems, particularly in terms of depending on private financing and markets to distribute oral healthcare. For example, approximately one in five Canadians report a cost barrier to care (see Table 6.3),[30] and Canada and the United States rank last among a select group of OECD nations in terms of cost barriers to care (see Table 6.1).[23]

There is also some interesting variability in the experience of cost barriers to oral healthcare in Canada. Historical data demonstrate clear and smooth income gradients in use and access-to-care barriers, yet by the start of the new millennium, these gradients were more variable (Figure 6.2).[29] This was first noticed in 2007, when it was shown that publicly insured Canadians reported more dental care visits than low-income uninsured Canadians.[1] This makes sense given that Canada attempts to meet need and demand for oral healthcare through public subsidies for low-income groups and through employment-based insurance for all other populations. Yet as labor markets changed, resulting in more precarious work environments, and as incomes stagnated due to global wealth trends, working poverty became an issue, and low- and middle-income uninsured families began to experience similar or worse cost barriers

• TABLE 6.3 Inequalities in Oral Health–Related Outcomes in Canada[9]

| | | DMFT > 0 (%) | Mean Number of Untreated Teeth With Coronal Caries | Mean Number of Filled Teeth | Edentulism (%) | Loss of Attachment of 6 mm or More (%) | Self-Reported Fair or Poor Oral Health (%) | Reporting Persistent Oral Pain (%) | Visited a Dental Professional in the Past 12 Months (%) | Avoided Visiting a Dental Professional Within the Last Year Due to Cost (%) | Declined Recommended Care Within the Last Year Due to Cost (%) |
|---|---|---|---|---|---|---|---|---|---|---|---|
| Gender | Male | 95.4 | 3.0 | 7.3 | 6.3 | 6.9 | 16.8 | 9.7 | 15.5 | 14.4 | 15.5 |
| | Female | 96.5 | 2.8 | 8.5 | 6.5 | 5.0 | 14.1 | 13.5 | 19.2 | 18.6 | 19.2 |
| Income | Lower | 94.7 | 3.2 | 6.5 | 10.9 | 9.0 | 24.6 | 16.0 | 34.5 | 29.7 | 34.5 |
| | Middle | 96.2 | 3.2 | 7.5 | 8.5 | 7.3 | 16.5 | 12.2 | 19.5 | 18.3 | 19.5 |
| | Higher | 96.8 | 2.4 | 8.9 | 3.2 | 3.6 | 10.9 | 9.1 | 8.8 | 9.9 | 8.8 |
| Dental insurance | Private | 95.5 | 2.3 | 8.3 | 3.0 | 4.7 | 12.9 | 10.2 | 8.6 | 10.9 | 8.6 |
| | Public | 96.9 | 3.7 | 8.3 | 13.3 | 7.8 | 26.3 | 17.8 | 8.9 | 18.1 | 8.9 |
| | None | 96.7 | 3.5 | 7.2 | 11.4 | 6.4 | 18.6 | 13.2 | 35.9 | 27.4 | 35.9 |
| Place of birth | In Canada | 96.7 | 2.9 | 8.1 | 6.9 | 3.8 | 14.7 | 11.6 | 15.8 | 15.4 | 15.8 |
| | Outside Canada | 93.5 | 2.9 | 7.3 | 4.8 | 12.4 | 18.3 | 11.8 | 22.8 | 20.3 | 22.8 |
| Indigenous status | Indigenous | 97.7 | 3.0 | 9.2 | NP | NP | 28.0 | 26.8 | NP | 15.8 | NP |
| | Non-Indigenous | 95.9 | 2.9 | 7.9 | 6.4 | 6.1 | 15.1 | 11.1 | 17.4 | 16.5 | 17.4 |

*NP, Estimate not provided because of extreme sample variability or small sample size.*

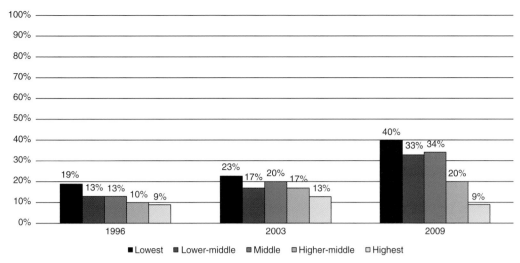

• **Figure 6.2** Prevalence of self-reported cost barriers to dental care by income, Canada, select years.[29]

to care as no- or low-income publicly insured families.[27,29] This is apparent when looking at trends in self-reported cost barriers to oral healthcare over time in Canada (see Figure 6.2).

## The Burden of Oral Disease

Oral diseases impose a burden on Canadians, their healthcare system, and society. It is well known that oral health conditions hold functional and psychosocial impacts for individuals, influencing such things as the ability to eat and speak, self-esteem, and social inclusion.[3,9,16] Here too, social gradients exist in terms dentition status, treatment needs, income, education, dental visiting patterns, dental insurance status, and the ability to afford care.[9,16,35] In fact, the greater in number and frequency with which Canadians report cost barriers to dental care, the worse the impacts on their clinical oral health status and oral health–related quality of life.[15,36] There is also the potential for Canadians with a compromised dental appearance (e.g., dental decay, stained and broken teeth) to experience discrimination.[19] For example, males, those who are older, those with more right-leaning political perspectives, and those with higher incomes are more likely to blame the poor for their oral health conditions, attributing such conditions to individual failings.[19]

In terms of the healthcare system, as in the United States, attention has been paid in Canada to the inappropriate use of physician offices and hospital emergency departments for dental problems that are preventable and best treated in dental settings.[3,11,14,24,26,28,29,31,34,42] This consumption of healthcare resources is generally viewed as inefficient and ineffective, as physicians and hospitals are for the most part ill equipped to diagnose and treat dental conditions. Worse, when hospitalization is required (again, for diseases that are preventable and easily and effectively treated in dental settings), the costs to Canada's publicly financed healthcare system can be significant.[28] Available data for emergency department use in Canada and the United States suggests that the issue is comparable between both countries. For example, in the first decade of the new millennium, the rate of emergency department visits associated with preventable dental problems was 3.4 and 3.7 in Ontario (Canada's most populated province) and the United States, respectively, and made 0.93% and 1.18% of all emergency department visits in the same.[14,26,34,42] And importantly, at least

in Canada, these visits are more common in adults, individuals without dental insurance, and those in the lower-middle income group, rather than those of lowest income.[24,26,28,31] As previously described, this makes sense when one considers that children and lower income groups may often be eligible for government dental care programs in Canada.

In terms of the societal burden of oral disease, this can be demonstrated through the indirect costs attributed to time lost from work, school, or normal activities due to dental problems and treatment. In 2007/09, approximately 40 million hours per year were lost in Canada due to dental problems and treatment, or 3.5 hours per person.[8] The amount of time lost was greatest for those experiencing oral pain, and experiencing such pain was the strongest predictor of both reporting time lost and the amount of time lost.[8] Ultimately, this is estimated to result in potential productivity losses to Canadian society of over $1 billion.[8]

## Comparing Income-Related Inequalities in Oral Health and Oral Healthcare Between Canada and the United States

As detailed in previous sections of this chapter, Canada and the United States share similarities in social, economic, and political contexts and in the structure of their oral healthcare systems. To this end, comparing oral health–related outcomes between both countries can provide insights into the contribution of contextual or other factors to the income-related inequalities (or differences in oral health–related outcomes between income groups) that have been described in this chapter. Although existing Canadian and American datasets limit this type of analysis due to a lack of comparable exposure and outcome data—in particular for contextual factors—comparisons can still be made based on select individual exposures (such as age, gender, income, education, and household/family size) and outcomes (prevalence of one or more decayed teeth, prevalence of one or more filled teeth, presence of edentulism, and prevalence of dental visits in the past 12 months). The final section of this chapter will thus provide a comparative case study of Canada and the United States in this regard, using a novel methodological approach, or a complex measure of inequality (i.e., the concentration index).

| • TABLE 6.4 | Income-Related Inequalities in Oral Health Outcomes in Canada and the United States[6] | | | |
|---|---|---|---|---|
| | | **CANADA** | | **UNITED STATES** |
| | | NCNS 1970/72 | CHMS 2007/09 | NHANES 1971/74 | NHANES 2007/08 |

| | | CANADA | | UNITED STATES | |
|---|---|---|---|---|---|
| | | NCNS 1970/72 | CHMS 2007/09 | NHANES 1971/74 | NHANES 2007/08 |
| Prevalence of one or more decayed teeth | Absolute difference (%) | 10.4 | 19.5 | 17.4 | 32.3 |
| | Relative difference | 1.22 | 2.21 | 1.50 | 4.08 |
| | Concentration index | −0.158 | −0.164 | −0.160 | −0.209 |
| Prevalence of one or more filled teeth | Absolute difference (%) | 12.2 | 10.7 | 30.0 | 21.5 |
| | Relative difference | 0.85 | 0.92 | 0.68 | 0.77 |
| | Concentration index | 0.076 | 0.053 | 0.227 | 0.106 |
| Presence of edentulism | Absolute difference (%) | 17.7 | 9.7 | 21.3 | 7.0 |
| | Relative difference | 3.64 | 7.46 | 3.69 | 3.69 |
| | Concentration index | −0.147 | −0.085 | −0.159 | −0.083 |
| | | JCUSH 2002/03 | CCHS 2012 | JCUSH 2002/03 | NHIS 2012 |
| Prevalence of dental visit in the past 12 months | Absolute difference (%) | 33.7 | 34.1 | 37.2 | 43.8 |
| | Relative difference | 0.57 | 0.57 | 0.54 | 0.46 |
| | Concentration index | 0.157 | 0.149 | 0.164 | 0.197 |

Notes: NCNS 1970/72, CHMS 2007/09, NHANES 1971/74, NHANES 2007/08 data are for adults 20 to 74 years. Joint Canada/United States Survey of Health (JCUSH) 2002/03, Canadian Community Health Survey (CCHS) 2012, and National Health Interview Survey (NHIS) 2012 data are for adults aged 20+. Original analysis of the JCUSH 2002/03, CCHS 2012, and NHIS 2012.

To begin, Table 6.4 outlines two simple measures and one complex measure of income-related inequality (absolute and relative differences and the concentration index, respectively) for several clinical oral health and utilization outcomes in Canada and the United States, comparing two periods (the early 1970s with the 2000s, and roughly the beginning and end of the first decade of the new millennium). As seen, the absolute and relative differences for each oral health–related outcome (or the absolute and relative difference between the lowest and highest income groups) reveal the following in general terms:

- There have been increases to inequalities in decayed teeth in both countries over time.
- There have been decreases to inequalities in filled teeth in both countries over time.
- There are greater inequalities in edentulism in Canada over time and in the 2000s.
- There are greater inequalities in decayed teeth and dental visits in the United States in the 2000s.

Despite these findings, the extent of income-related inequality in oral health–related outcomes at the population level cannot be inferred. These simple measures of inequality really only assess these outcomes at the individual and not population level. For example, simple measures of inequality do not incorporate the oral health outcome experiences for the population as a whole, nor do they capture the size of each income group in a given population or address its changes over time.[41] This makes it difficult to compare changes to inequalities over time or between different countries.

To do this, one needs a complex measure on inequality. The concentration index is an econometric approach that measures the magnitude (or the size) of socioeconomic differences in health status between social groups at the population level.[40] It provides an overall value for the relationship between a health outcome and a ranked (from lowest to highest or vice versa) socioeconomic variable in a given population, in this case income.[39] Unlike comparisons of proportions and means between groups (as with simple measures of inequality), the concentration index accounts for the number of people in each income group and in the entire population. The value of the concentration index ranges from −1 to +1, with values of 0 indicating total equality in the distribution of a health outcome across the income spectrum, and values closer to ±1 indicating greater income-related inequality (or greater differences across income groups). In this analysis, socioeconomic status was ranked from lowest to highest income, which means that a value of −1 is "pro-poor" (the outcome concentrates mostly in the poor) and a value of +1 is "pro-rich" (the outcome concentrates mostly in the rich).[40]

Thus, looking back to Table 6.4, the concentration index values reveal the following:

- Pro-poor inequalities in decayed teeth and edentulism in both countries at both time points.
- Pro-rich inequalities in filled teeth and dental visits in both countries at both time points.
- Greater increases in pro-poor inequalities in decayed teeth in the United States over time.
- Increases in pro-rich inequalities in dental visits in the United States over time.

One can hypothesize what changes in social, economic, and political contexts may have played a role here. In terms of empirically evaluating the contributors to these income-related inequalities, the concentration index is useful as it can also be broken down or "decomposed" to identify such contributors.[37] As described, understanding the role of any given factor depends on the available

| • TABLE 6.5 | **Percent Contribution to Income-Related Inequalities in Oral Health Outcomes in Canada and the United States[6]** | | | | |
|---|---|---|---|---|---|

| | | CANADA | | UNITED STATES | |
|---|---|---|---|---|---|
| | | **NCNS 1970/72** | **CHMS 2007/09** | **NHANES 1971/74** | **NHANES 2007/08** |
| Prevalence of one or more decayed teeth | Age | −0.003 | −0.006 | 0.003 | 0.002 |
| | Sex | −0.004 | 0.013 | 0.004 | 0.002 |
| | Age × Sex | 0.004 | −0.002 | 0.001 | 0.002 |
| | Income | −0.014 | −0.161 | −0.092 | −0.128 |
| | Educational attainment | −0.006 | −0.012 | −0.014 | −0.023 |
| | Household/family size | 0.001 | 0.029 | 0.011 | 0.006 |
| Prevalence of one or more filled teeth | Age | 0.001 | 0.001 | 0.000 | 0.004 |
| | Sex | −0.001 | −0.001 | −0.001 | −0.001 |
| | Age × Sex | 0.008 | −0.002 | 0.001 | 0.000 |
| | Income | 0.008 | 0.008 | 0.038 | 0.017 |
| | Educational attainment | 0.005 | 0.000 | 0.017 | 0.003 |
| | Household/family size | 0.000 | −0.002 | −0.006 | −0.001 |
| Presence of edentulism | Age | −0.025 | −0.096 | −0.107 | 0.017 |
| | Sex | −0.058 | −0.021 | −0.002 | −0.003 |
| | Age × Sex | 0.000 | 0.014 | 0.000 | 0.003 |
| | Income | 0.010 | −0.084 | −0.07 | −0.102 |
| | Educational attainment | −0.028 | −0.005 | −0.043 | −0.019 |
| | Household/family size | −0.002 | 0.000 | −0.003 | −0.018 |
| | | **JCUSH 2002/03** | **CCHS 2012** | **JCUSH 2002/03** | **NHIS 2012** |
| | Age | 0.009 | 0.026 | 0.016 | −0.002 |
| | Sex | −0.023 | −0.014 | −0.013 | −0.009 |
| Prevalence of dental visit in the past 12 months | Age × Sex | 0.006 | −0.007 | −0.005 | 0.003 |
| | Income | 0.322 | 0.370 | 0.333 | 0.351 |
| | Educational attainment | 0.113 | 0.056 | 0.109 | 0.114 |
| | Household/family size | 0.004 | 0.002 | −0.009 | 0.001 |

Notes: Aggregate results presented for each variable. Values further away from 1 indicate greater contribution to inequality. Negative values indicate contribution to pro-poor inequalities. Positive values indicate contribution to pro-rich inequalities. An age × sex interaction term was included to account for variation in effect of age on the outcome based on sex. NCNS 1970/72, CHMS 2007/09, NHANES 1971/74, NHANES 2007/08 data are for adults 20 to 74 years. JCUSH 2002/03, CCHS 2012, and NHIS 2012 data are for adults aged 20+. Original analysis of the JCUSH 2002/03, CCHS 2012, and NHIS 2012.

variables in each data set; as such, it is not possible here to determine the contribution of things like social, economic, and political context, nor dental insurance and oral health behaviors. Nevertheless, Table 6.5 details the results of a decomposition analysis using the available variables, which reveals the following:
• A greater contribution of income to inequalities in filled teeth in the United States compared to Canada (as indicated by larger ± percent contributions).
• A greater contribution of age to inequalities in edentulism than to other outcomes.
• Increases in the contribution of income to inequalities in decayed teeth, edentulism, and dental visits over time.
• Increases in the contribution of educational attainment to inequalities in decayed teeth in Canada and the United States and dental visits in the United States over time.

• Decreases in the contribution of educational attainment to inequalities in dental visits in Canada over time.

## Conclusion

Healthcare in Canada is not socialized, meaning while it publicly finances the great majority of hospital and physician care, delivery is mixed, combining public and private care. Further, oral healthcare is not actually included in Canada's national system of health insurance, as many believe, and it was not incorporated for a variety of social, political, and economic reasons. And, although Canada spends less than the United States on a per capita basis for publicly financed dental care, having a homologous albeit simpler oral healthcare system in general terms, the oral health status of the populations is similar. Yet it appears that affordability issues may be worse in the United States in terms of access to care, as are income-related inequalities in a variety of oral health–related outcomes. It also appears that over time income and education have played a stronger role in shaping the American population's experience of oral health–related inequalities than in Canada.

In closing, we hope such comparisons prove beneficial for understanding the dynamics of oral healthcare in both countries and provide a window into potential solutions to the challenges that face each country in terms of population oral health and oral healthcare.

# References

1. Bhatti T, Rana Z, Grootendorst P. Dental insurance, income and the use of dental care in Canada. *J Can Dent Assoc.* 2007;73(1):57.
2. Canada Nutrition. *Dental Report.* Ottawa, ON: Health and Welfare Canada; 1977.
3. Canadian Academy of Health Sciences. *Improving Access to Oral Health Care for Vulnerable People Living in Canada.* Ottawa, ON: Canadian Academy of Health Sciences; 2014.
4. Department of Health and Human Services. DHHS Publication No. (PHS) 81-1673. In: *Decayed, Missing and Filled Teeth Among Persons 1-74 Years, Data from the National Health Survey Series 11, No. 223.* Washington, DC: U.S. Department of Health and Human Services, Public Health Service, Office of Health Research, Statistics, and Technology, National Center for Health Statistics; 1981.
5. Dye BA, Tan S, Smith V, et al. Trends in oral health status: United States, 1988–1994 and 1999–2004. *Vital Health Stat.* 2007; 11(248):1–92.
6. Farmer J, McLeod L, Siddiqi A, et al. Towards an understanding of the structural determinants of oral health inequalities: a comparative analysis between Canada and the United States. *SSM Pop Health.* 2016;2:226–236.
7. Finkelstein A. The effect of tax subsidies to employer-provided supplementary health insurance: evidence from Canada. *J Public Econ.* 2002;84(3):305–339.
8. Hayes A, Azarpazhooh A, Dempster L, et al. Time loss due to dental problems and treatment in the Canadian population: analysis of a nationwide cross-sectional survey. *BMC Oral Health.* 2013;13(1):17.
9. Canada Health. *Summary Report on the Findings of the Oral Health Component of the Canadian Health Measures Survey, 2007–2009.* Ottawa, ON: Health Canada; 2010.
10. Kelsall D, O'Keefe J. Good health requires a healthy mouth: improving the oral health of Canada's seniors. *CMAJ.* 2014;186(12):893.
11. LaPlante NC, Singhal S, Maund J, et al. Visits to physicians for oral health-related complaints in Ontario, Canada. *Can J Public Health.* 2015;106(3):127–131.
12. Lasser KE, Himmelstein DU, Woolhandler S. Access to care, health status, and health disparities in the United States and Canada: results of a cross-national population-based survey. *Am J Pub Health.* 2006;96(7):1300–1307.
13. Leck V, Randall GE. The rise and fall of dental therapy in Canada: a policy analysis and assessment of equity of access to oral health care for Inuit and First Nations communities. *Int J Equity Health.* 2017; 16(1):131.
14. Lee HH, Lewis CW, Saltzman B, et al. Visiting the emergency department for dental problems: trends in utilization, 2001 to 2008. *Am J Pub Health.* 2012;102(11):e77–e83.
15. Locker D, Maggirias J, Quiñonez C. Income, dental insurance coverage, and financial barriers to dental care among Canadian adults. *J Public Health Dent.* 2011;71(4):327–334.
16. Locker D, Quiñonez C. Functional and psychosocial impacts of oral disorders in Canadian adults: a national population survey. *J Can Dent Assoc.* 2009;75(7):521.
17. Marshall K. Benefits of the job. *Perspect Labour Income.* 2003;4 (5):5–12.
18. Mathu-Muju KR, Friedman JW, Nash DA. Saskatchewan's school-based dental program staffed by dental therapists: a retrospective case study. *J Public Health Dent.* 2017;77(1):78–85.
19. Moeller J, Singhal S, Al-Dajani M, et al. Assessing the relationship between dental appearance and the potential for discrimination in Ontario, Canada. *SSM Popul Health.* 2015;1:26–31.
20. Nash DA, Friedman JW, Mathu-Muju KR, et al. A review of the global literature on dental therapists. *Community Dent Oral Epidemiol.* 2014;42(1):1–10.
21. Naylor D. *Private Practice, Public Payment: Canadian Medicine and the Politics of Health Insurance, 1911–1966.* Montreal, QC: McGill-Queen's Press; 1986.
22. O'Connor JS, Orloff AS, Shaver S. *States, Markets, Families: Gender, Liberalism and Social Policy in Australia, Canada, Great Britain and the United States.* Cambridge, UK: Cambridge University Press; 1999.
23. Osborn R, Squires D, Doty MM, et al. In new survey of eleven countries, US adults still struggle with access to and affordability of health care. *Health Aff.* 2016;35(12):2327–2336.
24. Quiñonez C. Self-reported emergency room visits for dental problems. *Int J Dent Hygiene.* 2011;9(1):17–20.
25. Quiñonez C. Why was dental care excluded from Canadian Medicare? *Network for Canadian Oral Health Research Working Papers Series.* 2013;1(1):1–5.
26. Quiñonez C, Gibson D, Jokovic A, et al. Emergency department visits for dental care of nontraumatic origin. *Community Dent Oral Epidemiol.* 2009;37(4):366–371.
27. Quiñonez C, Grootendorst P. Equity in dental care among Canadian households. *Int J Equity Health.* 2011;10(1):14.
28. Quiñonez C, Ieraci L, Guttmann A. Potentially preventable hospital use for dental conditions: implications for expanding dental coverage for low income populations. *J Health Care Poor Underserved.* 2011; 22(3):1048–1058.
29. Ramraj C, Sadeghi L, Lawrence HP, et al. Is accessing dental care becoming more difficult? Evidence from Canada's middle-income population. *PLoS One.* 2013;8(2):e57377.
30. Ramraj C, Weitzner E, Figueiredo R, et al. A macroeconomic review of dentistry in Canada in the 2000s. *J Can Dent Assoc.* 2014;80(1): e55.
31. Ramraj CC, Quiñonez CR. Emergency room visits for dental problems among working poor Canadians. *J Public Health Dent.* 2013; 73(3):210–216.
32. Schneider E, Sarnak D, Squires D, et al. *Mirror, Mirror 2017: International Comparison Reflects Flaws and Opportunities for Better U.S. Health Care.* New York, NY: The Commonwealth Fund; 2017.
33. Shaw J, Farmer J. *An Environmental Scan of Publicly Financed Dental Care in Canada: 2015 Update.* Toronto, ON: Faculty of Dentistry, University of Toronto; 2016.
34. Singhal S, McLaren L, Quiñonez C. Trends in emergency department visits for non-traumatic dental conditions in Ontario from 2006 to 2014. *Can J Public Health.* 2017;108(3):e246.
35. Thompson B, Cooney P, Lawrence H, et al. Cost as a barrier to accessing dental care: findings from a Canadian population-based study. *J Public Health Dent.* 2014;74(3):210–218.
36. Thompson B, Cooney P, Lawrence H, et al. The potential oral health impact of cost barriers to dental care: findings from a Canadian population-based study. *BMC Oral Health.* 2014;14(1):78.
37. van Doorslaer EV, Koolman X, Jones AM. Explaining income-related inequalities in doctor utilisation in Europe. *Health Econ.* 2004; 13(7):629-47.
38. Vujicic M, Bernabé E, Neumann DG, et al. Dental care. In: Scheffler R, ed. *World Scientific Handbook of Global Health Economics and Public Policy. Vol 2: Health Determinants and Outcomes.* Singapore: World Scientific Publishing Co.; 2016:83–121.

39. Wagstaff A, Doorslaer EV. Overall versus socioeconomic health inequality: a measurement framework and two empirical illustrations. *Health Econ.* 2004;13(3):297–301.

40. Wagstaff A, O'Donnell O, Van Doorslaer E, et al. *Analyzing Health Equity Using Household Survey Data: a Guide to Techniques and Their Implementation.* Washington, DC: World Bank Publications; 2007.

41. Wagstaff A, Paci P, Van Doorslaer E. On the measurement of inequalities in health. *Soc Sci Med.* 1991;33(5):545–557.

42. Wall T, Nasseh K. Dental-related emergency department visits on the increase in the United States. In: *Health Policy Resources Center Research Brief.* Chicago, IL: American Dental Association; 2013.

# 7

# Financing Dental Care

VICTOR M. BADNER, DMD, MPH

DAVID ALBERT, DDS, MPH

PETER DAMIANO, DDS, MPH

## CHAPTER OUTLINE

According to the World Health Organization, healthcare financing is that aspect of a health system that is "concerned with the mobilization, accumulation and allocation of money to cover the health needs of the people, individually and collectively, in the health system."[95] Healthcare generates costs or expenses that must be equal to the payments received for delivering that care. The costs of providing healthcare are categorized in the same manner as any business operation and can be fixed or variable and direct or indirect (Box 7.1).[70] All costs must be accounted and paid for or the healthcare system cannot continue to function. Some costs or charges are paid by the recipients of care, while others are borne by governmental entities via taxes or by third parties (e.g., health insurance, employers, charitable organizations). A variety of systems have been created to distribute the costs and charges as well as the payments made for healthcare.

## Background

In the United States, the traditional methodology for paying for healthcare (especially dental care) is called fee for service (FFS). Under fee for service, the provider receives payments based on the services that are provided to a specific patient. Customarily these payments come directly from the patient, but they may also come from intermediaries (e.g., insurance companies or third parties). Regardless of the source of the funds, the charges and payments under this system are based explicitly on the procedures or care provided. While fee-for-service payment by individuals (i.e., out-of-pocket payment) was once the traditional methodology for paying for healthcare expenses in the United States, assistance provided by third parties to pay for healthcare has mostly replaced individual out-of-pocket payments. This began with the enactment of the Social Security Act of 1935. Third-party payments expanded when employer-based insurance began during World

---

### • BOX 7.1   Direct and Indirect Costs

Direct costs are related to the product and the amount of the expense that is easily assignable/traceable to the product. These costs are assigned to the product based on a cause-and-effect relationship. Total variable cost changes in proportion to the change in output, such as material costs. Per-unit variable cost remains fixed. Total fixed cost is cost that does not change in proportion to the change in output, such as the monthly salary cost of a supervisor. Per-unit fixed cost is variable. Indirect costs are related to the product, but the amount of expense is not traceable in an economically feasible manner. These costs are allocated to the product based on some reasonable basis.

War II and continued with the development of government programs during the mid-1960s when the national "War on Poverty" gained traction.[50]

The third party in these payment arrangements is often called the carrier, insurer, underwriter, or administrative agent. The purchaser of the plan can be an organized private group such as a union, or it can be an employer, a union-employer welfare fund, a governmental agency, or an individual. It has been argued that this arrangement should most properly be called prepayment rather than insurance, particularly for dental insurance, because it does not fulfill the traditional definitions of insurance as discussed later in this chapter. Be that as it may, the term dental insurance has entered the lexicon, and the terms dental prepayment and dental insurance as commonly used are virtually synonymous.

There is also the question of who ultimately bears the cost of nongovernment–supported care paid through a third party. The most widely accepted answer is employers, because they often pay for insurance directly or provide reimbursement for employees who purchase coverage. Of course, the employers' payments for employee coverage come from the employees in foregone wages. This is particularly evident during unions' collective bargaining negotiations on behalf of employees, though it is true for all employees with healthcare benefits. These costs are also passed along to consumers as a cost of doing business. Reference to the third-party agency as the payor for services, although common, is therefore incorrect, because these costs are defrayed by employer, employee, and consumer; neither are employees receiving "free" care, even if they do not pay for care directly out of pocket. When the government is involved in the payment of healthcare expenses, the term commonly used is public financing of care. The best-known public health insurance programs are Medicare, Medicaid, and the Children's Health Insurance Program (CHIP); programs that cover military members and their dependents; and those that finance community health centers, federally qualified health centers, and many other healthcare programs.

Over time, private dental insurance expanded, particularly after passage of the Taft-Hartley Act in 1947, which allowed labor unions to seek fringe benefits, in addition to wages, through collective bargaining. Since then, healthcare insurance has been the primary employee fringe benefit. One of the reasons for its popularity is that because of the Taft-Hartley Act, healthcare premiums paid by an employer are exempt from income and payroll taxes. Each dollar of earnings taken in the form of health insurance therefore buys more healthcare than cash wages would, because cash wages are taxed. In addition, large employers can deduct the cost of the insurance from their taxes; in effect, a government subsidy designed to encourage employer-sponsored insurance. Health insurance as a tax-protected fringe benefit thus subsidizes the insurance and healthcare industries in the United States.[23]

There have been frequent unsuccessful attempts at the federal level to limit the amount of these health insurance premiums that are protected from taxes. For example, President George W. Bush's tax commission recommended limited deductibility of overly generous benefit packages, or "Cadillac" plans.[41] Then again in the 2010 Patient Protection and Affordable Care Act (ACA), "Cadillac" plans were deemed taxable, currently scheduled to begin in 2022. In times of budgetary difficulty, we may expect periodic attempts to tax employer-sponsored health insurance.[8] If taxed, employer-sponsored health insurance premiums would have yielded as much as $250 billion in taxes 2016 alone.[26] During debates for President Trump's tax overhaul in 2018, some suggested that the employer-paid healthcare premiums should be taxable. This was not ultimately included in the version of tax reform that passed, but this proposal would have been a fundamental change and may have incentivized employers to eliminate or reduce this funding.

## Insurance Principles and Dental Care

To understand the relationship between dentistry and third-party payment, a review of insurance principles is helpful. As medical care grew rapidly in the years following World War II, dental care was one of the "fearful four" areas of healthcare considered uninsurable by commercial insurers (the other three were psychiatric care, prescription drugs, and long-term care), based on an assumption that the nature of dental need violated the basic principles of insurance,[22] which state that to be insurable, a risk event must be:

1. Precisely definable,
2. Of sufficient magnitude that, if it occurs, it constitutes a major loss,
3. Infrequent,
4. Of an unwanted nature, such as destruction of a home through fire,
5. Beyond the control of the individual, and
6. Without "moral hazard," which means that the presence of insurance itself should not lead to additional claims.

Although there are many similarities between medical and dental insurance, there are also many differences. While the costs and use of medical care are for the most part unpredictable, the costs for dental care for a group can be predicted accurately and planned. Dental benefit plans are not insurance plans but are prepayment plans. The concept of insurance—a benefit to be used infrequently—must be abandoned in dental benefit plans. For a dental benefit plan to affect oral health positively, it must be used regularly. Delaying treatment increases the disease's severity over time and the costs for required treatment. In a well-designed dental benefit plan, there are no deductibles or copayments for diagnostic, preventive, and emergency services, and they are reimbursed at the 100% level. In contrast to general health, most oral diseases are preventable, which is the key to cost control in dental benefit plans, not reduced utilization.[29]

Dental prepayment plans began in the 1954 when the state of California enacted legislations enabling dental insurance products. Employer-based plans gained popularity in the 1970s. These private third-party insurance plans are available in two distinct types. The first is the fully insured plan. In the fully insured plan, the insurance company assumes financial risk and establishes premiums through the evaluation of health status and historical utilization patterns in a given population or group seeking coverage. The second is the self-insured plan, or administrative services only (ASO) plan, sometimes referred to as administrative services contract (ASC). In the self-insured plan, the third party only serves as the processing agent for the insurance product and thus the company/employer group is taking the financial risk for the cost of claims. Many large companies elect to be self-insured and seek relationships with traditional insurance companies to provide administrative services for a fee. The costs for administration of self-insurance contracts are often below 5%, whereas fully insured plans may have administrative costs over 20% of the overall healthcare expenditures provided by a plan sponsor.[21,94] In addition to costs, regulatory complexity is further reduced for self-insured plans because they can avoid variable state-level insurance regulations under provisions in the Employee Retirement Income Security Act (ERISA).

In 2014, self-insured plans represented 41% of health plans, while 52% were fully insured and 7% were a blend of funding. Large groups select the self-insured option more frequently and represent 46% of all covered lives; 37% of those covered are in mixed plans and the remaining 17% are in fully insured plans.[7] Consumers are usually unaware of whether they are members of a fully insured, self-insured, or mixed insurance product. In a self-insured plan the employer determines which services are covered, and in a fully insured plan the insurance company determines coverage. An employee with a denied service in a self-insured plan can query their human resources (HR) department and ask for a review of the denial of a procedure by the third-party carrier. To improve employee satisfaction, the HR department of a self-insured product can elect to cover a previously denied service. In a fully insured plan, appeals are adjudicated by the insurance company. The primary incentive to expand services in this arrangement is to reduce employee complaints and dissatisfaction, which might put the employer's renewal of the contract at risk.

All health insurance violates some of the basic principles of insurance. For example, many benefits paid by health insurance represent relatively small amounts of money (violates the second principle), and people with insurance are more likely to use care than those without it (violates the sixth principle above).[46,62] Third-party companies offering dental insurance have circumvented the increased risks when insurance principles are violated in several ways, such as:

- Having patients pay a share of the costs,
- Limiting the range of services covered,
- Offering coverage only to groups,
- Including waiting periods after enrollment before benefits became payable,
- Using preauthorization and annual expenditure limits, and
- Creating networks of providers who accepted a prenegotiated care delivery arrangement.

Requiring patients to pay part of the cost of some services—thereby creating an economic disincentive to overutilization of care—is one way in which insurers reduce the moral hazard associated with insurance. Three systems commonly used to influence cost sharing by members for a portion of their care costs are the deductible, coinsurance, and copayment. A deductible is a set amount of money that the patient must pay toward the cost of treatment before full benefits of the program go into effect.[2] A familiar example of a deductible is the up-front payment of a claim under automobile or home insurance. Coinsurance means that the insured pays a percentage of the total cost.[2] For example, if the insured person's coinsurance is 20%, then their personal responsibility for the service is 20% of the charged amount, and therefore the amount paid will vary depending on the fee. A copayment is a fixed amount that a member pays for a visit or service (e.g., $10 payment for a dental visit of any kind or $10 for filling any prescription drug).

Insurance carriers can also control costs by setting a maximum fee for each procedure. Other ways carriers control costs to purchasers of dental coverage are by setting annual maximums, limiting the range of services covered, and requiring preauthorization of procedures. Annual maximums for dental coverage are very common, and many plans currently have a $1500 annual maximum. Insurance carriers typically consider offering coverage for services that have a supporting evidence base for clinical effectiveness. This range of covered services is termed coverage, covered charges, scope of benefits, or schedule of benefits. Examples of services that are not usually covered in dental insurance policies are newer or high cost techniques and procedures (for example: silver diamine fluoride, dental implants, cosmetic procedures, and extensive treatment for temporomandibular joint disorder). For patients, a common point of confusion is over coverage denial. That is, when a service is not covered by (or is denied by) insurance, the patient may still seek the service, but the patient, rather than the insurer, will be responsible for the payment.

A preauthorization (also called predetermination, precertification, pretreatment review, or prior authorization)[2] is required by some carriers (and advised by others) when the costs of treatment are expected to exceed some preestablished limit. In these scenarios, the dentist must submit the treatment plan to the insurer for review before the treatment begins. This review has several functions, including guaranteeing that the patient's insurance covers the planned treatment (and to what extent) and confirming the appropriateness of the care by a consultant who works for the insurer.

Ostensibly, preauthorization ensures that the proposed treatment is reasonable and that the same quality of care could not be achieved for lower cost. These reviews directly reduce the cost of care, because treatment plans are often revised after discussion with a consultant. Preauthorization requirements also reduce costs indirectly, because dentists soon learn that insurers are unlikely to allow expensive treatment when less expensive alternatives appear reasonable. In general, insurance carriers provide payments based upon the principle of the least expensive acceptable alternative treatment/dental service (LEAATS), also called the least expensive professionally acceptable treatment (LEPAT). That is, if the provider plans to provide multiple fixed partial dentures in an arch where a removable partial denture would suffice, the carrier may reimburse the provider based on the fee of a removable partial denture.

Health insurance was at first offered only to preexisting groups, such as member of associations or unions, because illness experience is reasonably predictable for a group but much less so for an individual. With groups, the risk of adverse selection—which means the inclusion of too many high-risk beneficiaries in the group of insured individuals—was reduced because insuring only large groups amortized or averaged out the risks. Although a large group would likely include people with high levels of need, there would also be many who had little need for care and who would still pay premiums. The fact that the cost of care required for a few people far exceeds the premiums paid for them is irrelevant as long as the total cost of care (plus the administrative costs) across the entire group is less than total amount of money collected from the premiums (see the section on Assumption of Risk later in this chapter).

The probability of adverse selection is further reduced by the use of waiting periods after enrollment. The waiting period ensures that people with current disease do not join the plan, receive treatment for their condition, and then drop out. As experience with the administration of health insurance grew and practices like waiting periods came into effect, carriers were able to offer individual policies. Many insurance carriers make individual policies available, although premiums are considerably higher and benefits can be more limited than for group policies. In light of the list of basic insurance principles, one can see why dental care was for so long considered uninsurable. Nearly everyone has dental treatment needs. Dental visits are frequent regardless if they are for diagnoses, prevention, or treatment (violating the third principle), and unlike the cost of hospital care the cost of dental treatment is rarely catastrophic (violating the second principle). Nevertheless, evaluation in the early 1950s of some of the earliest group prepayment plans indicated that dental care was indeed insurable because cost was found to be only one of the barriers to dental care.[73-75]

Although utilization of dental service increased after dental insurance became available, even when the cost barrier was lowered or removed completely, the percentage of insured people who came for dental care was lower than expected. In other words, although all members of the group may have need for dental care and all were paying a premium toward it, only some members sought treatment. Unlike medical insurance plans, which were established primarily to supply coverage for catastrophic events, dental care plans were founded on the principle of prevention and as a benefit for employee recruitment and retention. Almost all types of dental plans feature full or nearly full coverage for preventive services. Consumer preference and cost-effectiveness assessments have moved the medical insurance marketplace into full or higher coverage for preventive services, bringing the medical and dental insurance marketplaces into alignment on coverage for preventive services.

## Expenditures for Healthcare

Expenditures for healthcare have risen sharply in all industrialized countries over the last several decades, but nowhere has this pattern been as pronounced as in the United States. Figure 7.1 shows that in 1960, expenditures in the United States for healthcare (including dental care) accounted for 5% of the gross domestic product (GDP).[82] Since 1960, the amount has gone steadily upward,

reaching 17.8% of GDP in 2015.[28,93] Predictions suggest that national spending for healthcare could approach 20% of the GDP in the next few years,[12,52] a level of expenditure that deepens the existing concern.[11,47]

Figure 7.2 shows how the per capita national health expenditures rose from an annual average of $2395 for private healthcare expenditure and $1089 for public coverage in 2010 to $3186 in 2016 for private coverage and $1704 for public coverage in 2016. Figure 7.2 also shows the increase in the portion of healthcare costs paid by public funds. In 2016, 53% of total national health expenditures were paid by public (government) funds compared to 45% in 2000.

Some of the reasons for increases in the cost of healthcare in the United States are the following factors:

1. **Valuation of labor:** Some believe that the incomes of healthcare professionals have risen faster than the incomes for many other workers.

2. **Difficult economies of scale:** It is harder to achieve economies of scale in healthcare than in many other sectors of the economy. For example, in many manufacturing industries, the production of an additional 10% of a product does not require a 10% increase in workers. However, some argue that it is difficult to provide expanded services in healthcare without a concomitant increase in the healthcare workforce.

3. **Practice of "defensive" medicine:** This leads some clinicians to order tests that are carried out to protect the provider against possible litigation rather than to treat the patient. Unnecessary tests lead to a rise in costs.

4. **Aging U.S. population:** Because older people need and use more healthcare services, this has contributed to an increase

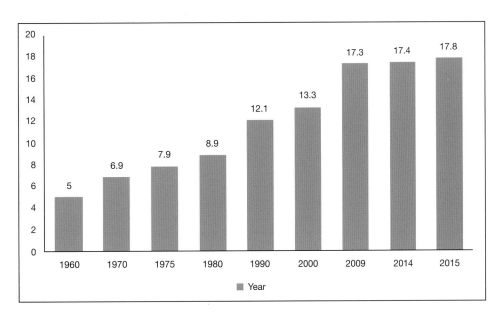

Centers for Medicare & Medicaid Services, Office of the Actuary, National Health Statistics Group, National Health Expenditure Accounts, National Health Expenditures Aggregate. Available from: https://www.cms.gov/Research-Statistics-Data-and-Systems/Statistics-Trends-and-Reports/NationalHealthExpendData/NationalHealthAccountsHistorical.html, accessed on January 5, 2017.

U.S Department of Commerce Bureau of Economic Analysis, National Economic Accounts, National Income and Product Accounts, Table 1.1.4, accessed on January 5, 2017. Available from: http://www.bea.gov/iTable/iTable.cfm?ReqID=9&step=1.

See Appendix I, National Health Expenditure Accounts (NHEA); National Income and Product Accounts (NIPA).

• **Figure 7.1**  National health expenditures as a percentage of gross domestic product in the United States, selected years, 1960–2015.[10]

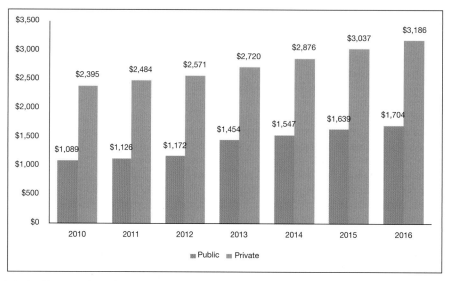

Does not Include worksite health care, other private revenues, Indian Health Service, workers' compensation, general assistance, maternal and child health, vocational rehabilitation, other federal programs, Substance Abuse and Mental Health Services Administration, other state and local programs, and school health.

• **Figure 7.2** Per capita national health expenditures, showing the proportionate expenditure of private and public funds in the United States, selected years, 2010–2016.[13]

in per capita healthcare costs. Thus the average cost of care will increase as the average age of the population increases. This is not true for dentistry, however, because lack of public funding for dental services for the elderly has limited the amount of services that older Americans can afford and therefore obtain.

5. **Developments in technology:** While some innovations reduce the costs of care because they are so much more effective than any available alternatives (antibiotics, for example, reduced the average length of a hospital stay when they were introduced in the 1940s and 1950s), others do not. In dentistry, for example, the use of dental cone beam CT scan may provide additional diagnostic information for some treatments, but if this image does not affect the treatment approach, it just increases the cost of care. Other technologies that might be regarded as preventive (or conservative) can also add to overall costs. For example, caries diagnosis devices that use laser fluorescence may lead to assessment of caries at an earlier stage before frank cavitation or painful symptoms, but with the use of topical fluorides and remineralization protocols, restoration of these lesions may be unnecessary. The dentist who has purchased these diagnostic devices may, however, have "moral hazard" and proceed to restore early lesions that can be more conservatively addressed. Other technologies that provide previously unavailable care can only add to aggregate costs. A medical example is treatment for end-stage renal disease for patients who would have died at earlier stages of the disease without recent advancements in care. With dialysis these patients now live, but at a cost of roughly $81,000 for hemodialysis per person per year, $75,000 for peritoneal dialysis per person per year, and $30,000 per person per year for kidney transplantation in 2012.[92] Examples in dentistry would be the use of dental implants to support removable dentures when dentures may be sufficient or an extraction and implant rather than endodontically treating the tooth.

6. **Third-party payment:** Insurance has funneled large amounts of money for care that would otherwise have been unavailable. For example, Medicare benefits pay for medical care and hospitalization for many elderly and/or poor members of the population who may otherwise be unable to seek treatment. Without this program, the total and per capita costs of care would undoubtedly be smaller. The same is true for private insurance; many customers facing large bills for hospitalization and other services would have been forced to go without treatment.

The spiraling costs of healthcare presents American society with a tradeoff dilemma and a clear indication that financial incentives alone cannot produce the most effective level of healthcare utilization. On the one hand, if the financial structure of a health plan leads its members to defer preventive care or go without healthcare that can improve or prolong their lives, both the individual and society suffer. On the other hand, the proportion of the GDP devoted to healthcare cannot increase indefinitely. As more available resources go to healthcare, fewer remain for housing, education, recreation, and other necessities that contribute to health, wealth, and happiness.

The dilemma is made even more difficult and pressing by the fact that the percentage of GDP going toward healthcare has risen; 10.3% of the nonelderly population were without health insurance in 2018. And studies repeatedly demonstrate that the uninsured are less likely than those with insurance to receive preventive care and services for major health conditions and chronic diseases. Moreover, 20% of the nonelderly adults without coverage say that they went without care in the past year because of cost compared to 3% of adults with private coverage and 8% of adults with public coverage.[30,40,52] So even while the expenditure is rising, a significant proportion of the population does not have coverage and access to care. There is justifiable outcry that some form of coverage should be provided for the entire population, but to do so would further increase national expenditures, at least in the short term.[31,62,93] The tension between an individual's healthcare and its societal cost may always exist.

Resolution of this dilemma is made even more complex by the inclusion of government and private third-party agencies. Because the total costs of care continue to climb and increase pressure on the economy, and because most healthcare costs are paid through third parties, the pressure for collective action to control these costs will continue—as will the current stream of proposals aimed at controlling or reforming the healthcare system. One example of an attempt to deal with the increasing costs of healthcare and the lack of coverage for a significant portion of the population is the ACA, which is described in detail later in this chapter.

## Expenditures for Dental Care

Although total expenditures for Americans' dental care are only a fraction of the total healthcare expenditures, they are nevertheless substantial. Figure 7.3 illustrates that the total expenditures for dental care in America grew from almost $2 billion in 1960 to an estimated $124 billion in 2016.[13,19,44,83] A review of the data presented in Figure 7.4 reveals that while dental expenditure per capita increased from 2000 to 2015 by 68% (from $220 to $371/person), medical expenditures increased by over 106% (from $4855 to $9994).[13]

Figure 7.5 shows that relative to the total cost of personal health-care expenditures, dental expenditures have fallen steadily from the 5% reported in 2000 to 3.7% in 2015.[15,92] This reflects the steep rise in the overall costs of medical care and the more modest rise in the costs of dental care. The percent of dental care as a component of the GDP has been remarkably steady, with 0.54% of the GDP represented by dental care in 1990 and 0.53% in 2015.[48]

## History and Trends of Third-Party Reimbursement in Dentistry

The history of dental insurance in the United States is depicted in Figure 7.12[20] and demonstrates an expanding involvement of third parties in the payment for healthcare services from the early part of the 20th century until today. Private fee-for-service payment, the two-party arrangement, is the oldest form of reimbursement for dental services in the United States. As shown in Figure 7.6, in 2000, 52% of all dental service payments (or $237 out of pocket of a total of $456) came directly from patients. In 2015, this decreased to 46% of payments ($307 out of pocket of a total of $664).[48] Dental care comprises about 4% of overall private health insurance expenditures which is considerably lower than physician services, prescription drugs, and hospital care (Figure 7.7).[11]

By the late 1960s, with some 85% of the American population covered by hospital and surgical expense insurance,[35] coverage for dental expenses emerged as a popular area for negotiation by labor groups seeking additional fringe benefits. The rapid growth of pre-payment since 1970 has changed the nature of dental practice. The proportion of the U.S. population covered by some sort of dental insurance increased from less than 5% in 1970 to well over 50% by the turn of the century. Since 2007, perhaps as a consequence of the 2008 stock market crisis, the robust growth in dental insurance

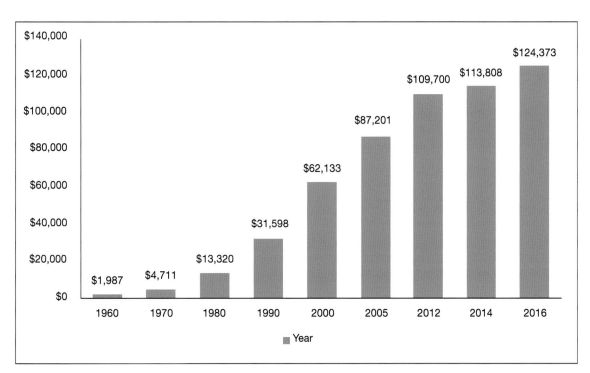

NOTE: Numbers and percentages may not add to totals because of rounding. Dollar amounts shown are in current dollars. Percent changes are calculated from unrounded data.

• **Figure 7.3** Total expenditures for dental care in the United States, selected years, 1960–2016.[11]

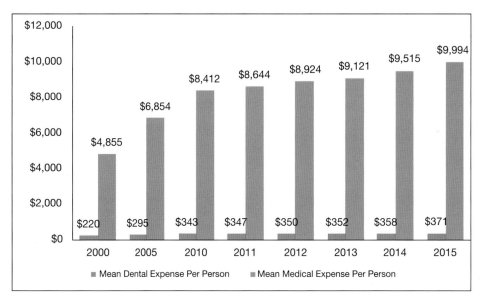

• **Figure 7.4** Mean per capita dental expense and mean per capita national health expenditures per year per person in the United States, selected years, 2000–2015.[13]

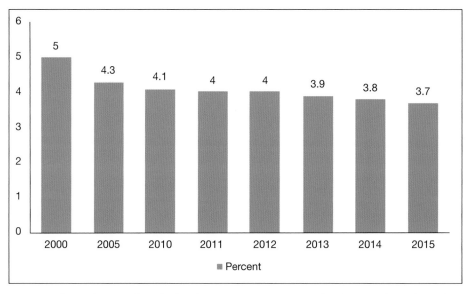

• **Figure 7.5** Per capita expenditure for dental care as a percentage of total health expenditures in the United States, selected years, 2000–2015.[13]

has leveled off (see Figure 7.6); private insurance coverage paid 44% of overall dental care expenditures in 2000 and 45% in 2015.

## Reimbursement of Dentists in Third-Party Plans

Major forms of third-party reimbursement currently in use are:
• Table of allowances/maximum plan allowance (used by most preferred provider organizations [PPOs])
• Usual, customary, and reasonable (UCR) fee
• Reasonable and customary (RC) fee
• Fixed fee schedules
• Capitation

### Table of Allowances

A table of allowances (or schedule of allowances) is often referred to as maximum plan allowances (MPA). This method lists covered services with an assigned dollar amount that represents the plan's total payment obligation, but an amount does not necessarily represent a dentist's full fee for that service.[2] A provider can receive reimbursement as the lesser amount of the billed charge or the MPA. For example, in a table of allowance fee method, if a participating network dentist's usual fee for a particular service is $20 and the plan lists a fee of $15 as payable for that service, the dentist will provide the service, collect $15 from the carrier, and may not charge the patient $5 to make up the difference. If the dentist

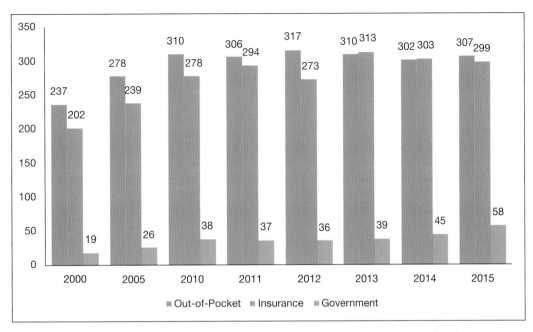

• **Figure 7.6**  Total dental care expenditures paid per year by consumers out of pocket, by private insurance, and by government funds in the United States, selected years, 2000–2015.[47]

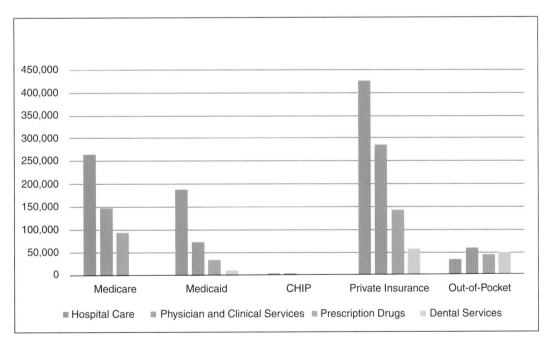

U.S. Bureau of the Census. Census resident-based population less armed forces overseas and population of outlying areas.

U.S. Department of Commerce, Bureau of Economic Analysis.

NOTE: Numbers and percentages may not add to totals because of rounding. Dollar amounts shown are in current dollars. Percent changes are calculated from unrounded data.

Centers for Medicare & Medicaid Services, Office of the Actuary, National Health Statistics Group; U.S. Department of Commerce, Bureau of Economic Analysis; and U.S. Bureau of the Census.

• **Figure 7.7**  Proportionate expenditures on various categories of health services by type of payment in the United States, 2016 (in millions of dollars).

charges only $13 for the same procedure, and the maximum fee on the schedule is still $15, the insurer will reimburse the provider only the $13. Table of allowance plans are used to reduce expenditures and therefore have lower reimbursement levels than some other mechanisms. These may not favored by dentists, but this is how most commercial PPO plans reimburse dentists today.

## Usual, Customary, and Reasonable Fee

*A usual fee* is the fee that an individual dentist most frequently charges for a given dental service. *A customary fee* is the fee level determined by the administrator of a dental benefit plan from actual submitted fees for a specific dental procedure to establish the maximum benefit payable under a given plan for that specific procedure. *A reasonable fee* is the fee charged by a dentist for a specific dental procedure that has been modified by the nature and severity of the condition being treated and by any medical or dental complications or unusual circumstances, which therefore may be higher than the dentist's "usual" fee or the benefit administrator's "customary" fee.[2] Insurance companies use proprietary algorithms to establish a usual, customary, and reasonable fee (UCR fee) that combines the three concepts. It is also known as reasonable and customary (RC).

Many dentists in the 1960s opposed the early implementation of third-party dental coverage on the grounds that they would be forced to adopt lower fees than those that they usually charged. The evolution of the UCR fee concept as an acceptable mechanism for both dentists and carriers has allowed the administration of third-party dental care while permitting individual dentists to charge what they believe their services are worth. Dental prepayment plans likely would not have been accepted by dentists without the UCR fee concept.[96]

UCR payment plans have fallen out of favor with purchasers of dental insurance because of rising costs and legal rulings pertaining to the establishment of UCR rates. UCR plans are regarded as inflationary because dentists submit their fee schedule to the insurance company and then are reimbursed based on a percentage of the UCR. If a dentist raises fees each year and the insurance payments continue to meet the dentist's fee, this signifies that the dentist's fees are lower than the UCR rate in the location of that practice. The dentist is therefore incentivized to raise fees annually to achieve the maximum UCR payment reimbursement level. As a result, to avoid these tendencies, some plans use a fixed table of allowances or a fixed fee schedule to determine the insurance payments.

Insurance companies have controlled the growth in expenses by requiring copayments from patients. Some copayments are fixed fees, but often copayments are based on a percentage of the charged fees and are called coinsurance. Copayment based on a percentage of the charged fees requires careful monitoring, as it is subject to fraud caused by a dentist's "waiving" of copayments. For insurers who base payments on the UCR rate, the copayment is part of the "usual" fee and often an important part of the cost-control mechanism. Furthermore, if dentists were allowed to raise their submitted "usual" fees so that the fee minus the copayment equaled the desired payment and then forgave the copayment, the cost-controlling effects of copayment would still be beneficial to the payor (the employer in most cases) but not to the individual or to societal cost containment. Concern over the effects of these billing practices has led to many strict state laws under which copayment-waiving practices are considered deceptive and fraudulent.

### Percentile Fees in UCR or RC Plans

To illustrate how percentiles are applied to dental fees, suppose 1000 dentists participate in a health plan. They each set their own fee for a particular service. In the data set of their 1000 fees, we can use percentiles to think about the distribution of observations, so that the 90th percentile of the data set is the value below which 90% of the observations lie. In this example, let us assume that the range of fees charged for the service runs from $40 to $85. If the fees are spread out in a cumulative frequency distribution from the lowest to the highest, the result might be like that shown in Figure 7.8. For this service, about 10% of dentists charge less than $60, 50% charge $65 or less, 80% charge $68 or less, and 90% charge $72 or less. For this service, therefore, $72 is the 90th percentile fee; 10% of dentists charge more than $72.

When payment on UCR fees is made at the 90th percentile, 90% of participating dentists receive their full fee for the service, and only 10% are paid less than their usual fee. Dentists who normally charge $65 receive $65, those who normally charge $70 receive $70, and so on up to $72, the 90th percentile. Those who normally charge more than $72 are paid $72. If nonparticipating dentists are paid at the 50th percentile, which

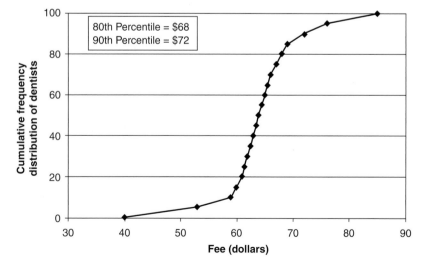

• **Figure 7.8** Cumulative frequency distribution of hypothetical fees for a given dental service to illustrate the 80th and 90th percentiles.

in this example is $65, they are paid whichever is lower of the fee that they actually charge or $65.

## Fixed Fee Schedule

A fee schedule is defined as a list of the charges established or agreed to by a dentist for specific dental services with a third-party coverage provider.[2] With a fee schedule, the dentist must accept the listed amount as payment in full and not charge the patient at all. Fee schedules for dental care are sometimes established by public programs, such as Medicaid in many states. Dentists' widespread opposition to fee schedules is based on: (1) the potential inflexibility of such schedules, meaning that the fees listed can fall below customary fees, particularly in times of rapid inflation; (2) the implicit assumption that all dentists' treatment is of the same quality and therefore worth the same fee; and (3) the fear that autonomy is threatened, especially if the fee schedule is not controlled by the dentists. A potential risk of the use of a fee schedule is that if fees paid are far below the usual rates, few dentists will be willing to treat the covered patients. The use of fixed fee schedules has been cited as one reason that many dentists either severely limit the number of their Medicaid patients or refuse to accept Medicaid patients altogether.[20,42]

## Capitation

The American Dental Association (ADA) defines capitation as a dental benefit program in which a dentist or dentists contract with the program's sponsor or administrator to provide all or most of the dental services covered under the program to subscribers in return for a payment on a per capita basis.[2] This capitation fee is usually a fixed monthly payment paid by a carrier to a dentist based on the number of patients assigned to the dentist for treatment. This is usually called the "per member per month payment." Capitation requires that patients be assigned to specific dentists or dental practices for care so that the capitation payment can be paid to the appropriate dentist or practice. This assignment is important, because the dentist receives a fixed sum of money per enrolled person regardless of whether the participants in the plan receive care during that month. The underlying assumption is that although some patients will need a lot of care, others will need little or none, and therefore the total amount of money paid to the dentist will be sufficient to cover the overall costs of care for the covered group.

The effects of capitation's financial incentives to participating dentists are mixed. Under capitation a dentist is contractually required to provide necessary services, while receiving only the fixed amount of funds provided through the contract. On one hand, the fixed funds incentivize dentists to provide preventive care and thereby reduce the need for expensive procedures. On the other hand, these limits may also compel dentists to reduce patient access to potentially necessary procedures to decrease their costs. In the early days of capitation post World War II, Dr. Max Schoen[70-72] argued that capitation works every bit as well as fee for service and that with proper planning it is a highly efficient method of financing group dental care, especially for less affluent groups. Despite Schoen's claims of success with capitation in his own group practice, many dentists and the ADA disagreed. The ADA is opposed to capitation and fee schedules as the sole forms of reimbursement in prepayment plans, arguing that where such mechanisms exist they should be on an equal footing with fee-for-service third-party dental plans so that prospective patients have a choice. Most capitation plans now include copayments, especially for more expensive services, and annual maximums, both of which limit the economic risks faced by the dentist. Ultimately, many dentists are resistant to capitation because it puts them at economic risk of unanticipated high utilization and expensive care.

The presumed advantages and disadvantages of capitation payment within a group practice or health maintenance organization context have been outlined by Carby[9] as provided in Box 7.2.

Despite some advantages, use of a capitation model of payment for reimbursement of dental care (i.e., a fixed dollar amount paid per member per month) is much less common than it is in medicine. Although capitated payment models became more common in dentistry during the 1980s and 1990s, overall use of capitation remains very low. In 2011 managed care plans comprised 8% of private dental insurance plans.[60] In recent years, less than 10% of dental third-party insurance plans have involved capitation payments.

## • BOX 7.2   Capitation Advantages/Disadvantages

### ADVANTAGES

1. Quality control. Consultation and peer review within group practices encourage the dentist to provide optimal dental care for the long-term benefit of the patient rather than the immediate benefit of earnings. Peer review is a condition for participation.
2. Prevention. Health education and prevention become strong incentives because dental group practices are paid on the basis of how many patients have enrolled. Early maintenance is to the advantage of the dentist and patient.
3. Capitation brings patients into a dental office who may never receive treatment if the service were not provided by an employer or union.
4. It eliminates incentives for dentists to provide certain services over others. Excessive x-rays are eliminated, and pressure to provide crowns rather than fillings would be reduced.
5. Claim forms are eliminated but not statements for services under copayments schedules.
6. Seasonal cash flow fluctuations may be less of a problem because capitation payment remains constant.

### DISADVANTAGES

1. It is conceivable that capitation programs could compromise a dentist's judgment of patient needs. The less treatment provided, the less overhead and the more profit.
2. Lack of choice of dentist. Patients must receive treatment from a doctor listed as a provider.[a]
3. Capitation is best suited for group practices; the solo practitioner may find it much harder to work as part of a network.
4. Dentists' services are subject to audit and review by the third-party payor.[a]
5. Poor access to a dentist within the capitation network may discourage patient utilization. Dentists are responsible for seeing that patients come to the office at least once a year, depending on the contract.
6. Substantial time may be required to bring patients up to maintenance level in the beginning of the program.[a]
7. Renewal capitation contracts may call for a reduced payment to the provider-dentist.

[a]These disadvantages may also occur when dental health insurance pays for benefits on a fee-for-service basis.

## Procedure and Diagnostic Codes

Dental procedure codes were developed in the early days of dental prepayment. With the advent of third-party involvement, an unambiguous method had to be developed to define which procedures would be covered and which would not and to facilitate the accurate reporting of which services were provided. There were various mechanisms for developing and maintaining these codes through the years, including the ADA Code on Dental Procedures and Nomenclature. The Health Insurance Portability and Accountability Act of 1996 (HIPAA) mandated a single set of codes; all dental insurers now use this standard set of procedure codes. The codes have syntax and are organized by specialty area for ease of use. The ADA maintains the dental codes, and every March the Code Maintenance Committee (CMC) reviews codes. Open meetings are held for input, and any interested party may submit requests for code revisions.[3] Code revisions can occur because new technologies need codes or because interpretation and utilization issues are identified. At the end of this process, the committee issues revised codes for implementation the following year on January 1.

In medical care, diagnosis codes (such as the International Classification of Diseases [ICD-10]) are required in addition to procedure codes when claims are submitted in medical practice for reimbursement.[38] If a submitted treatment code does not correspond to the appropriate diagnosis code, the insurance carrier will not provide payment for the procedure. However, in dentistry, diagnosis codes are not generally used in submitting claims for reimbursement. The absence of diagnosis codes from dental practice limits quality assurance activities and other types of clinical validations; it is difficult to assess in aggregate the appropriateness of procedures without information on treatment based on specific diagnoses.

## Not-for-Profit Dental Plans

The most prevalent type of not-for-profit dental insurance plans are called dental service corporations (DSC). A DSC is a corporation that is organized without capital stock and not for profit for the purpose of establishing, maintaining, and operating a not-for-profit dental service plan. Delta Dental was the first and is the largest dental insurance company of this type in the United States, operating in all 50 states. The Delta Dental Plans Association represents 39 of the state-level Delta Dental organizations. Delta Dental plans began in California, Oregon, and Washington during the early 1950s when health insurance was first becoming more prevalent as a way for dentists to work more directly with employers on expanding dental coverage—similar to the way that Blue Cross Blue Shield plans were developed by coalitions of medical providers and hospitals concurrently.[90] Today Delta Dental plans operate very similarly to for-profit insurance plans in the United States.

## For-Profit Dental Plans

### Commercial Insurance Plans

Once it was clear in the 1970s that prepaid dental plans were viable and likely to become a significant part of the health insurance market, commercial for-profit insurance companies began to view dental insurance as a viable area to develop new products. Commercial dental insurance plans are often underwritten and marketed by the same companies that provide medical insurance (e.g., Aetna, CIGNA, Blue Cross Blue Shield, UnitedHealthcare).

## Managed Care

Managed care is a term that is in widespread use but for which there is no precise definition. The Health Insurance Association of America defined managed care as:

> Systems that integrate the financing and delivery of appropriate healthcare services to covered individuals by means of arrangements with selected providers to furnish a comprehensive set of health-care services to members; explicit criteria for the selection of health-care providers; formal programs for ongoing quality assurance and utilization review; and significant financial incentives for members to use providers and procedures associated with the plan.[32]

Simply stated, what has come to be called managed care is an arrangement through which members receive all or most of their healthcare from providers (hospitals, physicians, and other personnel) who are formally linked to the organization. It is estimated that in 2017 about 97% of all insured individuals in the United States were enrolled in some type of medical managed care plan.[61] At the same time, there has been a push to move Medicaid and Medicare enrollees from traditional fee for service to managed care. The effect of these trends on medicine has been profound, as managed care has come to dominate the practicing life of many physicians.

Medicaid managed care for medical care grew rapidly in the 1990s. In 1991, 2.7 million beneficiaries were enrolled in some form of managed care. By 2004, that number had grown to 27 million, an increase of 900%. Of the total Medicaid enrollment in the United States in 2009, almost 72% were receiving Medicaid benefits through managed care. With the exceptions of Alaska and Wyoming, all states enroll at least a portion of their Medicaid population in a managed care organization (MCO). The primary stimulus for the growth of managed care is concern over the continual increases in medical treatment costs. The intention—or at least the way managed care is marketed—is that overall costs and patients' out-of-pocket expenditures will be substantially lower than they would be for care sought outside of an MCO. The widespread supposition is that managed care can somehow help control the costs and assess and maintain the quality of medical care.[53]

## Dentistry in Managed Care

The financing methodologies that influence the practice of medicine affect dentistry as well. Virtually all of the innovations tried in medicine are evident in dentistry. Some of this has occurred because purchasing groups have demanded the same system for their dental coverage that they are using for their medical coverage. Some has come from entrepreneurs both inside and outside dentistry who see managed care as an opportunity to earn profits by managing the practice of dentistry. Certain distinctions between medicine and dentistry make it unlikely that managed care will play as significant a role in dentistry as it has in medicine, however.

In 2016, the most important difference was the fact that about 91% of the population had medical insurance and only 77% had coverage for dental care. Historically, the percentage of patients with dental insurance coverage has been considerably lower, with 60% of the U.S. population insured in 2012. The increase to 77% in 2016 was in large part because of the expansion of Medicaid dental benefits.[34,59] Because insured patients account for nearly all of the income of physicians and hospitals, physicians and hospitals are extremely vulnerable to the influence of large purchasing groups. Conversely, large numbers of dental patients are not covered by insurance, so individually and as a whole, dentists, are less susceptible to pressure from large purchasers.

## Health Maintenance Organizations

Although the concept behind health maintenance organizations (HMOs) is not new and they are known to have existed since the turn of the 20th century, the Health Maintenance Organization Act of 1973 (Public Law 93-222) formally required HMOs to be offered as part of employer-based plans in the United States. This act made federal funds available under certain conditions for the development of HMOs. These funds were intended to provide an acceptable alternative to the fee-for-service private practice system.

One of the principal advantages of HMOs as a method of distributing healthcare is the relatively lower cost of healthcare for participants and insurers. These savings are purportedly due to the emphasis on ambulatory care (and consequently, reductions in hospital use) and the carefully disbursed coverage for costly services (and consequently, reductions in "unnecessary" hospitalization, such as for routine diagnostic tests and minor surgery). Dental care, however, is almost exclusively ambulatory, because few dental procedures require inpatient hospitalization. The major advantage of HMOs—the reduction of hospitalizations—therefore has little application to dentistry, but the close monitoring of utilization of costly services (e.g., hospitalization for medicine and implants or prosthetics in dentistry) emphasized in HMOs is an important concept of HMOs.

The 1973 act defined an HMO as "a legal entity which provides a prescribed range of health services to each individual who has enrolled in the organization in return for a prepaid, fixed, and uniform payment."[81] Usually, but not always, an HMO looks like a large group practice with a number of services available under one roof. An HMO is described as having five essential elements: a managing organization, a delivery system, an enrolled population, a benefit package, and a system of financing and prepayment.[58] HMOs use a prepaid capitation system of financing medical services. Enrollment in HMOs grew rapidly after their introduction in 1973, peaking at 80.8 million in 1999.[33] Since that time enrollment has begun to decline, likely due to consumer resistance to what has been seen as restrictive access to some services. The decline in HMO enrollments have been more than balanced by rapid growth in PPOs and point-of-service arrangements described later.[3]

### Dental Personnel in Health Maintenance Organizations
Only a small proportion of HMOs offer dental services. When dental services are offered, they are financed through the primary capitation premium, a separate premium, or fee for service. Dental care in HMOs is provided according to one of the four basic organizational models of HMOs:

**Staff model:** Dentists, dental hygienists, and dental assistants are salaried employees of the HMO. The staff model is the only one of the four models that affects auxiliary personnel directly; in the other three, the terms of employment do not differ from those of traditional private practices.

**Group model:** The HMO contracts directly with a group practice, partnership, or corporation for the provision of dental services. The group receives a regular capitation premium from the HMO.

**Independent practice association (IPA):** The IPA is an association of independent dentists (or physicians in medical practice) that develops its own management and fiscal structure for the treatment of patients enrolled in an HMO. An IPA thus is not a distinct form of practice but instead a legal arrangement through which individual dental offices participate as providers for groups of patients enrolled in HMOs. Dentists continue to practice in their own offices. The IPA receives its capitation premium from the HMO (or other prepayment agency) and in turn reimburses individual dentists on either a modified fee-for-service basis or a capitation basis.

**Capitated network or direct contract model:** The network is similar to the IPA, except that the HMO contracts directly with individual providers for the provision of services. This is the most common form of capitation arrangement in dentistry. Dental insurers who wish to offer a capitation product recruit and contract with dental offices that are willing to have patients assigned to them.

## Preferred Provider Organizations

In both medical and dental insurance markets, preferred provider organizations (PPOs) have expanded rapidly. A schedule of benefits is the foundation of the PPO plan design. Unlike UCR plans, PPOs control for inflationary rises in cost by limiting increases in the payment schedules for dental services. Most PPOs—medical and dental alike—allow patients to visit providers outside of the PPO panel. However, to encourage use of PPO providers and thus maintain expected cost savings, patients receiving care outside of the network are usually required to pay for a larger portion of their care. As a result of the continuing push to control healthcare costs, some PPOs now cover no out-of-network care except emergency care. This form of PPO is usually referred to as an exclusive provider organization. PPOs now comprise the majority of dental plans: 85% in 2017.[60] This represents a rapid growth in PPO dental market share from 2002, when PPOs constituted 44% of dental plans.

## Point-of-Service Plans

Point-of-service (POS) plans are managed care plans that allow enrollees to receive some of their care if they wish from providers who are outside of the managed care providers. Members who elect to receive care outside of the POS panel pay a larger part of the costs of that care. The recent increase in enrollment in POS plans indicates that many individuals are willing to pay extra for the increased flexibility that these plans offer over more restrictive managed care arrangements.[60]

## Concerns Regarding Managed Care
### Assumption of Risk
The concept of assumption of financial risk is important in healthcare. In the case of patients who pay for their own care, the situation is uncomplicated. If a patient accepts the treatment proposed by the dentist, the patient is responsible for payment. With the advent of traditional fee-for-service insurance, insurance companies typically agreed to assume financial risk. The fee-for-service arrangement includes a set of covered services—usually subject to some copayments and an annual maximum—but the insurance company is responsible for paying for the covered care with the money it has collected from the premiums. The insurer carefully evaluates each

group to estimate how much the group's care will cost so that it can be sure to set the premiums at a level that is sufficient to cover the costs of care but not so high that a competitor will make a lower bid. In any case, with traditional insurance, the insurance company is "at risk" for most excess costs. Acceptance of this risk is part of the product the insurer sells.

In principle, one of the main features of the capitation method is that the risk (which in fee-for-service insurance is assumed by the insurer) shifts to the provider, because the provider receives a previously agreed-on sum per patient enrolled regardless of whether the patient seeks care. In return, the provider agrees to provide specified services as necessary for a predetermined period. Clearly, the concern of the provider is that the payment received (known before a contract is signed) will suffice to cover services needed (which are unknown, although they often can be reasonably estimated, especially across a large group of patients). If the cost of services required exceeds the income received through the contract, the provider incurs the financial losses. Conversely, if the cost of services required is less than the income provided by the contract, the provider profits. It follows that under some capitation contracts, there is the potential for undertreatment and discouragement of service utilization, which raises concerns about ethics and quality of care.[15]

Therefore, it is understandable that both the ADA and individual dentists are cautious about assumption of risk. Of course, an HMO assumes risk when it establishes its monthly premium for enrollees, just as any insurer of a prepaid care plan assumes risk. Capitation, however, brings the assumption of risk directly to the dentist. Features such as patient copayments and annual maximums—both standard cost-control mechanisms in fee-for-service plans—have become common in capitation plans as ways to reduce the dentist's risk. The pressure for innovative approaches to control the costs of medical care has in turn caused purchasers to demand—and insurers to provide—similar approaches for financing dental care. The basis of capitation is that the contracting provider, whether an HMO, group practice, IPA, or individual dentist, receives a fixed sum, usually monthly, for each eligible patient. The money is paid regardless of whether patients use care. In return, the patient is entitled to receive covered services as needed. As of 2002, the National Association of Dental Plans estimated that about 23.5 million individuals were enrolled in dental HMOs (sometimes referred to as DHMOs),[33,59] and over the past 15 years, enrollment in DHMOs has declined by over 50% as this type of benefit plan becomes less and less popular.[59]

### Capitation Versus Fee for Service Versus Pay for Performance in Managed Care

For some, the primary concern with capitation is that it might encourage undertreatment. Under pure capitation, the dentist receives the same payment whether or not treatment is provided; this incentivizes undertreatment and neglect. Others argue that consistency is a virtue of capitation, because the dentist is assured a predictable income and is thus able to make decisions about treatment without worrying about revenues if treatment need is low. Many think that the fee-for-service system, in which dentists are paid only if they find treatment to provide, incentivizes overtreatment. In the current era of relatively low disease levels, the chances of overtreatment increase. PPO arrangements may also encourage overtreatment because agreed-on fees are discounted, incentivizing providers to perform multiple services per visit to make each patient visit more remunerative.

These concerns have led to increasing pressure on insurers to develop new ways to pay for healthcare so that patients receive precisely the amount of care they need or want. Payors—whether for-profit, not-for-profit, or government—want assurances that the care they are paying for provides the most extensive benefits possible to the patients they cover. Thus, a new method of payment has been developed and implemented recently for some medical care that rewards healthcare providers for better patient outcomes or for achieving defined healthcare standards. This methodology is called pay for performance (P4P). The Medicare program was an early adopter of P4P to improve quality and reduce healthcare costs. The Centers for Medicare & Medicaid Services (CMS) implemented 10 hospital quality measures that if achieved would result in increased payments to hospitals. These performance metric domains include avoidable utilization of emergency departments, primary care access, mental health medication adherence, mental health screening and treatment, and patient evaluations of the healthcare experience as assessed through surveys.[15]

Payors of healthcare have developed sophisticated ways to monitor the quality and quantity of care. Ideally purchasers and individual patients should be confident that the care they pay for is appropriate and of acceptable quality, regardless of the payment method. These efforts are generally part of performance improvement and utilization review programs. To assure purchasers that the quality of care is high and the patterns of care provided are reasonable, some insurers conduct analyses of claims data to detect patterns that could be signs of substandard or fraudulent care.[4] These programs and efforts are reviewed in more detail in the Quality Assurance/Performance Improvement sections of this text.

The ADA in 2006 developed principles for P4P or other third-party financial incentive programs, including: (1) improvement in quality; (2) no interference with the patient–doctor relationship; (3) reward for both the achievement of desired quality levels and significant improvement in quality; (4) no limits on access to care; (5) exact, clear, and measurable goals; (6) reporting to the public must be fair; (7) voluntary participation; (8) cost savings should not accrue to plans but rather to patients; and (9) regular assessment for plans must include input from dentists.[28]

## Direct Reimbursement

Direct reimbursement is a payment alternative to dental care insurance that plays a minor role in the dental finance market. Direct reimbursement involves an agreement between an employer and its employees in which the employer agrees to reimburse the employees for some part of their expenses for dental care. Employees can go to any dentist they choose for care. The patient is responsible for paying the dentist, and the dentist has no responsibility to an insurer (third party) for such things as scope of covered services or limits on frequency of services. All treatment decisions are made by the patient and the dentist in a traditional two-party manner. After treatment has been provided and paid for, the patient takes the receipt to the employer and is reimbursed for these expenses according to the rules of the agreement. Reimbursement is usually on a percentage basis, and annual limits are common.

Even though this payment methodology has been around for many years, it remains an uncommon method of dental coverage. Direct reimbursement accounted for less than 1% of dental plans in 2018.[60] The ADA actively promotes direct reimbursement as an alternative to the more common forms of dental insurance[49] because it keeps third parties out of care decisions such as available services, care frequency, fees, and provider selection. Direct reimbursement also minimizes administrative costs, although the employer, or a hired administrator, still must process these reimbursements and keep track of annual limits.

Purchasers of health insurance, accustomed to the more conventional forms of third-party insurance, have not readily embraced direct reimbursement in part because they have come to expect and value direct payment from the insurer to the dentist, so that patients face lower cash requirements and fewer monetary transactions. Purchasers also expect that insurers, by protecting their own interests, will actively ensure that the scope, quantity, and quality of services are reasonable. Direct reimbursement purposely attempts to keep third parties out of these areas, but many purchasers consider third-party involvement a valuable part of dental insurance.

## Discount Dental Plans

Discount dental plans, a form of dental benefits that constitutes neither prepayment nor insurance, have arisen within the last 20 to 30 years because of carriers' attempts to capture markets (especially the individual market) beyond the traditional large groups. Carriers curate panels of dentists who agree to lower-than-average fees, similar to PPO panels, and agree to charge these discounted fees to patients who present a discount card. The carrier charges the patient a small monthly fee for the card. The major difference from other forms of coverage is that the patient is responsible for the entire discounted fee; the patient's monthly fee for the discount card buys access to the panel of dentists' discounted rate. The discount dental plan is a rapidly evolving product with some dentists selling these out of their own offices. Currently about 5% of all commercial plans involve a discount plan.[60]

## Health Savings Accounts and Flexible Savings Accounts

There are several mechanisms for providing tax-free or tax-reduced ways to subsidize out-of-pocket costs and make relatively limited insurance more attractive. Medical savings accounts (MSAs) were one of the first government-subsidized healthcare spending options that were established in 1996 as a part of HIPAA. The MSA, discontinued in 2005, was a precursor to the health savings account (HSA), which was established in 2003 as a component of the Medicare Prescription Drug, Improvement, and Modernization Act of 2003.[27] HSAs allow a person to establish and contribute tax-protected funds to a special savings account to be used as needed to cover medical expenses.[27,88,89] In 2018, the annual HSA contribution maximum was $6900 for families. Each HSA must be combined with a high-deductible health plan (HDHP). The HDHP is considered a mechanism for lowering healthcare costs by making the consumer take a relatively active stake in the cost of each healthcare service because of the higher initial out-of-pocket costs required by this type of plan. The HSA is used to pay expenses incurred before the annual deductible is met. In theory, when individual patients are responsible for the actual cost of routine medical expenses, they will be more prudent users of care. In 2016 HDHPs were offered as an enrollment option in approximately 28% of the medical insurance marketplace.[40]

HDHPs and HSAs have been infrequently used to pay for dental care. However, the HSA can be used to pay healthcare bills, including those for dental services. HSAs can be invested, and unused funds roll over year to year. In addition, there are also flexible spending accounts (FSAs), or flex plans, which allow employers to set up individual accounts for their employees into which employees make contributions that are not subject to income tax. In 2018 the annual maximum individual contribution was $2650. These funds can then be used during the tax year for qualifying healthcare expenses that are not covered by insurance. FSAs differ from HSAs in two key ways: They need not be created in conjunction with an HDHP, and any funds in the account not used for medical care in the year are forfeited by the employee, so the employee must carefully plan how much income to allocate to the account.[87]

## Forces Affecting Third-Party Dental Care Programs

Most mechanisms for controlling the costs of medical care also affect the way that dental care is provided and financed. For instance, HMOs and PPOs include substantial financial incentives for patients to seek care from a participating provider. Low out-of-pocket payments and a wider range of covered services are common methods to encourage beneficiaries to choose managed care options. Even though the many forms of insurance options can seem bewilderingly complex, the underlying forces are consistent: Purchasing groups want to buy sufficiently easy and convenient access to care at the lowest possible price. For some groups, wider access is worth higher premiums; for other groups it is not. In an increasing number of cases, the cost of acceptable access is more than an employer can afford, and employees are being asked to pay an increasing share of the premiums. In some cases, employers require employees to pay the entire premium; in these cases, coverage is voluntary. In this case, the sole benefit to the employee, if they must pay with after-tax money, is the chance to buy insurance coverage through a group that might not otherwise be available for individual coverage. The continual pursuit by these groups of the best balance between access to care and cost will continue to put pressure on providers to keep costs under control. To many dentists, the expression *"cost control"* is synonymous with administrative harassment, red tape, and poor quality of care. However, appropriate methods of cost control do not demand the use of inferior materials or techniques. Cost control should be based on the concepts of evidence and cost effectiveness, that is, how can a purchasing group best spend the available money to gain maximum dental health benefits for its members?

Most dental practices have a vital stake in the continued economic health of the third-party payment system because it represents a substantial share of their income. At the same time, purchasers of care are experiencing the growing cost of providing dental insurance.[6,25,63] A number of cost-containment mechanisms have been described and are in common use; others are continually under development. If cost controls are not routinely and successfully incorporated, individual dental plans will simply not succeed in the marketplace. The challenge is to find ways of keeping the costs of dental care within a range that purchasers are willing to pay while at the same time providing a level of care and access to providers that both dentists and patients find acceptable. Although cost-control mechanisms are numerous and evolving and can thus be confusing and frustrating to providers and patients alike, the underlying principles are simple.

The challenge for those who design dental insurance products is to find the best balance between access and price. At one extreme, if insurance coverage will pay for whatever care the patient and dentist choose with few and small patient copayments, the cost to employer/purchaser will tend to be relatively high. Less expensive for the employer/purchaser will be a plan that limits payments only to dentists who have agreed to provide services at low or discounted fees or a plan that requires substantial deductibles or patient copayments. Perhaps least expensive for the employer/purchaser of all would be a plan that provides the beneficiary with a discount card that ensures that participating dentists will charge discounted fees, but these fees will be paid entirely by the patient.

Ongoing changes in product design are attempts by the various insurance companies to find a balance between access and cost to create products that will be attractive to customers. This balance can be especially critical for dental insurance because, unlike medical insurance, the risks of going without dental insurance are not large. Therefore, dental insurance companies must not only meet the competition posed by other insurers but also the challenge of customers deciding to go forward with no dental insurance at all. A prepayment system for dental care that cannot continue to provide a group with a desirable level of coverage (or access) at an acceptable price risks the group's decision to do without dental coverage—to leave the market—altogether. In this scenario, no party benefits.

Because of annual limits and cost-sharing requirements, third-party plans do not entirely remove the cost barrier to dental care; they merely change it. The amount of care a plan can finance is still finite; the object of controls is to try to use the available financing to the best advantage. The more that dentists accept this philosophy, the better they can work with purchasers and administrators to devise mutually acceptable methods of cost control. The continual push and pull of the prepayment marketplace is a manifestation of the unrelenting pressures of the marketplace to stay within the range of acceptable access and price balance.

## Public Financing of Healthcare

### Public Expenditures for Dental Care

The federal government has been involved in the direct financing of healthcare almost from the founding of the United States. In 1798, Congress established the Marine Hospital Fund, the forerunner of the U.S. Public Health Service, to provide medical care for merchant seamen. The federal government gradually accepted responsibility for providing healthcare to other groups; the care received by military and Coast Guard personnel, American Indians, Alaska Natives, and inmates of federal penitentiaries is financed with federal funds and often provided at federal facilities. This limited, carefully defined role of the federal government was seen for a long time as its right and proper function in healthcare provision.

The relationship between the various levels of government in the United States was permanently changed in 1935 with the passage of the first Social Security Act. This act, passed during the Great Depression, sought to alleviate the unprecedented problems caused by mass unemployment and widespread poverty. The Social Security Act of 1935 provided no funds expressly for the provision of healthcare; before the end of the Great Depression, however, people's difficulty with purchasing healthcare in the traditional fee-for-service way was recognized as a major social problem. As a result, a system of grants-in-aid was developed to supply federal finances for needed healthcare services without disturbing the established federal-state separation. Grants-in-aid were federal funds allocated to the states according to specific formulas. To receive these grants, states had to expend their own funds for

the same objectives as those supported by the grant-in-aid, often in the ratio of $1 from state or local sources to $2 from federal sources. Grants-in-aid were available in the 1940s only for support of specific demographics, such as dependent children, blind individuals, elderly individuals, or permanently and totally disabled individuals.

A significant change in the method of federal financing for healthcare came with the passage of the Kerr-Mills Act in 1960. This legislation developed into the Medicaid bill 5 years later. The legislation, supported by both the ADA and the American Medical Association, linked healthcare needs to the general welfare of low-income seniors through a program known as Medical Assistance for the Aged. Although the effects of this program were relatively lackluster,[77] the Kerr-Mills Act introduced the use of vendor payments for healthcare, meaning payments (in this case, by the federal government) directly to service providers rather than to care recipients. Vendor payments ensured that allocated funds would be used exclusively for healthcare.

In the early 1960s, growing public awareness of the problems of poverty, ill health, and the lack of health insurance coverage for many of society's most vulnerable set the stage for the 1965 amendments to the Social Security Act that established the Medicare and Medicaid programs. These amendments were landmark pieces of legislation just as the original act had been 30 years earlier. Title XVIII, later known as Medicare, provided for the receipt of healthcare services by all persons aged 65 and over, regardless of their ability to pay, and Title XIX, known as Medicaid, was intended to bring access to healthcare to indigent and medically indigent segments of the population. The term medically indigent refers to those who are not dependent on public welfare to meet the necessities of life but who do not have sufficient income to purchase healthcare through private channels. (This concept is limited, because highly expensive treatments can make almost anyone medically indigent.) In 1997 the Social Security Act was further amended through Title XXI, which created the State Children's Health Insurance Program (SCHIP). SCHIP allocates federal funds to states to pay for healthcare for children in families whose income is too high to qualify for Medicaid but too low to afford health insurance. As in Medicaid, these federal funds are provided on the condition that the states also supply funds.

A marked difference between medical and dental care is the degree of government involvement in payments for care. In 2017, government funds accounted for about half of all medical care expenditures but only about 18% of dental expenditures.[12] Thus, if government attempts to curb expenditures for healthcare are to be successful, medical care costs must be addressed, as dental care costs are so small they are relatively unimportant to this effort. Because it controls such a large portion of medical reimbursement, the government can exert an enormous influence over providers. In dental care, however, this is not the case. For example, since Medicaid reimbursement levels routinely have been well below what many dentists deem reasonable, dentists have refused to participate without affecting their economic well-being—an impossibility for many practitioners in medicine.

### Medicare

Medicare was designed to provide a safety net for the high costs of acute medical conditions rather than comprehensive insurance coverage. As originally conceived in the early 1960s, it was designed to remove financial barriers for hospital and physician services for persons age 65 and over. Medicare has two parts: Part A, hospital insurance, which people receive regardless of financial means in conjunction with Social Security benefits (some disabled people or those with kidney failure) and Part B, voluntary supplemental medical insurance which they may choose to purchase (and 93% make that choice).[79] Both parts contain a highly complex series of service benefits and require some copayment by the individual. Apart from these copayments, Medicare is financed completely from a Social Security trust fund supported by payroll taxes. Because Medicare covers some of the sickest, highest users of care in the United States, program costs have grown beyond estimations almost from its inception. In the 1980s, cost controls were instituted through diagnosis-related groups (DRGs) for inpatient hospital treatment (Part A) and relative value units (RVUs) for Part B payments to healthcare providers.

Dental care has never been a significant part of the Medicare program. Medicare's oral health services are limited to services requiring hospitalization—usually surgical treatment for fractures or oral cancer—and hence constitute a negligible part of the program. This is partly because Medicare was never intended to provide comprehensive insurance coverage and partly in response to successful lobbying by the ADA. In 1964 the ADA sent Dr. Lawrence I. Kerr to testify before the Senate and House of Representatives against dental inclusion in the Medicare program. Dr. Kerr presented the ADA viewpoint that those working in the 1960s and retiring in the 1980s and 1990s would receive lifetime oral healthcare benefits from their prior employers, so the government need not provide dental insurance for older Americans. These predictions, although ultimately incorrect, led Congress to pass the Medicare Amendment without dental benefits.

Medicare was created because the health insurance system was unable to adequately provide for people over age 65 (or seniors). This is in part because health insurers collect premiums sufficient to cover anticipated payouts, and the risk of adverse selection in those over age 65 is high, which forces premiums higher. What's more, while younger people usually receive medical insurance through an employer, older people are less likely to be working enough time to receive coverage from employer-sponsored health insurance programs. In addition, in 1965, because the income of persons aged 65 and older was considerably less than that of the employed population, seniors had relatively limited funds to spend on healthcare. Between 1966 and 2010, the proportion of seniors below the poverty line declined significantly, from 17.9% to 7.7, although this proportion has been inching upward more recently. In 2017, 11.8% of seniors lived below poverty level.[18,80] The uproar from the health professions that surrounded Medicare's birth in 1965 ("socialized medicine") subsided as the public realized that it filled a necessary gap in the financing of healthcare. It also subsided once providers realized they had a source of payment for treatment that previously was unreimbursed and reduced uncompensated care.[56] CMS in 2018 showed that more than 53.4 million Americans—about 16.4% of the population—were enrolled in Medicare. Federal expenditures for the program were estimated to be approximately $342 billion, or $10,000 per capita, in 2016.[84] In 2006, legislation was enacted to add prescription drug benefits to Medicare as Medicare Part D.[14] In 2016, while $38.9 billion was spent on the Medicare Part A and B drug benefit, $89.8 billion was spent on the Medicare part D (Box 7.3).[14] Medicare also covers some people who are disabled and some younger people with permanent kidney failure.

Because Medicare does not cover most dental care, on average, Medicare beneficiaries cover nearly three-fourths of the costs of dental services out of pocket (OOP). The portion covered by a

**• BOX 7.3  Medicare Prescription Drug Benefit**

People with Medicare may get drugs as part of their inpatient treatment during a covered stay in a hospital or skilled nursing facility (SNF). Generally, Part A payments made to the hospital, SNF, or other inpatient setting cover all drugs provided during a covered stay. Part B covers drugs that usually aren't self-administered. These drugs can be given in a doctor's office as part of their service. In a hospital outpatient department, coverage generally is limited to drugs that are given by infusion or injection. Part D offers outpatient comprehensive prescription drug coverage for a formulary of medications to people with original Medicare (Part A and Part B).[55]

third party is primarily the result of some retirees having dental insurance that they are allowed to keep into retirement or of being "dual eligible" for Medicare and Medicaid and residing in a state whose Medicaid program covers adult dental care. While inflation-adjusted dental costs increased from 2002 to 2012, the percentage of OOP spending on dental services by Medicare beneficiaries remained consistent, even across key sociodemographic characteristics such as age, gender, and education.

To some degree to address this gap in coverage, a growing number of Medicare Advantage plans include dental services to entice seniors to enroll with a particular Medicare managed care or third-party plan.[65] It is important to note that the dental benefit in these Medicare Advantage plans is usually very limited, covering items like an exam, dental cleaning, and radiographs. These are usually not comprehensive dental coverage. Medicare Advantage plans try to differentiate themselves from others by offering the dental coverage. Attempts to expand Medicare coverage for oral healthcare have not succeeded to date, although there are continuous efforts to move toward a dental benefit in Medicare.[17]

## Medicaid

Title XIX of the Social Security amendments of 1965, commonly referred to as Medicaid, is a public program that was originally designed primarily to finance care for low-income populations, particularly mothers and children. Over time, this program has expanded to be a major payor of care for individuals with disabilities and special needs and for low-income adults in long-term care facilities. Medicaid differs from Medicare in several important ways. Whereas Medicare is funded federally from payroll taxes through a trust fund, Medicaid costs are shared jointly by the federal and state governments. The portion of support provided by the federal government varies by state, and federal allocations are made according to a formula based on the ratio of the state's per capita income to the national per capita income.[89] States may develop their own Medicaid provider networks in accordance with federal requirements or contract with a managed care entity to establish the provider network. Managed Medicaid has grown significantly—between 1999 and 2012, the proportion of Medicaid beneficiaries enrolled in managed care increased from 64% to 89%.[1] In fiscal year 2016, the federal government's portion of the cost for state Medicaid programs averaged 63%, ranging between 50% and 74% for each state.[69] The Medicaid expenditure totaled $574.2 billion, including administrative costs, accounting adjustments, and expenditures in the U.S. territories. These costs have a significant impact on total spending at both the state and federal level.[68]

Medicaid programs generally pay for services through fee for service to providers or capitated arrangements with managed care entities. To change the way they pay Medicaid providers, states must submit a state plan amendment (SPA) to get a waiver from CMS. There are several options for waivers to allow states to be more creative with their Medicaid programs, including incorporating managed care options. One program is called an 1115 waiver, under which many states have operated managed care programs. These waivers were available prior to the ACA and are generally approved for 5 years (renewable). A second type of Medicaid waiver is the "1332" waiver (also called state innovation waivers); "1332" waivers were established by the ACA and allow for even more flexibility than the 1115 waivers. Both of these waiver programs have to be budget neutral, and the 1115 waivers have to have an evaluation component to assist other states with the potential generalizability.

As of October 2018, 66.3 million people (or just over 20% of the population) in the United States had healthcare coverage under the Medicaid program.[37] Medicaid eligibility criteria are established by the states and vary widely, as do expenditures on authorized services. Expenditures for the overall Medicaid program were relatively level for most of the decade prior to the implementation of the ACA in 2010. Since then there has been an expansion of Medicaid enrollment and a concomitant growth in overall expenditures, as indicated by Figure 7.9.[10] States are required to provide dental care for Medicaid-enrolled children through the Early and Periodic Screening, Diagnosis and Treatment (EPSDT) program, but dental care for adults is considered an optional service; states determine the comprehensiveness of their adult dental benefit. Dental care is a relatively small portion of all Medicaid costs. In 2016, $28 billion was spent on Medicaid fee-for-service dental services, representing approximately 2% of overall Medicaid expenditures. As Figure 7.10 indicates, increases in Medicaid expenditures for dental care have been relatively steady, although Figure 7.11 shows a small increase in the proportion of dental expenditures

for Medicaid and State Health Insurance Programs from 2000 through 2016.[10]

While most Medicaid waivers relate to medical care, there have been innovative small-scale demonstration programs that include dental care in some states. For example, in Oregon (Box 7.4) an 1115 waiver demonstration program is seeking to transform their Medicaid delivery system with a stronger focus on the integration of physical, behavioral, and oral healthcare through a performance-driven system aimed at improving health outcomes and managing costs.[64] Minnesota is another state that has filed an 1115 waiver and also operates an innovative Medicaid program.[57] The majority of the Medicaid population in managed care are at lower risk and nondisabled, and the share of Medicaid spending attributed to payments for managed care only rose from 15% to 37% during that period.[68]

The effectiveness of the EPSDT program in providing dental care for Medicaid-enrolled children has been called into question.

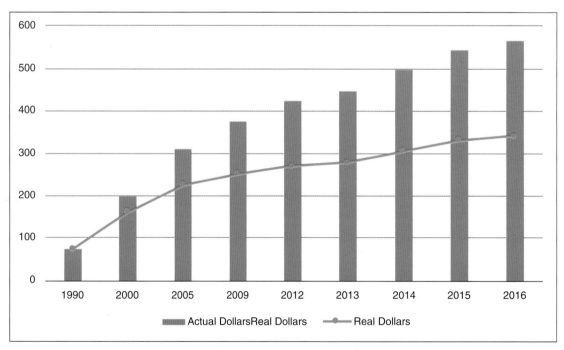

• **Figure 7.9** Total Medicaid and Child Health Insurance Program expenditures in actual dollars and adjusted to constant 1990 dollars (real dollars) in the United States, selected years, 1990–2016 (in billions of dollars).[11]

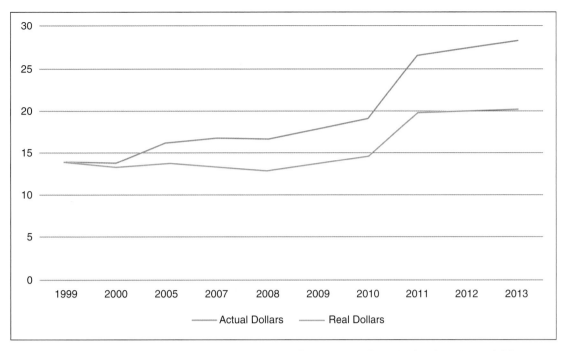

• **Figure 7.10** Medicaid and Children's Health Insurance Program expenditures for dental care in actual dollars and adjusted to constant 1999 dollars (real dollars) in the United States, selected years, 1999–2013 (in billions of dollars).[10]

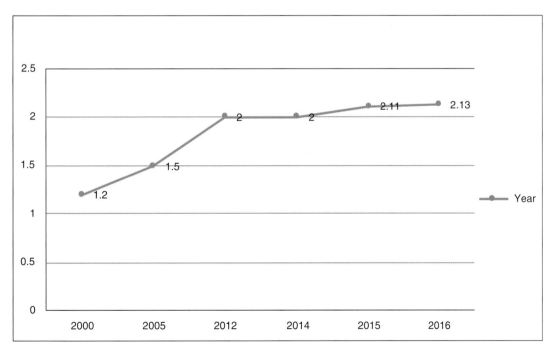

• **Figure 7.11** Medicaid expenditures for dental care as a percentage of total Medicaid expenditures in the United States, selected years, 2000–2016 (in billions of dollars).[10]

Although the EPSDT dental benefit package of covered services is better than that for most private dental insurance plans, actual utilization of services is relatively low. Of the slightly less than 40 million children under the age of 21 who were eligible for EPSDT services for more than 90 days in FY 2016, just over 19 million received any dental services, with 17.5 million (just under 50%) receiving preventive services.[10] This does, however, represent a significant improvement in the use of preventive services over the last 35 years (in 1993, only 20% of eligible children received preventive services).

### Medicaid for Children

As mentioned, for states to qualify for the federal government's share of Medicaid funds, every state Medicaid program is required to cover a set of basic services for all children receiving federally supported financial assistance though the EPSDT program. EPSDT was instituted in 1968, and requires that states offer a comprehensive benefit package of early and periodic screening, diagnosis, and treatment services, including comprehensive dental care, to all children in Medicaid through age 20.

### Medicaid for Adults

States have considerable discretion in defining the level of adult dental benefits they will cover for their Medicaid population. Forty-six states and Washington, DC, currently provide some dental benefits for adults in Medicaid. However, the comprehensiveness of dental services covered varies significantly by state, as does the per-person annual maximum allowed for dental care. As of February 2016, 15 states provided extensive adult dental benefits (defined as a comprehensive mix of services including more than 100 diagnostic, preventive, and minor and major restorative procedures) with a per-person annual expenditure cap of at least $1000. Nineteen states provided limited dental benefits (defined as including fewer than 100 procedures) with a per-person annual expenditure cap of $1000 or less. The remaining 13 states with any adult dental benefits covered only dental care for pain relief or emergency care for injuries, trauma, or extractions. Four states provided no dental benefits at all.[62] Even in states that provide some dental benefits, adult Medicaid beneficiaries may face high out-of-pocket costs for dental care, making it difficult or impossible to afford.

Under the ACA, states were given the option of expanding access to Medicaid coverage to adults previously not eligible for Medicaid (i.e., primarily nondisabled single adults), up to 138% of the federal poverty level, as part of the mechanism for reducing the number of uninsured adults in the United States. While adoption of the Medicaid expansion was slow in some traditionally conservative portions of the country, by the end of 2018 all but 14 states had opted to expand their Medicaid programs.[43] Adult dental benefits for the expansion population remained a state option under the ACA as it was for the traditional Medicaid population. As of 2018, 9.8 million adults gained dental benefits in the 23 states that expanded Medicaid and had adult dental benefits.[36] All but two of these states (Montana and North Dakota) provide the same dental benefits for expansion adults as they do for the traditional adult Medicaid population.

There is evidence that the expansion of Medicaid has the potential to have a significant impact the oral health status of low-income adults. Research in Iowa found that a dentally uninsured population had much lower oral health status and greater problems accessing dental care than an adult Medicaid population (this uninsured population later became the foundation for Iowa's Medicaid expansion population). Oral health problems were the most common chronic health condition among the uninsured adults, and their self-reported oral status was much lower—and their dental unmet need much higher—than their traditional adult Medicaid

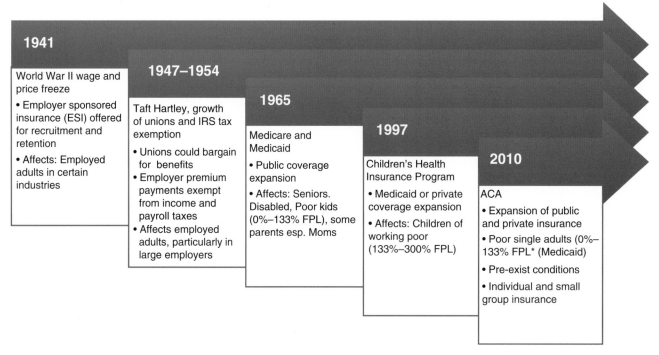

**1941**

World War II wage and price freeze
• Employer sponsored insurance (ESI) offered for recruitment and retention
• Affects: Employed adults in certain industries

**1947–1954**

Taft Hartley, growth of unions and IRS tax exemption
• Unions could bargain for benefits
• Employer premium payments exempt from income and payroll taxes
• Affects employed adults, particularly in large employers

**1965**

Medicare and Medicaid
• Public coverage expansion
• Affects: Seniors. Disabled, Poor kids (0%–133% FPL), some parents esp. Moms

**1997**

Children's Health Insurance Program
• Medicaid or private coverage expansion
• Affects: Children of working poor (133%–300% FPL)

**2010**

ACA
• Expansion of public and private insurance
• Poor single adults (0%–133% FPL* (Medicaid)
• Pre-exist conditions
• Individual and small group insurance

• **Figure 7.12** Insurance coverage in U.S. over time: Filling the gaps.

counterparts.[66] Research has also shown that when states reduce or eliminate adult dental benefits, unmet dental care needs increase, preventive dental service use decreases, and emergency department use for dental problems increase.[43,45,78,91] The ADA's Health Policy Institute has estimated that adding an extensive adult dental benefit would cost, on average, 1.1% of total state Medicaid spending.[36]

## Children's Health Insurance Program

The Children's Health Insurance Program (CHIP), established in 1997, was the first new federal health insurance program for children since the EPSDT defined pediatric Medicaid coverage almost 30 years earlier. Originally known as the State Children's Health Insurance Program (SCHIP), this program was intended to provide coverage to children of the "working poor" (i.e., families with incomes above those eligible for Medicaid but too low to enable them to afford conventional health insurance). CHIP covers children in families with incomes up to at least 200% of the federal poverty level (FPL), a federally established level of income used to define poverty for government purposes,[24] although states may choose to extend CHIP coverage to children in families with incomes up to 300% of the FPL. By 2003 about 5.8 million children in the United States—a bit over 7% of the child population of the country and about one-half of the uninsured children that SCHIP initially intended to reach—were enrolled in CHIP.[58] As of 2016, CHIP provides coverage to more than 8 million children and 370,000 pregnant women.[51]

States have more flexibility in the design of their CHIP programs than they do of their Medicaid programs. State CHIP programs vary from a simple expansion of the state's Medicaid program to a completely separate program with a different set of rules, potentially contracted out to a managed care entity. States are required to cover dental care as part of their CHIP programs, but unlike state Medicaid programs under the EPSDT guidelines, these separate CHIP programs may require patient copayments, monthly premiums, and annual payment limits for dental care for CHIP members. In January 2018, after extensive public advocacy and congressional debate, Congress passed a 6-year extension of CHIP funding as part of a broader continuing resolution to fund the federal government. The extension provides stable funding for states to continue their CHIP coverage.

## The Affordable Care Act

As has been mentioned throughout this chapter, the Patient Protection and Affordable Care Act (ACA), enacted in 2010, is quite broad in its impact, affecting both health insurance coverage and the delivery of care. The ACA actually refers to two separate pieces of legislation—the Patient Protection and Affordable Care Act (P. L. 111-148) and the Health Care and Education Reconciliation Act of 2010 (P.L. 111-152).[67] Regarding the impact on coverage, the ACA expands health insurance through a combination of public and private components; part through a Medicaid expansion for those up to 138% of FPL and part by subsidizing the purchase of private insurance for adults from 100% to 400% of FPL through the health insurance marketplace (www.healthcare.gov). The delivery of care is affected primarily through the development of accountable care organizations and value-based purchasing arrangements, initially for Medicare beneficiaries and then expanding to Medicaid and private insurance plans.

As has been discussed, the ACA is only the latest in the attempts made in the United States to support health insurance coverage through the involvement of the government since the 1940s. First, tax benefits were provided to employers to encourage employer-based insurance. Medicare and Medicaid were then introduced to cover the most vulnerable populations at the time: seniors, people with disabilities, and low-income mothers and children. CHIP expanded coverage to children of the working poor; the ACA was intended to fill the largest gap in 2010 low-income single adults who didn't qualify for Medicaid and people with preexisting conditions in the individual and small group insurance market. The ACA improved the quality of insurance plans by establishing a set of 10 essential health benefits for plans offered through the health insurance marketplace (i.e., ACA-compliant plans) and eliminated annual and lifetime dollar caps on coverage and changed the rating process to make the plans more affordable to those with a preexisting condition, older individuals, and women.

By 2017, the insurance expansions under the ACA resulted in about 17 million nonelderly people gaining public or private insurance.[40] The primary reasons for being uninsured remain that the cost is too high and the loss of health insurance benefits due to a change in job status. The greatest number of uninsured people are in states that opted not to participate in the Medicaid expansion (e.g., Texas, Florida). Some changes have been made by the current (2018) executive administration to the rules governing the individual insurance market that could result in an increase in the number of uninsured and/or the number of individuals in non–ACA-compliant plans, but it is too early to tell the long-term implications of these changes. Additionally, there are several judicial challenges to the ACA, for example, in December 2018 a Texas court judge ruled that the ACA was unconstitutional, so the structure of this program could change.

As has been mentioned, about 10 million adults gained dental coverage through the expansion of Medicaid in states that provide comprehensive coverage. The ACA also enshrined oral health as a critical component of children's overall health, with children's dental care listed as one of the 10 essential health benefits, which was intended to require that pediatric oral health coverage be offered in most private insurance packages nationwide, including on the newly created health insurance marketplaces. Although oral health as an essential health benefit for children has not been enforced, through Medicaid, CHIP, and the ACA, 90% of children have some form of dental coverage. An unspecified but proportionally smaller number of adults and children have gained private dental coverage through the purchase of individual dental policies through the health insurance marketplace. (Figure 7.12)

In doing so, the ACA effectively made dental coverage more like a true insurance product. Prior to the ACA, purchasing coverage was often very confusing and unaffordable for many people. In addition to integration of coverage, the ACA created opportunities for integration of care. Among the ACA's preventive services that must be offered at no cost to consumers are oral health services provided by pediatricians, including an oral health risk assessment, fluoride varnish, and referral to dentist.

## Future Considerations and Concerns

Although Medicaid reaches a large number of people, many remain without health insurance. Efforts to limit Medicaid expenditures have persisted throughout its history.[16] The economic recessions of the early 21st century sharply increased the number of people eligible for Medicaid, and because this happened during periods of rapidly increasing medical care costs, many states viewed the higher costs of the Medicaid program as excessive. As a result, during that period some states cut back on eligibility, reducing the availability of services and the payment amounts to providers. Dental services were often among the first of these cutbacks, and Medicaid-funded services for adults were hit especially hard. Many dentists, frustrated by rapidly changing eligibility standards for prospective patients, reductions in available services, changes in percentile fees paid, and delays in payment for services rendered, have refused to treat Medicaid patients.

Following the enactment of the Affordable Care Act in 2010, some of those rollbacks were reversed as government funds aided in state expansions of Medicaid coverage. While the ACA expanded Medicaid from 2012 to 2016 and the rate of uninsured people declined from 15.4% to 9%, during the following 2 years the rate of uninsured people increased to just over 12%. The impact on pediatric dental care, now mandated an essential service, was considerable; the ACA also expanded coverage for adults in states that had an existing adult program before the ACA implementation.

Medicaid is constantly changing. Budget constraints create pressure to reduce government spending at both the federal and state levels. Social service programs such as Medicaid are a prime target for reductions, partly because they do not have a vocal constituency. The ACA helped states expand their Medicaid coverage, but with the efforts to constrict the ACA, these expanded benefits may not persist. Whatever the outcome, Medicaid recipients who are threatened with loss of access to health services, particularly adults, stand to lose the most.

The shift of social welfare program implementation from the federal government to the states will cause continuing loss of needed services if funding is not also made available to already stretched state budgets. State governments, unlike the federal government, are unable to operate at a deficit. If tax revenues and other sources of funds are not sufficient to meet budget needs, programs must be reduced or eliminated. There have been proposals to fund the program through block grants to the states, through which the federal government disburses previously categorical funds (evolved from the grant-in-aid days) in lump sums to be allocated to specified programs at a state's discretion. With block grant funding, the total sum of federal funds received by the state is known and fixed and there are heavy political pressures to use the funds for health-related purposes other than dental care.

In an effort to control costs of Medicare and Medicaid, the government has made a major effort to encourage enrollment in managed care plans. This movement has made it more difficult to access and track data on the amount of funds devoted to dental services, as dental benefits are imbedded in the funds transferred to managed care plans. Although the movement of beneficiaries to managed care appears somewhat successful, especially in Medicaid, it remains to be seen whether costs are actually controlled and whether access and other quality indicators will be at satisfactory levels.

## Examples of Public Financing Programs for Dental Care

Government, whether federal, state, or local, is involved in the financing of healthcare in many ways. Programs include support for undergraduate and graduate education; direct service in schools, clinics, and Head Start programs; public health clinic construction; and healthcare personnel salaries. The following are some examples of those financing programs.

## Medicare GME

Medicare's share in funding teaching hospitals includes residency training support under Part A (hospital services), commonly referred to as graduate medical education (GME). Medicare GME has two components: direct graduate medical education (DGME) and indirect medical education (IME). Medicare DGME payments cover costs related to the training of residents, such as resident stipends and fringe benefits, supervising faculty salaries and fringe benefits, and allocated overhead for direct costs (malpractice) and institutional (maintenance and utilities) items. IME was created to compensate for factors that make teaching hospitals' costs relatively high, such as treating a more severely ill patient population, offering a wider range of services and technology, providing more diagnosis and therapeutic services to certain types of patients, and allowing clinical inefficiencies (such as the ordering of more tests than is standard) as residents learn their profession.

As a result of GME funding, dental and medical residency programs have grown in number, and interns and residents and have become increasingly important to the services delivered. The funding is a major source of revenue for teaching hospitals, which has expanded access to care for underserved patients by supporting the hospitals that provide that care. In 2011, total funds disbursed to teaching hospitals under Medicare GME were $15 billion ($3.5 billion under DGME).[54]

Medicare has shared in the cost of approved education activities that take place in teaching hospitals. Residencies provide important training for dental graduates pursuing careers in general dentistry, the dental specialties, hospital dentistry, and geriatric dentistry. Well over 65% of graduates enroll in postdoctoral training. As of 2017, more than 38% of graduates were enrolled in hospital-based residencies supported by GME.[5]

## The Indian Health Service[39,86]

The Indian Health Service (IHS), an agency within the Department of Health and Human Services, is responsible for providing federal health services to American Indians and Alaska Natives. The provision of health services to members of federally recognized tribes grew out of the special government-to-government relationship between the federal government and Indian tribes. This relationship, established in 1787, is based on Article I, Section 8 of the Constitution, and has been given form and substance by numerous treaties, laws, Supreme Court decisions, and executive orders. The IHS is the principal federal healthcare provider and health advocate for Indian people. The IHS provides a comprehensive health service delivery system for approximately 2.2 million American Indians and Alaska Natives who belong to 537 recognized Indian tribes in 37 states. The Division of Oral Health of the IHS is responsible for direct care through its own clinics and contract care through private dental offices for a large portion of this population. Federal funds also are provided for some tribes to run their own program.

## The Ryan White Comprehensive AIDS Resources Emergency (CARE) Act[85]

Another program with federal involvement that includes a dental care component is the Health Resources and Services Administration, which provides funds for academic centers that provide dental care to individuals with human immunodeficiency virus infection through the federal Ryan White CARE Act Part F and other Ryan

White programs. These funds amounted to approximately $10 million in fiscal year 2018. While these funds, specifically earmarked for treatment of HIV-infected patients, help provide support for care, the support is minimal and the funding level has remained stagnant over the past 10 years.

### RYAN WHITE

Ryan White was a teenager with hemophilia who was infected with HIV after a transfusion with contaminated blood. He was denied readmission to school out of fear that he would infect other children. He fought that decision and became the poster child for the rights of people infected with HIV. In 1990 the Ryan White Care Act was adopted to help fund care for low income, uninsured and under insured people infected with HIV.

## Conclusion

As described in this chapter, the financing of dental care in the United States has evolved over several decades. The trend shows that as the cost of healthcare—both medical and dental—continues to escalate, the financing of this care will continue to evolve with innovative models and delivery systems developed to meet the future need and demand.

## References

1. American Dental Association. *HPI Infographic—Medicaid Expansion and Dental Benefits.* Available from: https://www.ada.org/en/science-research/health-policy-institute/dental-statistics/dental-benefits-and-medicaid.
2. American Dental Association, Council on Dental Benefit Programs. CDT. *Current Dental Terminology.* Chicago, IL: ADA; 2019.
3. American Dental Association, Council on Dental Benefit Programs. *Code on Dental Procedures and Nomenclature.* Available from: https://www.ada.org/en/publications/cdt.
4. American Dental Association, Council on Dental Care Programs. *Policies on Dental Care Programs.* Chicago, IL: ADA; 1991.
5. American Dental Association. *Education.* Available from: https://www.ada.org/en/science-research/health-policy-institute/data-center/dental-education.
6. Bailit HL, Bailit JL. Corporate control of health care: Impact on medicine and dentistry. *J Dent Educ.* 1988;52:108–113.
7. Brien MJ, Panis CWA. *Annual Report on Self-Insured Group Health Plans 2017 Appendix B. Advanced Analytic Consulting Group/Deloitte.* Available from: https://www.dol.gov/sites/default/files/ebsa/researchers/statistics/retirement-bulletins/annual-report-on-self-insured-group-health-plans-2017-appendix-b.pdf.
8. Cadillac Tax Delayed Till 2022. Available from: http://www.hrworks-inc.com/article/cadillac-tax-delayed-until-2022. https://www.brookings.edu/blog/usc-brookings-schaeffer-on-health-policy/2018/02/01/how-to-interpret-the-cadillac-tax-rate-a-technical-note/.
9. Carby C. Institute of Medicine Public Policy Options for Better Dental Health Dec. In: *Is Capitation a Threat.* National Academy Press; 1980.
10. Centers for Medicare & Medicaid Services, Centers for Medicaid and CHIP Services. *Medicaid Statistical Information System (MSIS), granular file.* MSIS data for 2013 accessed October 5, 2016. Available from: https://www.cms.gov/Research-Statistics-Data-and-Systems/Computer-Data-and-Systems/MSIS.
11. Centers for Medicare & Medicaid Services, Office of the Actuary, National Health Statistics Group. *National Health Expenditure Accounts, National Health Expenditures Aggregate.* Available from: https://www.cms.gov/Research-Statistics-Data-andSystems/Statistics-Trends-and-Reports/NationalHealthExpendData/NationalHealthAccountsHistorical.html.
12. Centers for Medicare & Medicaid Services, Office of the Actuary, National Health Statistics Group. *Table 6 Personal Health Care Expenditures.* Available from: https://www.cms.gov/Research-Statistics-Data-and-Systems/Statistics-Trends-and-Reports/NationalHealthExpendData/NationalHealthAccountsHistorical.html.
13. Centers for Medicare & Medicaid Services, Office of the Actuary, National Health Statistics Group. *Table 2, National Health Expenditures; Aggregate and Per Capita Amounts, by Type of Expenditure.* Available from: https://www.cms.gov/Research-Statistics-Data-and-Systems/Statistics-Trends-and-Reports/NationalHealthExpendData/NationalHealthAccountsHistorical.html.
14. Centers for Medicare & Medicaid Services (CMS). *Medicare Part D Drug Spending Dashboard & Data.* Available from: https://www.cms.gov/Research-Statistics-Data-and-Systems/Statistics-Trends-and-Reports/Information-on-Prescription-Drugs/MedicarePartD.html.
15. Centers for Medicare & Medicaid Services (CMS). *Hospital Value-Based Purchasing Program Results for Fiscal Year 2019.* Available from: https://www.cms.gov/newsroom/fact-sheets/cms-hospital-value-based-purchasing-program-results-fiscal-year-2019.
16. Chang D, Holahan J. Medicaid spending in the 1980s: The access-cost containment trade-off revisited. In: *Urban Institute Report 90-2.* Washington, DC: Urban Institute Press; 1990.
17. Chávez EM, Calvo JM, Jones JA. Dental homes for older Americans: The Santa Fe Group call for removal of the dental exclusion in Medicare. *Am J Public Health.* 2017;107(suppl 1):S41–S43.
18. Cornfield J. *Bankrate study: Seniors' incomes in 47 states don't go far enough. Bankrate.* May 23, 2016; Available from: https://www.bankrate.com/retirement/bankrate-study-seniors-incomes-in-47-states-dont-go-far-enough.
19. Cooper BS, Worthington NL. National Health Expend, 1929–72. *Soc Secur Bull.* 1973;36(1):3–19.
20. Damiano PC, Brown ER, Johnson JD, et al. Factors affecting dentist participation in a state Medicaid program. *J Dent Educ.* 1990;54:638–643.
21. Douglas B. Sherlock. *Administrative Expenses of Health Plan.* Available from: http://s3.amazonaws.com/zanran_storage/www.bcbs.com/ContentPages/25302966.pdf
22. Faulkner EJ. The role of health insurance. In: Gregg DW, ed. *Life and Health Insurance Handbook.* Homewood, IL: Irwin; 1959: 523–532.
23. Field MJ, Shapiro HT. *Employment and Health Benefits: A Connection at Risk.* Institute of Medicine (US) Committee on Employment-Based Health Benefits. National Academies Press; 1993. Available from: https://www.ncbi.nlm.nih.gov/books/NBK235989/.
24. *Federal Poverty Level.* Healthcare.gov United States Census Bureau Available from: https://www.healthcare.gov/glossary/federal-poverty-level-fpl/.
25. Garrison J. Purchasers and payers: Who's driving the market? *J Dent Educ.* 1996;60:356–359.
26. Goodman D, Flaherty S. *Federal subsidization of health insurance: the "Cadillac Tax" and tax credits in the affordable care act and beyond Goodman D. ECO 490 5/17.*
27. Goodman JC, Musgrave GL. *Patient Power: Solving America's Health Care Crisis.* Washington, DC: Cato Institute; 1992.
28. Guay Albert H. *Understanding pay for performance.* 2007. Available from: http://www.ada.org/prof/resources/pubs/asanewsarticle.aso?articleid=2344.
29. Guay JA. The differences between dental and medical care: implications for dental benefit plan design. *J Am Dent Assoc.* 2006;137:801–806.
30. Hadley J. Insurance coverage, medical care use, and short-term health changes following an unintentional injury or the onset of a chronic condition. *JAMA.* 2007;297:1073–1084.
31. Hadley J, Steinberg EP, Feder J. Comparison of uninsured and privately insured hospital patients. Condition on admission, resource use, and outcome. *JAMA.* 1991;265:374–379.
32. Health Insurance Association of America. *Source Book of Health Insurance Data, 1995.* Washington, DC: HIAA; 1995.
33. Health Insurance Association of America. *Source Book of Health Insurance Data, 2002.* Washington, DC: HIAA; 2002.

34. *Health Insurance Coverage in the United States: 2016.* September 12, 2017. Report Number P60-260 Jessica C. Barnett and Edward R. Berchick. Available from: https://www.census.gov/library/publications/2017/demo/p60-260.html.

35. Health Insurance Institute. *Source Book of Health Insurance Data, 1977–78.* Washington, DC: HII; 1978.

36. Health Policy Institute. *Medicaid Expansion and Dental Benefits Coverage.* Health Policy Institute Infographic. American Dental Association; 2018. Available from: https://www.ada.org/~/media/ADA/Science%20and%20Research/HPI/Files/HPIgraphic_1218_3.pdf?la=en.

37. Health Policy Institute. Medicaid Expansion and Dental Benefits Coverage. Health Policy Institute Infographic. American Dental Association. Available from: https://www.ada.org/~/media/ADA/Science%20and%20Research/HPI/Files/HPIgraphic_1218_3.pdf?la=en. Accessed December 29, 2018.

38. *International Classification of Diseases, Tenth Revision, Clinical Modification (ICD-10-CM).* CDC National Center Health Statistics. Available from: https://www.cdc.gov/nchs/icd/icd10cm.htm.

39. Indian Health Service (IHS). *Part 5: Patient Care Statistics.* IHS Tribal Health Contract, Grant, and Compact Awards. Available from: HTTPS://WWW.IHS.GOV/SITES/DPS/THEMES/RESPONSIVE2017/DISPLAY_OBJECTS/DOCUMENTS/TRENDS%20PART%205-PATIENT%20CARE%20STAT.PDF.

40. Kaiser Family Foundation. *Key Facts About the Uninsured Population.* Available from: https://www.kff.org/uninsured/fact-sheet/key-facts-about-the-uninsured-population/?utm_campaign=KFF-2018-December-Uninsured-People-ACA&utm_source=hs_email&utm_medium=email&utm_content=68185283&_hsenc=p2ANqtz–6eal3lgI0PVApBe-ujBTYdqgFjOjd94x2WKFfcAdZEjoG6hzjPsMxojTJO70lxF0S-ubk1TsJ8THEnqiIS5VBUhPNGA&_hsmi=68185283; 2018.

41. Kronenfeld JJ, Parmet WE, Zezza MA. *Taxing High-Cost (Cadillac) Plans Debates on U.S. Health Care.* https://doi.org/10.4135/9781452218472.n21. Available from: http://sk.sagepub.com/reference/ushealthcare/n21.xml.

42. Lang WP, Weintraub JA. Comparison of Medicaid and non-Medicaid dental providers. *J Public Health Dent.* 1986;46:207–211.

43. Laniado N, Badner VM, Silver EJ. Expanded Medicaid dental coverage under the Affordable Care Act: an analysis of Minnesota emergency department visits. *Public Health Dent.* 2017;77(4):344–349. https://doi.org/10.1111/jphd.12214.

44. Levit KR, Lazenby HC, Braden BR, et al. National health expenditures, 1995. *Health Care Finance Rev.* 1996;18(1):175–202.

45. Lewis CW, et al. Visits to U.S. emergency departments by 20–29-year-old with toothache during 2001–2010. *J Am Dent Assoc.* 2015;146(5):295–302.

46. Manning WG, Bailit HL, Benjamin B, et al. The demand for dental care: Evidence from a randomized clinical trial in health insurance. *J Am Dent Assoc.* 1985;110:895–902.

47. Manski RJ, Rohde F. *Dental Services: Use, Expenses, Source of Payment, Coverage and Procedures. Research Findings #38: Dental Services: Use, Expenses, Source of Payment, Coverage and Procedure Type, 1996–2015.* Agency for Healthcare Research and Quality.

48. Manski RJ, Rohde F. *Dental Services: Use, Expenses, Source of Payment, Coverage and Procedure Type, 1996–2015: Research Findings No. 38. National Income and Product Accounts Tables, Table 1.1.5, Nominal GDP.* Rockville, MD: Agency for Healthcare Research and Quality; 2017.

49. Marcus M. Managed care and dentistry: promise and problems. *J Am Dent Assoc.* 1995;126:439–446.

50. Martin PP, Weaver DA. Social Security: a program and policy history. *Social Security Bulletin.* 2005;66(1).

51. Teeth Matter. *Children's Dental Health Project. A special month, a special program.* Available from: https://www.cdhp.org/blog/335-a-special-month-a-special-program.

52. McMorrow S, Kenney GM, Goin D. Determinants of receipt of recommended preventive services: implications for the Affordable Care Act. *Am J Public Health.* 2014;104(12):2392–2399.

53. Medicaid Managed Care Enrollment and Program. https://www.medicaid.gov/medicaid/managed-care/enrollment/index.html. Accessed December 29, 2018.

54. Medicare Payments for Graduate Medical Education. *What Every Medical Student, Resident, and Advisor Needs to Know.* AAMC Tomorrow's Doctors, Tomorrow's Cures; January 2003. Available from: https://www.aamc.org/data-reports/faculty-institutions/report/medicare-payments-graduate-medical-education-what-every-medical-student-resident-and-advisor-needs.

55. *Medicare Drug Coverage Under Medicare Part A, Part B, Part C, & Part D.* Available from: https://www.cms.gov/Outreach-and-Education/Outreach/Partnerships/downloads/11315-P.pdf.

56. Millenson LM. *Medicare, Fair Pay, and the AMA: The Forgotten History.* Available from: https://www.healthaffairs.org/do/10.1377/hblog20150910.050461/full/.

57. Minnesota Department of Human Services. *Federal Health Care Waivers.* Available from: https://mn.gov/dhs/partners-and-providers/news-initiatives-reports-workgroups/minnesota-health-care-programs/federal-waivers.jsp.

58. Myers BA. Health maintenance organizations: Objectives and issues. *HSMHA Health Rep.* 1971;86:585–591.

59. National Association of Dental Plans (NADP). *Research Commission Post 2019 Industry Research Schedule.* National Associations of Dental Plans. Available from: https://www.nadp.org/dental_benefits_basics/dental_bb_1.aspx.

60. National Association of Dental Plans (NADP). *State of Dental Benefits Market, March 2013, Enrollment Trends—NADP 2018 Dental Benefits Report: Enrollment, September 2018, pg 13; 2012.* Dallas, TX.

61. National Conference of State Legislatures. *Managed Care, Market Reports and the States.* http://www.ncsl.org/research/health/managed-care-and-the-states.aspx; July 1, 2017.

62. Oberg CN, Lia-Hoaberg B, Hodkinson E, et al. Prenatal care comparisons among privately insured, uninsured, and Medicaid-enrolled women. *Public Health Rep.* 1990;105:533–535.

63. Olsen ED. Dental insurance: a successful model facing new challenges. *J Dent Educ.* 1984;48:591–596.

64. Oregon Demonstration Factsheet. Medicaid.gov. https://www.medicaid.gov/medicaid-chip-program-information/by-topics/waivers/1115/downloads/or/or-health-plan2-fs.pdf.

65. Pope C. *Supplemental Benefits Under Medicare Advantage.* Available from: https://www.healthaffairs.org/do/10.1377/hblog20160121.052787/full/; January 21, 2016.

66. Peter C. Damiano, Suzanne E. Bentler, Elizabeth T. Momany, Ki H. Park, Erin Robinson. Evaluation of the IowaCare Program. *Information About the Medical Home Expansion.* University of Iowa, Public Policy Center; June 2013. Available from: https://ir.uiowa.edu/ppc_health/81.

67. Patient Protection and Affordable Care Act (PL 111-148), 42 U.S.C. § 18001 (2010). Available from: https://www.congress.gov/111/plaws/publ148/PLAW-111publ148.pdf.

68. Report CBO. *Exploring the Growth of Medicaid Managed Care, Nov 2, 2017.* Available from: https://www.cbo.gov/publication/53264.

69. Rudowitz Robin. *Understanding How States Access the ACA Enhanced Medicaid Match Rates. Kaiser Family Foundation.* Available from: https://www.kff.org/medicaid/issue-brief/understanding-how-states-access-the-aca-enhanced-medicaid-match-rates/; 2014.

70. Sanjay BB. *Types of Costs and Relationship of Direct & Indirect Costs with Fixed & Variable Costs.* Harold Averkamp. Available from: https://www.accountingcoach.com/blog/direct-indirect-fixed-variable-costs. Accessed February 21, 2020.

71. Schoen MH. Group practice and poor communities. *Am J Public Health.* 1970;60:1125–1132.

72. Schoen MH. Group practice owned by a partnership using some salaried dentists and contracting directly with purchasers of group dental care. *J Am Dent Assoc.* 1961;62:392–398.

73. Schoen MH. Methodology of capitation payment to group dental practice and effects of such payment on care. *Health Serv Rep.* 1974;89:16–24.

74. Smith QE, Pennell EH, Bothwell RD, et al. Dental care in a group purchase plan: a survey of attitudes and utilization at the St. Louis Labor Health Institute. In: *PHS Publication No. 684.* Washington DC: Government Printing Office; 1959.

75. Smith QE, Mitchell GE, Lucas GA. *An experiment in dental prepayment: the Naismith Dental Plan. PHS Publication No. 970.* Washington, DC: Government Printing Office; 1962.

76. Smith QE, Pennell EH. Service requirements in dental prepayment: Predictability and adverse reaction. *Public Health Rep.* 1961;76:11–18.

77. Stevens R, Stevens R. Medicaid: anatomy of a dilemma. *Law Contemp Probl.* 1970;35:348–425.

78. Sun BC, Chi DL, Schwarz E, et al. Emergency department visits for nontraumatic dental problems: a mixed-methods study. *Am J Pub Health.* 2015;105(5):947–955.

79. Ben Umans, Lynn Nonnemaker K. *The Medicare Beneficiary Population.* AARP Public Policy Institute. Available from: https://assets.aarp.org/rgcenter/health/fs149_medicare.pdf

80. United States Census Bureau. *Historical Poverty Tables: People and Families 1959–2017, Table 15: Age Distribution of the Poor: 1966–2017.* Available from: https://www.census.gov/data/tables/time-series/demo/income-poverty/historical-poverty-people.html.

81. United States Congress, Senate. In: *Health Maintenance Organization Act of 1973; Public Law 93-222. 93rd Congress, 2nd Session.* Washington, DC: Government Printing Office; 1974.

82. U.S. Bureau of Economic Analysis, National Income and Product Amounts, Table 1.1.4 Price Indexes for Gross Domestic Product Accounts, Assessed January 5, 2017.

83. United States Department of Health and Human Services. Centers for Medicare and Medicaid Services. In: *Highlights—National Health Expenditures*; 2002.

84. United States Department of Health and Human Services, Centers for Medicare and Medicaid Services. *2017 Annual Report of the Boards of Trustees of the Federal Hospital Insurance and Federal Supplementary Medical Insurance Trust Funds;* July 13, 2017.

85. United States Department of Health and Human Services, Health Resources and Services Administration, HIV/AIDS Bureau. *2004 Ryan White CARE Act Grantee Conference Information.*

86. United States Department of Health and Human Services, Indian Health Service. *Medical and Professional Programs: IHS Division of Oral Health.* https://www.ihs.gov/doh/documents/New%20Dental%20Provider%20Orientation%20Presentation.pdf. Accessed February 21, 2020.

87. United States Department of Labor, Bureau of Labor Statistics. *Health Spending Accounts.* Available from: https://www.bls.gov/opub/mlr/cwc/health-spending-accounts.pdf.

88. United States Department of the Treasury. *Treasury Secretary Snow Statement on Health Savings Accounts.* Available from: https://www.treasury.gov/press-center/press-releases/Pages/js101423.aspx.

89. United States Public Health Service, Health Care Financing Administration. *Medicare and Medicaid Data Book, 1988.* HCFA Publication No. 03270. Washington, DC: Government Printing Office; 1989.

90. United States Public Health Service. *The Dental Service Corporation: A New Approach to Dental Care.* PHS Publication No. 570. Washington, DC: Government Printing Office; 1961.

91. Thomas Wall MA, Marko Vujicic. Emergency Department Use for Dental Conditions Continues to Increase, Health Policy Institute; American Dental Association April 2015. http://www.ada.org//media/ADA/Science%20and%20Research/HPI/Files/HPIBrief_0415_2.ashx.

92. United States Renal Data System *Chapter 11; National Institute of Diabetes and Digestive and Kidney Diseases.* Available from: https://www.usrds.org/2013/view/v2_11.aspx.

93. Weissman J, Epstein AM. Case mix and resource utilization by uninsured hospital patients in the Boston metropolitan area. *JAMA.* 1989;261:3572–3576.

94. *Where Does Your Health Care Dollar Go?* Available from: https://www.ahip.org/wp-content/uploads/2017/03/HealthCareDollar_FINAL.pdf.

95. World Health Organization. *Health Systems Financing.* Available from: https://www.who.int/healthinfo/systems/WHO_MBHSS_2010_section5_web.pdf.

96. Zatz M, Landay M, LeDell JD. Dental Benefits and reimbursements. *Dent Clin North Amer.* 1987;31(2):193–207.

# 8

# The Oral Health Workforce

ELIZABETH MERTZ, PhD, MA

KARL SELF, MBA, DDS

JEAN MOORE, DrPH, FAAN

HANNAH MAXEY, PhD, MPH, RDH

## CHAPTER OUTLINE

## The Oral Health Team

*Dental team* is more of a concept than a precise term, although the dental profession in the United States has long recognized that multiple categories of personnel are fundamental to the efficient provision of oral healthcare. Virtually all dentists employ at least one staff person, 86.3% of general practitioners employ at least one full- or part-time chairside assistant, and 77.5% employ at least one full- or part-time hygienist.[12] The dental team is becoming increasingly interprofessional, working collaboratively with medical, social, and mental health professionals. This chapter defines the types of personnel involved in the provision of oral healthcare services, explores the evolution of individuals engaged in oral healthcare delivery, and assesses the factors that influence workforce supply and distribution.

## Dentists

A dentist is a person who is permitted to practice dentistry under the laws of the relevant state, province, territory, or nation. These laws are intended to ensure that a prospective dentist has satisfied certain requirements such as (1) completion of a specified period of professional education in an approved institution, (2) demonstration of competence, and (3) evidence of satisfactory personal qualities such as ethics and professionalism. Dentists are trained in the prevention and control of the diseases of the oral cavity and the treatment of pathologic conditions or trauma or inherent malformations. A dentist is legally entitled to diagnose and treat patients, to prescribe certain drugs, and to employ and supervise other dental personnel. The mechanisms for fulfilling these requirements differ among nations. In the United States and Canada, for example, professional education is separate from the additional testing required for licensure.[9] In many other countries, these two functions are combined under the authority of the educational institutions.

## General Practice

As of 2016, the American Dental Association (ADA) estimated that there were 196,000 professionally active dentists in the United States.[12] From 1920 until the early 1980s, 1% to 3% of dentists were women,[65] but since the early 1980s this percentage has increased. In 2001, over 16% of dentists were women, and almost one-third of dentists who had graduated within the previous 10 years were women.[5] In 2016, first-year dental school enrollees were 48.7% women compared with 39.1% women in 2000.[89] Not only are the numbers of women increasing, but dentistry is becoming more racially and ethnically diverse. Approximately 90% of dentists in practice as of 1995 reported themselves to be white non-Hispanic,[4] whereas in 2016, 51.4% of first-time dental school enrollees identified as white and 24.1% identified as Asian.[89] Despite this increasing racial/ethnic diversity, African-American, Hispanic/Latino, and American Indian/Alaska Native populations continue to be significantly underrepresented in the field.[58]

## Dental Postgraduate Training and Specialties

The early development of dental specialists was informal, and as such specialists did not require certification.[45] Varying patterns of formal training and certification developed as each specialty grew and matured relatively independently. Examining boards that certified specialty competence came into being, as did specialty societies, such as the American Association of Public Health Dentistry, American Academy of Pedodontics (now Pediatric Dentistry), and the American Association of Orthodontists, which maintained educational and experiential qualifications for membership. In addition, some states established specialty licensure following examination by the state board of dental examiners.

Under guidelines originally set by the ADA House of Delegates and the Council on Dental Education and Licensure, examining boards were established in nine areas of specialty practice: dental public health, endodontics, oral and maxillofacial pathology, oral and maxillofacial radiology, oral and maxillofacial surgery, orthodontics and dentofacial orthopedics, pediatric dentistry, periodontics, and prosthodontics. The ADA recognized dental public health as a specialty of dentistry in 1950,[2] with the establishment of dental public health divisions in state health departments following closely thereafter and the founding of the Oral Health Unit in the World Health Organization in 1953.[81] There are currently 15 accredited dental public health residency programs with a total enrollment of 65 residents in the 2017–18 academic year,[10] though as of 2018, there were only 174 board-certified public health dentists.[1] Currently, minimum criteria for being an ADA-recognized specialist are the completion of at least 2 years of approved advanced education through a Commission on Dental Accreditation (CODA)–accredited program and full-time limitation of practice to that specialty area. Certification as a diplomate by one of the specialty boards is not a prerequisite for specialty practice. The stated purpose of specialty boards is to provide leadership in elevating standards for the practice of the specialty and, through examination and certification, to recognize those individuals who have demonstrated competence.

More recently, numerous additional dental specialty groups such as anesthesiology, oral implantology/implant dentistry, oral medicine, and orofacial pain were established. Although these are not officially recognized as specialties by the ADA, in 2016, the organization made revisions to the Code of Ethics regarding dentist announcement and advertising of specialties not included in the nine ADA-recognized dental specialty groups. As of 2017, dentists may advertise being specialists in any of the nine recognized dental specialties "and in any other areas of dentistry for which specialty recognition has been granted under the standards required or recognized in the practitioner's jurisdiction, provided the dentist meets the educational requirements required for recognition as a specialist adopted by the American Dental Association or accepted in the jurisdiction [state] in which they practice."[8]

Unlike the situation in medicine, in which by 2015 more than 60% of practitioners were practicing in a specialty outside of primary care, 21% of dentists were specialists in 2016 (i.e., 79% of dentists were in general practice).[11] This general ratio has stayed steady in both medicine and dentistry since 1990.[21] From the 1970s until 2015, there was modest growth in the number of first-year specialty training positions from about 1200 to about 1600.[12] About 43% of specialists work in orthodontics or oral surgery, the two longest established specialties. From 2001 to 2016 (Figure 8.1), pediatric dentistry saw the largest growth in share of dental specialties, from 12% of dental specialists being pediatric dentists in 2001 to 18% in 2016.[12]

One area of postgraduate training with recent growth is in general practice residency (GPR) and advanced education in general dentistry (AEGD) programs. As of 2015, there were just over 1000 GPR and 785 AEGD residency positions, these numbers having increased from 943 GPR positions and 535 AEGD positions in 2005.[13]

## Supply, Distribution, and Education of Dentists

Dentists were first enumerated separately in the 1850 census. It listed 2900 dentists serving a population of 23 million,[46] or 12.6 dentists per 100,000 population. In 2016, there were approximately 60.8 active dentists per 100,000 people in the United States.[12] This number is nearly unchanged since the year 2000. These dentists, however, were not evenly distributed throughout the country. For example, in terms of dentists relative to each state's population in 2016, the figures ranged from 88.5 dentists per 100,000 people in the District of Columbia to 41.6 per 100,000 in Arkansas.[12]

There are a number of reasons for this uneven distribution of dentists. Personal preference such as attachment to a hometown,

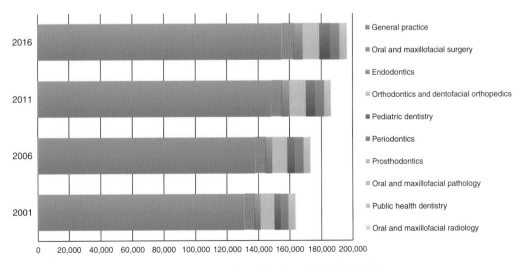

• **Figure 8.1** Dentist Supply by Specialty (2001–2016).

presence of good schools, or convenience to social, cultural, or recreational facilities affects where dentists choose to set up a practice.[72] Second is market capacity, meaning that the availability of dentists reflects demand for services. Areas of high income and education where demand for services is highest, such as affluent suburbs, have more dentists than do poorer areas. Finally, the location of dental schools also influences distribution, and the 66 American dental schools are located in only 38 states (plus the District of Columbia and Puerto Rico).[16] Many dental schools are in state universities, at which tuition usually is less for state residents than for out-of-state residents.

After many years of expansion, applications and enrollments in the late 1980s dipped in response to a slow period in the US economy and with a public perception that there was an oversupply of dentists. During the late 1980s and through the 1990s, six dental schools closed, and most others reduced their class size. The first-year capacity declined from its peak of 6301 in 1978 to approximately 4000 by 1990. Since 1990, applications and enrollments have recovered considerably.[89] In 2007, the number of dental school applicants peaked at 13,742, with about three applicants for every one dental school enrollment spot. From 2007 to 2016, the number of applicants to dental school declined to 12,058, with about two applicants for every one dental school enrollment spot.

From 2001 to 2016, the number of first-time enrollees in dental training programs grew from 4267 to 6100. This growth in enrollees can be attributed to an increasing number of dental schools in the United States and an increase in class size. Since 1997, there has been a net gain of 12 dental schools (13 opened, one closed), 10 of which have opened since 2008, bringing the current total to 66 dentals schools.[14] These new schools added nearly 1200 new dental student enrollees in 2017. Due to the growth of dental schools and expansion of first-year slots since the year 2000, the supply of dentists has also increased. In 2001, there were about 57.3 dentists per 100,000 population in the United States. This number grew to 60.8 per 100,000 in 2016.[12] Additionally, dentists have been retiring at older ages. In 2001, the dentists' average age at retirement was 64.8, and by 2013 this number has increased to 68.7 years.[22] There is no agreed upon target for the number of dentists or ratio of dentists to the population, and projections show that the supply of dentists is likely to keep growing through 2037.[61]

The most recent international comparisons of Organization for Economic Cooperation and Development (OECD) countries dentist:population ratios showed a wider range (from 10–127 per 100,000). At 60, the United States was just below the OECD average of 61, and between 1990 and 2007 the ratio in the United States had stayed constant, growing by only 0.1%.[69]

Foreign-trained dentists (FTDs), in contrast to foreign-trained medical graduates, have never been present in large numbers in the United States, making up less than 8% of dentists added to the workforce between 2005 and 2010, and they are projected to decrease in proportion as the number of US dental graduates grows.[62] Of the 28,407 dentists entering the workforce from 2008 to 2013, only 2079 were FTDs.[25] CODA ensures that US dental schools and graduates meet certain quality standards, as do other countries, but there is no universal international accreditation body.[24] FTDs' qualifications were assessed through a certification examination by individual states until the late 1970s, when most states began requiring FTDs to obtain a dental degree from a CODA-accredited dental program. Dental schools initially adopted an approach in which they evaluated and placed each FTD into a particular point in the curriculum depending on his or her skills and background.

Since that time, two pathways for gaining educational qualification have emerged: pre-doctoral international dental programs or advanced standing (IDP/AS) programs and postgraduate dental residency training.[51] These programs generally share similar admissions criteria, consist of repeating 2 to 3 years of dental school, and result in FTDs gaining a CODA-accredited dental degree. Immigration laws affect the pipeline of FTDs as well, for those with citizenship or permanent residency will be able to work once licensed, whereas those without it must be sponsored in their work as part of the pathway to citizenship. As of 2016, there were 41 dental schools offering IDP/AS programs to FTDs, a nearly 400% increase in the number of FTDs who were admitted to IDP/AS programs from the mid-1980s to 2015.[1,8] FTDs can also complete postdoctoral specialty programs to qualify for licensure in some states.[73] However, only about 15% of residency positions are filled by FTDs, though this ranges by specialty: nearly 71% of dental public health (DPH) residents enrolled in 2017 and 2018 were FTDs.[12]

## Dental Hygienists

Dental hygienists primarily work in clinical roles where they assess, diagnose, plan, implement, evaluate, and document treatment for control, prevention, and intervention of oral diseases.[17,18,29] They may also work in corporate or entrepreneurial roles, education, public health, and research. The clinical duties of a dental hygienist are similar in most countries. These generally include sealant placements, application of fluorides and other preventive agents, provision of patient education, nutrition and tobacco cessation counseling, and removal of calcified deposits (scaling and root-planning), irrigation of sulcus, and placement of localized antibiotic therapies.[47]

Estimating the supply of hygienists is done in various ways, including counting individual licensees, estimating full-time equivalent from total supply, and estimating number of dental hygiene jobs. The US Bureau of Labor Statistics (BLS) Occupational Employment and Wages Survey estimates the number of jobs, which may vary from actual workforce supply because dental hygienists may work part-time, may job share, or may work multiple jobs. A 2018 analysis of American Community Service data identified 177,817 individuals,[32] while in 2012 HRSA estimated an FTE count of 153,600,[77] and in May 2018 BLS estimated 215,150 dental hygiene jobs in the United States.[83] Regardless of counting method, the occupation has experienced considerable growth over the last half century, from an estimated 15,000 dental hygienists in the 1970s to 120,000 in the early 2000s to currently over 200,000.[83] This growth, however, was not consistent across the years. Declines in enrollment occurred through the late 1980s, roughly parallel to the enrollment declines for dentists, but rebounded by the turn of the century. Dental hygiene workforce projections generated by the Department of Health and Human Services (HHS) and Department of Labor (DOL) suggest continued growth, although the magnitude of estimated growth varies. HHS estimates growth of up to 10% by 2025 whereas DOL estimates projected growth of up to 20% by 2026.[77,83]

As with dentists, the dental hygiene workforce is not evenly distributed across the United States, nor is it demographically representative of the population. As is the case with many healthcare workers, dental hygienists are clustered in urban/metropolitan areas.[76] Additionally, there is little diversity in the dental hygiene profession. Dental hygiene is a predominantly female occupation;

females account for approximately 95.8% of dental hygienists.[32] The majority (86.1%) of dental hygienists self-identify as white. Black or African American is the second most common race (5.2%) reported by dental hygienists.[32]

The entry-level education requirement for dental hygiene is currently an associate's degree, although dental hygiene programs available at the bachelor's level are increasing. The majority of dental hygiene programs are located in schools of allied health sciences, and in 2018, there were a total of 331 programs in all 50 states, the District of Columbia, and Puerto Rico. This number has grown from 202 programs in 1990.[30]

Educational requirements for dental hygiene are standardized nationally through CODA accreditation, but the clinical practice of dental hygienists varies by state. Since the mid-1980s, dental hygiene practice has been evolving to be more independent of dentist supervision, allowing them to work independently mostly in community settings, and expanded to include a greater scope of practice, allowing them to do more procedures. As of 2010, state Medicaid regulations in 15 states allowed dental hygienists to be paid directly for dental hygiene services provided by them.[19] This and other areas of hygiene practice are associated with state statute, administrative code defining clinical practice, and professional supervision requirements and are highly variable despite national training standards.

## Dental Therapists

The addition of dental therapists to the oral healthcare team is relatively new in the United States. A dental therapist is a primary care oral health professional who works under the supervision of a dentist. They are educated to provide evaluative, preventive, restorative, and minor surgical dental care. The concept of dental therapy, originally called dental nurses, was introduced in New Zealand in 1921 as a way to address the poor oral health status of the youth in New Zealand.[59] Today, dental therapists provide care in more than 50 countries including Australia, Canada, the Netherlands, New Zealand, and the United Kingdom.[63] Throughout the world, the primary reason for authorizing dental therapists is to improve access to oral healthcare.

The first attempt to introduce dental therapists into the US oral healthcare team occurred in 1949 through the Forsyth Dental Infirmary in Massachusetts. The law authorizing the project was eventually rescinded in 1950 with the strong urging of the ADA.[54] In the early 1970s, there were other attempts to either introduce dental therapists or educate allied dental providers to prepare and place fillings. These efforts were also discontinued due to pressure from organized dentistry.[53]

Dental therapy ultimately took root in the United States with tribal communities in Alaska. Specifically, since 2005, dental health aide therapists (DHATs) practice under the auspices of the Indian Health Services Act.[62] In 2009, Minnesota became the first state to authorize the education and practice of dental therapists. Its state statute limits dental therapists to primarily practicing in settings that serve low-income, uninsured, and underserved patients or in a dental health professional shortage area (DHPSA).[66] Maine became the next state to authorize dental therapy in 2014, Vermont followed in 2016, and Arizona and Michigan in 2018. There are now more states in 2019: New Mexico, Idaho, Nevada, Montana, Connecticut. Additionally, in 2016, Washington passed legislation supporting the ability of tribal communities in their states to use dental therapists, and in 2011, Oregon passed legislation allowing for pilot projects of new dental providers, under which dental

therapists are being tested in Oregon tribes. In the United States, the role of the dental therapist is to help increase underserved populations' access to oral healthcare, and it is promoted as one workforce solution to the shortage/maldistribution of dentists.

The scope of practice of a dental therapist, like that of dental hygienists and dental assistants, varies by authorizing jurisdictions, but minimally, it is designed to allow for the provision of oral screenings and assessments, preventive care, direct restorations, and some level of extractions. Studies have estimated that up to 75% of procedures performed by a general dentist in the United States could be delegated to a dental therapist.[36]

In 2018, there were three dental therapy education programs.[23] One, a collaboration between the Alaska Native Tribal Health Consortium and Iḷisaġvik College, educates DHATs who currently practice in Alaska, Oregon, and Washington. Minnesota is home to the other two programs, one operated by the Minnesota State Colleges and Universities and the other by the University of Minnesota School of Dentistry. A fourth program is slated to be opened at Vermont Technical College with additional educational programs are being developed. The establishment of dental therapy educational standards by CODA in 2015 was widely seen as beneficial to educational programs and established guidelines to facilitate employment portability between states, although as of October 2019 none of the existing programs are CODA accredited.

The profession of dental therapy in the United States is still in its infancy, with only 150 licensed/certified practitioners in 2019. Similar to dental hygiene, dental therapy is a female-dominated profession with 84% of all graduates being women. Nationally, dental therapists practice in a variety of settings and locations, with 40% in private practice and not-for-profit metropolitan area clinics, 32% in tribal clinics, and 28% in private practice and not-for-profit rural area clinics. Maine and Arizona and Connecticut and New Mexico require dental therapists to be dual trained as hygienists (except in Tribal communities), whereas Minnesota and Vermont provide this option but it is not mandatory.

Authorizing the practice of dental therapy remains controversial in the United States. Opponents of the new profession often express concerns about the impact of dental therapists on oral health outcomes.[92] Proponents note that global and domestic studies document the quality of care provided by dental therapists as well as their effectiveness in expanding access to care.[63] Recently, a long-term study demonstrated the effectiveness and acceptability of dental therapists in an Alaskan tribal community. It noted that in communities with care provide by a dental therapist, children had lower rates of tooth extractions and more preventive care than children did in communities without a dental therapist.[26,28] Thanks to studies documenting both the safety and effectiveness of this approach to care delivery and a strong national movement in favor of the new provider,[86] state regulatory agencies and legislative bodies are increasingly beginning to accept the concept of dental therapy, and is likely that in the future more states will pass enabling legislation.

## Dental Assistants

Dental assistants work closely with dentists, dental hygienists, and dental therapists providing chairside assistance in the provision of clinical care and performing administrative duties. Dental assistants prepare patients for treatment, dental examinations, and procedures; sterilize instruments; educate patients about good oral healthcare; and schedule appointments and bill for services.

The dental assisting workforce is adaptable, which is reflected in the variety of their practice settings, which include private dental offices, group specialty and multispecialty dental practices, public and community health clinics, school programs and clinics, mobile clinics, and hospitals.

There are a variety of educational pathways into dental assisting, from on-the-job training to formal education programs offered by high schools, vocational training programs, or postsecondary institutions, especially community colleges. Many formal education programs also offer continuing education for dental assistants wishing to gain competencies in *expanded functions* such as anesthesia, orthodontics, or restorative services. Currently, there are approximately 270 CODA-approved dental assisting programs in the United States.[30] Voluntary certification for dental assistants has been available since 1948, and Dental Assisting National Board (DANB) certification is accepted by some states as qualification to practice expanded functions defined in the state-specific dental practice act. Presently, about 37,000 dental assistants are DANB certified.[33] There is a wide variation in qualifications for entry to dental assisting, range of allowable services, and job titles for dental assistants and expanded function dental assistants (EFDAs) across states.[20]

Estimating dental assistant workforce supply mirrors the challenges discussed about dental hygienists. There are estimated to be nearly 346,500 active individual dental assistants in the United States.[80] This dental assisting workforce is mainly female (94%), with an average age of 37.[80] Just 62% of dental assistants identify as white (non-Hispanic), and more than 23% identify as Hispanic, making this workforce more diverse than either dentists or dental hygienists in the United States.[80] The BLS Occupational Employment and Wages Survey estimates the number of dental assisting jobs; dental assistants may work part-time, may job share, or may work multiple jobs. In 2017, BLS data indicated that there were 337,160 dental assisting jobs in the United States.[75] Between 1990 and 2012, the number of chairside assistants per dentist has stayed consistent at around 1.8.[12]

## Dental Laboratory Technicians

The dental laboratory technician's task is to fabricate crowns, bridges, dentures, and orthodontic appliances based on the prescription of a dentist. Many of these tasks require high precision, and the technician's skill weighs heavily on the ultimate success of the treatment. Laboratory technicians are trained on the job or in formal education programs. In 2018, there were 15 dental technology programs in the United States accredited by CODA.[30] The programs have dropped in number from the 1990s, reducing annual graduates from over 600 to just 300 in 2016.[15] Technicians also may become certified dental technicians in one or more of the areas of complete dentures, partial dentures, crowns and bridges, ceramics, and orthodontics.

Traditionally, technicians were directly employed by dentists and worked in a laboratory in the same office as the dentist. Over time, however, this arrangement became less cost-effective for most dentists. Most technicians now are employed by independent commercial laboratories, which provide their services to dentists. Customarily, dental prostheses were made by hand by technicians using wax, acrylic, or other dental materials, but with the creation of computer-aided design and computer-aided manufacturing (CAD/CAM) of dental prostheses and outsourcing internationally, the use of dental laboratory technicians may be in decline as seen in their trends of employment.[70] The BLS estimated that in 2017 there were 35,630 dental technician jobs in the United States, a 38% reduction from about 60,000 technician jobs in 1996.[74]

## Denturist

During the 1970s and early 1980s, some dental laboratory technicians tried to change state dental practice acts to allow them to treat the public directly for the fabrication of dentures. These technicians call themselves denturists and their occupation denturism. This activity came at approximately the same time as similar movements in Canada. Denturists are now legally recognized in most Canadian provinces/territories and six states (Arizona, Idaho, Maine, Montana, Oregon, and Washington).[64] The requirements for licensing vary among the states but usually include some educational component.

## Community Dental Health Workers

Community health workers (CHWs) have long been part of the medical workforce and are now being deployed in the dental field as well. In some cases, this involves integrating oral health information within traditional lay CHW work, also known as "promotores de salud," who have long been used in the Hispanic community.[27,35] One long-standing model is in the Indian Health Service, where the Community Health Representative (CHR) Program was established in 1968 under the authority of the 1921 Snyder Act (25 USC 13). IHS CHRs, many of whom are American Indians/Alaska Natives, are paraprofessionals who serve as a link between the clinical setting and the community to facilitate access to services and improve the quality and cultural competence of service delivery. They assist by increasing health knowledge of patients and communities through a broad range of activities such as transportation to health visits, outreach, community education, informal counseling, social support, and advocacy. Many CHRs have received specialized training and experience in oral health and, working under the indirect supervision of a dentist or dental hygienist, provide oral health education to patients, apply topical fluorides, and in some locations, oral health assessments.[73] In 2006, the ADA launched a program to formally train a new provider called a community dental health coordinator (CDHC).[3] The focus of the CDHC is on oral health education, disease prevention, and helping patients navigate the healthcare system. Although we have few formal evaluations of these new providers based on the success in medicine they hold promise to increase oral health literacy and access to care.

## Health Professional Workforce for Oral Healthcare

In recent years, there has been a push toward interprofessional education and practice and an acknowledgement that other health professionals can have an impact on their patients' oral health through guidance and preventive treatments. Importantly, with training, primary care providers can assess and evaluate their patients' oral health, incorporate oral health education into their practice, provide prevention and limited treatment, and develop and enhance referral networks and systems.[40] Providers who are increasingly engaged in oral health include primary care physicians, pediatricians, nurses, nurse practitioners, dietitians, and physician's assistants, just to name a few. Primary care providers are increasingly integrating oral healthcare into their primary care service lines. These services include oral health risk assessment, dental screenings, patient education, fluoride and other preventive therapies, and care coordination. Professional organizations have partnered to develop educational resources aimed at equipping nondental professionals with basic oral health knowledge,[34] and payors in about 36 states now reimburse nondental health providers for services such as fluoride varnish application.[85]

## Oral Health Workforce Policy Issues

The US Surgeon General's Call to Action[78] following the first ever report on oral health[79] recommended increasing the diversity, capacity, and flexibility of the workforce to better meet the oral health needs of the nation. The supply, demand, distribution, and quality of the oral health workforce is affected by a country's education, workforce, and payment policies and the organization of the delivery system—all of which in concert have an impact on access to high quality, affordable oral healthcare.

## Healthcare Education Policy

The United States is notably different from most other countries, where national governments directly determine how many practitioners, and of what type, will be produced. The US federal government lacks direct control over dental education, but it can provide incentives to programs to address the *supply of dental personnel* in the form of financial incentives to dental education programs and loan repayment to students or graduates of the programs. For example, the Health Professions Educational Assistance Act of 1963 was designed to alleviate the perceived shortage of health personnel, including dentists. This legislation subsidized existing schools, provided funds for new construction and renovation, and provided direct aid to students. An intended effect of this legislation was the sharp increase in the number of dental graduates. The Comprehensive Health Manpower Training Act of 1971 continued financial aid to schools but with specific provisions for the use of the money attached. This act was followed by a period of financial recession, inflation, slower population growth, and growing belief in some

dental circles that the perceived shortage of dentists had been alleviated and was tending toward an oversupply.

Between the mid-1970s and mid-1980s, there were substantial reductions in federal support to dental education, and since then no major changes have taken place. Today, the Health Resources & Services Administration (HRSA) grants support pre- and post-doctoral training in primary care dentistry, while graduate medical education (GME) funds are available for any hospital-based dental postgraduate training. These sources of federal support are not evenly distributed, and although public institutions may also receive state funding, the rising cost of education has largely been met with tuition increases.

Between 2000 and 2018, tuition for dental education increased exponentially for both public and private institutions. Average educational debt (standardized to 2017 dollars) has risen from $60,000 in 1990 to over $287,000 in 2017 (Figure 8.2), with an increasing rate of growth of this debt burden over time.[88] It needs to be noted that this debt, although called "educational debt," is the total borrowing by a student and includes living expenses in addition to tuition.

There are a number of options to help oral health professional students manage their debt. Pregraduation programs include scholarships, tuition assistance through the National Health Service Corps (NHSC) or the various branches of the armed forces, and federal loans with flexible repayment options. Other available programs following graduation are in return for service obligations and include loan forgiveness and repayment programs through the NHSC, the Indian Health Service, the armed forces, and individual state-administered programs.

Accreditation evolved as a voluntary, self-regulatory means of establishing and maintaining nationally acceptable standards of educational quality and to ensure *high quality of education* in the absence of federal control. Accreditation is the voluntary process by which an agency or organization evaluates and recognizes a program of study or an institution as meeting certain predetermined qualifications or standards.

CODA currently serves as the accrediting body for all training in dentistry in the United States. The commission is a semi-autonomous agency recognized by the United States Department of Education, and its membership includes 30 commissioners, consisting of dental providers, members of the public, and

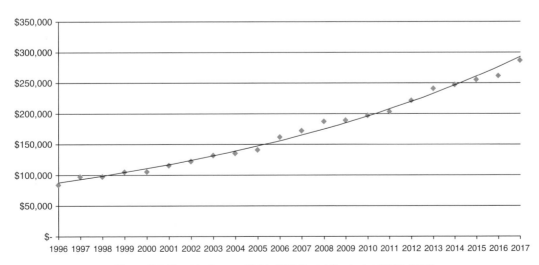

• **Figure 8.2** Trend in Average Debt of US Dental Graduates (1996–2017).

students.[30] In summary, the supply and quality of the oral health-care workforce is generally left to market forces and self-determination within a set of incentive structures provided by state and federal agencies. This arrangement has not resulted in an adequate distribution through the free movement of dentists.

## Policies Addressing Distribution and Composition of the Workforce

In contrast to earlier federal legislation focused on increasing supply, the Health Professions Educational Assistance Act of 1976 concentrated on improving the distribution of primary care personnel. Part of the act's requirements was that dental schools could qualify for federal support funds only if they either (1) increased enrollment of first-year students by a specified proportion, or (2) provided off-site training for dental students. Those grants set the agenda for an alleviation of the maldistribution of health personnel and lack of access to care for underserved populations, which continues to be a concern today.[77] In 2017, it was estimated that the United States had 5866 dental care health professional shortage areas (DHPSA) designations affecting a population of close to 63 million individuals and requiring 10,802 dentists to meet the needs in these areas.[44] At the same time, economic projections show a possible surplus of overall dentists,[37] indicating that more needs to be done to address the current distribution of providers.

The policies and programs developed to influence the distribution of dentists can be grouped into those that focus on the applicant pool, on dental education, and on the practice environment.[56] Mentoring programs and educational support programs such as postbaccalaureate programs help to prepare a diverse applicant pool.[31,91] This preparatory work is further enhanced through holistic admissions.[90] Dental education today includes externship programs[55] and many postgraduate dental clinical training opportunities to expose students to a variety of work settings and populations. Once in practice, providers can be enticed to service in underserved areas through such employment opportunities as federally qualified health centers (FQHCs) or look-alikes, rural and Indian health centers, and dental service organizations (DSOs). Often, private, state, and federal scholarship and loan repayment is available in these settings for immediate service of 2 to 4 years after training.

A key federally sponsored program aimed directly at easing the maldistribution of healthcare providers for which dentists and dental hygienists are eligible is the NHSC. The NHSC provides scholarships and loan repayment in return for obligated service at eligible facilities located in federally designated health professional shortage areas. Authorized in 1970, the NHSC is administered by HRSA within HHS.[43] The scholarship program supports students attending medical schools, dental schools, physician assistant programs, and advanced practice nursing programs. The loan repayment program targets all providers eligible for scholarships along with dental hygienists and behavioral health providers. According to HRSA data, as of August 2018, there were nearly 8000 NHSC providers, the majority of whom were in the loan repayment program, with more than 1000 dentists and more than 265 dental hygienists.[82]

Other incentives around licensure, such as mandatory postgraduate year-1 (PGY-1) or visa programs for foreign-trained dentists, have been explored but are not yet widely implemented.[56] Not surprisingly, the same patterns of maldistribution tend to hold true for hygienists and other dental care professionals who are required by state laws to work under the supervision of a dentist. Changing the scope of practice laws to allow reduced supervision for more flexibility of the current workforce such as dental hygienists and the development of new providers like dental therapists can be seen as additional strategies to address the maldistribution of providers.

## State Health Professions Practice Acts

State licensure is a labor market entry and practice requirement for dentists, hygienists, dental therapists and, in some states, dental assistants, laboratory technicians, and denturists. Licensing is the most robust form of occupational regulation, protecting both the use of an occupational title and a defined scope of practice. Licensure is enacted by states to certify baseline competency, protect public safety, and ensure quality of services. As a regulatory policy, licensing is enacted through state practice acts by the general assembly with rules and regulations generally promulgated by state boards. Such regulatory policy includes entry requirements (such as educational and examination) and practice definition (allowable tasks and supervisory requirements). Although licensure offers a robust mechanism for ensuring safety and quality at a state level while allowing for local innovations, variations in regulatory approaches threaten interstate mobility of the workforce and have resulted in varying practice environments. Regulatory reforms aimed at addressing these issues are challenging and require an onerous legislative process.[41] This approach also creates regulatory barriers for new types of providers and for innovative care delivery systems.[42]

To improve ease of movement of providers, *licensure by credentials* has been adopted by many states to allow providers who have passed a licensing examination in one state to present their credentials to another state to which they want to move; if the credentials meet the criteria, the board grants a license. The actual process and requirements vary widely but generally include requirements for some minimum time in practice and no evidence of existing or pending disciplinary or legal actions. In 2014, 46 states plus the District of Columbia and Puerto Rico allowed some form of licensure by credentials.[7] Encompassed within this concept is *reciprocity*, by which two or more states agree to honor each other's licenses.

This reciprocity among states and movement of providers has been made somewhat easier by the development of four regional examining boards. A dentist passing the clinical licensing examination in any participating state can apply, usually within 5 years of the original examination, for license in any state in the same region without having to take another clinical examination. By 2016, all states except New York and Delaware (which require a 1-year GPR or AEGD residency for licensure) were involved in one or more of these four regional examining boards.[41] To a lesser extent, the same systems of reciprocity and regional or national licensing are in place for hygienists, technicians, and assistants. But unlike for dentists, the scope of practice for these providers is so highly variable that movement to another state may be met with an increased or decreased set of allowable tasks or supervision requirements (Box 8.1). For dental therapists, the movement among states is much more complicated, with only a few states so far approving licensure, and those that do vary in their requirements.

Scope of practice law changes are necessary as clinical practice and technology evolve, but the current political system for making these evidence-based decisions is quite an onerous process. In most states, dental therapists, hygienists, technicians, and assistants are

World Dental Federation (FDI) Definitions

ADOPTED by the FDI General Assembly November 2000 in Paris, France REVISED September 2015 in Bangkok, Thailand

Dentist: Leader of the dental team with sole responsibility for diagnosis, treatment, organization and management, and the supervision of allied dental personnel, with the aim of providing the highest quality of oral healthcare to patients.

Allied Dental Personnel: Member of the dental team, to whom the dentist may delegate certain tasks pertaining to the delivery of oral healthcare. The functions, duties and roles of the allied dental personnel are regulated in accordance with the current legislation of the country and/or local regulations.

Delegation: Where permitted by law, assignment of specific tasks (under constant supervision and by keeping full responsibility) to another appropriately trained and qualified member of the dental team by the dentist.

Supervision: To oversee, direct or take charge of a person's activities to ensure that tasks are performed properly and safely; supervisory responsibility etc.

Monitoring: The observation, supervision or review of duties or functions performed by allied dental personnel under the supervision of a dentist; to keep under observation; to measure or test at intervals, esp. for the purpose of regulation or control.

Referral: The direction of a patient for treatment to a doctor, usually a dentist or dental specialist.

---

licensed and regulated by state boards of dentistry whose membership is mostly made up of dentists, with varying dental hygiene representation. Requests for greater scope of practice or reduced supervision levels have met conflict in this arena because organized dentistry generally opposes such moves. State regulatory structures have come under scrutiny as the Federal Trade Commission has investigated several antitrust cases involving state boards of dentistry, leading to the expansion of separate licensing boards for dental hygiene[24] and/or increased representation of hygienists and consumer/public members on dental licensing boards. Some states allow pilot projects to test new models before they are proposed in the legislative process.[25,68]

States that use expanded evidence-based scope of practice changes can improve access to care by enabling a more flexible workforce with greater capacity to serve where they are employed (Figure 8.3). It is becoming increasingly common for dental hygienists to practice without direct supervision in public health settings, schools, health centers, nursing homes, and similar types of facilities. In 1986, Colorado became the first state to permit the *independent practice* of dental hygiene, followed by California in 1997 and New Mexico in 1999. As of late 2019, the majority of states had provisions enabling dental hygienists to assess and treat patients without specific authorization by a dentist.[19]

Moves toward utilization of EFDAs were given impetus during the 1960s. Federal funds became available for dental schools to operate dental auxiliary utilization programs, which trained dental students in four-handed dentistry, and later for training in expanded auxiliary management programs, which taught dental students to work with auxiliaries who carried out an even wider range of functions, including packing and carving amalgams in cavities prepared by the students. The studies with EFDAs were carried out in a variety of special institutional settings, although considerable effort was made to simulate the characteristics of the private office. Limited studies in private offices also have been conducted,[60,71] and although they found some difficulties in adjustment of office routines, they confirmed that EFDAs can be successfully used there. EFDAs are routinely used in the Indian Health Service and military and Department of Veterans Affairs facilities and by some private practitioners in states where they are permitted.[51,60]

Today, many states regulate dental assisting practice using a tiered approach to task permissions based on the education, training, and experience of the dental assistant.[20] Some offer as many as five levels and job titles for those working in dental assisting within

their jurisdiction. This regulatory approach has created a career ladder for those in dental assisting that permits practice in a variety of EFDA roles. In those states recognizing EFDAs, additional training and/or passing a competency exam is required to practice in expanded roles. In a few states, the tasks (Box 8.2) that may be delegated by a dentist to a dental assistant mostly remain at the discretion of the supervising dentist. In other states, only tasks prohibited or not permitted to the dental assistant are enumerated in legislation or regulation.

The interest of government in promoting EFDAs and new workforce models is in increased productivity and the subsequent presumed lower cost of care to the public. In fact, the US General Accounting Office, in a 1980 report, urged states to develop practice acts that permitted expanded functions and recommended that all federal programs make wider use of EFDAs.[84] Additionally, the Federal Trade Commission has been active in addressing anticompetitive state dental regulations as a way to increase the output of basic dental services, reduce costs, and expand access to dental care.[39]

## Collaborative Practice, Interprofessional and Intraprofessional Models

The model of small private dental practice for care delivery is declining proportionally as new, larger, integrated organizational structures for oral health service delivery emerge and practice settings expand, enabled by new technology and care modalities.[52] Today, the oral health team has an increasing variety of practice options both for the traditional dental team and for interprofessional and public health practice. With the expanded number of professions and practice organizations comes new ways of working together outside the employment hierarchy of a traditional dental office. Collaborative practice can be described in terms ranging from philosophical to practical including common, clinical, and legal definitions.[57]

Although more common in medicine, in dentistry, a wide range of practices fall under the rubric of activities that make up collaborative practice with the goals of improving access and quality while reducing cost. For example, dental therapists and dental hygienists in alternative, public health, or direct access practice often must work under collaborative practice agreements with their supervising dentists that stipulate the specifics of their supervision and practice authority. Barriers exist to expanding collaborative practice in oral health, including prohibitive state policy (for example, state laws on who can own dental practices or supervise various staff), a lack of collaborative education, health IT interoperability,

# Variation in Dental Hygiene Scope of Practice by State

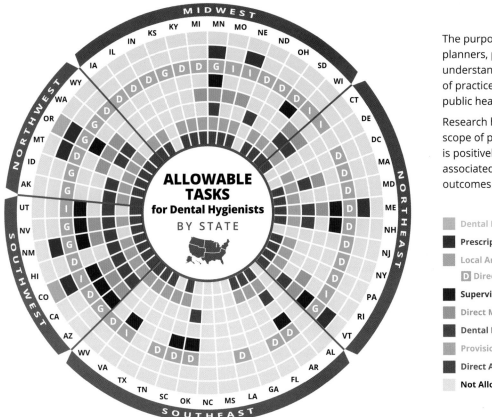

The purpose of this graphic is to help planners, policymakers, and others understand differences in legal scope of practice across states, particularly in public health settings.

Research has shown that a broader scope of practice for dental hygienists is positively and significantly associated with improved oral health outcomes in a state's population.[49,50]

Dental Hygiene Diagnosis

**Prescriptive Authority**

Local Anesthesia

D Direct  I Indirect  G General

**Supervision of Dental Assistants**

Direct Medicaid Reimbursement

**Dental Hygiene Treatment Planning**

Provision of Sealants

**Direct Access to Prophylaxis**

Not Allowed / No Law

## Dental Hygiene Diagnosis

The identification of oral conditions for which treatment falls within the dental hygiene scope of practice, as part of a dental hygiene treatment plan.

## Prescriptive Authority

The ability to prescribe, administer, and dispense fluoride, topical medications, and chlorhexidine.

## Local Anesthesia

The administration of local anesthesia.

### LEVEL OF SUPERVISION

**D  Direct:** The dentist is required to be physically present during the administration of local anesthesia by the dental hygienist.

**I  Indirect:** The dentist is required to be on the premises during the administration of local anesthesia by the dental hygienist.

**G  General:** The dentist is required to authorize the administration of local anesthesia by the dental hygienist but is not required to be on the premises during the procedure.

## Supervision of Dental Assistants

The ability to supervise dental assistants when performing tasks within the dental hygiene scope of practice.

## Direct Medicaid Reimbursement

The direct Medicaid reimbursement of dental hygiene services to the dental hygienist.

## Dental Hygiene Treatment Planning

The ability of a dental hygienist to assess oral conditions and formulate treatment plans for services within the dental hygiene scope of practice.

## Provision of Sealants Without Prior Examination

The ability of a dental hygienist working in a public health setting to provide sealants without prior examination by a dentist.

## Direct Access to Prophylaxis from a Dental Hygienist

The ability of a dental hygienist working in a public health setting to provide prophylaxis without prior examination by a dentist.

## Not Allowed / No Law

Sources: 1. Langelier M, Baker B, Continelli T. *Development of a New Dental Hygiene Professional Practice Index by State, 2016.* Rensselaer, NY: Oral Health Workforce Research Center, Center for Health Workforce Studies, School of Public Health, SUNY Albany; November 2016. 2. Langelier M, Continelli T, Moore J, Baker B, Surdu S. Expanded Scopes of Practice for Dental Hygienists Associated With Improved Oral Health Outcomes for Adults. *Health Affairs.* 2016;35(12):2207-2215.

http://www.oralhealthworkforce.org/wp-content/uploads/2017/03/OHWRC_Dental_Hygiene_Scope_of_Practice_2016.pdf

This work was supported by the Health Resources and Services Administration (HRSA) of the U.S. Department of Health and Human Services (HHS), under the Health Workforce Research Center Cooperative Agreement Program (U81HP27843). The content and conclusions presented herein are those of the authors and should not be construed as the official position or policy of, nor should any endorsements be inferred by HRSA, HHS or the U.S. Government.

This graphic describes the highest level of practice available to a dental hygienist in a state, including dental hygiene therapy. The graphic is for informational purposes only and scope of practice is subject to change. Contact the applicable dental board or your attorney for specific legal advice.

Last Updated January 2019.

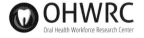

• **Figure 8.3** Allowable Tasks for Dental Hygienists by State.[67]

---

**• BOX 8.2**  **Examples of Duties Permitted to be Carried Out by Expanded-Duty Dental Personnel in the United[6] States**

- Applying topical fluorides
- Applying desensitizing agents
- Applying pit-and-fissure sealants
- Placing, carving, and polishing amalgam restorations
- Perform coronal polishing
- Placing and finishing composite restorations
- Placing and removing matrix bands

- Placing and removing rubber dams
- Monitoring nitrous oxide use
- Taking impressions for study casts
- Exposing and developing radiographs
- Removing sutures
- Removing and replacing ligature wires on orthodontic appliances

---

and evidence-based care protocols. Collaboration can exist under any financing model but may be facilitated best when providers are not competing for a fee for any particular service but are working under global budgets.

## State and Federal Dental Care Payment Policy

The final and critical component of workforce policy as discussed in this chapter is how we pay for dental care services. No matter the distribution, composition, or quality of the workforce, they must be paid in some way for providing care. As a country, the United States made progress on covering children through Medicaid, the Children's Health Insurance Program, and the Patient Protection and Affordable Care Act,[48] but a large number of adults remain uninsured, in large part because Medicaid does not mandate adult coverage and Medicare does not cover dental care at all. Therefore, it is not surprising that cost remains the most reported barrier to care, even over workforce availability.[87] Further, as the traditional private practice model is unsustainable in many low-income and underserved areas, these workforce efforts need to be complemented with institutions and payment systems that can be more flexible and cost effective for the populations that remain in need.[58] Federally qualified health centers, the Indian Health Service, and the Veterans Health Administration are all examples of how government funding policy can lead to alternative arrangements that employ dentists in areas where they might not be able to set up a practice.

Policy drives not only the population covered but, importantly, who can get paid for providing services and what services they can bill for. State laws cover not only the fee schedules in public programs but also which providers are billable providers and what modalities, such as telehealth, are acceptable for billing. This set of policies affects the ability of the workforce to sustainably address oral health needs.

## Conclusion

In summary, the oral healthcare workforce is evolving toward team-based care and expanding to include new types of dental providers and other health professionals who can address oral health in nondental settings. Regardless, access to dental care in the United States continues to be a large problem, and further workforce efforts are needed to improve the flexibility, diversity, and capacity of the oral health team. Health workforce policy plays a critical role in ensuring the quality, supply, distribution, and composition of the workforce.

## Acknowledgments

The authors would like to thank Dr. Jean Calvo and Aubri Kottek for their research assistance on this chapter.

## References

1. American Board of Dental Public Health. *Active Diplomates of the American Board of Dental Public Health. 2017–2018*; 2018. Available from: https://aaphd.memberclicks.net/assets/ABDPH/Active%20Diplomates%20of%20the%20American%20Board%20of%20Dental%20Public%20Health%202017-2018%20-1.pdf.
2. American Board of Dental Public Health. *Bylaws of the American Board of Dental Public Health*; 2018. Available from: https://aaphd.memberclicks.net/assets/ABDPH/ABDPH-Bylaws-2018-01-20.pdf.
3. American Dental Association. About community dental health coordinators. *Action for Dental Health*; 2016. Available from: http://www.ada.org/en/public-programs/action-for-dental-health/community-dental-health-coordinators.
4. American Dental Association. *Distribution of Dentists in the United States by Region and State, 1995*. Chicago, IL: ADA; 1997.
5. American Dental Association. *Distribution of Dentists in the United States by Region and State*. Chicago, IL: ADA; 1998. 2000.
6. American Dental Association. *Expanded Functions for Dental Assistants*; 2011. Available from: http://www.aapd.org/assets/1/7/StateLawsonDAs.pdf.
7. American Dental Association. *Licensure by Credentials*; 2017. Available from: http://www.ada.org/en/education-careers/licensure/licensure-dental-students/licensure-by-credentials.
8. American Dental Association. *Principles of Ethics and Code of Professional Conduct*; 2018. Available from: https://www.ada.org/en/about-the-ada/principles-of-ethics-code-of-professional-conduct.
9. American Dental Association. *State Dental Boards: Clinical Exams for Initial Dental Licensure*; 2017. Available from: http://www.ada.org/~/media/ADA/Education%20and%20Careers/Files/clinical_test_states_accept.pdf?la=en.
10. American Dental Association Health Policy Institute. *2017–18 Survey of Advanced Dental Education (Tables in Excel)*. Chicago, IL: ADA; 2019.
11. American Dental Association Health Policy Institute. *Employment of Dental Practice Personnel: Select Results from the Survey of Dental Practice (Tables in Excel) Table 1*; 2015. Available from: http://www.ada.org/~/media/ADA/Science and https://success.ada.org/en/practice-management/survey-of-dental-practice.
12. American Dental Association Health Policy Institute. *Supply of Dentists in the United States: 2001–2016 (Tables in Excel)*. Chicago, IL: ADA; 2017.
13. American Dental Association Health Policy Institute. *Survey of Advanced Dental Education*. Chicago, IL: ADA; 2016.
14. American Dental Association Health Policy Institute. *Trends in U.S. Dental Schools*; 2018. Available from: https://www.ada.org/~/media/ADA/Science%20and%20Research/HPI/Files/HPIGraphic_1218_2.pdf?la=en.
15. American Dental Education Association. *Dental Laboratory Technology Graduates, 1990 to 2016*. Available from: https://www.adea.org/data/students/; 2017.
16. American Dental Education Association. *ADEA. Snapshot of Dental Education 2017–18*. Available from: https://www.adea.org/snapshot/.
17. American Dental Hygienists' Association. *Career Paths*; 2018. Available from: http://www.adha.org/professional-roles.

18. American Dental Hygienists' Association. *Standards for Clinical Dental Hygiene Practice*. Revised. Chicago, IL: ADHA; 2016:2016.

19. American Dental Hygienists' Association Division of Governmental Affairs. *Dental Hygiene Practice Act Overview: Permitted Functions and Supervision Levels by State;* 2018. Available from: https://www.adha.org/resources-docs/7511_Permitted_Services_Supervision_Levels_by_State.pdf.

20. Baker B, Langelier M, Moore J, et al. *The Dental Assistant Workforce in the United States*. Rensselaer, NY: Center for Health Workforce Studies, School of Public Health, SUNY Albany; 2015.

21. Barbey C, Sahni N, Kocher R, et al. Physician workforce trends and their implications for spending growth. *Health Affairs (Millwood);* 2017. Available from: https://www.healthaffairs.org/do/10.1377/hblog20170728.061252/full/.

22. Bradley Munson, Marko Vujicic. *Supply of Dentists in the United States Is Likely to Grow.* American Dental Association Health Policy Institute; 2014.

23. Brickle CM, Self KD. Dental therapists as new oral health practitioners: increasing access for underserved populations. *J Dent Educ.* 2017;81(9):eS65–eS72.

24. California Department of Consumer Affairs. *Dental Hygiene Committee of California;* 2018. Available from: https://www.dhcc.ca.gov.

25. California Office of Statewide Health Planning and Development. *Health Workforce Pilot Projects Program;* 2018. Available from: https://oshpd.ca.gov/workforce-capacity/health-workforce-pilot-projects/.

26. Chi DL, Hopkins S, Zahlis E, Randall CL, Senturia K, Orr E, Lenaker D, et al. Provider and community perspectives of dental therapists in Alaska's Yukon-Kuskokwim Delta: A qualitative programme evaluation. *Community Dentistry and Oral Epidemiology;* 2019.

27. Centers for Disease Control and Prevention. *Promotores de Salud/Community Health Workers.* Health Equity, Minority Health, Public Health Practice. 2019. Available from: https://www.cdc.gov/minorityhealth/promotores/index.html.

28. Chi DL, Lenaker D, Mancl L, et al. Dental therapists linked to improved dental outcomes for Alaska Native communities in the Yukon-Kuskokwim Delta. *J Public Health Dent.* 2018;78(2):175–182.

29. Commission on Dental Accreditation. *Accreditation Standards for Dental Hygiene Education Programs.* Effective January 1, 2013. Chicago, IL: CODA; 2018.

30. Commission on Dental Accreditation. *Dental Programs;* 2018. Available from: https://www.ada.org/en/coda/find-a-program.

31. Davies TA, Kaye E, Stahlberger M, et al. Improving diversity of dental students through the Boston University master's of oral health sciences postbaccalaureate program. *J Dent Educ.* 2019;83(3):287–295.

32. Deloitte. Data US: Dental Hygienists. 2018; Deloitte report produced using ACS PUMS 1 year estimates. Available from: https://census.gov/programs-surveys/acs/technical-documentation/pums.html. Available from: https://datausa.io/profile/soc/292021/.

33. Dental Assisting National Board. *About DANB;* 2018. Available from: https://www.danb.org/About-DANB.aspx.

34. Douglass AB, Gonsalves W, Maier R, et al. Smiles for Life: a national oral health curriculum for family medicine. A model for curriculum development by STFM groups. *Fam Med.* 2007;39(2):88–90.

35. Edelstein BL. Pediatric dental-focused interprofessional interventions: rethinking early childhood oral health management. *Dent Clin North Am.* 2017;61(3):589–606.

36. Edelstein BL. Training new dental health providers in the United States. *J Public Health Dent.* 2011;71(suppl 2):S3–S8.

37. Eklund SA, Bailit HL. Estimating the number of dentists needed in 2040. *J Dent Educ.* 2017;81(8):eS146–eS152.

38. FDI World Dental Federation. *Supervision of Allied Dental Personnel.* Adopted by the FDI General Assembly November, 2000 in Paris, France. Revised September, 2015 in Bangkok, Thailand. 2015. Available from: https://www.fdiworlddental.org/resources/policy-statements-and-resolutions/supervision-of-allied-dental-personnel.

39. Federal Trade Commission. Letter to Honorable Senator Peggy Lehner re: SB330. In: Plannng OoP, ed. FTC; 2017. Available from: https://www.ftc.gov/system/files/documents/advocacy_documents/ftc-staff-comment-ohio-state-senate-regarding-competitive-effects-sb-330-increasing-access-quality/v170003_ftc_staff_comment_to_ohio_state_senate_re_ohio_sb_330_re_dental_therapists_and_hygienists.pdf.

40. Fisher-Owens SA, Mertz E. Preventing oral disease: alternative providers and places to address this commonplace condition. *Pediatr Clin North Am.* 2018;65(5):1063–1072.

41. Friedrichsen SW. Moving toward 21st-century clinical licensure examinations in dentistry. *J Dent Educ.* 2016;80(6):639–640.

42. Gavil AI, Koslov TI. A flexible health care workforce requires a flexible regulatory environment: promoting health care competition through regulatory reform. *Wash Law Rev.* 2016;91(1):147–197.

43. Heisler EJ. *The National Health Service Corps (CRS Report R44970).* Washington, DC: Congressional Research Service; 2017.

44. Henry J. Kaiser. *Family Foundation. Dental Care Health Professional Shortage Areas (HPSAs).* Available from: https://www.kff.org/other/state-indicator/dental-care-health-professional-shortage-areas-hpsas/?currentTimeframe=0&sortModel=%7B%22colId%22:%22Location%22,%22sort%22:%22asc%22%7D.

45. Hillenbrand H. The necessity for trained advanced dental professionals. *J Dent Educ.* 1981;45(2):76–87.

46. Historical Statistics of the United States, Colonial Times to 1957: A Statistical Abstract Supplement. Prepared by the Bureau of the Census with the Cooperation of the Social Science Research Council. (Washington, D. C.: U. S. Department of Commerce, Bureau of the Census. 1960. Pp. xi, 789. $6.00.). The American Historical Review. 1961.

47. Johnson P. Dental hygiene practice: international profile and future directions. *Int Dent J.* 1992;42(6):451–459.

48. Kranz AM, Dick AW. Changes in pediatric dental coverage and visits following the implementation of the affordable care act. *Health Services Research.* 2019;54(2):437–445.

49. Langelier M, Baker B. *Development of a New Dental Hygiene Professional Practice Index by State, 2016.* Rensselaer, NY: Oral Health Workforce Research Center, Center for Health Workforce Studies, School of Public Health, SUNY Albany; November 2016.

50. Langelier M, Continelli T, Moore J, et al. Expanded scopes of practice for dental hygienists associated with improved oral health outcomes for adults. *Health Aff (Millwood).* 2016;35(12):2207–2215.

51. LeGallee-Byle B. Trends in dental assistant utilization: a comparative study. Part II. *Dent Assist.* 1989;58(2):17.

52. Lo Sasso AT, Starkel RL, Warren MN, et al. Practice settings and dentists' job satisfaction. *J Am Dent Assoc.* 2015;146(8):600–609.

53. Lobene RR, Kerr A. *The Forsyth Experiment: an Alternative System for Dental Care.* Cambridge, MA: Harvard University Press; 1979.

54. Mathu-Muju KR. Chronicling the dental therapist movement in the United States. *J Public Health Dent.* 2011;71(4):278–288.

55. Mays KA. Community-based dental education models: an analysis of current practices at U.S. dental schools. *J Dent Educ.* 2016;80(10):1188–1195.

56. Mertz E, Anderson G, Grumbach K, et al. *Evaluation of Strategies to Recruit Oral Health Care Providers to Underserved Areas of California.* San Francisco, CA: Center for California Health Workforce Studies, UCSF Center for the Health Professions; 2004.

57. Mertz E, Lindler V, Dower C. *Collaborative Practice in American Dentistry: Practice and Potential.* UCSF Center for the Health Professions; 2011.

58. Mertz EA, Wides CD, Kottek AM, et al. Underrepresented minority dentists: quantifying their numbers and characterizing the communities they serve. *Health Aff (Millwood).* 2016;35(12): 2190–2199.

59. Moffat SM, Foster Page LA, Thomson WM. New Zealand's School Dental Service over the decades: its response to social, political, and economic influences, and the effect on oral health inequalities. *Front Public Health.* 2017;5:177.

60. Mullins MR, Kaplan A, Bader JD, et al. Summary results of the Kentucky dental practice demonstration: a cooperative project with practicing general dentists. *J Am Dent Assoc.* 1983;106(6):817–825.

61. Munson B, Vujicic M. *Supply of Full-Time Equivalent Dentists in the U.S Expected to Increase Steadily.* Chicago, IL: American Dental Association Health Policy Institute; 2018.

62. Nagel RJ. The development and implementation of dental health aide therapists in Alaska. *J Calif Dent Assoc.* 2011;39(1):31–35.

63. Nash DA, Friedman JW, Mathu-Muju K. *A Review of the Global Literature on Dental Therapists.* Battle Creek, MI: W.K. Kellogg Foundation; 2012.

64. National Denturist Association. *Affiliates Map.* Available from: http://nationaldenturist.com/affiliates

65. Niessen L, Kleinman D, Wilson A. Practice characteristics of women dentists. *J Am Dent Assoc.* 1986;113:883–888.

66. Office of the Revisor of Statutes. Minnesota statutes: Dental Therapist and Advanced Dental Therapist. In. Pub.L.No.150A.105 and 106. St. Paul, MN: Office of the Revisor of Statutes; 2017.

67. Oral Health Workforce Research Center. *Variation in Dental Hygiene Scope of Practice by State*; 2019. Available from: http://www.oralhealthworkforce.org/resources/variation-in-dental-hygiene-scope-of-practice-by-state/.

68. Oregon Health Authority. *Dental Pilot Projects*; 2018. Available from: https://www.oregon.gov/oha/PH/PREVENTIONWELLNESS/ORALHEALTH/DENTALPILOTPROJECTS/Pages/index.aspx.

69. Organisation for Economic Co-operation and Development. *Dentists.* Paris: OECD Publishing; 2009.

70. Poticny DJ, Klim J. CAD/CAM in-office technology: innovations after 25 years for predictable, esthetic outcomes. *J Am Dent Assoc.* 2010;141:5S–9S.

71. Redig D, Snyder M, Nevitt G, et al. Expanded duty dental auxiliaries in four private dental offices: the first year's experience. *J Am Dent Assoc.* 1974;88(5):969–984.

72. Rephann T, Wanchek T. Filling the gaps: explanations for disparities in the distribution of dentists among U.S. counties. *Journal of Regional Analysis and Policy.* 2016;46(1):60–71.

73. Ricks T, Mork N. *Personal Communication.* Indian Health Service, 2018.

74. U.S. Bureau of Labor Statistics. *Occupational Outlook Handbook: Dental and Ophthalmic Laboratory Technicians and Medical Appliance Technicians*; 2016. Available from: https://www.bls.gov/ooh/production/dental-and-ophthalmic-laboratory-technicians-and-medical-appliance-technicians.htm.

75. U.S. Bureau of Labor Statistics. *Occupational Outlook Handbook: Dental Assistants*; 2016. Available from: https://www.bls.gov/ooh/healthcare/dental-assistants.htm.

76. U.S. Bureau of Labor Statistics. *Occupational Outlook Handbook: Dental Hygienists*; 2016. Available from: https://www.bls.gov/ooh/healthcare/dental-hygienists.htm.

77. U.S. Department of Health and Human Services. *National and State-Level Projections of Dentists and Dental Hygienists in the U.S. 2012–2012.* Rockville, MD: National Center for Health Workforce Analysis, Health Resources and Services Administration; 2015.

78. U.S. Department of Health and Human Services. *National Call to Action to Promote Oral Health.* Rockville, MD: U.S. Department of Health and Human Services, National Institute of Dental and Craniofacial Research, National Institutes of Health; 2003.

79. U.S. Department of Health and Human Services. *Oral Health in America: A Report of the Surgeon General.* Rockville, MD: U.S. Department of Health and Human Services; 2000.

80. United States Census Bureau. *American Community Survey 2012–2016 (5 year average).* In:2018.

81. University of Michigan. *History of the Dental Public Health Program.* Available from: https://dent.umich.edu/about-school/department/crse/history-dental-public-health-program.

82. US Department of Health and Human Services. *HRSA Data Warehouse: Grants - FY; 2017.* 2017. Available from: https://data.hrsa.gov/.

83. US Department of Labor. *Occupational Employment and Wages, May 2018: 29-2021 Dental Hygienists*; 2017. Available from: https://www.bls.gov/oes/current/oes292021.htm#nat.

84. US General Accounting Office. *Increased use of expanded function dental auxiliaries would benefit consumers, dentists, and taxpayers.* In Publication No. HRD-80-51. Washington, DC: Government Printing Office; 1980.

85. Veschusio CN, Probst JC, Martin AB, et al. Impact of South Carolina's Medicaid fluoride varnish reimbursement policy on children's receipt of fluoride varnish in medical and dental settings. *J Public Health Dent.* 2016;76(4):356–361.

86. W.K. Kellogg Foundation. *Dental Therapy Resource Library*; 2018. Available from: http://dentaltherapyresourceguide.wkkf.org/.

87. Wall T, Nasseh K, Vujicic M. *Most Important Barriers to Dental Care Are Financial, Not Supply Related.* American Dental Association; 2014.

88. Wanchek T, Cook BJ, Valachovic RW. Annual ADEA survey of dental school seniors: 2017 graduating class. *J Dent Educ.* 2017;81(5):613–630.

89. Wanchek T, Cook BJ, Valachovic RW. US dental school applicants and enrollees, 2016 entering class. *J Dent Educ.* 2017;81(11):1373–1382.

90. Wells A, Brunson D, Sinkford JC, et al. Working with dental school admissions committees to enroll a more diverse student body. *J Dent Educ.* 2011;75(5):685–695.

91. Wides CD, Brody HA, Alexander CJ, et al. Long-term outcomes of a dental postbaccalaureate program: increasing dental student diversity and oral health care access. *J Dent Educ.* 2013;77(5):537–547.

92. Wright JT, Graham F, Hayes C, et al. A systematic review of oral health outcomes produced by dental teams incorporating midlevel providers. *J Am Dent Assoc.* 2013;144(1):75–91.

# 9

# Infection Prevention and Control

EVE CUNY, MS

KATHY EKLUND, RDH, MPH

## CHAPTER OUTLINE

## Introduction

The foundation of infection control lies in the principle of standard precautions. The primary goal is to prevent transmission of infectious diseases. In healthcare settings, including dental healthcare settings, the primary objective is to prevent healthcare-associated infections (HAIs) in patients and occupational injuries and illnesses in personnel.

Standard precautions are a set of infection prevention and control precautions that when used consistently ensure the safe delivery of oral healthcare. Standard precautions apply to contact with (1) blood; (2) all body fluids, secretions, and excretions (except sweat), regardless of whether they contain blood; (3) nonintact skin; and (4) mucous membranes.[29] Standard precautions include hand hygiene, personal protective equipment, respiratory hygiene, sharps safety, safe injection practices, sterilization, and disinfection of contaminated clinical surfaces.[18]

## Guidelines for Infection Control

Infection prevention and control guidance for dental healthcare settings has evolved from the early 1980s to the present. In the early 1980s human immunodeficiency virus (HIV) emerged in the

United States. HIV infection was not the only infectious disease to raise concerns about infectious risks associated with dental treatment. The risk of hepatitis B virus (HBV) infection was already acknowledged in dental practice settings, but the concern of HIV infection was a key driver for infection-control guidance in the 1980s.

The American Dental Association (ADA) published an infection-control guidance in the pre-HIV era,[2] mostly concerned with hepatitis, but the advent of HIV in the early 1980s led to more detailed guidance. Guidelines were developed by the ADA,[3] and the American Association of Public Health Dentistry produced its guidelines in 1986.[1]

As HIV transmission became a concern in healthcare settings, agencies began developing guidance on how to prevent transmission from patient to healthcare personnel (HCP), HCP to patient, and patient to patient. The Centers for Disease Control and Prevention (CDC) issued definitive guidelines initially in 1986 with an update in 1993, and a considerably extended version was released in December of 2003.[29,30,31] The CDC also developed infection-control guidelines for field examinations for surveys or research studies based on the 1993 CDC guidance.[18]

In 2016, the CDC published *Summary of Infection Prevention Practices in Dental Settings: Basic Expectations for Safe Care.*[28] The information presented is primarily from the previously published *Guidelines for Infection Control in Dental Health-Care Settings—2003.* This summary document represents infection-prevention expectations for safe care in dental settings and contains a two-part checklist for dental practice settings to evaluate compliance with the recommendations.[28] In addition to recommendations for infection control in dentistry, there are also specific, broader recommendations for sterilization, disinfection, and healthcare worker immunizations.[16,32]

## Infection Prevention and Control: Regulatory and Guidance Agencies

Numerous agencies and organizations develop standards and regulations related to infection control (Table 9.1). Among these, four agencies of the US government play key roles in infection prevention and control in the United States. Guidelines and regulations developed by these four agencies have established national standards for infection prevention and control related to patient care, patient care equipment and materials, employee safety, and the environment. In addition to federal agencies, many state, county, and city government agencies have regulations that apply to

**• TABLE 9.1 Agencies That Provide Guidance or Regulations for Infection Control and Prevention**

| Agency/Organization and Website | U.S. Federal Agency | Regulatory Authority Yes/No | Key Document or Activity That Affects Infection Prevention and Control in Dentistry |
|---|---|---|---|
| Centers for Disease Control and Prevention (CDC) http://www.cdc.gov | U.S. Department of Health & Human Services (HHS) https://www.hhs.gov/ | No—Develops evidence-based guidelines and develops and applies disease prevention and control, environmental health, and health promotion and health education | CDC Guideline for Infection Control in Dental Healthcare Settings—2003 / Other CDC guidelines and guidance for healthcare settings and healthcare personnel |
| National Institute for Occupational Safety and Health (NIOSH) http://www.cdc.gov/niosh/ | HHS https://www.hhs.gov CDC http://www.cdc.gov | No—Conducts research and makes recommendations to prevent dental healthcare provider injury and illness | Personal Protective Equipment http://www.cdc.gov/niosh/topics/PTD/ Eye safety Respirators Protective clothing / Selecting Sharps Containers http://www.cdc.gov/niosh/docs/97-111/ / Sharps Injury Prevention http://www.cdc.gov/niosh/topics/bbp/safer/step1b.html |
| Occupational Safety and Health Agency (OSHA) https://www.osha.gov | U.S. Department of Labor https://www.dol.gov | Yes—Employers in the private sector for the health and safety of employees | OSHA Bloodborne Pathogens Standard / Hazards Communication Standard |
| Environmental Protection Agency (EPA) https://www.epa.gov | EPA | Yes—Variety of public and private sector regulations | Hospital Antimicrobial Disinfectant Registration / Hazardous Waste Regulations—RCRA, etc. |
| U.S. Food & Drug Administration (FDA) https://www.fda.gov/ | HHS | Yes—Regulates through pre-market clearance for safety and efficacy | Medical Device Clearance / Medical Product Clearance / Medical device safety and reporting MAUDE |
| American National Standards Institute (ANSI)[a] https://www.ansi.org | | No | Standards for protective clothing, eyewear, etc. |
| Association for the Advancement of Medical Instrumentation (AAMI)[a] https://www.aami.org | | No | ST79 Comprehensive Guide to Steam Sterilization |
| International Standards Organization (ISO)[a] http://www.iso.org/iso/home.html | | No | ISO 9000 Series Quality Management |
| American Dental Association (ADA) Standards Committee[a] http://www.ada.org/en/science-research/dental-standards/us-tag-for-iso-tc-106-dentistry | | No | Sub-TAG 3: Dental Terminology, Sub-TAG 4: Dental Instruments, Sub-TAG 6: Dental Equipment, |
| Organization for Safety, Asepsis and Prevention (OSAP) www.osap.org | | No | Credible resources and tools for infection prevention and control in dentistry |

[a]Standard setting organization

infection control. These include state boards of licensure, state health departments, and city and county health departments, among others.

**The Centers for Disease Control and Prevention (CDC)** is one of eight federal public health agencies within the U.S. Department of Health and Human Services. Its mission is to increase the health security of our nation. As the nation's health protection agency, the CDC saves lives and protects people from health threats. To accomplish this mission, the CDC supports and conducts critical science, provides health information to protect our nation against expensive and dangerous health threats, and responds when health crises arise. The CDC develops guidelines and recommendations; among these are infection-control recommendations for healthcare settings. The CDC is not a regulatory agency and does not enforce the guidelines it develops. Box 9.1 provides CDC guidance documents specific to dental healthcare settings and Box 9.2 contains CDC guidance documents applicable to all healthcare settings.

Many state licensing boards and department of public health have adopted the CDC's *Guidelines for Infection Control in Dental Health-Care Settings – 2003* recommendations, in part or in total, as regulation for licensees and facilities that provide dental services. Even though the CDC uses terminology such as *should*, in those states that regulate compliance with the recommendations the *should* is considered a *must*. Even in states that do not regulate compliance, CDC recommendations are considered a standard of care.

**The Occupational Safety and Health Administration (OSHA)** is an agency of the U.S. Department of Labor. With the Occupational Safety and Health Act of 1970, Congress created

the OSHA to ensure safe and healthful working conditions for working men and women by setting and enforcing standards and by providing training, outreach, education, and assistance. In December 1979, congress established OSHA as an agency within the U.S. Department of Labor. Congress passed additional amendments to the 1970 act in November 1990. OSHA is responsible for establishing standards for safe and healthy working conditions for workers in the private sector and regulating maintenance of these standards. OSHA has regulatory authority to enforce its workplace safety regulations.

OSHA's standards cover most industries: mining, shipping, construction, logging, food service, healthcare, and many others. OSHA also has standards that are specific to workers handling hazardous or potentially hazardous substances and materials, so the reach of this federal agency is considerable. In approximately half of the states, there are state-administered OSHA agencies. The remainder of the states are regulated by federal OSHA. State agencies may institute their own unique requirements that are separate from the federal OSHA regulations but must be at least as stringent as federal requirements.

Employers of dental healthcare settings are subject to occupational health and safety laws and regulations to protect the health and safety of their employees. The OSHA standard that is most closely associated with infection prevention and control is the Bloodborne Pathogen (BBP) Standard.[20] This standard first became effective in March 1992 and was revised in January 2001.[20] It applies to all work activities in which employees have contact or potential contact with human blood or other potentially infectious materials (OPIM). The BBP standard applies to

---

**• BOX 9.1    CDC Infection Prevention and Control Recommendations for Dental Settings**

*CDC Infection Prevention & Control Recommendations for Dental Settings* https://www.cdc.gov/oralhealth/infectioncontrol/guidelines/

*Summary of Infection Prevention Practices in Dental Settings: Basic Expectations for Safe Care* https://www.cdc.gov/oralhealth/infectioncontrol/pdf/safe-care2.pdf

*Recommendations from the Guidelines for Infection Control in Dental Health-Care Settings—2003* https://www.cdc.gov/oralhealth/infectioncontrol/pdf/recommendations-excerpt.pdf

*Guidelines for Infection Control in Dental Health-Care Settings—2003. MMWR. 2003;52(RR-17).* https://www.cdc.gov/mmwr/PDF/rr/rr5217.pdf

*CDC Screening and Evaluating Safer Dental Devices* https://www.cdc.gov/oralhealth/infectioncontrol/forms.htm

---

**• BOX 9.2    Additional Centers for Disease Control and Prevention Infection Prevention and Control Guidelines**

**Additional CDC Infection Prevention and Control Guidelines**

*Dental Infection Prevention Guidelines for Infection Control in Dental Health-Care Settings—2003* https://www.cdc.gov/mmwr/PDF/rr/rr5217.pdf

*General Infection Prevention Guidelines 2007 Guideline for Isolation Precautions: Preventing Transmission of Infectious Agents in Healthcare Settings* https://www.cdc.gov/infectioncontrol/guidelines/isolation/index.html

*Guideline for Disinfection and Sterilization in Healthcare Facilities, 2008* https://www.cdc.gov/infectioncontrol/pdf/guidelines/disinfection-guidelines-H.pdf

*Guideline for Hand Hygiene in Health-Care Settings, 2002* https://www.cdc.gov/mmwr/PDF/rr/rr5116.pdf

*Guidelines for Environmental Infection Control in Health-Care Facilities, 2003* https://www.cdc.gov/infectioncontrol/pdf/guidelines/environmental-guidelines-P.pdf

*Guidelines for Preventing the Transmission of Mycobacterium Tuberculosis in Health-Care Settings, 2005* https://www.cdc.gov/mmwr/pdf/rr/rr5417.pdf

*Immunization of Health-Care Personnel: Recommendations of the Advisory Committee on Immunization, 2011* https://www.cdc.gov/mmwr/pdf/rr/rr6007.pdf

*Management of Multidrug-Resistant Organisms in Healthcare Settings, 2006* https://www.cdc.gov/infectioncontrol/pdf/guidelines/mdro-guidelines.pdf

**Key Links for Additional Information**

*CDC Division of Oral Health* https://www.cdc.gov/oralhealth

*CDC Webpage on Hand Hygiene* https://www.cdc.gov/handwashing

*CDC Webpage on Influenza* https://www.cdc.gov/flu

*CDC Webpage on Injection Safety* https://www.cdc.gov/injectionsafety

**OSHA Resources: Bloodborne Pathogens and Needle Stick Prevention**

*OSHA's Bloodborne Pathogens Standard* (29 CFR 1910.1030) https://www.osha.gov/pls/oshaweb/owadisp.show_document?p_table=STANDARDS&p_id=10051

*Bloodborne Pathogens - OSHA's Bloodborne Pathogens Standard.* OSHA Fact Sheet (January 2011). https://www.osha.gov/OshDoc/data_BloodborneFacts/bbfact01.pdf

Bloodborne Pathogens and Needlestick Prevention: Evaluating and Controlling Exposure. https://www.osha.gov/SLTC/bloodbornepathogens/evaluation.html

Occupational Exposure to Bloodborne Pathogens; Needlestick and Other Sharps Injuries; Final Rule (PDF). *OSHA Federal Register Final Rules.* 2011;66:5317–5325. OSHA revised the Bloodborne Pathogens standard in conformance with the requirements of the Needlestick Safety and Prevention Act. https://www.osha.gov/pls/oshaweb/owadisp.show_document?p_table=FEDERAL_REGISTER&p_id=16265

*Bloodborne Pathogens and Needlestick Prevention* https://www.osha.gov/SLTC/bloodbornepathogens/index.html

*Most Frequently Asked Questions Concerning the Bloodborne Pathogens Standard. OSHA Standard Interpretation* (February 1, 1993; updated November 1, 2011). Responses to common questions about the bloodborne pathogens standard. https://www.osha.gov/pls/oshaweb/owadisp.show_document?p_table=INTERPRETATIONS&p_id=21010&p_text_version=FALSE

*Quick Reference Guide to the Bloodborne Pathogens Standard.* OSHA; 2011. Provides answers to frequently asked questions regarding bloodborne pathogen hazards. https://www.osha.gov/SLTC/bloodbornepathogens/bloodborne_quickref.html

*Reducing Bloodborne Pathogens Exposure in Dentistry: an Update* http://www.dir.ca.gov/DOSH/REU/bloodborne/REU_BBPdent1.html

*FDA, NIOSH and OSHA Joint Safety Communication on Blunt-Tip Surgical Suture Needles* (May 30, 2012). https://www.fda.gov/media/83834/download

---

hospitals, outpatient medical and dental facilities, paramedical and ambulance services, blood banks, research facilities, and any workplace settings with potential exposure to blood and OPIM.[21] In addition to the BBP, OSHA has several other regulations that apply to dental practice settings. The OSHA.gov website has industry-specific portals to access relevant standards, regulations and resources. Box 9.3 contains some relevant OSHA documents and resources.

**The U.S. Food and Drug Administration (FDA)** along with the U.S. Environmental Protection Agency (EPA) provides regulatory oversight of products and devices used in the application of infection-control procedures. Established as the Food and Drug Act in 1906, today's FDA mission statement contains three key activities:

- Promoting and protecting the public health by helping safe and effective products reach the market in a timely way
- Monitoring products for continued safety after they are in use
- Helping the public obtain accurate, science-based information needed to improve health

The FDA regulates medical devices and adjuncts to medical devices, from simple items such as tongue depressors and thermometers to complex technologies such as heart pacemakers and dialysis machines. Different levels of registration or clearance are required based on the complexity and use of products or devices. These differences are dictated by regulations and the relative risks that the products pose to patients. Many products, such as new drugs and complex medical devices, must have scientific evidence of safety and effectiveness before manufacturers may legally sell and distribute in the United States. The FDA only regulates the manufacturers of medical products and devices and does not regulate the end user.

It is the responsibility of manufacturers of reusable medical and dental devices to provide detailed and validated instructions for reprocessing items for use on multiple patients. Reprocessing directions are critical to the safe delivery of patient care. In 2015, the FDA released updated guidance for reprocessing medical devices in healthcare settings.[26] The guidance gives manufacturers of reusable medical devices recommendations on how to write and scientifically validate reprocessing instructions. Reusable devices that received FDA clearance before 2015 might not have reprocessing instructions that meet the requirements of the 2015 guidance. According to the FDA, "reprocessing instructions for some older,

legally-marketed, reusable devices may not be consistent with state-of-the-art science and therefore may not ensure that device is clean, disinfected, or sterile." It is incumbent on the device manufacturer to provide sufficient instructions on how to prepare devices for use on the next patient.[26]

The FDA requires that medical device manufacturers provide end users in healthcare facilities with specific instructions for use (IFU). The IFU contains specific directions for cleaning and sterilization of the device. Different instruments and devices may have conflicting instructions for sterilization cycle times and temperatures, making it imperative for individuals responsible for reprocessing devices to carefully review IFUs. Clinicians should collect and maintain this information for every reusable device processed at their clinics or healthcare facility. If a manufacturer fails to provide this information, the healthcare facility should document and report the problem through MedWatch, the FDA Safety Information and Adverse Event Reporting Program.[25]

The CDC also recommends that dental healthcare settings use FDA-cleared products and devices for numerous infection-control practices including hand hygiene, personal protective equipment (PPE), instrument processing materials and devices (e.g., instrument cleaning devices, packaging material, chemical monitors, biologic monitors, sterilizers).[18,31]

**The Environmental Protection Agency (EPA)** was established in 1970. The EPA's regulatory mission is to protect human health and the environment. Areas of the EPA's regulatory authority that affect infection prevention and control include regulation and registration of hospital germicides used in healthcare.[13] The CDC recommends that dental healthcare settings use EPA-registered hospital disinfectants.[18,31]

The EPA also regulates the disposal of medical waste and hazardous waste.[23,24] EPA regulations apply to the transport and disposal of the waste, and OSHA has separate regulations on the handling of regulated waste by employees and the storage of the waste.[20] State and local environmental protection regulations must minimally meet the federal EPA regulations and may exceed the federal regulations.

## Hepatitis B and C viruses

Because most dental procedures generate spray, spatter, or aerosol that may contain patient body fluids, there is a risk of bloodborne disease transmission when treating patients infected with one of the viruses that cause these infections. Infected healthcare workers may pose a risk of transmitting bloodborne infections to their patients if they do not apply appropriate infection-control precautions. HIV was previously discussed and was a motivation for dental healthcare providers (DHCPs) adopting infection-control precautions. Hepatitis viruses may also be transmitted in dental healthcare settings, and these transmissions have been documented with greater frequency than healthcare-associated HIV transmission.

## Hepatitis B Virus

HBV transmission occurs through contact with the body fluids of a person with either an active or a chronic HBV infection. Transmission can occur when there is contact of infected body fluids that the HBV replicates in the liver of an infected individual and then circulates through the body fluids, including blood, semen, vaginal fluids, and saliva. This is particularly significant in healthcare because it is known that transmission may occur in dental care settings from patient to healthcare worker, healthcare worker to patient, and patient to patient.[4,14,15] Transmissions may be due to percutaneous injury, such as needle sticks, mucous membrane or nonintact skin contact with contaminated body fluids, improper sterilization practices, mishandling of multidose medication vials, and contaminated medical or dental equipment.[33]

In great part due to widespread adoption of the HBV vaccine, there has been a dramatic decrease in new cases of HBV in the past several decades, declining an estimated 81% between 1991 and 2009. Despite the decline in new cases of HBV, chronic HBV remains a major public health challenge, with an estimated 700,000 to 1.4 million persons in the United States chronically infected (and therefore capable of transmitting HBV to others) and at risk for HBV-associated complications, including liver cancer and cirrhosis.[34,38]

HBV may be spread by having unprotected sex with an infected individual, from an infected mother to her infant at birth, by contact with the blood or open sores of an infected person, through needle sticks and other contaminated exposures, and by sharing household items such as razors and toothbrushes with an infected person. The virus can survive for 7 days outside of the body and still be capable of transmitting an infection. Proper disinfection and sterilization procedures and the use of appropriate personal protective attire are important measures to prevent the transmission of HBV in the dental office setting.[30,31]

## Hepatitis C Virus

Hepatitis C virus (HCV) is the most common chronic bloodborne infection in the United States, with an estimated 3.2 million people chronically infected. Chronic infection means that the virus is actively replicating in the liver and circulates in the blood and other body fluids of the chronically infected person. Chronically infected individuals may transmit HCV to others. The most common means of transmission in the United States is through illegal injection drug use. It is estimated that approximated one-third of young injecting drug users (age 18–30 years) are HCV infected.[22] Other means of transmission include blood and blood product transfusions and organ transplantation. Rarely, HCV may be transmitted sexually or by sharing personal items contaminated with blood. Rare outbreaks associated with healthcare have also been documented.[35] Screening of blood and tissues for transfusion and transplants became available in 1992, resulting in a significant decline in the number of healthcare-associated transmissions, although cases do continue to occur sporadically. Sharps injuries in healthcare have also resulted in transmission of HCV, although transmission via this route is less likely with HCV than it is with HBV.[35]

## Infection Prevention and Control in the Clinic Environment

Infection prevention and control refers to a comprehensive, systematic program that, when consistently applied, prevents the transmission of infectious agents among persons who are in direct or indirect contact with the healthcare environment. The goal of infection prevention and control is to create and maintain a safe clinical environment to eliminate or significantly reduce the potential for disease transmission from clinician to patient, patient to clinician, or patient to patient. The risk of infectious disease transmission occurs when an infectious agent has a viable portal of entry to a susceptible host.

Although transmission of infectious agents among patients and DHCPs in dental settings is rare, noncompliance with infection-prevention procedures increases the likelihood for transmission to occur.

There are no work restrictions recommended for DHCP infected with HIV, HBV, or HCV who perform routine dental procedures. There are work restrictions recommended by the CDC for healthcare providers who harbor or may be incubating certain transmissible diseases (Table 9.2).

## Policy and Program Management

Developing site and program-specific infection prevention and control programs require integration of the relevant guidance, regulations, and standards into a written and operational infection-prevention program. Policies and standard operating procedures (SOPs) guide implementation of effective and efficient infection prevention and control practices.

All dental care facilities should have policies consistent with the CDC guidelines and all applicable regulations and conduct training at initial assignment to jobs where there will be contact with patients or contaminated patient care materials, such as equipment and instruments. Facilities should provide periodic training to ensure DHCP continue to adhere to evidence-based infection-prevention practices and provide additional information or precautions as they become available. In addition, evaluation of infection-prevention practices should be an integrated element of every program. Regular assessment, feedback, and modification of practices is an ongoing effort. Tools for assessment and self-inspection are available from a variety of sources (Box 9.4). Results of monitoring and evaluation help document compliance and identify gaps in policies, procedures, education, and training. Program evaluation is part of a continuing quality improvement program. The goal is to create and maintain a culture of safety for patients/populations, personnel, and environmental protection.

CDC recommendations include assigning an infection-prevention coordinator to oversee the development of written policy and assess infection-prevention practices. Policies should be reviewed and updated regularly, reflect the current regulatory requirements, and take in account the types of services provided at the facility, the patient population served, and current evidence-based recommendations.[9] Assigning a dedicated coordinator to

• TABLE 9.2 Recommended Work Restrictions for Healthcare Workers

| Disease/Problem | Work Restriction | Duration |
|---|---|---|
| Conjunctivitis | Restrict from patient contact and contact with patient environment | Until no discharge |
| Cytomegalovirus infection | No restriction | |
| Diarrheal disease | Restrict from patient contact, contact with patient's environment, and food handling | Until symptoms resolve |
| Enteroviral infection | Restrict from care of infants, neonates, and immunocompromised patients and their environments | Until symptoms resolve |
| Hepatitis A | Restrict from patient contact, contact with patient environment, and food handling | Until 7 days after onset of jaundice |
| Hepatitis B | No restriction[a]; refer to local regulations; standard precautions should always be followed | |
| Hepatitis C | No restrictions on professional activity[a]; HCV-positive healthcare personnel should follow aseptic technique and standard precautions | |
| Herpes simplex (hands) | Restrict from patient contact and contact with patient's environment | Until lesions heal |
| Herpes simplex (orofacial) | Evaluate need to restrict from care of patients who are at high risk | |
| Human immunodeficiency virus; personnel who perform exposure-prone procedures | Do not perform exposure-prone invasive procedures until counsel from an expert review panel has been sought; panel should review and recommend procedures that personnel can perform, taking into account specific procedures as well as skill and technique; standard precautions should always be observed; refer to local regulations or recommendations | |
| Measles (active) | Exclude from duty | Until 7 days after the rash appears |
| Measles (postexposure of susceptible personnel) | Exclude from duty | From fifth day after first exposure through 21st day after last exposure or 4 days after rash appears |
| Meningococcal infection | Exclude from duty | Until 24 hours after start of effective therapy |
| Mumps (active) | Exclude from duty | Until 9 days after onset of parotitis |
| Mumps (postexposure of susceptible personnel) | Exclude from duty | From 12th day after first exposure through 26th day after last exposure or until 9 days after onset of parotitis |
| Pediculosis | Restrict from patient contact | Until treated and observed to be free of adult and immature lice |
| Pertussis (active) | Exclude from duty | From beginning of catarrhal stage through third week after onset of paroxysms or until 5 days after start of effective antibiotic therapy |
| Pertussis (postexposure-asymptomatic personnel) | No restriction; prophylaxis recommended | |
| Pertussis (postexposure-symptomatic personnel) | Exclude from duty | Until 5 days after start of effective antibiotic therapy |
| Rubella (active) | Exclude from duty | Until 5 days after rash appears |
| Rubella (postexposure-susceptible personnel) | Exclude from duty | From seventh day after first exposure through 21st day after last exposure |
| Staphylococcus aureus infection (active, draining skin lesions) | Restrict from contact with patients and patients' environment or food handling | Until lesions have resolved |
| Staphylococcus aureus infection (carrier state) | No restriction unless personnel are epidemiologically linked to transmission of the organism | |

*(Continued)*

**• TABLE 9.2  Recommended Work Restrictions for Healthcare Workers—Cont'd**

| Disease/Problem | Work Restriction | Duration |
|---|---|---|
| Streptococcal infection Group A | Restrict from patient care, contact with patient's environment, and food handling | Until 24 hours after adequate treatment started |
| Tuberculosis (active) | Exclude from duty | Until proven noninfectious |
| Tuberculosis (PPD converter) | No restriction | |
| Varicella (active) | Exclude from duty | Until all lesions dry and crust |
| Varicella (postexposure-susceptible personnel) | Exclude from duty | From 10th day after first exposure through 21st (28th day if varicella-zoster immune globulin [VZIG] administered) after last exposure |
| Zoster (localized, in healthy person) | Cover lesions, restrict from care of patients[b] at high risk | Until all lesions dry and crust |
| Zoster (generalized or localized in immunosuppressed person) | Restrict from patient contact | Until all lesions dry and crust |
| Zoster (postexposure-susceptible personnel) | Restrict from patient contact | From 10th day after first exposure through 21st day (28th day if VZIG administered) after last exposure or, if varicella occurs, when lesions crust and dry |
| Viral respiratory illness, acute febrile | Consider excluding from the care of patients at high risk or contact with such patients' environments during community outbreak of respiratory syncytial virus and influenza | Until symptoms resolve |

[a]Unless epidemiologically linked to transmission of disease.

[b]Those susceptible to varicella and who are at increased risk of complications of varicella (e.g., neonates and immunocompromised persons of any age).

Adapted from Bolyard EA. Hospital Infection Control Practices Advisory Committee. Guidelines for infection control in health care personnel, 1998. *Am J Infect Control.* 1998;26:289–354.

Modified to reflect changes in hepatitis B work restriction guidelines found in Holmberg SD, Suryaprasad A, Ward JW. Updated CDC Recommendations for the management of hepatitis B virus-infected health-care providers and students. *MMWR.* 2012;61(RR03);1–12

**• BOX 9.4  Resources for Monitoring and Evaluating an Infection Prevention and Control Program**

CDC. *Summary of Infection Prevention Practices in Dental Settings: Basic Expectations for Safe Care.* Atlanta, GA: Centers for Disease Control and Prevention, US Department of Health and Human Services; 2016. https://www.cdc.gov/oralhealth/infectioncontrol/pdf/safe-care2.pdf and Infection Prevention Checklist for Dental Settings (fillable form) https://www.cdc.gov/oralhealth/infectioncontrol/pdf/dentaleditable_tag508.pdf

OSAP. OSAP Infection Control Checklist for Dental Programs Using Mobile Vans or Portable Dental Equipment. http://www.osap.org/resource/resmgr/Checklists/Final.checklist.pdf

OSAP. *Incorporating the CDC Guidelines Into Your Dental Practice.* https://cdn.ymaws.com/www.osap.org/resource/resmgr/ICIP_Issues/ICIP.jan04.cklist.pdf

Joint Commission Resources. *The APIC/JCR Infection Prevention and Control Workbook,* 3rd ed. http://www.jcrinc.com/the-apic-jcr-infection-prevention-and-control-workbook-third-edition/

ensure written programs are appropriate and providing training will help address the issue of lack of knowledge and implementation of infection-prevention practices in private dental offices.[9]

## Infection Control in Public Health Programs

There is an ever-increasing need to provide oral healthcare to populations who have difficulty gaining access to the traditional dental care delivery system. These groups include a variety of people with special needs such as those who reside in residential facilities or are homebound, people who live in isolated areas or where there are no dental offices, and children who do not have regular access to preventive services.

There are private dend public health dental delivery models that provide dental services using a mobile vehicle dental clinic, portable

dental equipment, or a hybrid of the two. These mobile/portable dental programs administered by agencies such as hospitals, community health centers, dental schools, health departments, and not-for-profit associations serve as a dental "safety net" for these underserved populations. The settings include schools, early learning centers, homeless shelters, transitional housing facilities, nursing homes, and community outreach settings.

In 2009, a cluster of acute HBV infections was reported among attendees of a two-day portable dental clinic in West Virginia.[36] Failure to adhere to CDC recommendations for infection control in dental settings likely led to the transmissions.[4,14] A charitable organization held the portable outreach program in a gymnasium staffed by 750 volunteers, including professional dental care providers who treated 1137 adults. Five acute HBV infections were identified by the local and state health departments involving three patients and two volunteers not involved directly with patient care. The three case patients underwent extractions; one received restorations and one a dental prophylaxis. The investigation by the CDC and the West Virginia Health Department revealed numerous infection-control breaches. The authors suggested that "all dental settings should adhere to recommended infection-control practices, including oversight; training in prevention of blood-borne pathogens transmission; receipt of HBV vaccination for staff who may come into contact with blood or body fluids; use of appropriate personal protective equipment, sterilization and disinfection procedures; and use of measures, such as high-volume suction, to minimize the spread of blood."[14]

The CDC *Guidelines for Infection Control in Dental Health-Care Settings—2003* recommendations are applicable to all settings in which dental treatment is provided. These settings include traditional fixed dental settings and a variety of nontraditional dental settings, such as schools, community settings, and nursing homes, using portable dental equipment, mobile vehicle dental clinics, or a hybrid combination.

To date, the CDC has not published official recommendations for infection prevention and control for these nontraditional settings using portable equipment or mobile clinics. In 1993, the CDC did publish some general principles for infection control that can be applied during oral health outreach and screenings and referenced the CDC's *Recommended Infection-Control Practices for Dentistry, 1993*.[31] The guiding principles of infection control outlined by the CDC include:

- Principle 1. Take action to stay healthy
- Principle 2. Avoid contact with blood and other potentially infectious body substances
- Principle 3. Make patient care items (instruments, devices, equipment) safe for use
- Principle 4. Limit the spread of blood and other infectious body substances

In 2003, the CDC further identified levels of anticipated contact between the DHCP or volunteer and the patient's mucous membranes, blood, or saliva visibly contaminated with blood to determine the suggested elements for the infection-control program.[31]

I. Anticipated contact with the patient's mucous membranes, blood, or saliva visibly contaminated with blood
II. Anticipated contact with the patient's mucous membranes but not with blood or saliva visibly contaminated with blood
III. No anticipated contact with the patient's mucous membranes, blood, or saliva visibly contaminated with blood

In 2008, the Organization for Safety, Asepsis and Prevention (OSAP) worked with stakeholders in academia and public health first to identify some of the infection-control challenges and considerations for portable and mobile dental programs and second to provide strategies and suggestions to facilitate compliance with the CDC recommendations. From this work, OSAP developed an infection-control site assessment tool and a checklist for portable and mobile oral health programs.[13] The checklist is based on the previously reported CDC *Guidelines for Infection Control in Dental Health-Care Settings—2003*, the 1993 Principles of Infection Control, and the 2003 Levels of Anticipated Contact.[30,31] There are a number of other resources for public health settings that include infection prevention and control information (Box 9.5).

## Environmental issues in dentistry

### Amalgam

Amalgam restorations have been used in dental practice since the mid-19th century, and it would be impossible to calculate how many have been placed since then. Today, millions of people around the world are carrying amalgam restorations in their mouths without apparent ill effects. Amalgam use has lasted so long because amalgam is stable in the complicated oral environment, it is easy to handle, and it is relatively cheap. Even with composite and bonding materials now in use, amalgam remains a basic restorative material. Vapors from elemental mercury do contain toxic properties, particularly in doses higher than generated by dental amalgams. Extensive research into these potential effects have concluded that doses found in humans related to dental amalgams do not pose a risk to adults or children over the age of 6.[27]

Mercury vapor is released from amalgams, and average daily intake of mercury from amalgam restorations is estimated to be 1.2 to 1.3 mcg when tested subjects have seven or eight restorations.[12,17] This amount constitutes 6% to 12% of total mercury intake from all sources.[11] Earlier estimates of up to 20 mcg/day from amalgam restorations have been criticized as being some 16 times too high because of the failure to account for the difference between the flow rate of the mercury vapor detector and that of human respiration.[11,22] However, opponents of amalgam use still insist that exposure to mercury from dental amalgams exceeds the sum of exposures from all other sources.[10]

The evidence against the use of amalgam restorations on health grounds is largely circumstantial. Among patients, intraoral measurements of mercury vapor show higher readings in adults with amalgam restorations than in those without, and the differential is higher after chewing.[19,36] Computer simulations based on these data have led to the estimate that long-term inhalation of mercury vapor from restorations results in an increasing mercury burden in the tissues.[37]

The FDA regulates amalgam for use in dentistry as a Class II medical device. The FDA has issued several statements regarding the safety of amalgam use in dentistry, saying in part, "FDA has reviewed the best available scientific evidence to determine whether the low levels of mercury vapor associated with dental amalgam fillings are a cause for concern. Based on this evidence, FDA considers

---

**• BOX 9.5  Resources With Infection Control Guidance for Public Health Programs**

*ASTDD Basic Screening Surveys 2017*
  https://www.astdd.org/basic-screening-survey-tool/#children
*Mobile-Portable Dental Manual*, a companion to the Safety Net Clinic Manual
  https://www.mobile-portabledentalmanual.com/
Organization for Safety Asepsis and Prevention (OSAP). *Site Assessment Worksheet and Worksheet* ©2010-2016 https://www.osap.org/page/PortableMobile

*Seal America. The Prevention Invention,* 3rd ed. 2016 https://www.mchoralhealth.org/seal/
Step 4 Selecting Supplies & Equipment https://www.mchoralhealth.org/seal/step-4-0.php
*Safety Net Dental Clinic Manual* https://www.dentalclinicmanual.com/index.php
Unit 6 Clinic Operations https://www.dentalclinicmanual.com/6-clinical/

dental amalgam fillings safe for adults and children ages 6 and above. The weight of credible scientific evidence reviewed by FDA does not establish an association between dental amalgam use and adverse health effects in the general population. Clinical studies in adults and children ages 6 and above have found no link between dental amalgam fillings and health problems."[27]

It is clear that research and public inquiry on this issue should continue, though as with many environmental questions the determination of cause and effect is extraordinarily difficult. Symptoms of mercury toxicity are general in nature, similar to those of dozens of other medical conditions. Threshold limits in occupational medicine are at best broad estimates, and extrapolation from animal studies to human conditions is always difficult. Improvements in alternative restorative materials are nevertheless to be encouraged, and the sealants and minimally invasive restoration procedures that are evolving are increasingly appropriate for restorations that eliminate the need to use amalgam.

The FDI World Dental Federation (FDI) and the World Health Organization (WHO) issued a consensus statement on dental amalgam in 1997, stating in part, "Dental amalgam is a frequently used material for restoring decaying teeth. It has been used successfully for more than a century and its quality has improved over the years. Amalgam restorations are durable and cost-effective; they are, however, not tooth-colored. While much research has been devoted to the development of dental restorative materials, there is currently no direct filling material that has the wide indications for use, ease of handling and good physical properties of dental amalgam. The restorative materials currently available as alternatives to dental amalgam significantly increase the cost of dental care."[6] Amalgam often remains the best option for restorative material used in low-resource settings because of the relatively low cost and the ability to be used without expensive equipment such as curing lights.

Concern regarding mercury continues, and in 2013, more than 130 countries agreed on the Minamata Convention on Mercury. This international treaty governs the mining, use, and trade in mercury. In 2014, the FDI adopted a policy statement, *Dental Amalgam and the Minamata Convention on Mercury,* in response to this treaty. This statement addresses the need to phase down the use of amalgam in dentistry as identified in the Minamata Convention and details the ways in which the FDI encourages the dental profession to use and dispose of amalgam responsibly, reduce the use of amalgam, and continue to serve the public health needs of all populations.[5] The disposal of amalgam responsibly requires preventing amalgam from entering the waste stream—particularly through the sanitary sewer, where it will eventually end up in aquafers and groundwater may pose a risk to aquatic life and to people who consume fish and other aquatic life. Due to environmental concerns linked to amalgam in dental wastewater, the EPA adopted regulations in 2017 that require all dental facilities to employ the use of amalgam separators that have at least a 95% removal efficacy by 2020.[7] The EPA estimates the implementation of effective amalgam separators will reduce the mercury effluent by 5.1 tons annually in the United States.[22]

## Hazardous Waste

The delivery of dental care may result in the generation of biohazardous waste such as used disposable sharps (e.g., needles and scalpel blades), human tissue, and items contaminated with blood and saliva during dental treatment, such as extractions and dental surgery.

Dental materials such as acid etch, liquid disinfectants, chloroform, bleach, cleaning agents, pesticides, ultrasonic cleaning solutions, isopropyl and ethyl alcohol are used for a variety of purposes in dental practice and may pose an occupational or environmental hazard if not handled and discarded appropriately. These materials have important practical and clinical applications in dentistry, and DHCP should be aware of the recommended precautions for safe use.

OSHA regulates the safe handling of chemicals in the workplace in its Hazard Communication Standard.[8] Recognizing that exposures to hazardous chemicals in the workplace account for numerous injuries and deaths each year, OSHA adopted the Hazard Communication Standard in 1983 and revised it in 2012 to reflect the adoption of a global harmonization system of classification and labeling of hazardous materials.[8] This regulation requires all employers to list the hazardous materials found in the workplace, ensure a safety data sheet (SDS) is available for each hazardous substance, develop a written program, and provide training to all employees. Management of the program includes maintaining an accurate list of hazardous materials in the workplace and ensuring all personnel who may have contact with the materials receive ongoing training when new hazardous materials are introduced to the workplace.[8] Assigning these tasks to the infection-prevention coordinator mentioned earlier in this chapter helps ensure program continuity and consistency.

## Summary

Dental professionals and patients may be exposed to a variety of hazards in the oral healthcare setting. Some of these hazards may also have potential environmental impacts. Government agencies and professional organizations provide a wide variety of resources, information, and guidance on how to perform dental services in a safe manner. Understanding the manner in which a hazard can cause harm—such as modes of disease transmission, inhalation of hazardous mercury vapors, and materials unsafe for discharge to the environment—is an important element in the responsible delivery of healthcare services that all oral healthcare professionals should aspire to, whether in private or public practice.

## References

1. American Association of Public Health Dentistry. The control of transmissible diseases in dental practice: a position paper of the American Association of Public Health Dentistry. *J Public Health Dent.* 1986;46:13–22.
2. American Dental Association Council on Dental Materials and Devices and Council on Dental Therapeutics. Infection control in the dental office. *J Am Dent Assoc.* 1978;97:673–677.
3. American Dental Association Council on Dental Therapeutics and Council on Prosthetic Services and Dental Laboratory Relations. Guidelines for infection control in the dental office and the commercial dental laboratory. *J Am Dent Assoc.* 1985;110:969–972.
4. Cleveland JL, Gray SK, Harte JA, et al. Transmission of blood-borne pathogens in US dental health care settings: 2016 update. *J Am Dent Assoc.* 2016;147(9):729–738.
5. FDI. *Dental Amalgam and the Minamata Convention on Mercury.* Available from: https://www.fdiworlddental.org/resources/policy-statements-and-resolutions/dental-amalgam-and-the-minamata-convention-on-mercury; 2014.

6. FDI. *WHO Consensus Statement on Dental Amalgam.* Also approved by the FDI General Assembly in September. 1997. Available from: https://www.fdiworlddental.org/sites/default/files/media/documents/WHO-consensus-statement-on-dental-amalgam-1997.pdf.

7. Federal Register. Code of federal regulations. *Protection of Environment. Dental Office Point Source Category. CFR.* 2017;40(1):N:441.

8. Register Federal. Final rule. *Hazard communication Rules and Regulations Pages.* 2012;77(58):17574–17896.

9. Laramie AK, Bednarsh HS, Isman BI, et al. Use of bloodborne pathogens exposure control plans in private dental practices: results and clinical implications of a national survey. *Compend Contin Educ Dent.* 2016;38(6):398–407.

10. Lorscheider FL, Vimy MJ, Summers AO. Mercury exposure from "silver" tooth fillings: emerging evidence questions a traditional dental paradigm. *FASEB J.* 1995;9:504–508.

11. Mackert JR Jr, Leffell MS, Wagner DA, et al. Lymphocyte levels in subjects with and without amalgam restorations. *J Am Dent Assoc.* 1991;122(3):49–53.

12. Mackert JR Jr. Factors affecting estimation of dental amalgam mercury exposure from measurements of mercury vapor levels in intraoral and expired air. *J Dent Res.* 1987;66:1775–1780.

13. Organization for Safety. *Asepsis and Prevention. Infection Control Checklist for Dental Settings Using Mobile Vans or Portable Dental Equipment;* 2012. Available from: https://cdn.ymaws.com/www.osap.org/resource/resmgr/Checklists/Final.checklist.pdf.

14. Radcliffe RA, Bixler D, Moorman A, et al. Hepatitis B virus transmissions associated with a portable dental clinic, West Virginia, 2009. *J Am Dent Assoc.* 2013;144(10):1110–1118.

15. Redd JT, Baumbach J, Kohn W, et al. Patient-to-patient transmission of hepatitis B virus associated with oral surgery. *J Infect Dis.* 2007;195:1311–1314.

16. Rutala WA. *Weber DJ, and the Healthcare Infection Control Practices Advisory Committee (HICPAC). Guideline for Disinfection and Sterilization in Healthcare Facilities.* Available from: http://www.cdc.gov/hicpac/pdf/guidelines/Disinfection_Nov_2008.pdf; *2008.*

17. Snapp KR, Boyer DB, Peterson LC, et al. The contribution of dental amalgam to mercury in blood. *J Dent Res.* 1989;68:780–785.

18. Summers CJ, Gooch BF, Marianos DW, et al. Practical infection control in oral health surveys and screenings. *J Am Dent Assoc.* 1994;125:1213–1217.

19. Svare CW, Peterson LC, Reinhardt JW, et al. The effect of dental amalgams on mercury levels in expired air. *J Dent Res.* 1981;60:1668–1671.

20. U.S. Department of Labor, Occupational Safety and Health Administration. 29 CFR Part 1910.1030. Occupational exposure to bloodborne pathogens; needlesticks and other sharps injuries; final rule. *Federal Register.* 2001;66:5317–5325. As amended from and includes 29 CFR Part 1910.1030. Occupational exposure to bloodborne pathogens; final rule. *Federal Register.* 1991;56:64174–64182. Available from: http://www.osha.gov/SLTC/dentistry/index.html.

21. U.S. Environmental Protection Agency. *Antimicrobials Products Tested or Pending Testing.* Available from: https://www.epa.gov/pesticide-registration/antimicrobials-products-tested-or-pending-testing and https://www.epa.gov/pesticide-registration/antimicrobial-testing-program.

22. U.S. Environmental Protection Agency. *Dental Effluent Guidelines;* 2017. Available from: https://www.epa.gov/eg/dental-effluent-guidelines.

23. U.S. Environmental Protection Agency. *Hazardous Waste.* Available from: https://www.epa.gov/hw.

24. U.S. Environmental Protection Agency. *Medical Waste.* Available from: https://www.epa.gov/rcra/medical-waste.

25. U.S. Food and Drug Administration. *MedWatch: The FDA Safety Information and Adverse Event Reporting Program.* US Food and Drug Administration, US Department of Health and Human Services. Available from: https://www.fda.gov/Safety/MedWatch/default.htm.

26. U.S. Food and Drug Administration. *Reprocessing Medical Devices in Health Care Settings: Validation Methods and Labeling. Guidance for Industry and Food and Drug Administration (FDA) Staff.* Silver Spring, MD: US Food and Drug Administration, US Department of Health and Human Services; 2015.

27. U.S. Food and Drug Administration. *About Dental Amalgam Fillings.* 2017. Available from: https://www.fda.gov/medicaldevices/productsandmedicalprocedures/dentalproducts/dentalamalgam/ucm171094.htm U.S. Food and Drug Administration. *About Dental Amalgam Fillings.* 2017. Available from: https://www.fda.gov/medicaldevices/productsandmedicalprocedures/dentalproducts/dentalamalgam/ucm171094.htm.

28. U.S. Public Health Service. *Centers for Disease Control and Prevention. Summary of Infection Prevention Practices in Dental Settings Basic Expectations for Safe Care;* 2016. Available from: http://www.cdc.gov/oralhealth/infectioncontrol/guidelines/index.htm.

29. U.S. Public Health Service, Centers for Disease Control and Prevention. Recommended infection-control practices for dentistry. *MMWR.* 1986;35:237–242.

30. U.S. Public Health Service, Centers for Disease Control and Prevention. Recommended infection-control practices for dentistry. *MMWR Recomm Rep.* 1993;42(RR-8):1–12.

31. U.S. Public Health Service, Centers for Disease Control and Prevention. Guidelines for infection control in dental health-care settings — 2003. *MMWR Recomm Rep.* 2003;52(RR-17):1–66. Available from: https://www.cdc.gov/mmwr/PDF/rr/rr5217.pdf.

32. U.S. Public Health Service. Centers for Disease Control and Prevention. Immunization of health-care personnel: recommendations of the Advisory Committee on Immunizations. *MMWR Recomm.* 2011;60(7).

33. U.S. Public Health Service. Centers for Disease Control and Prevention. *Hepatitis B Information for Health Professionals.* Available from: http://www.cdc.gov/hepatitis/HBV/HBVfaq.htm#overview.

34. U.S. Public Health Service. Centers for Disease Control and Prevention. Prevention of hepatitis B Virus infection in the United States: recommendations of the Advisory Committee on Immunization Practices. *MMWR Recomm Rep.* 2018;67(1):1–25.

35. U.S. Public Health Service. *Centers for Disease Control and Prevention. Hepatitis C Information for Health Professionals;* 2013. Available from: http://www.cdc.gov/hepatitis/HCV/HCVfaq.htm#b1.

36. Vimy MJ, Lorscheider FL. Serial measurements of intra-oral air mercury: estimation of daily dose from dental amalgam. *J Dent Res.* 1985;64:1072–1075.

37. Vimy MJ, Luft AJ, Lorscheider FL. Estimation of mercury body burden from dental amalgam: computer stimulation of a metabolic compartmental model. *J Dent Res.* 1986;65:1415–1419.

38. Wasley A, Kruszon-Moran D, Kuhnert W, et al. The prevalence of hepatitis B virus infection in the United States in the era of vaccination. *J Infect Dis.* 2010;202:192–201.

# 10

# Reading the Dental Literature

BRIAN BURT, BDS, MPH, PhD[†]

THAYER SCOTT, BS, MPH

ANA KARINA MASCARENHAS, BDS, MPH, DrPH, FDS RCPS (Glasgow)

*The literature* is the generic name given to the body of writing in books, journals, reports, and other sources that makes up the sum of knowledge in a branch of science. In the case of dentistry we refer to the *dental literature*. However, the literature is more than just our compendium of knowledge and our scientific base; it is our very identity. It defines who we are and what we do; it charts the progress of dentistry to its present status and provides guidelines for future directions.

Technologic and social developments, in dentistry as elsewhere, are proceeding at a speed that is both bewildering and overwhelming. Although dental and dental hygiene graduates learn enough in professional school to begin practice, "keeping up" is absolutely essential for professional growth. Attendance at continuing education courses is one way to do so (such attendance is required in most states), but the literature is the primary source of new knowledge. Therefore it follows that dentists and hygienists must keep familiar with those sections of the literature that most concern them if they are to function properly. To do this, they need to be able to locate the literature they need and read it critically; they need to distinguish front-line from mediocre journals and be aware of how to distinguish good from poor research. Acquiring these skills requires some time and practice, but confidence with them will pay off in helping practitioners use their time efficiently while they grow professionally. Professional training, unfortunately, does not usually include critical reading. The usual progression begins with accepting the veracity of reports unquestioningly and without conscious thought, because "if it weren't true, it wouldn't be printed." After being misled a few times, readers can become increasingly skeptical. In the extreme, they can move full circle from believing everything they read to believing nothing. The ideal course is between the two extremes, somewhere between blind acceptance and blanket mistrust.

This is the first of two chapters on how to efficiently locate and interpret information that is needed for effective clinical practice. This chapter deals with assessing the quality of an individual report in the literature, whereas Chapter 11 is devoted to evidence-based dentistry and assessment of a body of literature to determine best clinical practices.

## Textbooks and Peer-Reviewed Journals

Textbooks are the most familiar source of information for students. Although good books may be the first source to be consulted on a subject, books soon become dated. The copy a student buys from the bookshop or electronically may be new, but if it was published 5 to 10 years ago then there is a risk that at least parts of it are obsolete and have been superseded by new information. That proviso accepted, the best textbooks present the state of the science, at least at the date of publication, and a sound foundation on which to build further information.

Journals are the basic source of current information in any science-based field, including dentistry. The number of journals in dentistry, as in most other disciplines, has exploded in recent years. It is virtually impossible for anyone to keep up with all journals, so selectivity is needed. There are good journals and not-so-good ones, and there are some clues to picking which is which. The most basic is that good journals are all peer reviewed.

## Peer Review

*Peer review* means that manuscripts, when first received by the journal editor, are sent out to be reviewed by several experts in the subject area of the manuscript. Usually two reviewers are selected, sometimes more, and the identity of the reviewers is concealed from the authors to promote candid reviews. Some journals, though not all, also mask the identity of the authors from the reviewers in an effort to remove any bias from the reviewers' judgment. The reviewers' task is to assess the manuscript critically for the quality of its science, relevance, its logic, its manner of presentation, and other features that might reflect on its value in the literature. Poor-quality manuscripts are rejected outright at this stage; others that are methodologically sound but have room for improvement are returned to the authors for revision. Most articles published in journals have been returned to the authors for revisions

[†]Deceased

at least once prior to acceptance. Many prestigious journals, such as the *New England Journal of Medicine*, reject far more manuscripts than they publish; their reviewing standards are extremely rigorous. The top dental journals publish less than one-fifth of the manuscripts they receive.

Peer review is a system that has evolved through the years, and there is no question that it has contributed to raising the standards of published material. However, it does have some limitations. For example, the process can suffer when the reviewers chosen are inappropriate, either because they are not sufficiently expert in the field of study or because their own prejudices get in the way of an objective review. More common are reviewers who simply do not give a manuscript the attention it deserves. An inherent problem is the tendency of the peer-review process to inhibit original research or creativity and to push imaginative thoughts into a safe middle ground. On balance, however, peer review has served to greatly elevate the quality of the literature.

## Judging the Quality of a Journal

The first step in judging a journal's quality is to find out whether it is peer reviewed. Some provide this information in their instructions to contributors, which are found on the journal's website. The second thing to find out is the journal's sponsorship, that is, who puts it out?

There are four broad categories of sponsorship:

*A Learned Society:* Learned societies frequently present the best and most important research papers—their reason for existing, after all, is to promote and disseminate research findings. Some, like the International Association for Dental Research, which publishes the *Journal of Dental Research* and *Advances in Dental Research*, promote dental research in all fields. Others advance research in specialized or semispecialized areas. Journals published by learned societies are invariably peer reviewed and have a strong emphasis on scientific rigor. These journals are characterized by a straightforward format with a relative absence of advertising, a strong editorial board, and explicit instructions to contributors. On the downside, a relatively small circulation to a specialized group often makes them expensive.

*A Professional Organization:* A professional organization is a dental or dental hygiene association, a specialty society, or any other professional group. The best journals in this category, such as the *New England Journal of Medicine, British Medical Journal,* and *Journal of the American Medical Association*, rank among the most prestigious in biomedicine. The majority of journals in this group are peer reviewed. In contrast to the journals published by learned societies, these can show some bias in choice of material. There can be a tendency to publish papers favorable to the organization's views and not to publish papers with contrary views, regardless of their quality. These journals can carry a fair amount of advertising, which together with wide distribution to the association's membership keeps the price moderate. In the better journals, advertising material must pass editorial scrutiny for factual content and taste.

*A Reputable Scientific Publisher:* Some journals are produced by publishers of medical and dental texts to fill a need: *Community Dentistry and Oral Epidemiology* and *Journal of Periodontal Research*, published by John Wiley & Sons, are examples. The best journals in this group are rigorously peer reviewed and generally are the equal of those issued by learned societies in terms of quality.

*A Commercial Publisher:* Journals issued by commercial publishers comprise a category often referred to as "throwaways,"

and some can be more accurately described as magazines rather than journals. They carry a lot of advertising, which often permits them to be distributed free of charge, and their articles are often written by professional in-house staff. Some do accept contributed papers, but peer review is unusual. The scientific quality of these journals is usually not high, as that is not their function. These journals fill a niche, as long as readers recognize them for what they are.

The third step in quality determination is to look for a listing of an editorial board, advisory board, or consultants. These terms can be used loosely and interchangeably, and the functions of these groups can vary widely, from taking an active role in journal policies to being little more than window dressing. The presence of such a list, however, suggests that the journal is at least trying to keep up standards.

As the fourth step, a reader should be able to judge the nature of the papers from a quick perusal: research reports, case reports, opinion pieces, reviews, political commentary. First and most important, the reader should be able to tell which is which. Looking over the editorials, in those journals that carry them, can give a feel for any particular political stance the journal may take.

The fifth step can be to scan the advertising for the products and services presented and the advertising style. Better-quality journals either have no advertising or a reasonably restrained advertising style. Look for some statement of advertising policy, such as is found in the advertising standards of the *Journal of the American Dental Association*.

Finally, the production standards should be checked. Typographical errors, lack of consistency, and inadequate citations in references can make a reader wonder what else is wrong that is less readily apparent.

The number of open access online journals has been multiplying exponentially over the past several years. In its best application, these journals' rapid research publishing, along with free access for readers, increases exposure to current scientific knowledge for all. While these journals are cost effective for readers, these journals remain economically viable by transferring the cost of online publication to the author. Reputable open access publishers function like traditional print publishers by employing a quality editorial board and performing robust peer review. Unfortunately, predatory online publishers exist with the primary purpose of profiting off the publication process, not to advance scientific knowledge. These journals may use editors and/or peer reviewers with little to no knowledge of the topic, providing a shaky foundation to inform current scientific knowledge and future research.[6]

In order to appear to have a high-quality editorial board, predatory publishers actively recruit researchers based on their prior publications or conference presentations, independent of whether their expertise corresponds with the journal's mission. Unknowing academics who agree to join these boards report that papers that they rejected for publication were subsequently published in the journal. In addition, researchers who attempt to remove themselves from the editorial board can be ignored, with some reports of being listed online as a peer reviewer over a year later. Hijacked journal websites, or having similar journal names to reputable journals (e.g., *Journal of Polymer Science* vs. *American Journal of Polymer Science*) are also mechanisms that predatory journals have employed.[2] This profitable business model has resulted in an explosion of predatory journals, reaching more than 10,000 predatory journals at the end of 2016, as reported by Beall's List of Predatory Open Access Publishers. Although this "blacklist" ceased functioning the beginning of 2017, an archived version exists along with a list of criteria for determining whether an open access publisher is predatory.[1]

Another potential resource is the "whitelist" Directory of Open Access Journals (DOAJ), which lists credible, high quality, peer-reviewed, open access journals based on review of information provided by the journal's publisher.[4]

A professional's ability to understand scientific reports in the literature demands some grasp of research design. Although the principles of research apply to all kinds of scientific inquiry, the details described in this chapter relate specifically to epidemiologic studies and to clinical trials.

## Critical Reading—Evaluating the Quality of a Published Paper

### Hierarchy of the Quality of Information

As far as possible, knowledge upon which treatment procedures and other actions are based should come from the results of carefully structured research designs, free of bias and confounding, minimizing random error, and carried out with human subjects. This is inherently impossible in some instances and simply lacking in others, so a reader needs to judge the source of information carefully when assessing the state of knowledge on any subject. It was this need, often frustratingly unresolved, that spawned the move toward evidence-based medicine (see Chapter 11).

The best-developed measuring scales for assessing the quality of information in a published report are for studies of therapeutic and preventive products and interventions. A number of such scales have been suggested. The first of these was developed by a Canadian panel that had the task of appraising the value of the routine physical examination in preventing morbidity.[3] The scale the panel constructed was used, more or less unchanged, by the U.S. Preventive Services Task Force a few years later and with some modification is still being used by that group.[5] These pioneering scales can be seen in retrospect as early steps in the growth of evidence-based medicine. The scale in Box 10.1 gives hierarchy for judging the quality of an individual study that tests the value of a therapeutic or preventive product or intervention.[8] This is a broad guide, with many overlaps, but provides a framework for judging the *internal validity* of a paper, that is, the extent to which its conclusions are supported by its methods and results. (Note that this scale is not applicable to judging papers on diagnosis, prognosis, appropriateness of policy, or economic analysis.)

Many questions regarding treatment or prevention in dentistry are simply not amenable to testing in randomized trials, either for ethical reasons (are amalgams harmful to human health?) or because of inherent difficulties (is group practice more efficient than solo practice?). In such instances, evidence from less rigorous study designs must do. Case studies can be helpful in guiding appropriate treatment, but individual patients may be atypical, and the treatment outcome therefore not generalizable; that is, case studies lack *external validity*—they cannot be generalized to the base population. The opinion of an acknowledged expert is always worth listening to, but experts are human too and subject to bias.

In many areas of basic science, animal studies and other laboratory experiments are a major source of information that can be applied to humans. The fundamentals of trials involving rats, hamsters, guinea pigs, dogs, monkeys, and other animals used in studies are the same as those for trials with humans. The reader should look for the special complications of animal studies: Was the strain of rat used susceptible to the disease? Were the results potentially biased by an undue number of deaths in one group? An ever-present difficulty with animal studies is the extent to which results should be applied to humans. The same concern applies to all laboratory procedures: Does the dental enamel in the test tube react the same way to fluoride as it does in the mouth? Are the bacteria produced from pure culture the same as those found in the oral environment? The ideal occurrence for reaching conclusions is when the results of laboratory studies are confirmed in humans, but again this happy circumstance often is not possible.

### Criteria for Judging the Quality of an Individual Paper

There are essentially four kinds of papers published in journals. These are broadly categorized as:

*Research reports*, which describe original clinical, basic, or epidemiologic research. A question is identified, a study is designed to test the question, the results are discussed, and some conclusions are reached.

*Case reports*, which are accounts by clinicians of unusual manifestations of disease conditions, treatment outcomes, or disease progression. In many areas of surgery, randomized trials will never be carried out because of the inherent difficulties, so case reports form the body of literature on many surgical procedures.

*Reviews* of the literature, which summarize knowledge in a particular area (the narrative review is referred to here; systematic reviews are discussed in Chapter 11). A *narrative review* is a traditional approach in which a knowledgeable person or persons collects the published information on a subject and reaches conclusions on what the literature collectively says about the issue in question. The best narrative reviews are superb additions to the literature, and when done well they can be among the most influential and valuable works in the literature; the poorest ones, narrow and biased.

*Commentaries*, in which some documented facts are used as a basis for urging program development, health policy, or some

---

**• BOX 10.1  Scale for Judging the Quality of Information in Reports on Therapeutic and Preventive Interventions in Human Studies, Ordered From Best Quality (I) to Weakest (III)[8]**

I. Properly powered and well-conducted randomized clinical trials in humans, in which all criteria described in Experimental Study Designs in Chapter 12 are met; well conducted systematic review or metaanalysis of homogeneous randomized controlled trials

II-1. Well-designed controlled clinical trials without randomization; the more that these elements are missing or the criteria inadequately satisfied, the greater the threat to internal validity

II-2. Well-controlled cohort and case-control analysis studies

II-3. Multiple time series, with or without the intervention; results from uncontrolled studies that yield results of large magnitude. Clinical trials without concurrent control groups, such as those using historical controls, and retrospective cohort studies. The better examples here can be considered equal to those in item II-2.

III. Descriptive studies or case reports; personal opinion, subjective impressions, and anecdotal accounts based on clinical experience other kind of action. Commentaries can vary greatly in quality, ranging from beautiful insights to hopelessly biased diatribes.

The essential features to look for when reading a paper in the literature can be presented in semichecklist form, and this is done for three types of reports in Boxes 10.2 to 10.4 (case reports do not fit this model). The list may seem rather long at first, but with practice, readers will soon be able to apply these criteria quickly and in due course almost unconsciously. The goal, in fact, is that their application becomes an automatic feature of reading reports in journals.

As evidence-based medicine developed, it quickly became apparent that a major stumbling block to synthesizing clinical trial reports from the literature was their lack of homogeneity. Vital information (e.g., method of subject allocation, control of exposure, data reliability) was often presented in vague terms or, worse, not mentioned at all. The response to this problem was the development of a protocol known as the CONSORT Statement (CONSORT is an acronym for Consolidated Standards of Reporting Trials), which journals adopted as a means of ensuring that all published clinical trials contain adequate detail on the methods used. The goal is to achieve homogeneity in reporting, which in turn permits metaanalysis (see Chapter 11) and improves the quality of systematic reviews.[7] When authors adhere to CONSORT standards their papers are easier to read, and it is easier for readers to judge the quality of the papers. Protocols for reporting other kinds of scientific study have been developed in the wake of CONSORT; these are discussed in Chapter 11.

---

## • BOX 10.2    Quality Issues in Judging Research Reports

### General Issues

- Nature of the journal in which the report appeared (see discussion on journals in the text).
- Qualifications of the authors. Is at least one a well-known researcher? Is there evidence of research training among the authors? Are they affiliated with a reputable institution?
- Research funding. If the work was commercially funded, is there any reason to believe that the sponsors might have influenced the results?
- Date of publication. Knowledge is moving rapidly in some fields, less so in others. Is the report likely to have been superseded by more recent work?

### Research Specifics

- Are the research question, purpose of the paper, and a hypothesis clear and succinctly stated? If not, is a hypothesis at least implied?
- Although the review of current knowledge must often be brief in a research report, is it a balanced summary of previous work? (The "selective" review to support a particular point of view is unfortunately not unknown.)
- Are the measurement variables and other terms specifically defined? If standard terms and measures are being used, are references given for their definition? If new measures are being introduced, are they clearly defined and is it made clear why existing ones cannot be used? (These questions are all aimed at checking internal validity.)
- If the study involves humans, is the population studied appropriate in view of the stated purposes? Does the report give details on participants in the study, such as the numbers of people approached, those who agreed to begin the study, and those who remained at the end?

- Is the research design appropriate to test the hypothesis and thus answers the underlying question?
- Are the materials and methods clearly detailed? Are measurements applied as described? Have the researchers taken steps to ensure that the measures are being recorded as reliably as possible? With regard to this latter point, if there are several examiners in an epidemiologic study, are they experienced in such research or have they been trained and their evaluations calibrated for this project? Are any checks made to ensure examiner reliability?
- Is the statistical analysis appropriate for the types of data collected? Have the authors presented sufficient data in the way of tables or graphics to permit the reader to check this question? Are the statistical tests used appropriate for testing the stated hypothesis?
- Does the discussion look critically at any limitations of the methods used? Are appropriate comparisons made with previous work and reasons discerned for similarities or differences? Is a fair assessment of the relevance of the work made, with some specifics given for the next steps?
- Are the conclusions clear and warranted by the results of the research? Have the authors made suitable distinction between statistical significance and clinical importance?
- Is the paper clearly and concisely written? Does the abstract give a clear profile of the study?
- Have the issues of informed consent and ethical research been dealt with adequately and clearly stated?
- If the report is a clinical trial, have the reporting requirements listed in the CONSORT (Consolidated Standards of Reporting Trials) Statement been met?

---

## • BOX 10.3    Quality Issues in Judging Narrative Reviews of the Literature

- Is the subject of the review clearly stated and are its boundaries delineated?
- As far as you can determine, is all appropriate work included in the review?
- Is there a fair but critical analysis of the reports reviewed, or does the author(s) seem to be emphasizing only one side of an issue?

- Does the review critically assess the value of different research reports, or are they all taken at face value and given equal merit? Lack of critical assessment weakens a review.

---

## • BOX 10.4    Quality Issues in Judging Commentaries

- Has the author used whatever factual basis is available to develop the case? (Hard data should always be used as much as possible, even though some conclusions must be reached with less information than is desirable.)

- Is there respect for various points of view?
- Are conclusions warranted by the argument made, or is there a sense of preconceived conclusions?

There are a few other aspects common to all reports in the literature. Reports should have a concise yet informative title that allows the reader to recognize the content and assists in electronic retrieval. A good abstract permits readers to quickly identify the basic contents of the paper. An abstract for a research paper should (1) state the objectives and scope of the investigation, (2) describe briefly the methods used, (3) summarize the most important findings, and (4) state the main conclusions. Some journals require that an abstract be written strictly to this format, whereas others request adherence to their own format. The wise author chooses words for the abstract that are similar to the Medical Subject Headings (MeSH) terms under which the paper will be indexed. Abstracts should never contain information or conclusions not stated in the body of the report. Brevity (no more than 250 words helps electronic storage and retrieval) requires that abstracts be objective, straightforward, and free of opinion or speculation.

## Finding the Reports You Need in the Literature

Practitioners often need to find information about a given subject: What is this material that a vendor is pushing? Do sealants work on primary teeth? Has this new cavity liner been adequately tested? Does silver diamine fluoride work? Are dental therapists safe, within their scope of practice? The list is endless. Dental professionals need to know how to search the vast literature efficiently to find the information they need to reach a conclusion. Fortunately, the rapidly developing electronic methods for searching the literature make this task much less arduous than it once was.

A useful start is the reference lists at the ends of textbook chapters, although the earlier caveats on obsolete material in textbooks pertains to the references too. Not only do they risk being dated, but such reference lists often are not complete or they can reflect an author's bias or incomplete grasp of a subject. These reference lists can be a good starting place, but usually more is needed. Good reviews of the literature on a related topic can be useful. Although the conclusions of the review may be enough for some purposes, the reader should follow up on some of the papers cited in the review.

The main repository of bibliographic information on the biomedical literature is the *Index Medicus*, a vast compendium managed by the National Library of Medicine (NLM), located on the campus of the National Institutes of Health in Bethesda, Maryland. Prior to the late 1990s a bibliographic guide to the dental literature for years was to be found in the bound copies of the *Index to Dental Literature*. Today, searching the biomedical literature involves a search of electronic databases and the Internet. All biomedical literature since 1966 indexed by the NLM is now searchable online through MEDLINE, biomedicine's primary database. MEDLINE indexes most, but not all, of the world's biomedical research literature, although EMBASE, another biomedical database, is stronger in non-English publications and the drug literature.

The most popular version of MEDLINE is PubMed, designed for quick and easy use by the busy practitioner. The Clinical Queries option in PubMed allows the clinician to quickly focus a large search on the question of interest. When one first begins to use MEDLINE, the effect can be overwhelming: a tidal wave of information gushes over the user, often far more than can be readily digested. Sometimes this reflects reality; there is just so much more published on an issue or topic than the user may have imagined. At other times it means that the search is too broad and that a lot of inappropriate material is included. Practice in the use of keywords and increasing familiarity with the MeSH terminology make searching much more efficient. It does not take long for even a technophobe to conduct an efficient search.

A dental practitioner with a computer in the back room of the practice can easily search an issue over a lunchtime sandwich and refine the search to a usable number of relevant references. Abstracts usually accompany the reference citation for most journals, making the search more efficient, with the full article available online for almost all biomedical journals. Online subscriptions are the norm; with a print subscription being a thing of the past and more expensive.

The result of a search is a stream of references, most with abstracts that flow across the screen; unless they are captured and stored, the search is a transitory thing. Therefore, to go along with the electronic searching procedures, bibliographic database software permits downloading of the search results into the storage database. The search is performed, the desired references are selected from among those perused, and these are downloaded into the database; then they are on hand permanently. Once we got accustomed to this way of searching the literature, it is difficult to know how we ever got along without it.

These days, searching beyond the traditional MEDLINE resources is important to achieve a fuller interprofessional understanding of current knowledge, starting with the dental literature. Also important is expanding to other allied professions, public health, psychology, and social sciences, to name a few. Some free resources of interest to the practitioner include Web of Science, which accesses multiple databases to search science, social science, and art and humanities publications; ClinicalTrials.gov for information about registered clinical trials and their results; the Cochrane Collaborative for systematic reviews; Popline, which searches reproductive, maternal, and child health; and the ADA Center for Evidence-Based Dentistry, which offers critical summaries, guidelines, and systematic reviews primarily oriented toward dental topics. For a fee, several other resources exist to broaden searches, including CINAHL (nursing and allied health database), PsycINFO (behavioral and mental health resource including information regarding attitudes toward a topic), and Academic OneFile (subscription-based database including peer-reviewed and professional journals, along with newspapers, magazines, podcasts and television/radio broadcasts). (Link, Alissa, Education and Informational Services Librarian, Boston University Alumni Medical Library. Personal communication, March 4, 2018.)

In the special instance of performing a systematic review, the practitioner needs to take the literature search to the next level by searching down the "gray literature" to obtain a complete picture of the current level of knowledge about a topic. The "gray literature" is research that has yet to reach publication in a traditional peer-reviewed journal, ranging from research that has not left the lab yet, to conference proceedings, symposia, white papers, program evaluation, and bulletins.

Best known of the search engines is Google, which can produce a large number of results if your search strategy is not refined enough by using the advanced options, but a disadvantage is that it is not peer reviewed. The Health Systems Evidence database, managed by McMaster University, focuses on providing evidence-based resources to inform governance, financial aspects and delivery of healthcare, and implementation strategies, which include policy briefs, completed systematic reviews and those planned and in process, and economic evaluations, descriptions of health systems, and their reforms   (https://www.healthsystemsevidence.org/about?lang=en).

In addition, the American Public Health Association operates the Policy Statement Database, which allows searching of their policy statements released between 1948 and the present.[7] Perhaps the most important tool to recommend is your local librarian, who is trained in advanced search strategies and knows all the avenues to explore to identify relevant literature. In addition, a good librarian can also identify free literature through interlibrary resources that you might not be able to easily access on your own.

The amount of useful information on the Internet continues to grow at a staggering rate. Although the web generally remains a delightfully anarchic affair, a lot of useful information can be found there. A vast amount of reputable health-related information can be found on the websites for the ADA, National Institutes of Health, Centers for Disease Control and Prevention, and World Health Organization. However, anyone can publish a website, and not all information on the web is reliable or true. As with journals, care should be taken to use Internet resources administered by trusted organizations with strong scientific expertise.

We live in interesting and exciting times, with a wealth of information available at our fingertips. Unfortunately, these days we can no longer automatically assume that a piece of information can be trusted when it is published in a journal or available on a website. We need to remember to use our knowledge to assess all information sources critically to evaluate their validity and usefulness.

## References

1. Beall J. *Criteria for Determining Predatory Open-Access Publishers.* 3rd ed; January 1, 2015. Archived version available from: https://web.archive.org/web/20170105195017/https://scholarlyoa.files.wordpress.com/2015/01/criteria-2015.pdf.
2. Bohannon J. Who's afraid of peer review? *Science.* 2013;342:60–65.
3. Canadian Task Force on the Periodic Health Examination. The periodic health examination. *J Can Med Assoc.* 1979;121:1193–1254.
4. DOAJ. *Directory of Open Access Journals.* https://doaj.org/.
5. Harris RP, Helfand M, Woolf SH, et al. Current methods of the US Preventive Services Task Force; a review of the process. *Am J Prev Med.* 2002;20(3 suppl):21–35.
6. Pisanski K, Sorokowski P, Kulczycki E, et al. Predatory journals recruit fake editor. *Nature.* 2017;543:481–483.
7. Schulz KF, Altman DG, Moher D, et al. CONSORT 2010 Statement: updated guidelines for reporting parallel group randomized trials. *PLoS Med.* 2010;7(3):e1000251.
8. US Preventive Services Task Force. *Procedure Manual*; 2015. Available from: https://www.uspreventiveservicestaskforce.org/Page/Name/procedure-manual.

# 11

# Evidence-Based Dentistry

AMIR AZARPAZHOOH, DDS, MSc, PhD, FRCD(C)

CHRISTOPHER OKUNSERI, BDS, MSc, MLS, DDPH RCSE (England), FFD RCSI (Ireland)

## CHAPTER OUTLINE

## Introduction

What do you do when a patient with periodontal disease says, "I read in a magazine that gum disease can cause a heart attack but that there is a drug available to prevent this. Should I be taking this drug?" Chances are that you don't know how to respond. You may have studied the relationship between periodontitis and cardiovascular disease, but you have never heard of the drug the patient describes. Your first instinct is probably to dismiss the whole thing, but you have a feeling that perhaps there is something to it. Another scenario is the challenge on how to work with policymakers to determine how health services can be provided, financially supported, implemented, and evaluated.[4,18,33]

These context-dependent decisions are usually complex and involve studying and considering several criteria before an option or a group of options are presented as the most suitable for an individual, a population, or a specific health system–level problem. To address concerns of this nature, this chapter provides a review of evidence-based dentistry (EBD) and evidence-based public health (EBPH) and a summary of the different tools and techniques available to clinical and public health practitioners. While this chapter describes what both EBD and EBPH are, increased attention is

given to EBD and how it will influence oral health professionals', policymakers', and program planners' decisions in the future. Additional information on the responsibilities that come with adherence to evidence-based practice and evidence-based public health are also provided.

## What Is Evidence-Based Dentistry?

EBD is sometimes described as doing the right thing, for the right patient, at the right time. This definition is succinct and hard to dispute, but it still leaves the practitioner with little concrete direction in the day-to-day, patient-by-patient decisions that must be made in a practice. What, in fact, is the right thing to do in each situation that presents itself, who is the right patient to treat with which procedure, and when is the time right? These are complex questions and usually do not have clear-cut answers.

In modern medicine, the EBD concept was formalized in the 1970s by Guyatt at McMaster University's Medical School, Hamilton, Ontario, Canada and has evolved in the last four decades. He actually coined the term "*evidence-based medicine*" to label a clinical learning strategy at his school that had been developing for over a decade. A more detailed definition of evidence-based medicine (EBM), from which EBD is derived, is:

> The conscientious, explicit, and judicious use of current best evidence in making decisions about the care of individual patients. The practice of evidence-based medicine means integrating individual clinical expertise with the best available external clinical evidence from systematic research.[45]

Inherent to this definition are three essential components of EBM: the scientific basis for any treatment decision a practitioner makes, the clinical expertise of the practitioner, and the patient's values. The integration of these three pillars would form a diagnostic and therapeutic alliance between the provider and recipient of care, an alliance that arguably optimizes clinical outcomes and ultimately the quality of life.[45] Dentistry has come to this field later than medicine and has for the most part adopted the same language and conventions. So the definition just given for EBM is applied to EBD, as are the three components, although this more detailed definition also requires interpretation before the clinician can be confident about how it applies in the day-to-day clinical practice of dentistry. Both EBM and EBD relate to patient care and are invoked when the practitioner is seeking to make the best treatment decision for a particular patient.

But hasn't dentistry always based treatment decisions on scientific evidence? Yes and no, as we'll discuss further. Clinical practice used to be based on experience and opinion. Although these are still relevant, clinical decision making is increasingly based on scientific evidence. The landmark Gies report of 1926 noted "the growth of quackery" during the 19th century,[20] and even the 1995 Institute of Medicine report on the future of dental education recommended greater development of the scientific base in dental practice.[32]

Empowering clinicians with the tools to distinguish good from poor science leads to evidence-based care. The modern evidence-based approach in medicine, which got underway during the 1970s, is now well established—one could almost say institutionalized. The years between the 1970s and the present day saw an evolution of the methods for the systematic collection of information in EBM and its application to clinical practice, so that today, as we develop EBD, we can benefit from the experience of our medical colleagues. Evidence to inform any clinical decision is abundant. Yet, not all evidence is trustworthy. Hence, evidence-based health care "⋯ takes place when decisions that affect the care of patients are taken with due weight accorded to all valid, relevant information".[24] Unbiased versus biased information can be considered after appropriate assignment of relative importance to the type of information (importantly all of the available information), and assessment of their validity and applicability to the decisions we make for improvements in our patient care. Therefore, what is now emerging in dentistry is the formal recognition that clinical decision-making requires the application of the rigorous rules of evidence. One sign of this increased attention is the establishment of two journals on the topic: *Evidence-Based Dentistry* first appeared as a supplement to the *British Dental Journal* in 1998 and became a standalone journal in 2000. The *Journal of Evidence-Based Dental Practice* began publication in the United States in 2001.

## The Art and Science of Dentistry

The phrase *the art and science of dentistry* means that when we care for our patients we combine our clinical acumen, experience, and human sensitivity with procedures that are based on the highest quality, most up-to-date science. Essentially, the "art" of dentistry is the acceptance of the individuality of each patient. We recognize that treatment we think is appropriate for one person will not necessarily be appropriate for another with the same condition. We use the art side of our practice to assess the patient's interest in his or her oral health when formulating a treatment plan. We also factor into the treatment plan the patient's age, existing state of oral and general health, and ability and willingness to pay for treatment. The art of dentistry also includes the clinician's individual experience in using certain materials or techniques. Sometimes a clinician will have a special knack for working with a material or procedure and so can make a given treatment perform better than the average clinician would.

In the context of EBD, this art aspect of clinical dentistry should remain: it will be our ability to '⋯ use clinical skills and past experience to rapidly identify each patient's unique health state and diagnosis, their individual risks and benefits of potential interventions, as well as personal values and expectations."[44] It is only out of place when the opinions, beliefs, and attitudes of the dentist—no matter how well intentioned—are allowed to override facts that are clearly demonstrated through science. There should be a mix of art and science in each treatment plan, but the procedures that we consider as treatment options should, as far as possible, be justified by science. There will be occasions in which a scientific base for a treatment option is nonexistent, and in these cases the practitioner must determine what the best practices are. In such cases it is up to the dental research community to see that resources are directed into these areas to ensure that the necessary scientific base is developed.

It is useful to distinguish between the principles of EBD and the methods that have been proposed for implementing it. Regarding the principles there is little dispute, because no one can argue against using evidence as the basis for care. This philosophical stance, however, is immediately followed by the practical issues of what qualifies as evidence and how that evidence is evaluated. With EBD, the traditional ad hoc and subjective approach to these issues is replaced by explicit and objective methods to evaluate the available evidence. We recognize that today it is more difficult than ever for clinicians to assess all the rapidly expanding treatment options before deciding on their value to their patients. Although the methods of EBD are not a panacea for the challenge of increased options, they do provide a framework for a systematic and unbiased approach to evaluating those options. Rather than requiring an ad hoc assessment by each individual clinician to determine the strength of the scientific evidence on each aspect of dental care, EBD uses a systematic process to assemble, evaluate, and summarize the evidence on particular treatment questions discussed in the next section.

## Rating the Quality of the Literature

If the quality of the scientific evidence is to form an important part of our clinical decision-making, then how do we judge the quality of that evidence? In Chapter 10, we looked at how to evaluate the quality of an individual paper. In terms of assembling components of the scientific base to support a treatment procedure, EBM and EBD extend that analysis by objectively measuring the quantity and quality of the *body of evidence* on a subject. The traditional process is by means of the *narrative review* (see Chapter 10) in which an expert or experts assess the literature on the subject and then reach conclusions. Again, as noted in Chapter 10, the quality of such reviews varies from brilliant to mediocre or even misleading. This range results from differences in the research attention the subject has received, the thoroughness of the literature search, and the ability and objectivity of the reviewer.

An inherent problem in any literature review is the variation in quality of research reports or studies on the subject. As stated in Chapter 10, to be of value, any review must be a critical review. That is, the variation in quality of the various research reports must be explicitly recognized. This variation in the quality of the literature was a problem facing a Canadian expert panel in the 1970s whose task was to assess the value of the annual physical examination in preventing mortality and morbidity.[18] To deal with the range in quality of papers on the subject, the Canadian group developed a hierarchical scale to give a quality score to each paper the members reviewed. This scale is shown in Table 11.1 and includes a hierarchy of evidence as the highest (Level I) being a properly randomized controlled trial, to the lowest (Level III) being opinions of respected authorities, based on clinical experience, descriptive studies, or reports of expert committees. These quality scores were the basis for the recommendations issued on the use or rejection of the procedure specific clinical preventive actions: Grades A–E, and I with Grade A showing good evidence to recommend the clinical preventive action to Grade E showing good evidence to recommend against the clinical preventive action, and

| TABLE 11.1 | Scale for Categorizing the Strength of Evidence for a Program or Procedure[4] |
|---|---|
| **Code** | **Criteria** |
| I | Evidence obtained from one or more properly conducted randomized clinical trials (i.e., one using concurrent controls, double-blind design, placebo, valid and reliable measurements, and well-controlled study protocols) |
| II-1 | Evidence obtained from one or more controlled clinical trials without randomization (i.e., one using systematic subject selection, some type of concurrent controls, valid and reliable measurements, and well-controlled study protocols) |
| II-2 | Evidence obtained from one or more well-designed cohort or case-control analytic studies, preferably from more than one center or research group |
| II-3 | Evidence obtained from cross-sectional comparisons involving subjects at different times and places, or studies with historical controls; dramatic results in uncontrolled experiments (such as the results of the introduction of penicillin treatment in the 1940s) could also be regarded as this type of evidence |
| III | Opinions of respected authorities, based on clinical experience; descriptive studies or case reports; or reports of expert committees |

Grade I showing insufficient evidence, in quantity and/or quality, to make a recommendation (Table 11.2).

This methodologic approach had sufficient appeal to be adopted a few years later by the US Preventive Services Task Force[19] and, in slightly modified form, by the Centers for Disease Control and Prevention for a major report on fluoride a few years later.[41] This approach does require some summary judgments by the review panel when the research reports on testing of a procedure are of mixed quality. Scaling the quality of a whole body of evidence as a unit still has some application, although the principal method now used for assessing the quality of a body of evidence is the *systematic review*, which is based on grading each of the individual reports selected and then reaching an overall conclusion.

| TABLE 11.2 | Scale for Strength of Recommendation on the Use or Rejection of a Procedure[9] |
|---|---|
| **Grade** | **Criterion** |
| A | There is good evidence to support the use of the procedure. |
| B | There is fair evidence to support the use of the procedure. |
| C | There is a lack of evidence to enable a specific recommendation to be made (i.e., the subject has not been adequately tested). This grade will also apply to mixed evidence (i.e., some studies support the use of the procedure and some oppose it). |
| D | There is fair evidence to reject the use of the procedure. |
| E | There is good evidence to reject the use of the procedure. |

## What is a Systematic Review?

Remaining updated in knowledge is challenging. It is well known now that a busy general practitioner needs to read at least 17 to 20 articles every day to remain up to date.[15] While the number may be lower, this might well be true for a dental practitioner. Thus, for most of us, the most convenient way to catch up with an often-overwhelming amount of information on a subject is to read reviews of the literature. There are two main types of synthesis articles: informal or narrative review and formal or systematic review.

The traditional format is the narrative review, which often takes the form of a paper given at a conference or symposium, in which the authors assess the information from published reports on etiology, diagnosis, prognosis, or therapy and management of a disease and then reach a conclusion based on the weight of evidence. One example of this would be the recent article on internal root resorption that reviewed the prevalence, etiology, pathogenesis, histological manifestations, differential diagnosis with cone beam computed tomography, and treatment perspectives.[40]

Narrative reviews have been around for ages and generally have served a valuable purpose, but they can have limitations. The first problem with any type of review is that not all research gets published. A significant number of clinical trials, in particular, do not find their way into scientific journals.[26] Corporate sponsors are generally reluctant to publish clinical trials with so-called negative results,[17] meaning that a benefit from the tested product or procedure could not be demonstrated, and accordingly, researchers tend not to submit reports with negative results.[39] This particular problem is called *publication bias.* Another aspect of publication bias is the fact that only two-thirds of published abstracts that cannot provide methodologic detail get into print as full publications within a 2-year period.[46] Furthermore, the narrative reviews are mostly opinion-based and do not contain critical assessments of the quality of the included studies.

What can be done about this? The response to these problems of bias and incomplete information in narrative reviews is the *systematic review*, which reduces the potential for bias at all levels. A systematic review is defined as "··· a review of a clearly formulated question that uses systematic and explicit methods to identify, select, and critically appraise relevant research, and to collect and analyze data from the studies that are included in the review".[25] There is a philosophical link between a systematic review and a scientific study. Just as a good report of an experiment carried out in the laboratory gives sufficient methodologic detail to let the reader know just how the results were achieved, the existence of written protocols in a systematic review lets the reader know just how the authors came to the conclusions they did. The word is *transparency.*

Systematic reviews are transparent in that the reader is given a priori all the details of the search strategy, inclusion and exclusion criteria, quality ratings, and the way final conclusions were reached. This is rarely the case with a narrative review. In a systematic review, the reader knows exactly how the authors arrived at their conclusions. An example of well-conducted systematic reviews (which would encourage the clinician to implement the practice in dental care) would be a series of publications by the Cochrane Oral Health Group (Box 11.1) that evaluate the effectiveness and safety of topical fluoride (e.g. varnishes or gels) for preventing dental caries in children and adolescents[29,30]. More examples of other well-conducted systematic reviews can be found in the Oral Health Group of the Cochrane library.

The systematic review was developed for judging the efficacy of preventive or therapeutic procedures and hence is best geared toward

The Cochrane Collaboration, launched in 1993 and named after the late British epidemiologist Archie Cochrane, is an international nonprofit organization whose mission is to make up-to-date information about the effects of healthcare readily available to clinicians. It was born from Cochrane's frequent observations that, although many clinical trials had been carried out in medicine, there was no systematic collection of these trials that a busy practitioner could consult. The main product of the Cochrane Collaboration is the *Cochrane Database of Systematic Reviews,* which forms part of the Cochrane Library.[11] Cochrane's 11,000 members and over 68,000 supporters come from more than 130 countries, worldwide.

Much of this success is a result of the rigorous standards that the Collaboration maintains at all levels: from registering a title with a Cochrane review group, to submission of a systematic review protocol and the final product for internal and external peer review. The reviews are to be updated periodically as new information comes out. Readers can then be assured that what they read in a Cochrane review represents the most up-to-date summation there is.

There is already an impressive list of completed Cochrane reviews. Although access to the full reviews in the Cochrane Library usually requires a subscription, detailed abstracts of the Cochrane reviews are available online without charge and are beginning to appear in other publications.

---

assessing the quality of randomized clinical trials (RCTs). It quickly became evident that judging the quality of an RCT could be frustrated when the original report was deficient in some essential details (e.g., group allocation procedures, control of the procedure, statistical methods). This issue is separate from the quality of the study itself—the study may or may not be of top quality, but the report is deficient. This problem led a group of concerned researchers and editors to develop criteria for what should be included in the report of an RCT so that the quality of the study could be determined. The result was a checklist known as the CONSORT Statement.[35] CONSORT is an acronym for Consolidated Standards of Reporting Trials. The more journals that subscribe to CONSORT principles, the more readily comparable RCT reports will become and the more precise systematic reviews will become.

The idea of standards to promote more uniform reporting has now spread to encompass other types of primary research [e.g. STARD (Standards for Reporting of Diagnostic Accuracy)[5], STROBE (Strengthening the Reporting of Observational Studies in Epidemiology)[50]], systematic reviews [e.g. PRISMA (Preferred Reporting Items for Systematic Reviews and Meta-Analyses),[42] MOOSE (Meta-analysis Of Observational Studies in Epidemiology)[49] PRISMA-DTA (Preferred Reporting Items for a Systematic Review and Meta-analysis of Diagnostic Test Accuracy Studies)[31]], guidelines [e.g. AGREE (International Appraisal of Guidelines, Research and Evaluation)[7] and RIGHT (Reporting Items for practice Guidelines in HealThcare)[13]] as well as study protocols [e.g. PRISMA-P checklist (Preferred Reporting Items for Systematic Review and Meta-Analysis Protocols)[36] and SPIRT checklists (Standard protocol items for clinical trials for clinical trials)[11]].

## Conducting a Systematic Review

The systematic review is the cornerstone of EBD. It is most valuable in informing clinical decision making, and constitutes a powerful tool to translate knowledge into action.[10] As such, here we present some detail on how to conduct a systematic review. Just as with a research proposal, all the protocols are written down before the search begins: making up the rules or acting on whims as one goes along is not allowed. Many journals now expect the authors of systematic reviews to register the protocol of the reviews. One platform for this is PROSPERO, an international database of prospectively registered systematic reviews at the Centre for Reviews and Dissemination, University of York, York, UK. This registry "⋯ provides a comprehensive listing of systematic reviews registered at inception to help avoid duplication and reduce opportunity for reporting bias by

enabling comparison of the completed review with what was planned in the protocol."[43] The following describes briefly the required steps in conducting systematic reviews.

### Step 1 - Question to Be Examined

The purpose of a narrative review is usually rather general, for example, to assess the effect of oral hygiene on the prevention of gingivitis. In a systematic review, the question is sharpened—just as in a research proposal a broad research question is honed into a hypothesis that can be tested experimentally. The oral hygiene and gingivitis question for systematic review would then become, for example, "Does toothbrushing once every 48 hours prevent gingivitis?" Or the time interval selected might be 24 hours, which could result in the inclusion of some different studies in the review and might lead to a different conclusion. Or the question could substitute dental flossing for toothbrushing, which again would change the direction of the search. The question to be examined in a systematic review *must* be stated precisely and explicitly. Defining PICOS—participants, interventions, comparisons, outcomes, and study design—helps to refine the question that is addressed in a systematic review and corresponds with the eligibility criteria outlined by the authors of the studies that are included in the review.[10]

### Step 2 - Inclusion and Exclusion Criteria

The inclusion and exclusion criteria follow from the question, and the criteria must be stated so the reader can be satisfied that there is little chance of inclusion bias, that is, that not all publications were considered or that inappropriate ones were included. To illustrate, one such criterion is language of publication. Americans tend to read only the English-language literature, but in some fields, this can be a source of inclusion bias. Another criterion is the range of the outcome. If the subject is the effect of fluoride varnish in preventing caries, for example, the reviewers must specify whether they intend to include root caries and coronal caries, caries in the primary and the permanent dentition, noncavitated lesions and cavities, secondary caries, and so on. Age of people and other key participant demographics such as socioeconomic status studied must also be considered.

### Step 3 - Search Strategy

Reviewers need to describe the comprehensive search for available evidence, and then screen the references' title, abstract, and then make a full report to establish the basis for inclusion/exclusion of the retrieved articles against the selection criteria.[10] Electronic searching is the logical starting point, and the reader needs to know which databases were searched. MEDLINE (Medical Literature Analysis and Retrieval System Online) is the principal database for reports in dentistry, but only about half the papers on most topics can be found readily in MEDLINE, mainly because of inappropriate indexing.[16] It may also take up to a year for recent papers to be indexed in MEDLINE. This is not a criticism of MEDLINE, because relevant reports are usually in the MEDLINE database somewhere, but if they are inappropriately indexed they will not be found with the usual keywords. Other databases can profitably be added to the search for many fields of study. The reviewers also must state the keywords used in the search[27] to make the search method as transparent as possible. To learn more about specific databases and their characteristics, the readers can refer to a previously published article, entitled "A Practical Approach to Evidence-Based Dentistry: How to Search for Evidence to Inform Clinical Decisions."[6] Electronic searching usually needs to be augmented by hand searching, largely because of the chances of missing improperly indexed reports in MEDLINE and other databases, as mentioned earlier. Hand searching is what we used to do all the time before there were electronic databases. It consists of going through the references listed at the ends of some publications and going through back copies of specific journals in which publications on the topic are most likely to have appeared. Hand searching is tedious and time consuming, but it is absolutely necessary if inclusion bias is to be avoided.

### Step 4 - Criteria for Study Quality

The step of developing criteria for study quality sets the attributes that a report must possess to be included in the final analysis. For example, with RCTs the reviewer wants a description of how subjects were allocated to groups. If the use of random allocation as an inclusion criterion results in the discarding of virtually all the studies because no trials used random allocation, then a less rigorous criterion would probably have to be written. Because one of the results of systematic reviews is identification of further research needs, in this instance a recommendation for true RCTs might be a logical conclusion.

### Step 5 - Development of Conclusions

Assessment of the final group of reports can be qualitative or quantitative. *Qualitative* means that no further statistical analysis is done by the reviewer; instead, the studies are grouped as being on one side of the question or another, and a conclusion is reached based on where most results lie. Further *quantitative* analysis can in some circumstances be carried out by combining the data from a number of studies to produce a single estimate of effect, a process called *metaanalysis.*[24] The rationale for metaanalysis is that the statistical power of the estimate can be increased by enlarging the sample size. The limitation to this procedure is that there must be design homogeneity among the studies to be combined; otherwise, the exercise loses validity.

## Examples of Evidence-Based Dentistry

Now that formal EBD approaches to evaluating the research literature have been developed, there is a rapidly growing body of such reviews. Many can be found in the Cochrane Library, an online catalog of systematic reviews to augment the published journals (Box 11.1). Two such reviews are outlined here as examples of how these reviews can help the clinician provide authoritative scientifically based information and treatment choices to patients.

## EBD Example: Are Powered Toothbrushes Superior to Manual Cleaning for Oral Health?

With the proliferation of powered toothbrushes that are marketed directly to the consumer, dentists are asked about them by patients. The analysis of a Cochrane review compares plaque removal and gingivitis in people using manual toothbrushes and in those using one of six different types of powered toothbrushes.[12] An early problem was that most of the studies in the literature were excluded from the review because of various shortcomings in their design, execution, or reporting. This immediately points out to the reader the importance of not being unduly influenced by individual literature reports that do not meet contemporary standards for quality research and reporting.

After carefully proceeding through the statement of the question, inclusion and exclusion criteria, the search strategy, and the criteria for judging quality, this systematic review reported the following primary findings:

- For powered toothbrushes with oscillation-rotation action, plaque and gingivitis scores were 7% to 17% lower than for manual toothbrushes.
- The studies were of insufficient duration to determine whether these reductions are relevant to the development of destructive periodontal disease.
- An insufficient number of high-quality studies were available to judge whether other types of powered toothbrushes were superior to manual toothbrushes.
- There was no evidence that powered toothbrushes were more likely to cause injury than manual toothbrushes.
- No information on durability, reliability, and cost of powered toothbrushes was provided by the available studies.

With this kind of information, the clinician is able to provide authoritative information to patients and can be confident that the information provided is realistic and does not promise more than can be supported by the best-quality research available.

## Current State of the Science

It will be a long and slow process to conduct the necessary RCTs and then mount the systematic reviews to cover even a small proportion of all the necessary details of modern dental practice. Even in some of the most widely researched areas, the available systematic reviews do not always provide clear direction for the clinician in choosing which patients to treat in which way. An example is found in a systematic review of professionally applied fluorides in which virtually all of the vehicles tested were shown to be effective, but the clinician was still left with no clear direction as to which patients should receive fluorides, what fluoride product to use, and how long they need to be provided to each patient.[28] The clinician must still rely on professional judgment in areas such as the tradeoff between the cost of treatment and the likelihood that the patient will develop caries in its absence.

It is also possible that the experimental subjects in the studies on which the systematic reviews are based are fundamentally different from the patients in a particular dentist's practice. Some patients may be at very low risk for certain conditions, so the appropriateness of using some preventive methods on a frequent basis may be questionable. Other patients may be at higher than average risk and may need more aggressive treatment. Evaluation of these types of subtle distinctions is not common in the current scientific literature, and thus recommendations by systematic reviews on these dimensions are rarely available. Nevertheless, the shortcomings of the literature that are identified in scientific reviews can help define the future research agenda and to address the current gaps in knowledge, so that the level of specificity possible in future systematic reviews will make them even more valuable to clinicians in the future.

## The GRADE Evidence-to-Decision Framework

The Grading of Recommendations, Assessment Development and Evaluation (GRADE) approach to assess the certainty in the evidence and grading the strength of recommendations, options, or decisions has been widely used since its inception in the 2000s.[2,3,21] Since then, a number of applications of its principles have been created in the areas of environmental and occupational health,[37] coverage decisions,[15] tests in clinical practice and public health,[47] and economic evidence.[9] One of the main developments of this approach was the creation of the evidence-to-decision (EtD) framework for health system and public health decisions.[34]

The main purpose of this framework is to assist panelists, policy makers, and managers with the process of informing their decisions using evidence, making sure that all key criteria for decision-making are considered, pros and cons of the options under evaluation are discussed, and their judgments are summarized in an explicit and transparent manner. This EtD framework includes three main sections described below:

### 1. Formulating the Question

In this first stage, the panel of policy makers, in collaboration with methodologists, formulate the questions that reflect the healthcare problem at hand. To guide this process, methodologist take the panel through the process of defining the population of interest, the options/interventions under consideration, the outcomes that will inform the decision, and the settings where the options would be implemented—always prioritizing a population or system-level perspective (e.g., ministry of health, state, province). When defining policy at the broadest level, there is a chance that the panel would unintentionally disregard subgroups of populations who would require special consideration when deciding among different options. To avoid this, and making sure that the methods team gathers the necessary evidence, panels require to define in advance which subgroups need to be acknowledged when making the recommendations (e.g., rural vs. urban, variability in access to care, elders vs. others). It is essential to define these questions carefully because they guide the whole policy-development process.

### 2. Making an Evidence-Informed Assessment

After the panel defines the questions to address a specific problem, the methodologic team works using evidence synthesis methods and other strategies to gather the necessary evidence to inform the decision. It is important to note when making health policy decisions that the evidence informing this process is of a different nature (e.g., systematic reviews of clinical or population studies, routinely collected data, local epidemiologic studies). In addition to the presentation of evidence, the EtD framework allows for the documentation of judgments and special considerations from the group.

Among the most important criteria included in the EtD framework are these questions[1,34]:

- Is the problem a priority?
- How substantial are the desirable anticipated effects?
- How substantial are the undesirable anticipated effects?
- What is the overall certainty of the evidence of effects?
- Is there important uncertainty about or variability in how much people value the main outcomes?

- Do the desirable effects outweigh the undesirable effects?
- How large are the resource requirements?
- Are the net benefits worth the incremental cost?
- What would the impact be on health equity?
- Is the intervention acceptable to key stakeholders?
- Is the intervention feasible to implement?

By answering these questions and documenting the judgements, the EtD framework guides the panel through the process of examining the available evidence before drawing conclusions and defining which would be the most favorable options to consider.

### 3. Drawing Conclusions

After the panel has carefully considered the criteria presented in the framework, the panel defines one or more courses of action to follow and the strength of those recommendations. The strength of a recommendation represents "the extent to which one can be confident that the desirable consequences of an intervention outweigh its undesirable consequences."[33] Recommendations can be graded as strong or weak/conditional. For policy makers, a strong recommendation means that the defined course of action "can be adopted as a policy in most situations. A strong recommendation implies that variability in clinical practice between individuals or regions would likely be inappropriate. Thus, for governments, institutions, provider groups, or third-party payers responsible for ensuring high-quality care, strong recommendations also constitute candidates for performance measures (quality of care criteria)."[33]

On the other hand, a weak or conditional recommendation means that "policy making will require substantial debate and involvement of many stakeholders. A weak recommendation implies that variability between individuals or regions may be appropriate, and the use of a quality of care criterion is inappropriate unless the criterion is about whether patients were properly informed and helped to make a decision consistent with their own values (such as by the use of a decision aid)."[33] In reality, policy makers may decide to implement a specific option and complement that process with an evaluation and monitoring of the impact of the decision over time across different subgroups or consider a stepwise approach to definitive implementation.

The EtD framework was created to provide policy makers and stakeholders with a structured process for policy development. By requesting panels to define specific healthcare problems (questions), making an evidence-informed assessment of explicit criteria, and documenting the panel's judgment, the framework brings transparency to the decision-making process.

## Evidence-Based Public Health

Evidence-based public health (EBPH) has been defined as the "conscientious, explicit, and judicious use of current best evidence in making decisions about the care of communities and populations in the domain of health protection, disease prevention, health maintenance and improvement (health promotion)."[27] A combination of scientific evidence and values, resources, and context are attributes in public health decision making.[8] EBPH components include using the best available peer-reviewed scientific evidence for making decisions, systematic use of data and information, application of program-planning frameworks, engagement of community in decision-making, conduction of sound evaluation, and dissemination of what is learned to key stakeholders and decision makers.[8]

Some of the barriers to implementing EBPH include political environment, lack of resources, and deficits in appropriate and timely research, leadership, information systems, and necessary competencies.[8] EBD and EBPH are somewhat different. EBD is more about treating an individual patient with a dental condition based on results from randomized controlled trials, which is likely to produce effects immediately or within days or weeks.[8] The training and educational requirement is considered formal and cohesive and tends to be clinician driven. EBPH requires a different type and volume of evidence, such as cross-sectional studies, quasi-experimental designs, and time-series analysis, with clear identification of the limitations when interpreting the results. Natural experiments are relevant in EBPH decision-making, such as a state adopting a new policy and comparing it with other states yet to adopt the policy.[8] EBPH involves one or the blending of several interventions within a community, and training is much more variable than in clinical disciplines. EBPH is multidisciplinary, and training can be acquired in state health agencies, local health departments, and community-based programs.[8]

The practice of EBPH in public health practice is a science and art, in which the science is built on epidemiology, behavioral and policy research indicating the size and scope of the public health problem, and the most appropriate intervention or interventions for the identified problem. Some of the tools employed in EBPH include surveillance, economic evaluation,[52] health impact assessment, and participatory approach.

## Future Actions to Support Evidence-Based Public Health

Evidence- based dentistry seems to face many obstacles. Difficulty in changing the current practice model, resistance and criticism from colleagues, and lack of trust in evidence or research have been perceived as common and challenging issues when implementing recommendations from EBD clinical guidelines.[48] In shifting paradigm from traditional dental practice to EBD, there are always concerns regarding obstacles and barriers which may be influential in clinicians, and their behavior on decision making.[23] A published systematic review in BMJ open discussed the barriers regarding to the uptake of evidence from systematic reviews and meta-analyses, and concluded that lack of use, lack of awareness, lack of access, lack of familiarity, lack of usefulness, lack of motivation and external barriers were the most barriers among studied.[51] Similarly, the barriers involved in the application of EBD principles, as reported by dentists, have been highlighted in a 2020 systematic review.[38] These barriers can be categorized into four domains: 1) self-related barriers (e.g. limited EBD training or skills, personal inaccurate views of EBD, resistance to change or lack of interest in EBD), 2) evidence-related barriers (e.g. difficulties inherent in research, literature and dental knowledge field, preference for other information sources), 3) context-related barriers (e.g. practical issues, unfavorable work conditions) and 4) patient-related barriers (e.g. attitudes or conditions). Some of the barriers to implementing EBPH include political environment, resources, deficits in appropriate and timely research, leadership, information systems and necessary competencies.[8]

The future of evidence-based public health would require actions in these areas:

- Expanding the evidence base studies for preventive intervention in community settings through reliance on well-tested conceptual frameworks that are aligned with dissemination and implementation

- Overcoming barriers to dissemination and implementation by acquiring and attaining more knowledge on effective mechanisms to translate evidence-based practice to public health settings.
- Engaging leadership, which is essential in promoting adoption of EBPH.
- Expanding training opportunities for public health practitioners on the rationale for EBPH; how to select intervention, how to adapt them, and how to monitor the implementations
- Enhancing accountability for public health expenditures through the direction of public funds to support evidence-based strategies
- Understanding how to identify and implement EBPH interventions to address health disparities by using systematic reviews that focus specifically on interventions that show promise in the reduction and elimination of health disparities

## Limitations of Evidence-Based Dentistry

EBD is an important evolution in the continuing drive to provide the right care, to the right patient, at the right time. It is not an infallible prescription for what to do in all clinical situations, and in many areas the underlying clinical research simply has not been done. Nevertheless, the research base will continue to develop, and the approach provides a workable method to give the busy clinician a rigorous review and balanced summary of the evidence available up to the present in a form that is readily accessible and digestible. This body of underlying evidence and systematic summaries will grow rapidly and should be an ever-increasing part of both clinical teaching and everyday clinical practice.

Systematic reviews are not always unambiguous, and they are always open to reinterpretation and revision.[35] As with all of science, new evidence or reinterpretation of current evidence may in the future change the conclusions of a review. It must further be remembered that there is not a single truth that, once discovered, will remain so forever. By its very nature, science is always open to revision and reevaluation. Therefore, EBD, based as it is firmly on science, is always open to revision. These facts place significant demands on the clinician. On the one hand, it is imperative that the current best practices, as supported by rigorous science and systematic reviews when available, be carefully considered when making treatment decisions. On the other hand, such practices emphatically must not be taken as immutable fact and used without further thought throughout a career. The competent clinician must constantly look for systematic reviews to find new evidence as it becomes available and watch for signs of changes in what had previously been considered the best evidence.

*It is paramount that educators "··· provide communication skills to aid decision making, address the technical dimensions of dentistry, promote lifelong learning, and close the gap between academics and dentists in order to create mutual understanding."*[22]

## Responsibilities of Practitioners and Educators

Individual dental practitioners are not expected to conduct systematic reviews on their own for each clinical question that they encounter. Conducting systematic reviews efficiently and effectively requires extensive training and practice well beyond what can be reasonably expected from all clinicians. The responsibility for most clinicians is thus to be aware of—and to use wherever applicable—the findings from systemic reviews carried out by others. An important step in this process is for the clinicians to learn how to critically read and appraise systematic reviews and assess their risk of bias, results, and applicability.[10] If the process were to stop when a review was completed, and the review were simply to gather dust on the library shelf, it would provide little benefit in improving oral healthcare. What obviously must follow the systematic review is a process to put the results into practice. Indeed, EBD explicitly incorporates both a research component (along with the systematic review) and the translation of that research into practice.[4]

Dental and dental hygiene education has at least two primary tasks. The first is to teach students the best available procedures and how to perform them competently, a process demanding an emphasis on manual skills. The second is to instill in students the recognition—indeed the certainty—that much of what they are learning will become obsolete during their lives in practice. The challenge for the busy clinician is to recognize when this has occurred, yet neither to replace the outmoded treatment with the latest inadequately tested fad nor to wait so long that patients are receiving outdated care.

At the very least, the concept of EBD should make it routine for the clinician to consider all options when treating each patient, rather than relying on comfortable habits and familiar procedures. The clinician must routinely ask, "Could I have misdiagnosed this condition?" and "What are the possible alternative diagnoses?" When preventive and restorative choices are made, the clinician must ask, "What is the state of knowledge concerning this procedure or material?" and "What is the likelihood that this patient will benefit from this procedure?" Also, "What are the possible risks associated with this procedure and is the probability of success sufficient to tolerate those risks?" Furthermore, "How does the balance among these considerations fit with the preferences of the patient and the costs involved?"

Although the process may at first seem cumbersome and involved, with routine use it will become second nature. Moreover, it is part of the fundamental responsibility of a healthcare professional to ensure that the best possible care is being provided to each patient. At the very least, EBD has made us aware of the continuing responsibility of every practitioner to be up to date on the most recent scientific literature. It further has shown us that simply providing the same service or set of services to virtually every patient is unlikely to be consistent with providing the best possible care.

The concepts of EBD also make it clear that the challenge for the clinician is never ending. The right thing, the right patient, and the right time will constantly evolve as change inexorably takes place in disease patterns, our understanding of oral diseases and conditions, the available therapies and materials, and patient preferences.

## Acknowledgments

Dr. Alonse Carrasco-Labra, DDS, MSc, PhD provided specific content to this chapter regarding the use of the GRADE approach to information health system and policy decisions informed by evidence.

## References

1. Alonso-Coello P, Schunemann HJ, Moberg J, et al. GRADE Evidence to Decision (EtD) frameworks: a systematic and transparent approach to making well informed healthcare choices. 1: Introduction. *BMJ*. 2016;353:i2016.

2. Andrews J, Guyatt G, Oxman AD, et al. GRADE guidelines: 14. Going from evidence to recommendations: the significance and presentation of recommendations. *J Clin Epidemiol*. 2013;66(7): 719–725.

3. Andrews JC, Schunemann HJ, Oxman AD, et al. GRADE guidelines: 15. Going from evidence to recommendation-determinants of a recommendation's direction and strength. *J Clin Epidemiol*. 2013;66(7): 726–735.

4. Bader J, Ismali A, Clarkson J. Evidence-based dentistry and the dental research community. *J Dent Res*. 1999;78(9):1480–1483.

5. Bossuyt PM, Reitsma JB, Bruns DE, et al. STARD 2015: an updated list of essential items for reporting diagnostic accuracy studies. *BMJ*. 2015;351.h5527.

6. Brignardello-Petersen R, Carrasco-Labra A, Booth HA, et al. A practical approach to evidence-based dentistry: How to search for evidence to inform clinical decisions. *J Am Dent Assoc*. 2014;145 (12):1262–1267.

7. Brouwers MC, Kerkvliet K, Spithoff K, Consortium ANS. The AGREE Reporting Checklist: a tool to improve reporting of clinical practice guidelines. *BMJ*. 2016;352.i1152.

8. Brownson RC, Fielding JE, Maylahn CM. Evidence-based public health: a fundamental concept for public health practice. *Annu Rev Public Health*. 2009;30:175–201.

9. Brunetti M, Shemilt I, Pregno S, et al. GRADE guidelines: 10. Considering resource use and rating the quality of economic evidence. *J Clin Epidemiol*. 2013;66(2):140–150.

10. Carrasco-Labra A, Brignardello-Petersen R, Glick M, Guyatt GH, Azarpazhooh A. A practical approach to evidence-based dentistry: VI: How to use a systematic review. *J Am Dent Assoc*. 2015;146(4): 255–265. e251.

11. Chan AW, Tetzlaff JM, Altman DG, et al. SPIRIT 2013 statement: defining standard protocol items for clinical trials. *Ann Intern Med*. 2013;158(3):200–207.

12. Chandler J CM, Thomas J, Higgins JPT, Deeks JJ, Clarke MJ. Chapter I: Introduction. In: Higgins JPT TJ, Chandler J, Cumpston M, Li T, Page MJ, Welch VA, ed. *Cochrane Handbook for Systematic Reviews of Interventions version 6.0 (updated August 2019)*: Cochrane; 2019.

13. Chen Y, Yang K, Marusic A, et al. A Reporting Tool for Practice Guidelines in Health Care: The RIGHT Statement. *Ann Intern Med*. 2017;166(2):128–132.

14. Cochrane Training. Chapter: Introduction. https://training.cochrane.org/handbook/current/chapter-i. Accessed May 13, 2019.

15. Dahm P, Oxman AD, Djulbegovic B, et al. Stakeholders apply the GRADE evidence-to-decision framework to facilitate coverage decisions. *J Clin Epidemiol*. 2017;86:129–139.

16. Dickersin K, Min YI. Publication bias: the problem that won't go away. *Ann N Y Acad Sci*. 1993;703:135–146; discussion 146-148.

17. Dickersin K, Scherer R, Lefebvre C. Identifying relevant studies for systematic reviews. *BMJ*. 1994;309(6964):1286–1291.

18. Examination CTFotPH. The periodic health examination. *Can Med Assoc J*. 1979;121(9):1193–1254.

19. Force UPST. *Guides to Clinical Preventive Services*. 2 ed. Washington DC: Department of Health and Human Services; 1996.

20. Gies WJ. Dental education in the United States and Canada. A report to the Carnegie Foundation for the advancement of teaching. 1926. *J Am Coll Dent*. 2012;79(2):32–49.

21. Guyatt GH, Oxman AD, Kunz R, et al. What is "quality of evidence" and why is it important to clinicians? *BMJ*. 2008;336(7651): 995–998.

22. Hannes K, Norre D, Goedhuys J, Naert I, Aertgeerts B. Obstacles to implementing evidence-based dentistry: a focus group-based study. *J Dent Educ*. 2008;72(6):736–744.

23. Hannes K, Staes F, Jo G, Bert A. Obstacles to the implementation of evidence-based physiotherapy in practice: A focus group-based study in Belgium (Flanders). *Physiotherapy theory and practice*. 2009;25: 476–488.

24. Hicks N. Evidence based thinking about health care. [online]. http://www.medicine.ox.ac.uk/bandolier/band39/b39-9.html. Published 2011. Accessed.

25. Higgins JaG S. Cochrane Handbook for Systematic Reviews of Interventions. In: Library TC, ed. Chichester. UK: John Wiley & Sons, Ltd.; 2006.

26. Ioannidis JP. We need more randomized trials in nutrition-preferably large, long-term, and with negative results. *Am J Clin Nutr.* 2016; 103(6):1385–1386.

27. Jenicek M. Epidemiology, evidenced-based medicine, and evidence-based public health. *J Epidemiol.* 1997;7(4):187–197.

28. Marinho VC, Higgins JP, Sheiham A, Logan S. Combinations of topical fluoride (toothpastes, mouthrinses, gels, varnishes) versus single topical fluoride for preventing dental caries in children and adolescents. *Cochrane Database Syst Rev.* 2004;1. CD002781.

29. Marinho VC, Worthington HV, Walsh T, Chong LY. Fluoride gels for preventing dental caries in children and adolescents. *Cochrane Database Syst Rev.* 2015;6. CD002280.

30. Marinho VC, Worthington HV, Walsh T, Clarkson JE. Fluoride varnishes for preventing dental caries in children and adolescents. *Cochrane Database Syst Rev.* 2013;7. CD002279.

31. McInnes MDF, Moher D, Thombs BD, et al. Preferred Reporting Items for a Systematic Review and Meta-analysis of Diagnostic Test Accuracy Studies: The PRISMA-DTA Statement. *JAMA.* 2018; 319(4):388–396.

32. Institute of Medicine. *Committee on the Future of Dental Education. Dental education at the crossroads.* Washington DC: National Academy Press; 1995.

33. Institute of Medicine. *Dental Education at the Crossroads: Challenges and Change.* Washington, DC: The National Academies Press; 1995.

34. Moberg J, Oxman AD, Rosenbaum S, et al. The GRADE Evidence to Decision (EtD) framework for health system and public health decisions. *Health Res Policy Syst.* 2018;16(1):45.

35. Moher D, Cook DJ, Eastwood S, Olkin I, Rennie D, Stroup DF. Improving the quality of reports of meta-analyses of randomised controlled trials: the QUOROM statement. Quality of Reporting of Meta-analyses. *Lancet.* 1999;354(9193):1896–1900.

36. Moher D, Shamseer L, Clarke M, et al. Preferred reporting items for systematic review and meta-analysis protocols (PRISMA-P) 2015 statement. *Syst Rev.* 2015;4:1.

37. Morgan RL, Thayer KA, Bero L, et al. GRADE: Assessing the quality of evidence in environmental and occupational health. *Environ Int.* 2016;92–93:611–616.

38. Neuppmann Feres MF, Roscoe MG, Job SA, Mamani JB, Canto GL, Flores-Mir C. Barriers involved in the application of evidence-based dentistry principles: A systematic review. *J Am Dent Assoc.* 2020;151(1): 16–25. e16.

39. Olson CM, Rennie D, Cook D, et al. Publication bias in editorial decision making. *JAMA.* 2002;287(21):2825–2828.

40. Patel S, Ricucci D, Durak C, Tay F. Internal root resorption: a review. *J Endod.* 2010;36(7):1107–1121.

41. Prevention CfDCa. *Recommendations for using fluoride to prevent and control dental caries in the United States.* Aug 17 2001. 1057-5987 (Print) 1057-5987 (Linking).

42. PRISMA. Transparent Reporting of Systematic Reviews and Meta-Analyses. http://www.prisma-statement.org/. Accessed October 1, 2018.

43. PROSPERO. International prospective register of systematic reviews. https://www.crd.york.ac.uk/PROSPERO/. Accessed.

44. Sackett DL, Rosenberg WM, Gray JA, Haynes RB, Richardson WS. Evidence based medicine: what it is and what it isn't. *BMJ.* 1996;312 (7023):71–72.

45. Sackett DLSS, Richardson WS, Rosenberg W, Haynes RB. *Evidence-Based Medicine: How to Practice and Teach EBM.* 2nd ed. Edinburgh: Churchill Livingstone; 2000.

46. Scherer RW, Dickersin K, Langenberg P. Full publication of results initially presented in abstracts. A meta-analysis. *JAMA.* 1994;272(2): 158–162.

47. Schunemann HJ, Mustafa R, Brozek J, et al. GRADE Guidelines: 16. GRADE evidence to decision frameworks for tests in clinical practice and public health. *J Clin Epidemiol.* 2016;76:89–98.

48. Spallek H, Song M, Polk DE, Bekhuis T, Frantsve-Hawley J, Aravamudhan K. Barriers to implementing evidence-based clinical guidelines: a survey of early adopters. *J Evid Based Dent Pract.* 2010; 10(4):195–206.

49. Stroup DF, Berlin JA, Morton SC, et al. Meta-analysis of observational studies in epidemiology: a proposal for reporting. Meta-analysis Of Observational Studies in Epidemiology (MOOSE) group. *JAMA.* 2000;283(15):2008–2012.

50. von Elm E, Altman DG, Egger M, et al. The Strengthening the Reporting of Observational Studies in Epidemiology (STROBE) statement: guidelines for reporting observational studies. *Ann Intern Med.* 2007;147(8):573–577.

51. Wallace J, Nwosu B, Clarke M. Barriers to the uptake of evidence from systematic reviews and meta-analyses: a systematic review of decision makers' perceptions. *BMJ Open.* 2012;2(5). e001220.

52. Weyant RJ. Short-term clinical success of root-form titanium implant systems. *Journal of Evidence Based Dental Practice.* 2003;3(3): 127–130.

# PART III

# Methods and Measurement of Oral Diseases and Conditions

# 12

# Epidemiology and Research Design in Dental Public Health

BRUCE A. DYE, DDS, MPH

## Epidemiologic Foundations

### Epistemology and Natural History of Disease

Understanding the etiology and natural history of a disease is critical to planning and implementing an effective disease-prevention strategy for populations. How a disease develops and progresses in the absence of an intervention is its natural history. Inherent to developing a keen understanding of the natural history of disease is the identification of who has the disease and who is at risk of developing the disease. Epidemiology is the discipline that provides the scientific methods we use to address these issues. The classic definition of epidemiology is the study of the distribution and determinants of disease or adverse health conditions in man. However, a more contemporary definition is the study of the distribution and determinants of health-related states or events (including disease), and the application of this study to the control of diseases and other health problems.[50] The contemporary definition brings into focus the importance of controlling adverse health conditions

as an essential component of epidemiology. Therefore, as our knowledge of the natural history of a disease improves, the aim of any intervention developed, therapeutic or preventive, is to change the natural course of disease in a way that improves the public's health. Equally important, these same concepts can be applied to other health problems, such as injury, addiction, and other adverse health conditions.

Epidemiology is about answering the who, the where, and the when to understand why an event occurred. We can visualize this as a classic triangle with "person," "place," and "time" at each point with each dependent on the other (Figure 12.1). Epidemiologic studies are generally classified as either descriptive, meaning that the data only describe the distribution of a condition in a population and no specific hypothesis is tested, or as analytic, meaning that the data collection and analysis are designed to answer a particular question. Descriptive and most analytic studies are observational; that is, they observe outcomes without intervening to affect them. Analytic studies in epidemiology look at people with and without the disease in question (the effect or outcome) and with and without exposure to the putative influences that may increase the risk of disease (the exposure). The clinical trial, an experimental design to test the efficacy of a preventive-control agent or treatment procedure in humans, is an aspect of analytic epidemiology sometimes classified separately as experimental epidemiology. The clinical trial is also an interventional design; that is, something is intervening in the natural history of a condition in an effort to give a beneficial outcome. Although observational studies are often viewed as having less scientific rigor compared to experimental studies, well-designed observational studies can provide valuable information that can lead to important health policy decisions, for example, the early case-control studies on smoking and lung cancer leading to the first US Surgeon General report on smoking and health.[47]

Observation had been an essential tool in a physician's toolbox for centuries. Medical diagnoses were made based on symptoms reported and what could be superficially observed, including bodily fluids. By the mid-19th century, physicians' powers of observation began to change with the introduction of new instruments like the stethoscope and the ophthalmoscope and the emergence of laboratory technologies to analyze biological specimens. Although the emergence of these new tools also required doctors to focus more on the process of a manual examination, observation remained an important aid in the diagnosis of an individual's ailment.

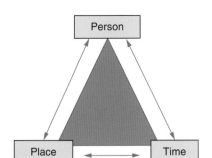

• **Figure 12.1** The Classic Epidemiology Triangle.

Interpreting observations is an essential practice in epidemiology as well. Epidemiology emerged as a scientific process to investigate large outbreaks of disease by examining a population as an individual. In the mid-19th century, cholera was rapidly spreading across the globe along the trade routes moving from parts of Asia to Europe and then to America. During this time, it was widely believed that the cause was due to miasma or "bad air." Because of high mortality, it was a feared disease and an outbreak could cause panic.

John Snow, a British physician in London, began his investigation of an outbreak of cholera in 1854 in Soho by trying to identify attributes common to those who died from the disease. Using a map of the local area, Snow plotted the residences of the deceased and identified a clustering effect ultimately leading him to determine that all of the victims had used water from the same source. That source was a public water pump on Broad Street. Snow concluded that restricting access to the water source was the best way to control the spread of the disease and advocated the removal of the pump handle to the local authorities.

In his rational process of investigation, Snow improved our understanding of the natural history of cholera, years before the germ theory of disease was understood. It would take another three decades before Robert Koch, a German microbiologist, identified how *V. cholerae* in intestines caused cholera with infected water as the source of transmission. Today, we recognize John Snow for applying a systematic approach to observation for population health; hence, he is often referred to as the "father of epidemiology."

As epidemiology grew into a scientific discipline, its concepts and methods were formed on two fundamental principles: "population thinking" and "group comparisons."[34] Morabia has characterized population thinking as a manner "of conceptualizing issues for a whole group of people defined in a specific way (for example, geographically, socially, biologically)."[34] Therefore, a population takes on attributes that are descriptive and unique, conveying a sense of individuality to that population. Analyzing what is observed in the existence of an exposure to what would have occurred in the absence of the exposure is the second fundamental principle: group comparisons. Thus, exposure drives the differences observed between groups. Recognizing and grouping characteristics based on patterns is foundational to the practice of epidemiology. We often group these characteristics based on: *biology* (age, sex, and race); *lifestyle* (tobacco use, dietary choices, physical activity, dental utilization, and oral hygiene practices); *social environment* (cultural influences, community and neighborhood characteristics, and family function); *physical environment* (sanitation, food and water supply, air quality, occupational hazards, and geography); and genetics (molecular inheritance, function and expression of genes).

Grouping characteristics also identifies potential targets for intervention to alter the natural history of disease. In the later part of the 19th century, when the bacterial agents in many infectious diseases were being identified, our ideas of disease control and prevention were more focused on evaluating and intervening on social and physical environments. It was during this period that we began to experience great improvements in life expectancy as a result of public health interventions affecting hygiene, water, and sanitation. The concept of disease at that time was dominated by acute, mortal infections with a single bacterial agent, and little thought was given to chronic conditions. Today we are more aware that disease is multifactorial, meaning that multiple causative circumstances can be defined for just about any disease. Heart disease, the leading cause of death in the United States, is associated with genetics, stress, diet, exercise, smoking, blood pressure, blood cholesterol levels, and systemic chronic inflammation often induced from putative bacteria. So what is the actual "cause" of heart disease? Dental caries is of bacterial origin but is also associated with sugar consumption, fluoride exposure, saliva quality, genetics, family education and income, and other factors in the physical and social environment. The complexity of all of these forces acting to cause dental caries has been detailed in a variety of conceptual models over the years, culminating with the Fisher-Owens model capturing the multiple pathways in which these factors operate.[15] So what is the "cause" of dental caries? Epidemiology is the scientific process we use to work through the multifactorial confusion to identify the risk factors and indicators associated with a disease and to determine which of them are the most important that offer an opportunity for intervention, whether therapeutic or preventive, to alter the natural history of that disease.

## Causality and Risk in Epidemiology

The causes of disease are often considered in terms of three factors: the host, the agent, and the environment, collectively known as the *epidemiologic triad*. In this context, disease is a result of an interaction between the person (host), the pathogen (agent), and the surroundings that promote the exposure (environment). For example, with chickenpox, the host is often a child, the agent is the varicella-zoster virus, and the environment provides the opportunity for susceptible individuals to be exposed to infectious persons. Nearly 50 years ago, the cause of dental caries was explained as the intersection of the tooth, the flora, and the substrate using a Venn diagram by Paul Keyes.[26] Keyes's approach in describing how tooth decay could occur used classic epidemiology (the epidemiologic triad) to better explain the cause of dental caries and where to intervene to prevent disease. However, for many diseases, a fourth factor, the vector, is a critical influencer for promoting disease (Figure 12.2).[16] For example, with malaria, the host (human), the

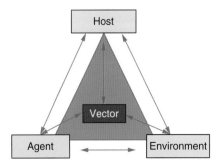

• **Figure 12.2** The Epidemiologic Triad of Disease.[16]

agent (the *Plasmodium* parasite), and the environment are all important, but the *Anopheles* mosquito acts as the vector by transmitting the parasite to the human host. The transmission of disease can occur directly or indirectly. As with chickenpox, the mode of transmission is direct, that is, person-to-person contact. With malaria, transmission is indirect, by means of the infected mosquito.

Multilevel factors operate at the host, the agent, and the environment levels. Host characteristics affect how an individual is able to adapt to the pressure exerted by the agent. A host's resistance is affected by a person's age, sex, genotype, health, lifestyle, nutritional status, social status (family, marital, cultural, and economic status), and their immune system. Agents of disease or illness can be grouped into several categories such as *biological* (e.g., bacteria, viruses, and some allergens), *chemical* (e.g., alcohol, smoke, and lead), *physical* (e.g., trauma, heat, and radiation), and *nutritional* (e.g., excessive consumption of nutrient-poor foods). Environmental factors can facilitate the likelihood that the contact between the host and agent leads to disease. Poor water, lack of sanitation, air pollution, bad weather, and contaminated food can make exposure to infectious diseases more likely. However, the environment also includes social, political, and economic factors such as crowding, neighborhood characteristics, discriminating policies, and economic chaos in society.

Causality, meaning that a certain exposure results in a particular outcome, can only be demonstrated unequivocally within the experimental study design. But it can also be difficult to extrapolate findings from a controlled experimental study to make an accurate conclusion of causality when studying disease in humans. Although *in vitro* study designs, such as using cell or tissue cultures, or a highly controlled clinical trial, can provide important foundational knowledge, these methods screen out the influences of the complex systems that encapsulate and support human life. Moreover, because clinical trials cannot be conducted on many topics for both practical and ethical reasons, causality in the study of disease usually must be derived from studies with nonexperimental designs.

To facilitate our understanding of causality, we typically evaluate the relationship between a factor and the disease as it appears in the causal pathway, which can be described as either being direct or indirect (Figure 12.3). When a factor causes a disease without any intermediate step(s), causation is considered to be direct. However, in indirect causation, intermediate step(s) must occur for that factor to cause disease.[16] Regardless of whether a factor directly or indirectly causes a disease, how that factor relates to disease can vary. Rothman's "causal pie model" provides a good basis for further understanding of this concept.[44,49] In the causal pie model, a *sufficient* cause is a group of component factors that make up a pie, or component cause, that leads to the outcome. In the absence of any one of the component factors making up the pie, the remaining component factors do not lead to the outcome.

This notion of a *sufficient* cause has led us to better explain how factors might function within causal relationships in epidemiology. There are four possible types of causal relationships: (1) sufficient and necessary, (2) sufficient but not necessary, (3) necessary but not sufficient, and (4) neither sufficient nor necessary.[16] A factor is both sufficient and necessary to induce disease when disease always develops in the presence of that factor (Figure 12.4). If multiple factors can induce disease and each factor is not dependent on the other(s) to produce disease, then the factors are sufficient but not necessary. If multiple factors are necessary to produce disease, but each factor independently cannot induce disease, then the factors are necessary but not sufficient. When a factor is neither sufficient nor necessary to independently induce disease, multiple components of factors become sufficient to produce disease. In this concept of multiple components, most chronic diseases, including dental caries and periodontitis, operate.

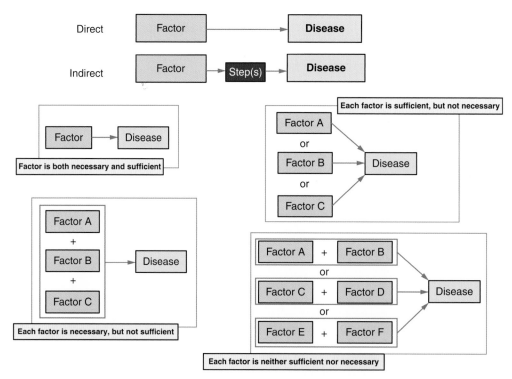

• **Figure 12.3** The Types of Causal Relationships With Disease.[16]

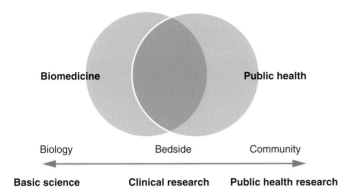

Biomedicine                    Public health

Biology          Bedside          Community

Basic science    Clinical research    Public health research

• **Figure 12.4** The types of research and their relationship with each other in improving health outcomes.

If a factor is identified as sufficient and or necessary to cause disease, what are the underlying criteria used to generate the evidence to support that conclusion? Originating from experimental studies in the late 19th century, Robert Koch outlined four postulates to establish causation (Box 12.1).[11] These criteria were designed to provide the evidence of a causal relationship between a pathogen and disease, and have greatly influenced microbiology and early epidemiology, especially around infectious diseases. But as epidemiology was transitioning in the early 20th century from predominately focusing on infectious diseases to being applied to understanding the etiology of chronic diseases, the influence of Koch's postulates became outmoded and unworkable.

With chronic diseases, a potentially causative factor cannot be grown in pure culture like a pathogen. As part of the early attempts to address this, Bradford Hill developed a set of guidelines in the 1950s for determining if the observed relationship between a factor and disease was causal.[29] These guidelines have substantially influenced the development of several Surgeon General's reports on smoking, tobacco, and health by providing the supporting evidence that has led to significant policy and societal changes since the first report on smoking in 1964.[47] Hill's criteria are summarized in Box 12.2.[16]

Some important considerations in the application of Hill's criteria are the presence of a factor (exposure) before the occurrence of the disease is central to establishing a temporal relationship. Not all observational study designs provide the opportunity to document exposure information before the outcome is observed. Consequently, exposure information would have to be obtained or derived from previous records or reported history, diminishing the potential strength of the findings. The magnitude of an odds ratio or relative risk ratio is a measure of the strength of the association; thus, the stronger the statistical association, the greater the likelihood the factor is causal. The evidence for causal relationship is also likely if a dose-response relationship is present. However, if an increasing exposure level does not yield a greater risk for disease, the exposure may operate at a specific threshold. Consequently, once an exposure level has surpassed the threshold, the outcome may be more likely. Consistency across observational studies is critical to establishing causality, but consistency with biological knowledge is essential to establishing plausibility and facilitating interpretation of the findings. Over the years the original Bradford Hill criteria have evolved and are summarized in Box 12.3 as they are usually understood today.[28]

Analytic studies, in contrast to descriptive studies, have the general aim of seeking out cause-and-effect associations. Because analytic observational studies cannot directly address cause and effect, they can seek to quantify the degree of disease risk in specified circumstances. Risk is the probability that an adverse or beneficial event will occur in a defined population over a specified time interval.[41] If researchers had to proceed with just the dichotomous judgment of whether a factor is or is not involved in causing a disease, our knowledge of disease causation and development would be seriously hindered. The concept of a risk factor permits quantification of the degree of importance of a particular factor in the development of a disease; some causal factors are more important than others.

A risk factor is broadly defined as an attribute or exposure that is known, from epidemiologic evidence, to be associated with a health condition considered important to prevent.[41] Although the term risk factor is applied loosely in the literature, modern usage ascribes a strong causal role to a risk factor: It is either part of the causal chain or is something that brings a person in contact with the causal chain. (An example of the latter situation is an occupation that requires handling toxic materials. The occupation itself is not a risk factor for toxicity, but because it brings a person into contact with toxic materials, which are the risk factors, it does increase the chance of disease.) Therefore, a factor that is causally related to a change in the risk probability of a relevant health outcome or condition is a risk factor. In practical application, a risk factor is an environmental, behavioral, or biological factor confirmed by temporal sequence, usually in longitudinal studies, which if present directly increases the probability of a disease occurring and if absent or removed reduces the probability.

Part of the concept of a risk factor is that it can be modified. People can stop smoking, lose weight, change to a healthier diet, or improve their oral hygiene. The identification of risk factors for a disease then allows the potential for prevention by removing or modifying the risk factors. As examples, smoking is a risk factor for lung cancer; poor oral hygiene is a risk factor for gingivitis. In both instances, removing or modifying the risk factor reduces the risk of disease, although neither exposure is a sole cause of the disease. As stated in this definition, a risk factor for a disease must be demonstrated as such longitudinally. This is because confirming the necessary time sequence—that is, ensuring that exposure to the risk factor occurs before the disease outcome—can nearly always be demonstrated only longitudinally. The ultimate test of a risk factor is that, if exposure to it is reduced, the risk of subsequent disease diminishes. As an example, quitting smoking reduces the risk of a heart attack.

What if a suspected risk factor cannot be confirmed as such because the necessary longitudinal studies are impractical or unethical? The factor may be classed as a risk indicator, defined as a factor shown to be associated with a disease in cross-sectional data and assumed, on theoretical grounds, to play some causal role.[31] Research experience has shown that risk indicators that emerge from cross-sectional studies can disappear in a more rigorous longitudinal analysis, so without longitudinal assessment it cannot be known whether a risk indicator is or is not a true risk factor. As would be expected, many more risk indicators for oral diseases have been identified than true risk factors.

A risk marker is an attribute or exposure that is associated with the increased probability of disease although it is not considered part of the causal chain. A risk marker can also be called a risk predictor when included in predictive statistical models. Some immutable characteristics of a person or group—namely, age, gender, and race or ethnicity—can influence disease occurrence, progression, or outcome. These attributes do not fit the concept of a risk factor because they are not modifiable. Although they can be useful in statistical models whose purpose is to predict disease occurrence, they clearly are of no use when considering disease prevention based on direct control of risk factors as they are either nonmodifiable or very difficult to modify due to complex social influences. Generally, many of these risk markers have been considered socio-demographic risk factors, but more recently we view some of them as social determinants of health, for example, low income or educational attainment and race/ethnicity.

## Estimating Risk in Epidemiology

When assessing the relationship between an exposure and the outcome (or event) of interest, the quantification of that association is an estimate of risk. Risk is typically estimated through the expression of a relative risk ratio or an odds ratio, and this is dependent on how time between exposure and outcome is accounted for in the study. Essentially, an association is when a risk factor or marker occurs in unison with the outcome more frequently than expected by chance alone. When risk is expressed as the probability of an event occurring over a specified period of time, it is mathematically equivalent to the number of people developing the outcome divided by the number of people available to develop the outcome when the period began. When exposure is factored into the calculation, risk is equal to the probability of the outcome if the factor is present divided by the probability of the outcome if the factor is not present. This calculation is known as relative risk and is most frequently used in studies with a prospective design.

An important element of calculating relative risk is knowing the number of times the outcome could have occurred in the ratio's denominator, which is dependent on incidence. If the incidence of the event in the exposed and unexposed cannot be assessed, the alternative estimate of risk that is calculated is known as an odds ratio. An odds ratio can be expressed in two ways: the odds of a person with the factor experiences the event divided by the odds of an unexposed person experiencing the event or the odds that an event occurred in a person exposed divided by the odds that an exposed person did not experience the event. The latter is the classic application for calculating odds ratios in a case-control study design. Odds ratios are also used to estimate risk in cross sectional studies and some cohort study designs. Measuring an estimate of risk can be expressed in a $2 \times 2$ table for both relative risk and the odds of experiencing the event (Figure 12.5). Both relative risk and odds ratios are the principal measures we use to quantify the strength of the association between a factor and the event.

## Using Epidemiology to Monitor Disease—Surveillance

Monitoring risk and disease at the population level is surveillance. The process of surveillance is the "systematic and continuous collection, analysis, and interpretation of data, closely integrated with the timely and coherent dissemination of the results and assessment to those who have the right to know so that action can be taken. It is an essential feature of epidemiologic and public health practice."[41] Surveillance performed on a routine basis is called passive surveillance. The cornerstone of any passive surveillance activity is the gathering of "reportable" disease reports generated from healthcare providers, hospitals, and laboratories. Many infectious diseases

|  | | Outcome (Event) | | |
|---|---|---|---|---|
|  | | Present | Absent | |
| **Factor** | Exposed | A | B | A + B |
|  | Unexposed | C | D | C + D |
|  | | A + C | B + D | |

Incidence in exposed = A / (A + B)
Incidence in unexposed = C / (C + D)
Relative Risk = [A / (A + B)] / [C / (C + D)]
Odds Ratio in Cohort Studies = (A / B) / (C / D)
Odds Ratio in Case Control Studies = (A / C) / (B / D)
Uniform Odds Ratio Calculation = AD / BC

• **Figure 12.5** Estimating Risk: Relative Risk and Odds Ratio.

make up the list of reportable diseases, for example, influenza and measles. Another activity that represents passive surveillance is the maintenance of a cancer registry. In the United States, the Surveillance, Epidemiology, and End Results (SEER) Program provides information on cancer statistics for the US population. Approximately one-third of the US population is covered by the current registry, which is supported by the Surveillance Research Program (SRP) at the National Cancer Institute. Information on the burden of oropharyngeal cancer in the United States comes from SEER.

Active surveillance involves contacting individuals directly either through periodic phone calls or personal visits. Although interviewing can be done in variety of ways, the most common method remains contacting people by telephone. Many of the large health surveys in the United States periodically collect information by phone. The oldest and one of the largest health surveys in the United States is the National Health Interview Survey (NHIS). This household survey was initiated in 1957 and typically collects information on more than 80,000 people in 35,000 households each year. Another passive surveillance activity is the Behavioral Risk Factor Surveillance System (BRFSS). Begun in 1984, this is the largest health-related telephone survey in the United States. The program collects state-level data from residents—focusing on lifestyle and risk behaviors, chronic health conditions, and use of preventive services, completing more than 400,000 adult interviews each year. Both the NHIS and BRFSS collect some oral health–related information.

Active surveillance that is designed around in-person visits is much rarer. In the United States, active surveillance at the state level often focuses on school-age children with periodic elementary school screenings to monitor dental caries and dental sealant prevalence. At the national level, the National Health and Nutrition Examination Survey (NHANES) is a series of health examinations and nutritional assessments involving children and adults. Initiated in 1960, NHANES is unique in that it combines interviews and physical examinations with laboratory tests. Each year, approximately 5000 individuals of all ages are interviewed in their homes and complete the health examination in a mobile examination center. Core information on the national prevalence of tooth loss, dental caries, and other oral health–related conditions in the United States is collected through NHANES. Active surveillance is more resource intensive and is challenging for many public health systems globally.

The science supporting the methodology and implementation of surveillance is rooted in epidemiology, but epidemiology is also the foundational science for public health research. This type of research is intended to contribute to generalizable knowledge and is best characterized by the following attributes: (1) intended benefits of the activity may or may not include study participants but always extends beyond the study participants, (2) data collected exceeds requirements for the care of the study participants, (3) project activities have rigorous study design, and (4) information is always collected under systematic procedures to reduce bias to promote generalizability beyond those receiving services or participating in routine programmatic activities.

Although all research is about discovery of facts that expand our knowledge of natural phenomena, not all research builds on that knowledge base in the same way. Basic research strives to uncover the fundamental relationships between health and disease at the molecular level, clinical research aims to extend this knowledge to the person level, and public health research expands it to the population level (Figure 12.6). Public health research is needed to:

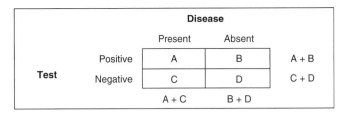

A = True Positives
B = False Positives
C = False Negatives
D = True Negatives
Sensitivity = A / (A + C)
Specificity = D / (B + D)
Positive Predicative Value = A / (A + B)
Negative Predicative Value = D / (C + D)
Accuracy = (A + D)/(A + B + C + D)

• **Figure 12.6** Sensitivity, specificity, and predicative values in screening and diagnostic testing.

- know what interventions lead to improvements in the public's health,
- understand how to change health behavior,
- know most effective (including cost-effective) interventions,
- identify best practices (evidenced-based healthcare), and
- know how to organize and deliver public health services.

## Using Epidemiology to Study Disease— Research

Good research demands careful, sometimes exhaustive planning. Every study, no matter how modest, needs a protocol, which is a written research plan encompassing the purpose and the detailed operation of the study. The essential elements of a protocol are listed in Box 12.4. A protocol demands careful thinking through of a project, a process that aids its design and helps the researchers anticipate potential problems. It also simplifies the writing of a final report, because key elements from the research plan form the basis of the report.

The rigor of any epidemiologic study begins with research design, which represents the framework and procedures that guide the process of collecting, managing, and analyzing data. Some research designs are appropriate for hypothesis testing, whereas others are more appropriate for hypothesis generation.[26] Although no research design is flawless, a good epidemiologic study design should (1) permit the comparison of an outcome variable (event occurrence) between two or more groups; (2) quantify the comparison in absolute or relative terms; (3) attempt to manage potential errors in data collection and later in the analyses, control for confounding; and (4) recognize the temporal relationship between the outcome variable and the main factor of interest.

## Epidemiologic Study Designs for Generating Hypotheses

A cross-sectional study is one in which both exposure to risk factors and the health outcomes in a group of people who are, or are assumed to be, a sample of a particular population (a "cross section") are assessed at the same time. Information is typically gathered by trained interviewers or examiners. There is no intervention

1. A precise definition of the research problem, the reasons for undertaking the research, and a review of pertinent literature.
2. Objectives of the study or hypotheses to be tested. A hypothesis is a conjecture cast in a form (the null hypothesis) that will allow it to be tested and refuted if it is false.
3. Population to be studied, including its selection, source, size, method of sampling, and method of allocation to groups (if a clinical trial).
4. Data to be collected, including a description of each item needed to accomplish the objectives or to test the hypotheses.
5. Procedures to be carried out, with details of exactly how the needed data will be obtained from the participants in the study and by whom.

6. Data collection methods, with examples of all data collection forms or computer methods of data collection and a list of all necessary supplies, equipment, and instruments.
7. Plans for data processing and analysis, including how the data get from field collection to computer, computer file organization, and statistical distributions to be examined.
8. Time schedule for planning, procurement of informed consent from study subjects, data collection and analysis, and report writing.
9. An assessment of any ethical issues involved in the study and certification that the necessary institutional human subjects clearance has been obtained.

and all information gathered is primarily for understanding current health status and factors associated with disease occurrence. Many national health surveys are designed as rigorous cross-sectional studies. This allows these studies to transition from a surveillance activity (descriptive epidemiology) to a hypothesis-generating (analytical epidemiology) study. With regards to large health studies that serve both a surveillance and hypothesis generating purpose, NHANES has been one of the most important for oral health research since the 1970s. Cross-sectional studies have several advantages and limitations. If selection for participation is through randomization, this can enhance the validity of the findings, especially if the sampling frame is designed to be representative of a particular group. If selection is based on a convenience sample, this weakens the generalizability of the findings. A major limitation of cross-sectional studies is the inability to effectively asses for temporal relationship between an event and the factor of interest.

An ecologic study is an analytic study in which data for both exposures and outcomes come from the population rather than from individuals. Often the exposure and outcome of interest occur in the same geographic area. For example, studies addressing the question of whether water fluoridation is related to hip fracture experience (i.e., suggesting that fluoridation is a risk factor for hip fracture) have used community data for both water fluoridation (the exposure) and for hip fractures (the outcome) to derive a relationship.[24,46] Such studies are relatively quick and inexpensive because they avoid sampling, interviewing, clinical examinations, or access to individual medical records. Their weakness, however, is that they cannot be certain that the people with the outcome condition (in this case, the hip fracture) are the same ones who had the exposure (drank fluoridated water). This weakness is often called the ecologic fallacy. Ecologic studies can be useful, although usually they are not definitive. They have a clearer role when a variable under consideration—for example, community income level—is by definition a group measure rather than an individual one.

## Epidemiologic Study Designs for Generating or Testing Hypotheses

The basic design of a case-control study centers on the identification of two groups: a group of persons with the outcome of interest (cases) and a group of people without the outcome (controls). Then, the frequency of past exposure is determined for each group. This can be accomplished by interview, health record review, lab tests, examination, etc. Because the exposures of interest are sought in the past of the study participants, the actual (relative) risk of the outcome cannot be determined. However, the relative risk can be estimated through the derivation of an *odds ratio,* a numerical statement of probability very similar to relative risk. Controls are minimally matched individually to cases on key sociodemographic characteristics (e.g. age, sex, and race/ethnicity). Case-control studies must be planned thoughtfully, because the characteristics on which the groups are matched (e.g., ethnic group) cannot be analyzed further as possible etiologic factors. Another concern with matching is the concept of overmatching. If a characteristic potentially in the causal pathway is serendipitously selected for matching cases and controls, this characteristic could not be evaluated as a risk indicator or "cause" of the outcome. In the landmark studies demonstrating an association between lung cancer and smoking,[7] if Richard Doll and Bradford Hill would have matched on smoking, they never would have found that exposure as a potential causal agent for lung cancer.

Case-control studies have some important advantages. They can be executed relatively quickly and are particularly useful for studying rare diseases. A limitation of this study design is the accurate assessment of exposure or key risk indicators that rely on recall or records as they exist in the past. Similar to cross-sectional studies, the temporal relationships between exposure and outcome and determined at the same time. Consequently, case-control studies can demonstrate risk indicators for a disease, but the retrospective design means that risk factors cannot be identified in this way. Risk factors for a disease can be confirmed only through rigorous cohort or experimental study designs.

In a cohort study design, participants are allocated to two groups: those exposed and those not exposed to one or more risk factors, and both groups are followed over time to determine who develops and does not develop the outcome of interest. Because new cases of disease (outcome of interest) are identified, incidence can be compared between exposure and nonexposure groups permitting estimation of actual (relative) risk for developing the outcome of interest in an exposed person compared to the risk among the unexposed.[41] A cohort can be organized for study in two general ways: prospectively and retrospectively. A prospective cohort study collects information on an exposure of interest and compares eventual outcomes at some point in the future. In a retrospective cohort study, the investigator looks back in time and identifies individuals exposed and nonexposed and selects them for follow-up to the present to determine who developed the outcome of interest. Although a retrospective cohort study design has many advantages, it has an important limitation: the inability to monitor and promote data quality assurance at the level that is possible for well-designed prospective studies.

All of these study designs are nonexperimental and noninterventional, meaning that they study conditions as they occur rather than manipulate conditions in the manner of a classical laboratory experiment. However, there are experimental designs in epidemiology that are used to test the efficacy or effectiveness of a therapeutic drug, a preventive material, or a treatment regimen.

## Epidemiologic Study Designs for Testing Hypotheses

There are several experimental study designs, but a well-conducted clinical trial is generally considered the "gold standard." A clinical trial is a controlled experimental study or group comparison based on epidemiologic principles and designed to test the hypothesis that a particular agent or procedure favorably alters the natural history of a disease. The group receiving the agent or regimen under study is the test group, sometimes called the experimental or study group, whereas a comparable group not subject to the agent or regimen is the control group. Clinical trials compare results in two or more samples of a single population, divided into groups that are essentially similar (in distribution of age, sex, race, socioeconomic status, and previous disease experience). The aim is to ensure that the only difference between the groups is the fact that the test group receives the treatment under study whereas the control group does not. Participants enrolled in a clinical trial do not know if they received the test or the nonexperimental intervention (process known as blinding). When assignment to an experimental agent is made through a randomization procedure, the study design is known as a randomized controlled trial (RCT). Although the study design of RCTs is based on the clinical trial approach, they can be applied in population-based research. When an RCT is implemented at the population level, they are referred to as a community or field RCT.

The National Institutes of Health defines a clinical trial as a "research study in which one or more human subjects are prospectively assigned to one or more interventions (which may include placebo or other control) to evaluate the effects of those interventions on health-related biomedical or behavioral outcomes."[38] Trials must follow good clinical practice (GCP) to promote safety, integrity, and quality of the study. The three main elements of GCP assurance are (1) ensuring the rights and well-being of human participants are protected; (2) facilitating appropriate design, conduct, and reporting of the study; and (3) producing valid and reliable data that supports analytical applications. When a new pharmacologic therapeutic agent is tested in humans, it typically proceeds through a series of clinical trials. The intent of a phase 1 trial is to determine if the agent is safe. In this study, only a few people receive the agent at low doses and are monitored for side effects. In phase 2 trials the aim is to determine if the agent works. The study group is larger, often including a few dozen upward to about 100 volunteers. Placebos are not given in both phase 1 and phase 2 trials. The primary aim of a phase 3 trial is to determine if the agent is better than what is customarily provided. The study group is much larger than a phase 2 trial, and treatment or intervention group(s) are formed along with a comparison group(s). Participants are randomized to a group, and a placebo may be used. Like all RCT studies, phase 3 trials are designed to ascertain efficacy. In phase 4 studies, the agent has already received approval for use but some questions require additional investigation to answer. Many of these questions look at outcomes beyond the efficacy of the agent, such as cost effectiveness, improved quality of life, and population effect. Phase 4 studies are designed to evaluate effectiveness.

Choosing a study population should be determined by the purpose of the trial. If the prime purpose of a clinical trial is to test the *efficacy* of a particular agent (i.e., whether it works), then the most favorable conditions should be created to show that it does work. For that reason, the project should be conducted with subjects who are selected for their susceptibility to the disease or condition. This means that a population of a specific age range is usually chosen deliberately, because many oral diseases are age specific. Sex, race, socioeconomic status, and geographic location are other factors considered in the choice of a study population for efficacy trials. If, however, the purpose is to assess the *effectiveness* of an agent under everyday conditions, then broad community populations—those with varying degrees of the disease or condition under study—should be chosen.[39] Confusing the purposes of trials can lead to the error of generalizing the results of efficacy trials conducted in special populations with unusual disease distributions, such as institutionalized people, to the general population.

The RCT is the cornerstone of evidence-based dentistry (see Chapter 11) and its rigor is derived from random allocation of participants to the study and control groups. Random allocation means that each participant has an equal chance of being assigned to either the study or the control group. Statistical probability is such that the assumption can then be made that bias is not intruding and that at the end of the trial any differences between the groups can be attributed only to the agent under study. Any uncontrolled variables influencing the outcome, which are usually undetected by the researchers, are likely to affect subjects in both groups equally and therefore not to affect the relative differences between the groups.

The principle of random allocation is simple, although it is a carefully planned and controlled procedure. Random allocation is not haphazard assignment or one based on volunteering or self-selection. A statistician can further improve the probability of establishing comparable groups by stratification, which means that before allocation the base population is separated by those factors known or thought to influence disease occurrence (usually age, gender, race, socioeconomic status, and previous disease experience). Subjects from each stratum are then randomly allocated to study and control groups. Another very important consideration affecting randomized allocation is sample size requirements and power. These concepts are discussed in detail in Chapter 13.

One of the challenges facing contemporary research into disease prevention and control is our increasing understanding of the role of multilevel risk factors, including social interactions, in disease initiation. This is especially relevant in health disparities research and why we need to evaluate interventions that operate at multiple levels in more real-world settings.[10] As such, tightly controlled trials, such as the RCT, often are not applicable to multilevel and community-based intervention projects. However, there are some study designs that can be used to address these issues and maintain rigor comparable to RCTs. The group or cluster randomized trial (GRT) is designed for interventions targeting groups rather than individuals, which allow a multilevel intervention to be delivered to communities or neighborhoods randomized to the intervention program.[8,35,36] GRTs are typically used to evaluate multilevel and community-based intervention programs.

Stepped wedge (SW) designs can also be used to study multilevel or community-based interventions.[21,22] In this design, the groups to be randomized are measured and one or more groups are selected at random to receive the intervention. After an appropriate interval, measurements are repeated and one or more groups are selected at random from those remaining to receive the intervention. This interval-selection process continues until all groups have received the intervention. There are a number of other options available, including some that are variations of the GRT and SW research design, such as sequential multiple assignment randomized trials (SMART).[4,5]

Nonrandomized trial designs are not uncommon in the dental literature.[42,43] Although they are weaker than randomized designs, sometimes practical considerations dictate their use. For example, the landmark Vipeholm study on diet and caries was a prospective study, but participants were assigned to groups on a convenience basis rather than by randomization.[18] This could have influenced the results to some extent. Some studies dispense with a control group altogether and determine efficacy by comparison with historical controls; that is, they use a before-and-after design in which disease levels at the end of the project are compared with those at the beginning.[20] The weakness in this design is that uncontrolled change could take place during the trial to invalidate results. For example, in a trial of a fluoride mouthrinse, children in sixth grade at the completion of a 3-year trial may have brushed with fluoride toothpaste more often than did the sixth-graders examined at the beginning of the trial. Without use of a concurrent control group it is impossible to tell if beneficial outcomes were due entirely to the mouthrinse or were due at least in part to the additional toothpaste use.

Before-and-after trials are often called demonstrations, intended to "demonstrate" the value of accepted preventive measures.[27] Presenting a case for the scientific validity of demonstrations can get complicated,[19,20] although it is worth noting that the pioneering Grand Rapids fluoridation trial used this design.[2,6] A major threat to the validity of a before-and-after design comes from undetected sociodemographic change in the population under study during the period of the trial.

Some studies have used a comparison group, defined as any group to which the study group is compared and a term that too often is used synonymously with control group.[41] It is less confusing, however, if the term control group is reserved for randomized controls and the term comparison group is used for nonrandomized comparisons. Examples of comparison groups are the control communities used in fluoridation field trials. Some comparison groups can be similar to study groups and thus permit fairly valid comparisons, but others are so far removed from the study group that they serve little purpose.

Certain types of trial use a crossover design, in which subjects serve as their own controls. Each subject receives an active treatment for a specific time and a placebo (or no treatment) during a control period. Crossover designs are useful in short-term trials (weeks or months, rather than years) for preventing reversible conditions like gingivitis or calculus accumulation but are unsuitable for caries prevention trials because the time needed for new lesions to develop is too long. They are also not appropriate for testing of regimens that have a carryover effect, because the effects of the treatment phase could influence responses during the nontreatment phase. Crossover designs are also inappropriate when the tested regimen may produce a permanent effect, when test agents may be retained at the site of action for prolonged periods, or when conditions may naturally undergo a rapid change in prevalence, incidence, or morbidity. The principal advantage of a crossover design is that results are not affected by variations in response among participating subjects.

## Placebos

The use of a placebo in experimental research designs has been considered essential for studying how well an agent fulfills its intended purpose, but there is debate about its ethical use.[17] A placebo is a material or formulation like the test product but without the active ingredient, such as a toothpaste that feels and tastes like a fluoride toothpaste but contains no fluoride. The purpose of using a placebo in a trial is to keep subjects unaware of whether they are in the test or control group (a blind study), so that their health behavior will not be consciously or unconsciously affected by group allocation. Bias, which is systematic though usually unconscious error, can affect examiners as well. An examiner who expects a product to be effective may unconsciously apply stricter criteria for caries in a control group if he or she knows which children are in which group. Examiners therefore also should not know the group allocation of subjects. When neither participants nor examiners know the group allocations, the trial is termed double blind.

Use of a placebo is inherently impossible in some instances, such as in trials of water fluoridation (where the fluoridating community is a matter of public record), fissure sealant (where sealant visibility determines the outcome), or dental health education (where the control at best is a comparable group that receives no program, a passive control). Placebos raise ethical issues, because it is usually considered unethical to deny established beneficial products to trial participants. If a manufacturer wants to test fluoride toothpaste with a stronger formulation than is standard, for example, the control group does not use a nonfluoride toothpaste but rather a standard-strength product. This is called a positive control; the results then compare the effects of the new product with the effects of the old one. Because the difference between these two groups would be expected to be less than if a placebo were used, the trial needs larger numbers of participants to allow any true difference to be shown.

This raises an important ethical issue. Do we increase enrollment substantially in trails to test marginal differences between a novel agent and currently used agent to demonstrate equivalency or noninferior efficacy? The weakness of efficacy trials without controls is that we never know if using a tested product in a public health program is any better than having no program. In an age of low caries experience and extensive fluoride exposure (apart from any that may be associated with the test product), that can be a fair question.

## Blinding

Randomized controlled trials designed to answer the question of whether a particular agent or regimen works must give the test agent every chance to succeed. Susceptible populations are chosen for the trial, and participants are randomly allocated to test and control groups not knowing if they are participating in the test or control group. This is known as a single-blind study. If examiners, observers, or others involved in delivering or assessing the agent are prevented from knowing who received the treatment or were assigned to a control group, then this trail is known as a double-blind study. Blinding is important in trials because it reduces bias and strengthens the application of a placebo and the evaluation for efficacy.

## Operational Control

Researchers need to be sure that the agent is used as intended in trials assessing efficacy. If it is a professionally applied agent or a treatment regimen, the protocol must specify precisely how the agent will be used, for how long, how often, at what concentration, and by whom.

A placebo, or positive control, would be applied the same way. If a self-applied agent is being tested, such as a mouthrinse, the protocol should call for the agent to be used under professional supervision. It is the researchers' task to ensure that the protocol is adhered to throughout the course of the study.

In an effectiveness trial, the agent or treatment can be used as it normally would. That means that professionals are given instructions in the use of a procedure or participants are given the rinse to take home and use as instructed. Therefore there is less certainty in an effectiveness trial that the material has been used as intended, but one of the aims of an effectiveness trial is to evaluate how the material works under everyday conditions. In operational control, as in other aspects of a trial, the purpose of the study must be kept in mind.

Clinical trials must be continued long enough to permit detection of new disease or extension of lesions already present. For caries trials, the minimum duration is usually 2 to 3 years, although precise timing depends on the purposes of the trial.[13] The longer the trial, the more expensive it is, so trade-offs are required. The FDI World Dental Federation suggested in 1977 that trials of plaque-inhibiting agents could be as short as 8 to 21 days,[14] but that guideline was for plaque measurements only. The FDI also recommended that studies of calculus-preventing agents should last at least 90 days for supragingival calculus and longer for subgingival calculus. The American Dental Association requires that plaque-inhibiting agents for which the association's seal of approval is sought demonstrate gingivitis reduction as well as plaque reduction; it requires such trials to be at least 6 months long.[1]

Loss of participants during a prospective clinical trial will occur and must be planned for. If the numbers of subjects in the groups are not large enough to begin with, at the end of the trial the researcher will be left with too few subjects to be able to show by statistical logic whether it is likely that an observed difference between the groups is real or a chance result. The result may then be that a real difference cannot be detected, and an agent that in fact is effective will not seem to be so. Statistical approaches are available for controlling loss of follow-up and analyzing findings. These issues are discussed in Chapter 13.

## Ethical Considerations

Group sizes in a clinical trial should not be unduly large, because it is unethical to involve participants in research when their involvement is scientifically unnecessary and needlessly exposes them to the inconvenience and possible risks of participation. Humans taking part in clinical trials must give informed consent, which means providing a written acceptance that the participant understands the conduct of the trial and the nature of any risks involved. Researchers must certify in the report of the trial that the study protocol has been accepted by their institution's review board, which any institution conducting research is required to maintain. If the study raises special issues or intends to include vulnerable populations (e.g., children, prisoners, people with intellectual disabilities, etc.), extra explanations seeking approval and description of protections are required. Other considerations, including how the rights of participants have been safeguarded, may also be needed if the study is conducted in a developing country that does not have the same rigorous standards for human subject protection as do the developed nations.

## Data Quality in Epidemiology

### The Concept of Measuring Disease

The good clinician thinks in qualitative terms. During a diagnostic examination, the dental practitioner not only looks for existing disease but also tries to look ahead to the possibility of future disease. Measuring the oral health of a population, however, requires a more standardized and objective approach. Specific diagnostic criteria, written explicitly for clinical, radiographic, microbiological, or pathologic examination, provide an objective framework for the practitioner's judgment. These criteria are applied to judge the condition of the oral tissues as they are at examination time, not as they might be in the future. This objective application of diagnostic criteria is the most important philosophical difference between the epidemiologic examination and the examination carried out for treatment planning.

Measurement, the quantification of observations, is the crux of science. Measurement variability is inherent in all fields of science; it is one reason why laboratory experiments are repeated before their findings can be accepted. In studies of oral disease, a count of carious lesions in a population is almost never duplicated; a repeat examination of the same group of patients frequently results in a different count of carious lesions. Any one count of disease in a group is therefore an estimate of conditions rather than absolute truth. As long as criteria are applied consistently, however, valid estimates will still result, because diagnostic drifts in one direction will be balanced by drifts the other way. Nevertheless, it is important that we try to ascertain these drifts and report them in a consistent and objective way.

Acute diseases such as measles are characterized by a sudden onset of symptoms, so the patient progresses rapidly from a state in which the disease is clearly absent to one in which the disease is clearly present. Remission of the acute phase of the disease is equally rapid, so little time is spent in the "gray areas." Chronic diseases, however, are usually characterized by a much slower onset. It is difficult to establish exactly when arthritis, alcoholism, mental illness, dental caries, and periodontitis become definitely established; there is a considerable gray area. In dentistry this problem is handled by counting as lesions only those that meet specific criteria.

Data quality is typically expressed in terms of *validity* and *reliability*. Validity is how well an instrument or protocol actually measures what it was intended to do. In the application of diagnostic testing, validity is how well the test can distinguish between those with and without disease. For epidemiologic applications, validity can also reflect accuracy, that is, how close a measurement is to a standard or the "truth." Reliability is how well repeated applications can give the same results, in other words, how reproducible is the test, instrument, or examination when conditions are the same. Reliability is very important to epidemiologic data collection. We measure reliability in several ways, ranging from sensitivity and specificity in diagnostic testing and screening to kappa statistics for the assessment of examiner performance.

### Measuring the Value of a Diagnostic Test

As previously discussed, the ultimate test for the efficacy of a preventive agent or procedure is the RCT, but this research design does not fit when the purpose is evaluation of a diagnostic test. The criteria for an ideal test are that it should be simple, inexpensive (relative to the direct or social cost of the disease), acceptable to the patient, valid, and reliable. A test should also be sensitive, which in this context means that it yields a positive result in those with the disease, and specific, meaning that it gives a negative result in those who do not have the disease. There are only a few tests that rate highly in both sensitivity and specificity, so the choice may be whether to use a test that is highly sensitive but not very specific (which would capture a lot of false positives—people who test positive but really don't have the disease), specific but not sensitive (which would lead to a lot of false negatives—people who test negative but really do have the disease), or not to test at all. Figure 12.7 summarizes how sensitivity, specificity, and related predictive values can be derived from the results of tests and subsequent disease outcome.

It is important to recognize that the purpose of a diagnostic test is different from the purpose of a screening test. Both are rooted in the same foundational concepts but are applied differently. Diagnostic tests have a clinical application, whereas screening tests are applied in population settings.

Understanding sensitivity and specificity is important for public health monitoring and research. We often identify large numbers of people in screening programs who screen positive for the disease or outcome of interest. This includes those who are *true positives* and those who are *false positives*. People who are screened positive for having the outcome of interest are generally directed to undergo more tests that have a higher degree of complexity and expense. This can create a number of concerns, including increased economic and utilization burden on the healthcare system and increased worry by the individuals who test positive. Alternatively, if screened people are identified as false negatives and the outcome of interest has substantial morbidity or mortality, these individuals would not be directed to life-altering care, especially if the disease is in its early stage.

In dentistry, screening tests have generally been problematic. A considerable number of predictive tests intended to identify caries-susceptible individuals have been explored through the years without much success. This is most likely due to the large number of factors that interact to initiate the disease. Nevertheless, caries risk assessment continues to be refined, especially for application in pediatric oral healthcare (see Chapter 14). Research aimed at finding tests for susceptibility to moderate-severe periodontitis is still a work in progress. There have been a number of indicators or markers promoted as possible uses for a screening test using (1) bacteriologic or biological tests such as measuring bacterial quality and load and inflammatory mediators; (2) clinical indicators such attachment loss, bleeding on probing, and suppuration; and (3) a constellation of environmental factors and socio-determinants. The only true risk factors established are tobacco use and diabetes, but the relationship between diabetes and periodontitis is most likely bidirectional. More recent attempts to identify a useful screening test for periodontitis have focused on the use of a questionnaire.[12] Another important improvement related to screening and surveillance of periodontitis (See Chapter 15).

Determining the effectiveness of a screening program is often more challenging than the practical implementation of it. At face value, a screening program may seem reasonable and beneficial, but the evidence for it may be lacking, especially in asymptomatic populations. This contrast is particularly evident for oral cancer screening. Oral and pharyngeal cancers include cancer of the lip, oral cavity, and pharynx, with the majority of all cancers classified as squamous-cell carcinoma (SCC). Given that more than 50% of persons with oropharyngeal SCC have regional or distant metastases at diagnosis,[37] screening for oral cancer should be beneficial if this cancer could be identified earlier and treated successfully. One challenge with developing a valid screening instrument is that oral and oropharyngeal cancer have different causes. Tobacco and alcohol use are strongly associated with oral cancer, whereas human papillomavirus (HPV) is an important risk factor for pharyngeal cancer (see Chapter 16). Currently, the US Preventive Services Task Service (USPSTF) has concluded the current evidence is insufficient to assess the balance of benefits and harms of screening for oral cancer in asymptomatic adults.[48] Although the USPSTF has determined there is inadequate evidence that screening improves morbidity or mortality, they also have determined there is inadequate evidence on harms from an oral cancer screening test from false-positive or false-negative findings. This is important because we continue to advocate for oral cancer screening even though the benefits and harms to screening have yet to be fully understood.

## Examiner Reliability

The validity of any study—cross-sectional to clinical trial—depends heavily on the reliability of the examiner(s) or rater(s). This factor is usually referred to as intraexaminer reliability (i.e., within-examiner consistency) or the ability of an examiner to record the same conditions the same way over time. Most examiners with training and experience can develop an acceptable degree of intraexaminer consistency. Consistency between different examiners, interexaminer reliability, is more difficult to achieve, even when the examiners train together from the same written criteria and with the same trainer. It is best to use one well-qualified examiner, but large-scale studies usually require more than one examiner, and multicenter trials certainly do. In such cases the examiners should undergo a period of training to bring their diagnostic standards as close together as can possibly be managed. This training procedure is referred to as standardization. When a single examiner serves as the reference examiner (sometimes referred to as the "gold standard" examiner), once training and standardization is achieved, all examiners are compared to the reference examiner through a process known as calibration.

Because one of the most significant contributors to data problems in epidemiologic studies can be a result of examiner error, a robust examiner training plan demonstrating knowledge and skill (calibration) prior to and during data collection is critical.[9] The issue of examiner reliability can make people uncomfortable, because to have one's inconsistencies exposed for the world to see can be humbling. (We stress that examiner reliability is totally unrelated to clinical skills or ability to care for patients.) Nevertheless, it is important to recognize that it is not unusual to find less-than-perfect agreement between readers, scorers, and examiners, and it is not unusual for an individual's interpretation of a condition or the data to be different from a previous observation. Intraexaminer reliability is quality that can be developed by most examiners with some training and experience. Interexaminer reliability—reaching agreement between two or more examiners—is usually more tedious. It requires initial agreement on interpretation of diagnostic criteria, then a period of training with repeated observations to ensure that examiners' judgments are comparable. Interexaminer reliability is rarely perfect, but when examination findings from two or more examiners are being pooled, a measure of interexaminer reliability training should be recorded.

Measuring agreement can be expressed in a $2 \times 2$ table (see Figure 12.6) when we want to assess reliability between a rater and the reference person. The most common expression of reliability is percent agreement. That is, when the examiner and the reference

| | | Reference Examiner | | |
|---|---|---|---|---|
| | | Positive | Negative | |
| **Examiner** | Positive | A | B | A + B |
| | Negative | C | D | C + D |
| | | A + C | B + D | |

Observed Agreement (Ao) = A + D

Maximum Agreement (N) = A + B + C + D

Overall percent agreement = (A + D) / (A + B + C + D)

Positive/Positive Agreement Expected by Chance (Aa): [(A + B)(A + C)] / N

Negative/Negative Agreement Expected by Chance (An): [(C + D)(B + D)] / N

Total Agreement Expected by Chance (Ac) = Aa + An

Kappa = (Ao − Ac) / (N − Ac)

• **Figure 12.7** Measuring Agreement Between Two Examiners (Interexaminer Reliability).

both agree that a condition exists or does not exist. Although percent agreement is useful, often it is an inadequate measure by itself to describe interexaminer reliability. In the literature, examiner reliability is sometimes vaguely dismissed with a statement like "the examiners achieved 96% agreement," which by itself is of little value because of its uncertain meaning (it usually seems to mean that one examiner's group mean score was 96% of the mean score of the other examiner's group). In addition, such a comparison does not account for decisions requiring little diagnostic judgment (e.g., inclusion of many obviously sound lower incisors in the denominator), nor does it account for agreement that would be expected by chance alone.[30] The measure most frequently used for expressing interexaminer reliability is the kappa statistic, a value between 0 and 1.0 that expresses the degree of agreement beyond that expected by chance alone.[23,30]

The kappa statistic is a more conservative measure of examiner reliability compared to a basic percent-agreement calculation. Because individuals could agree on an observation just by guessing, the kappa test essentially allows us to quantify any improvement in agreement. The kappa statistic is ratio and the numerator represents the improvement in agreement between the examiners over what guessing (chance) would have produced. The denominator is the maximum possible improvement over chance agreement.[25] The ratio ranges from a negative 1 to a positive 1. A zero represents agreement by chance, a positive 1 represents perfect agreement, and a negative 1 is perfect disagreement. The statistic is often presented as a percentage and is interpreted using thresholds (although arbitrary) recommended by Landis and Koch where "poor agreement" is 0 or less, "slight agreement" is 1% to 20%, "fair agreement" is 21% to 40%, "moderate agreement" is 41% to 60%, "substantial agreement" is 61% to 80%, and "almost perfect agreement" is 80% or higher.[30] An alternate, more user-friendly approach to interpreting kappa is the use of 0.60 as a threshold, where any kappa below 0.60 suggests inadequate reliability between an examiner and the reference.[32] When the outcome is not dichotomous (present or absent) and involves three or more categories, a weighted kappa test is used.[25] A weighted test acknowledges that some credit should be given for agreement when the difference between examiners may only be off by one category. Interpretability of weighted kappa works better when the categories are ordinal.

Correlation statistics and specified percent agreement, along with kappa, give a good picture of interexaminer reliability in a

study. However, it is frequently not clear in the literature that a rigorous training and evaluation plan has been implemented in most studies. When any measurements of disease are made over a period of time, conclusions reached are based on the comparison between two sets of results. Equally important, when measurements are made by multiple examiners during the same period, the pooling of data is used to calculate findings. It follows that the diagnostic criteria must be applied the same way at different times and by all examiners, because if they are not, the comparisons of data or the use of pooled data have little value. Reporting statistics demonstrating examiner performance with regards to data quality is critical for any study, whether it is an observation study or a clinical trial. This conforms with STROBE (Strengthening the Reporting of Observational Studies) guidelines for reporting data reliability and with the CONSORT (Consolidated Standards of Reporting Trials) Statement, a set of criteria for explicit reporting of clinical trials, which lists "any methods used to enhance quality of measurements" as one of the elements to be reported.[33,40,45]

## Epidemiology and Dental Public Health

Epidemiology is about studying the patterns of occurrence of diseases or conditions over time in people. It not only joins the basic sciences and clinical studies to increase our understanding of diseases using tools applied in clinical epidemiology, it also advances our understanding of how diseases and adverse health conditions exist in communities using epidemiologic principles developed for surveillance and population-based research. More importantly, epidemiology is the practice of identifying, implementing, and evaluating approaches that can control diseases and improve public health. Epidemiology has provided significant contributions to the field of dental public health. Earlier "discoveries" of the association between fluoride and dental caries, the impact of smoking on periodontal disease, and the interaction of common risk factors and their role in the relationship between overall health and oral health have mostly originated from epidemiologic studies. The importance of epidemiology continues today, with expanding our understanding of the factors that contribute to health disparities, interventions that reduce health disparities, and assessment of healthcare systems and policies that are intended to lead to improvements in health for all.

## References

1. American Dental Association, Council on Dental Therapeutics. Guidelines for acceptance of chemotherapeutic products for the control of supragingival plaque and gingivitis. *J Am Dent Assoc.* 1986;112:529–532.
2. Arnold FA Jr, Dean HT, Knutson JW. Effect of fluoridated public water supplies on dental caries prevalence. *Public Health Rep.* 1953;68(2):141–148.
3. Brian A, Burt and Stephen A, Eklund. *Dentistry, Dental Practice, and the Community.* 6th ed. St. Louis, Missouri: Elsevier Saunders; 2005.
4. Collins LM, Murphy SA, Strecher V. The multiphase optimization strategy (MOST) and the sequential multiple assignment randomized trial (SMART): new methods for more potent eHealth interventions. *Am J Prev Med.* 2007;32(suppl 5):S112–S118.
5. Collins LM, Nahum-Shani I, Almirall D. Optimization of behavioral dynamic treatment regimens based on the sequential, multiple assignment, randomized trial (SMART). *Clin Trials.* 2014;11(4):426–434.

6. Dean HT, Arnold FA Jr, Jay P, et al. Studies on mass control of dental caries through fluoridation of the public water supply. *Public Health Rep.* 1950;65(43):1403–1408.

7. Doll R, Hill AB. Smoking and carcinoma of the lung. *BMJ.* 1950; 2(4682):739–748.

8. Donner A, Klar N. *Design and Analysis of Cluster Randomization Trials in Health Research.* London, UK: Arnold; 2000.

9. Dye BA, Goodwin M, Ellwood RP, et al. Digital epidemiology - Calibrating readers to score dental images remotely. *J Dent.* 2018;74(suppl 1):S27–S33.

10. Dye BA, Duran DG, Murray DM, et al. The importance of evaluating health disparities research. *Am J Public Health.* 2019;109(S1): S34–S40.

11. Causation Evans AS. *Disease: A Chronological Journey.* New York, NY: Plenum; 1993:13–39.

12. Eke Pl, Dye BA, Wei L, Slade GD, Thornton-Evans GO, Beck JD, Taylor GW, Borgnakke WS, Page RC, Genco RJ. Self-reported measures for surveillance of periodontitis. *J Dent Res* 2013;92:1041–7.

13. Fédération Dentaire Internationale, Commission on Oral Health, Research and Epidemiology. Principal requirements for controlled clinical trials of caries preventive agents and procedures. *Int Dent J.* 1982;32:292–310.

14. Fédération Dentaire Internationale, Commission on Classification and Statistics for Oral Conditions. Principal requirements for controlled clinical trials in periodontal diseases. *Int Dent J.* 1977;27:62–76.

15. Fisher-Owens SA, Gansky SA, Platt LJ, et al. Influences on children's oral health: a conceptual model. *Pediatrics.* 2007;120(3):e510–e520.

16. Gordis L. *Epidemiology.* 5th ed. Philadelphia, PA: Elsevier Saunders; 2014.

17. Gupta U, Verma M. Placebo in clinical trials. *Perspect Clin Res.* 2013;4(1):49–52.

18. Gustaffson BE, et al. The Vipeholm dental caries study: the effect of different levels of carbohydrates intake on caries activity in 436 individuals observed for five years. *Acta Odont Scand.* 1954;11:232–364.

19. Horowitz HS, Meyers RJ, Heifetz SB, et al. Eight-year evaluation of a combined fluoride program in a nonfluoride area. *J Am Dent Assoc.* 1984;109:575–578.

20. Horowitz HS, Meyers RJ, Heifetz SB, et al. Combined fluoride, school-based program in a fluoride-deficient area: results of an 11-year study. *J Am Dent Assoc.* 1986;112:621–625.

21. Hughes JP, Granston TS, Heagerty PJ. Current issues in the design and analysis of stepped wedge trials. *Contemp Clin Trials.* 2015; 45(Pt A):55–60.

22. Hussey MA, Hughes JP. Design and analysis of stepped wedge cluster randomized trials. *Contemp Clin Trials.* 2007;28(2):182–191.

23. Hunt RJ. Percent agreement, Pearson's correlation, and kappa as measures of inter-examiner reliability. *J Dent Res.* 1986;65:128–130.

24. Jacobsen SJ, Goldberg J, Cooper C, et al. The association between water fluoridation and hip fracture among white women and men aged 65 years and older. A national ecologic study. Ann Epidemiol. 1992;2:617–626.

25. Jekel JF, Katz DL, Elmore JG, et al. *Epidemiology and Biostatistics and Preventive Medicine.* 3rd ed. Philadelphia, PA: Elsevier Saunders; 2007.

26. Keyes P. Present and future measures for dental caries control. *JADA.* 1969;79:1395–1404.

27. Klein SP, Bohannan HM. *The First Year of Field Activities in the National Preventive Dentistry Demonstration Program. Rand Report No. R-2536/1-RWJ.* Santa Monica, CA: Rand Corporation; 1979.

28. Kleinbaum DG, Kupper LL, Morgenstern H. *Epidemiologic Research: Principles and Quantitative Methods.* Belmont, CA: Lifetime Learning Publications; 1982:25–34.

29. Lilienfeld AM. Bradford Hill's influence on epidemiology. *Stat Med.* 1982;1:325–328.

30. Landis JR, Koch GG. The measurement of observer agreement for categorical data. *Biometrics.* 1977;33:159–174.

31. Locker D, Leake JL. Risk indicators and risk markers for periodontal disease experience in older adults living independently in Ontario, Canada. *J Dent Res.* 1993;72:9–17.

32. McHugh ML. Interrater reliability: the kappa statistic. *Biochem Med.* 2012;22:276–282.

33. Moher D, Schultz KF, Altman DG, for the CONSORT group. *Revised Recommendations for Improving the Quality of Reports of Parallel Group Randomized Trials;* 2001. Available from: http://www.consort-statement.org.

34. Morabia A. *History of Epidemiologic Methods and Concepts.* Therwil, Switzerland: Springer Basel AG; 2004.

35. Murray DM. *Design and Analysis of Group-Randomized Trials.* New York, NY: Oxford University Press; 1998.

36. Murray DM, Pennell M, Rhoda D, et al. Designing studies that would address the multilayered nature of health care. *J Natl Cancer Inst Monogr.* 2010;(40):90–96.

37. National Cancer Institute. *SEER: Oral Cavity and Pharynx.* Available from: https://seer.cancer.gov/statfacts/html/oralcav.html.

38. National Institute of Health. *NIH's Definition of a Clinical Trial.* Available from: https://grants.nih.gov/policy/clinical-trials/definition.htm.

39. O'Mullane DM. Efficiency in clinical trials of caries preventive agents and methods. *Community Dent Oral Epidemiol.* 1976;4: 190–194.

40. PLOS Medicine Editors. Observational studies: getting clear about transparency. *PLoS Med.* 2014;11(8): e1001711.

41. Porta MA. *Dictionary of Epidemiology.* 6th ed. New York, NY: Oxford University Press; 2014.

42. Ringleberg ML, Conti AJ, Webster DB. An evaluation of single and combined self-applied fluoride programs in schools. *J Public Health Dent.* 1976;36:229–236.

43. Ripa LW, Leske GS, Levinson A. Supervised weekly rinsing with a 0.2% neutral NaF solution: results from a demonstration program after two school years. *J Am Dent Assoc.* 1978;97:793–798.

44. Rothman KJ. Causes. *Am J Epidemiol.* 1976;104:587–592.

45. *STROBE Statement.* Available from: https://www.strobe-statement.org/index.php?id=strobe-home.

46. Suarez-Almazor ME, Flowerdew G, Saunders LD, et al. The fluoridation of drinking water and hip fracture hospitalization rates in two Canadian communities. *Am J Public Health.* 1993;83:689–693.

47. US Department of Health, Education, and Welfare. *Smoking and Health. Report of the Advisory Committee to the Surgeon General.* Washington, DC: Public Health Service; 1964.

48. US Preventive Services Task Force. *Final Recommendation Statement. Oral Cancer: Screening.* Available from: https://www.uspreventiveservicestaskforce.org/Page/Document/RecommendationStatementFinal/oral-cancer-screening1.

49. Wensink M, Westendorp RGJ, Baudisch A. The causal pie model: an epidemiological method applied to evolutionary biology and ecology. *Ecol Evol.* 2014;4(10):1924–1930.

50. WHO. *Epidemiology.* Available from: http://www.who.int/topics/epidemiology/en.

# 13

# Application of Biostatistics in Dental Public Health

DEBORAH V. DAWSON, PhD, ScM

DEREK R. BLANCHETTE, MS, PStat

BRUCE L. PIHLSTROM, DDS, MS

## Statistical Foundations

Data collection lies at the heart of scientific advancement. The mathematical discipline known as statistics is concerned with scientific methods for data collection, organization, summarization, and presentation, as well as the statistical analysis of data. Statistical analysis uses mathematical methods to describe characteristics of a population and to draw inferences or conclusions about population characteristics from sample data. Since the entire research process from data collection to data analysis is governed by statistical principles, the design of a research study and the planning of a statistical analysis are interrelated and, in fact, inseparable.

The statistical analysis of any study depends on its design. Unless research design and statistical analysis are considered together at the beginning of a study, it may be impossible to accomplish the goals of the study. Poor study design and poor conduct of research interfere with the ability to successfully analyze data, draw valid inferences, and answer the questions of interest. Simply stated, statistical analysis cannot correct a poorly designed or conducted study. Study planning must consider the research design, measurements of disease and outcomes, data collection, and the analytic methods to be used.

## Data Analysis: Estimation and Hypothesis Testing

### Population Estimates and Confidence Intervals

Descriptive studies are often conducted to estimate some unknown quantity in a population, such as prevalence of disease or fluoride concentration in a water supply. A quantitative characteristic of a population is generally called a *parameter*. Statistical methods are used to provide a single estimate or "point estimate" of an unknown parameter, such as when the mean of a sample from a population is used to estimate the mean in a population or a sample proportion is used to estimate prevalence in a population. A point estimate is the "best guess" of the true value of the population parameter. However, its measurement always involves some error, and a *confidence interval* is typically calculated that reflects the magnitude of the measurement error. Confidence intervals may be one-sided or two-sided, although the latter are most commonly used. For two-sided confidence intervals, a lower *confidence limit* and an upper *confidence limit* are provided according to some specified level of desired confidence, often 90%, 95%, or 99%.

Confidence intervals are routinely provided for many types of parameters, such as population means, odds ratios, and regression coefficients derived from multivariable modeling. Confidence intervals are typically based on the desired level of confidence (e.g., 95%), the point estimate (e.g., sample mean), and the standard error of the point estimate, which reflects the precision with which we are estimating the parameter. The true value of a parameter such as the population mean is a fixed constant; it is either in the interval or it is not. Confidence intervals are so constructed because they are expected to "capture" the true parameter value a certain percentage of the time. For example, when this procedure is used to construct a 95% confidence interval for a population mean, the procedure will provide an interval that will include the true mean value 95% of the time.

## Hypothesis Testing

The scientific method begins with a research question and a hypothesis. Researchers use their research question to develop a hypothesis that is framed in terms of population parameters that can be estimated, so that the hypothesis can be tested using statistical methods. For example, statistical hypothesis testing can be used to compare two or more groups with respect to the means of a quantitative measures or the proportion of persons having a certain population characteristic. Hypothesis testing can also be used to assess whether there is a correlation between two variables in a population or to test more complex associations among various measures in a population by using statistical models.

After establishing a hypothesis, the researcher tests it by checking it against "reality," that is, empirical evidence. Observational or experimental data are collected and, depending upon whether the data are consistent with the hypothesis, the hypothesis is accepted or rejected. It is important to understand that when data are gathered, random processes are at work. Because of variability, even if a hypothesis is true, data cannot be expected to fit the hypothesis perfectly. For example, one could make a hypothesis that when a fair coin is tossed, it would come up heads and tails an equal number of times. However, if such a coin were tossed 10 times, it would not be expected to come up exactly five times heads and five times tails. Under a given hypothesis, researchers are faced with the task of sorting out whether differences between what is observed and what is expected are due to chance or to a false hypothesis. *Statistical inference* is used to help researchers test their hypothesis so that they have a good chance of correctly answering their research question. Statistical tests of hypothesis are used to assess whether the observed data do or do not support a hypothesis.

## Null Hypothesis, Type I, and Type II Errors

An important concept is that of the *null hypothesis*, often denoted by $H_0$. The null hypothesis is typically stated in terms of *no effect*, for example, there is no difference between the means of two populations, no correlation between two quantitative measures, or a parameter does not differ from a specified value, as in the assertion that the fluoride level in a population does not differ from a designated target value. When testing a hypothesis, one chooses the probability of erroneously rejecting the null hypothesis, that is, rejecting the null hypothesis when it is true. This quantity is often denoted by the Greek letter $\alpha$ and is known by a variety of names: level of statistical significance, level of significance, probability of Type I error, and the significance level. It is very desirable to avoid making a Type I error, that is, we do not wish to assert that there is a difference or relationship where none exists (Box 13.1).

Figure 13.1 shows the four possible outcomes in statistical hypothesis testing. Let us assume we wish to assess whether the prevalence of caries differs in two populations; our null hypothesis ($H_0$) is that there is no difference in the prevalence of caries in the populations. As noted in the upper right box of this figure, if the null hypothesis is false (e.g., the prevalence of caries in the two populations truly differ), and, following statistical evaluation of the data, we reject $H_0$, then we have made the correct inference. On the other hand, as illustrated in the lower left box of the figure, if the prevalence in the two populations is actually the same, and the null hypothesis of no difference is not rejected, then a correct

## • BOX 13.1 Considerations in Hypothesis Testing: A Simple Example

Suppose an investigator wishes to test the fairness of a coin, that is, that the probability of obtaining heads when the coin is flipped is 1/2. The null hypothesis is that the probability of obtaining a head when the coin is flipped is 1/2. To test the null hypothesis, a coin is flipped 20 times and the number of times it comes up heads and tails is recorded.

If the coin comes up heads all 20 times, there are two possible interpretations: (1) although unlikely, a rare chance event of getting 20 consecutive heads has occurred, or (2) the results, while possible, are not probable. In the latter case, the null hypothesis of a fair coin (equal probability of heads and tails) would be rejected and the investigator would conclude that the coin is not fair—perhaps because it is unbalanced so it comes up heads more times than tails. However, there is still a small chance that the null hypothesis of no difference in the number of heads and tails was rejected in error.

When testing a hypothesis, we can control the risk of rejecting that hypothesis when it is in fact true (i.e., of making a Type I error). We can choose ahead of time the probability boundary defining rarity below which we will call a study outcome "possible but not probable" and reject the hypothesis under consideration. We do this by specifying the level of statistical significance $\alpha$, specifying the level of Type I error that is acceptable to us.

THE FOUR POSSIBLE OUTCOMES
IN STATISTICAL HYPOTHESIS TESTING

| "DECISION" (based on data) | "REALITY" | |
| --- | --- | --- |
| | $H_0$ IS TRUE | $H_0$ IS FALSE |
| REJECT $H_0$ | TYPE I ERROR | CORRECT DECISION |
| DO NOT REJECT $H_0$ | CORRECT DECISION | TYPE II ERROR |

• **Figure 13.1** The four possible outcomes in statistical hypothesis testing.

decision has again been made. However, just as there are two ways to be right, there are also two ways to be wrong (i.e., Type I and Type II errors). A type I error or $\alpha$, as shown earlier, occurs when the null hypothesis is rejected when it is actually true. That is, the true prevalence in the relevant populations was indeed the same, but it was erroneously asserted that they were different. The other type of error, called Type II error, occurs when the null hypothesis is false, but it is not rejected. This corresponds to the situation where the prevalence of disease actually does differ in two populations, but for whatever reason, our sample was such that we failed to detect that difference and did not reject the null hypothesis of no difference. The probability of Type II error is denoted by $\beta$, which is the probability that the null hypothesis is not rejected when it is, in fact, false.

As previously mentioned, $\alpha$ is determined by setting the probability boundary that corresponds to statistical significance. An $\alpha$ of 0.05 is a commonly specified level of statistical significance. However, $\beta$ is determined by a number of factors, some of which are not under the control of the researcher. These factors are considered in detail under the section in this chapter that discusses sample size estimation and *statistical power*. Statistical power, defined as $1 - \beta$, is the probability that the null hypothesis is correctly rejected, as when differences in disease prevalence are correctly identified in two populations. Clearly, it is desirable to have high power, that is, have a high probability of detecting a departure from the null hypothesis should it exist.

Statistical hypothesis testing involves: (1) formulating the null hypothesis, (2) specifying the desired level of statistical significance ($\alpha$), (3) using appropriate statistical procedures for data analysis, and (4) calculating a *test statistic* that is used to evaluate the sample data to decide whether to accept or reject the null hypothesis. It is critical that the sample characteristics, research design, and any related assumptions be considered when selecting and using statistical methods to test a hypothesis. The test statistic can be viewed as an index of disparity, which reflects the difference between the observed result based upon the sample data, and what would be expected if the null hypothesis were true. Some examples of test statistics are chi-square and t-statistics. Once the test statistic is used to evaluate the sample data, the decision is made to reject or accept the null hypothesis. As part of this process, a probability statement is made about the results based on sample data by calculating the significance probability, also called the descriptive level of significance or the "p-value." It is the probability of obtaining a result as rare as that based upon the observed data, or one even less likely, if the null hypothesis is true. If the p-value is less than the prespecified value of $\alpha$, the null hypothesis is rejected. The smaller the p-value, the stronger the evidence that there is a departure from the null hypothesis. See Box 13.2 for an illustration.

The approach to inference described here, in which both confidence intervals and hypothesis testing are used, is generally referred to as *frequentist inference*. Alternative inferential frameworks include *Bayesian inference* and *fiducial inference*, which are not addressed in this chapter.

## Meaning and Misuse of the P-Value

The meaning of the p-value is often confused. Several misinterpretations exist, but perhaps the most common is that the p-value represents the probability that a particular hypothesis is true.[35] In fact, the p-value reflects the strength of evidence *against* the null hypothesis. It should always be cited when reporting results of statistical data analysis for this reason. The p-value serves as a way of determining how unusual the observed result is, taking into account such factors as variability and sample size, relative to what would be expected under the null hypothesis. The specified value of

statistical significance ($\alpha$) is arbitrary, but $\alpha = 0.05$ is commonly used. It is important to emphasize that there is nothing particularly sacred about the significance value of 0.05; it is simply a kind of general consensus of what constitutes an unusual event. Indeed, it has been suggested that, in view of concerns about reproducibility of results, smaller significance levels, such as $\alpha = 0.005$, should be adopted as the threshold for significance.[35] Of course, if the p-value is provided, readers can apply whatever criterion for significance they wish. Further discussion of these issues may be found in the statement of the American Statistical Association on p-values.[58]

## The Problem of Multiple Testing

An important concern in hypothesis testing occurs when multiple statistical tests are performed. For example, researchers may wish to determine if any one of a number of genetic biomarkers is associated with a disease in a sample of patients. In studies evaluating the effectiveness of three or more treatments, multiple pairwise comparisons are typically carried out to determine which treatments are different from each other. If each statistical test of a possible association or treatment comparison were performed using a 0.05 level of significance, the chance of a Type I error occurring among the multiple tests would be much higher than 0.05, that is, the probability of finding a significant result, even if there are no true underlying departures from the null hypothesis, will be much greater than that specified level of significance. Simply stated, the more times that one tests for statistical significance, the more likely it is that a Type I error will occur. There are various approaches that can be used to control for the increased likelihood of a Type I error when multiple statistical testing is done; all basically set more stringent criteria for rejection of the null hypothesis.

The Bonferroni method provides one straightforward way to adjust the level of statistical significance when multiple statistical tests are performed. The number of tests $k$ to be performed and the desired overall (study-wise) level of significance $\alpha$ must be specified in advance. This method of adjustment for multiple testing specifies that a particular test will be considered statistically significant only if the associated significance probability $p < \alpha/k$. This adjustment insures that the overall probability of a Type I error, that is, of claiming a departure from the null hypothesis where none exists, is no greater than $\alpha$, regardless of whether the tests are independent. The Bonferroni method, though broadly applicable and widely used, is rather conservative; there are other approaches to adjust for multiple hypothesis testing, some of which are more appropriate or more powerful in specific situations.[24-26] See Box 13.3 for an illustration.

## Clinical and Statistical Significance

There is a natural progression from hypothesis testing to estimating parameters or effect sizes, especially if $H_0$ is rejected. Whereas the

---

**• BOX 13.2 Illustration of Hypothesis Testing: Comparing Prevalence in Two Populations**

Suppose a researcher wishes to determine if there is a difference among two populations in the prevalence of a disease such as dental caries. To do so, an investigator might independently select a random sample of 200 subjects from each of the two populations. After evaluating each subject for the presence of dental caries, the investigator finds that 45 subjects in Population 1 and 20 subjects in Population 2 have dental caries. Therefore, the estimated disease prevalence in the two populations is 22.5% and 10.0%, respectively.

These data can be appropriately analyzed using either the chi-square test of homogeneity or the equivalent statistical test of two independent proportions. Both statistical tests will yield identical results and inferences. In this instance, the p-value of the test statistic is 0.0007. If a value of $\alpha = 0.05$ had been specified, the null hypothesis of no differences in prevalence of dental caries between the two populations would be rejected and it would be concluded that there is greater prevalence of dental caries in Population 1. Further, the small p-value indicates that these data provide strong evidence of a true difference between the proportions of people who have dental caries in the two populations.

---

**• BOX 13.3 Illustration of the Bonferroni Method of Adjustment for Multiple Comparisons**

A researcher wishes to test 50 different biomarkers for possible associations with a particular disease in a sample of patients. The investigator sets the overall level of significance for the study at $\alpha = 0.05$. To use the Bonferroni method to adjust for the increased chance of a Type I error due to performing 50 tests, the investigator will consider a result significant only if the significance probability for the test of that particular biomarker $P < \alpha/k$, that is, if the associated significance probability $P < .05/50 = 0.001$. This will ensure that the overall probability of claiming a difference where none exists is no greater than $\alpha = 0.05$.

significance probability (p-value) derived from hypothesis testing gives an indication of the *strength* of the evidence against the null hypothesis, the point estimate and its associated confidence interval provide information about the *magnitude* of the parameter or effect and the *precision* associated with the estimate. There may be a statistically significant difference between two groups, but is it *clinically significant?* Is the difference large enough to be of practical importance? Would the magnitude of the difference be likely to change clinical practice or have an influence on public health policy? Whereas statistical analysis is helpful, it cannot directly answer questions of clinical significance; rather, results from statistical analysis assist researchers, clinicians, and policy makers in making judgments about clinical significance.

## Statistical Power and the Determination of Sample Size

The goal of study planning is to ensure that the planned investigations have a reasonable chance of achieving their objectives, and one of the most critical elements of such planning is to provide for appropriate statistical power. Power is the probability of rejecting the null hypothesis when it is false. That is, it is the probability that existing departures from the null hypothesis can be detected—that the investigator can find the existing difference between the outcome of two treatments, that an existing correlation between two quantitative measures is discovered, that true differences in caries prevalence between two populations are identified. Power is therefore the *complement* of the probability ($\beta$) of a Type II error: Power $= 1 - \beta$. As the power increases, the probability of making a Type II error decreases.

### Factors Affecting Statistical Power

Statistical power depends on several things, including: (1) the magnitude of the departure from the null hypothesis (effect size), (2) the variability (e.g., standard deviation) associated with the response or endpoint being studied, (3) $\alpha$, the specified level of Type I error (false positive) rate, (4) $\beta$, the specified level of Type II error (false negative) rate, and (5) sample size. Power is greater if the magnitude of the effect size or departure from the null hypothesis is larger; smaller, more subtle effects are harder to detect. As illustrated in Figure 13.2, it is easier (power will be greater) to detect a larger difference between two means (Figure 13.2A) than a smaller mean difference (see Figure 13.2B), all other things being equal. The impact of the second consideration, variability of the outcome of interest, is illustrated through the comparisons of Figure 13.2C and 13.2D. Although the mean difference is the same in both examples, an identical design will provide greater power to detect the difference in Figure 13.2C, where there are lower variability and clearer distinctions between the two distributions. In contrast, it will be more difficult to detect a mean difference of the same magnitude in the case depicted in Figure 13.2D. The "signal to noise ratio"—the ratio of the effect size to variability—is simply much greater in Figure 13.2C. Although it may be possible to reduce the measurement portion of the variability somewhat, such as through improved instrumentation or calibration of examiners, there is typically little that can be done to affect variation of the outcome in the population. It is simply another reflection of the true state of nature beyond the control of the researcher. It is through the last of these factors affecting power, the sample size, that it is possible to affect power: More information translates into more power!

### Determining Sample Size Requirements

The importance of having adequate sample size and sufficient statistical power when designing a research study cannot be overstated. The wastefulness and futility of expending resources on a project with little chance of success are obvious. However, such a course has other implications. For example, it would be unethical

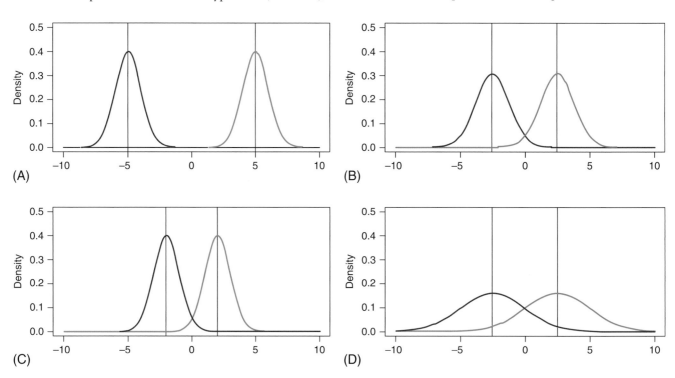

(A)

(B)

(C)

(D)

• **Figure 13.2** Factors Influencing Power. All else being equal, it is easier (power will be greater) to detect larger differences (A) than smaller differences (B); similarly, there will be greater power to detect an effect size of a given magnitude if the variability is lower (C) than if it is greater (D).

to expose participants in a clinical trial to risk if the study were too small to have sufficient power to detect differences between the interventions being tested or to identify a better treatment for a disease. In animal studies with a small sample size, low statistical power may result in false negative findings, needless sacrifice of animals, and little hope of scientific discovery. Moreover, publication of research findings that are not statistically significant because of low sample size and insufficient statistical power may discourage other investigators from pursuing further research in that area. It is important to emphasize that insufficiently powered studies may result in a loss of valuable scientific knowledge and abandonment of therapies for disease that may actually have important benefits.

Generally speaking, the first steps in the process of determining the appropriate sample size are the development of the study question, the formulation of the null and alternative hypotheses, and the selection of an appropriate statistical test.

Three basic questions are part of every sample size estimation:
1. What is the departure from the null hypothesis that the investigator would like to be able to detect (i.e., what is the effect size)?
2. How variable is the outcome of interest?
3. How sure the investigator wants to be—the level of Type I error ($\alpha$) and the desired level of power ($1-\beta$) must be specified.

Several factors need to be considered in determining the effect size that is used in estimating sample sizes for clinical studies. An important consideration is whether the anticipated effect size would likely be of clinical or practical significance. That is, what is the size or magnitude of the main outcome of a study that would likely change clinical practice or public health policy? In studies of a new drug or treatment, there may be useful indications of its potential effect size from the literature or from preliminary pilot investigations. In other instances, a percentage difference from the treatment effect of a widely accepted standard therapy, material, or population may be used to determine the anticipated effect size. For example, it has been proposed that a new chemotherapeutic agent for control of gingivitis should be expected to provide a 20% improvement over use of a control agent.[34] It is also important to emphasize that power calculations are estimated based on the main outcome or primary outcome variable of a study. Generally, studies are powered for only one primary outcome variable. If more than one primary outcome is specified for a study, the required sample size to achieve statistical significance may increase considerably. Secondary outcomes may be included in a study, but it must be borne in mind that the study was not designed or powered for the secondary outcome variables.

### Setting Parameters for Sample Size Estimation

Estimates of the variability (e.g., standard deviation) may be similarly obtained from the literature or pilot studies. It may be as straightforward as estimating the standard deviation of a quantitative outcome or it may be more complex. The variability of proportions, for example, depend upon the value of the proportion involved. It may be very difficult to estimate the variability of change in measures or scores, commonly used in studies involving a baseline measurement. Consultation with a statistician can provide guidance in such matters.

The levels of Type I error ($\alpha$) and power ($1-\beta$) are set by the investigator. Values of $\alpha = 0.05$ and 80% or 90% power are commonly used. Type I error rates greater than 0.05 and less than 80% power are generally not looked upon favorably, and some situations call for even more stringent specifications. For example, when there

are many treatments and multiple pairwise comparisons are of interest, the Type I error level should be adjusted to take account of this multiple testing. Moreover, if a clinical trial is very expensive, of high clinical importance, and unlikely to be repeated, having at least 90% power may be advisable.

Once the required information is available, sample size can be determined using appropriate tables or software. One caution about using sample size tables, such as those of Cohen,[12] is that they may express the effect size in standard deviation units, that is, desired effect size (difference between the means) divided by the standard deviation. This ratio may be referred to in reference works as the *standardized effect size* or simply as the *effect size,* so care must be taken when using these tables. This approach is used in tabulated approaches because it translates a wide variety of possible situations to a common solution. This does not need to be considered when software is used to calculate sample size.

Table 13.1 illustrates the impact of these factors on sample size for the comparison of two population means, which is one of the most commonly performed sample size calculations. It is equally applicable to the comparison of a quantitative response between two treatments, two materials, two populations, or two other groups from which independent random samples of observations are collected. If it is assumed that the outcome of interest is normally distributed in each group, and the variance is the same in the two groups, the appropriate statistical procedure to assess the

**• TABLE 13.1  Illustration of the Impact of Various Design Parameter Choices on Sample Size, Based on the Comparison of Two Means Using the Two-Sided Student's T-Test for Two Independent Samples and Equal Allocation of Sample Size**

| Effect size ($\Delta = \mu_1 - \mu_2$) | Standard Deviation ($\sigma$) | Probability of Type I error ($\alpha$) | Power ($1-\beta$) | n (per group) |
|---|---|---|---|---|
| A. Illustration of the impact of the desired effect size ($\Delta = \mu_1 - \mu_2$) | | | | |
| 1.5 | 6 | .05 | 0.80 | 253 |
| 4.5 | 6 | .05 | 0.80 | 29 |
| 6.0 | 6 | .05 | 0.80 | 17 |
| B. Illustration of the impact of the standard deviation ($\sigma$) | | | | |
| 4.5 | 3 | .05 | 0.80 | 9 |
| 4.5 | 6 | .05 | 0.80 | 29 |
| 4.5 | 9 | .05 | 0.80 | 64 |
| C. Illustration of the impact of the specification of Type I error probability ($\alpha$) | | | | |
| 4.5 | 6 | .05 | 0.80 | 29 |
| 4.5 | 6 | .01 | 0.80 | 44 |
| D. Illustration of the impact of the specification of power | | | | |
| 4.5 | 6 | .05 | 0.80 | 29 |
| 4.5 | 6 | .05 | 0.90 | 39 |

REQUIRED SAMPLE SIZES (N) PER GROUP FOR SPECIFIED DESIGN PARAMETERS difference between the two means is the (two-sided) Student's t-test for two independent samples. The effect size represents the difference between the two means the investigator wishes to be able to detect, and an estimate of the standard deviation of the outcome of interest supplies information about variability. This illustration assumes an equal sample size in the two groups. In the first calculation, having a desired effect size of 4.5 units, a standard deviation of 6 units, $\alpha = 0.05$ and 80% power yielded estimated required sample size of 29 *per group*. Note that in this case, the specified effect size corresponds to a 0.75 (4.5/6) standard deviation difference between the means. As seen in Table 13.1, sample size requirements increase as the desired effect size ($\Delta$) gets smaller, variability ($\sigma$) increases, specified level of Type I error ($\alpha$) decreases, and the desired level of power ($1-\beta$) increases.

### Equal Versus Unequal Allocation

Generally, allocation of equal sample size in comparison studies is considered optimal because a 1:1 sample size allocation typically results in the smallest total sample size. This is illustrated in Table 13.2 for a simple example comparing the means from two independent samples. As the ratio between the two sample sizes deviates farther from one, the estimate of the total required sample size increases. Nevertheless, there may be compelling reasons to use unequal sample sizes in some studies. The number of subjects for one group may be limited, as when a disorder is rare, or it may cost more to recruit subjects or acquire data from one of the groups. Unequal allocation of subjects is also frequently encountered in research that uses preexisting data or subjects, such as a nested case-control study making use of an existing cohort. In such instances, sample size estimates can be derived by specifying the size of one group or by specifying the desired ratio of the number of subjects in one group to the number of subjects in the other group.

If sample sizes are constrained because of time, resources, subject availability, or other reasons, it is still possible to estimate power and detectable effect size. For example, there may be only 150 subjects (75 in each of two comparison groups) available for a study in which the meaningful clinical difference is at least 4 units. Assuming standard normality and equal variance when comparing two means, if $\alpha$ is 0.05 and the standard deviation is 10 units, we would anticipate having about 68% power to detect the specified mean difference of 4 units. The investigator would have to decide if such a low power is acceptable. If not, a larger detectable effect size would have to be anticipated. In this example of 150 subjects, the estimated minimum detectable effect size

associated with at least 80% power is 4.6 units. Again, the investigator would then have to decide if it is acceptable to have a minimum effect size of 4.6 units to achieve 80% power. This illustrates why design and analysis must go hand in hand. Clearly, sample size cannot be estimated without considering the statistical issues involved. This highlights the critical need for investigators to consult with statistical collaborators in the early stage of planning their research.

Similar sample size estimation procedures apply to studies whose primary purpose is not to test hypotheses but to obtain an estimate of some population parameter. A common example is when the purpose of a study is to estimate disease prevalence. In such instances, the investigator must specify the level of confidence desired, provide an estimate of the variability, and indicate the precision with which the particular parameter is to be estimated, for example, it is desired to estimate prevalence within 2%.

### Sensitivity Analyses

Often the investigator does not have a firm idea of what parameter values are likely to be. After all, if the topic of interest is well known, there would be little point in studying it. Quantities taken from modest pilot studies, however valuable, are not likely to be well estimated, and values, such as standard deviations, taken from the literature may vary considerably from study to study. For this reason, a *sensitivity analysis* is often done: Power and/or sample size calculations are performed for a range of effect sizes or over a range of possible values for a parameter such as a measure of variability. The estimates in sections A and B of Table 13.1 represent examples of such sensitivity analyses, which are often demanded by reviewers or members of data and safety monitoring boards.

Practical considerations also have an impact on the determination of the final sample size. Attrition must be taken into account. Subjects may choose to drop out of the study or may become lost to follow-up. Specimen samples for determining the primary outcome may not be measurable or may be otherwise lost. The targeted sample size must account for attrition so that the desired levels of power will still be attained with the remaining sample. In addition, degradation of treatment response as a result of nonadherence may need to be considered. The anticipated effect size may need to allow for its possible attenuation due to subject noncompliance.

### Special Considerations

Special considerations apply to time-to-event studies, where the outcome of interest is survival time or the length of time from the beginning of the study until some event occurs. In such studies, the ability to distinguish between the merits of different treatments will depend on the number of events expected during the study period, **not** simply the number of subjects entered into the study. Thousands of enrolled subjects provide little power if few events occur during the study period. Such power and sample size calculations may be quite complex. Since many studies of this type use rolling enrollment over time, the investigators must consider not only the nature of the time-to-event distributions and the patterns of anticipated loss to follow-up, but also the rate of subject accrual and the amount of associated follow-up time, which may differ considerably for those enrolled at different times.

Special approaches to power and sample size estimation are needed for special designs such as matched designs, cluster sampling, longitudinal studies, genetic studies, and equivalence studies, all beyond the scope of this discussion. It is worth noting that sample size requirements can be influenced by the particular

| • TABLE 13.2 | Illustration of the Effect of Unequal Sample Allocation on Total Sample Size Based on the Comparison of Two Means Using the Two-Sided Student's T-Test | | |
|---|---|---|---|
| | $\alpha = 0.05$, 80% POWER | | |
| | Effect size $\Delta = \mu_1 - \mu_2 = 4.5$, S = 6 | | |
| Allocation ($n_2/n_1$) | $n_1$ | $n_2$ | N (Total) |
| Equal (1:1) | 29 | 29 | 58 |
| 2:1 Ratio | 22 | 44 | 66 |
| 4:1 Ratio | 18 | 72 | 90 |
| 9:1 Ratio | 16 | 144 | 160 |

statistical method used—some statistical techniques are "more powerful" than others and require a smaller sample size to give the same assurance (power) of detecting an effect of a specified magnitude. There are also instances where an investigator might use statistical procedures that require larger sample sizes, such as nonparametric tests that do not require parametric statistical assumptions. There are methods for estimating sample size and power for commonly used nonparametric procedures. However, while these are fairly straightforward if sufficient preliminary data are available, estimating effect size for nonparametric statistical tests is often less than intuitive and may be challenging for the investigator to articulate in the absence of such pilot information. For this reason, procedures associated with common parametric tests often serve as approximations, possibly in conjunction with normalizing transformations, if appropriate. In complex situations, simulation approaches in collaboration with a statistician may be needed.

## Selecting the Appropriate Statistical Method

The selection of the appropriate statistical test for a given situation depends on a number of factors. A first consideration is the data type, illustrated in Table 13.3. In the case of *categorical* or *discrete* data, observations can be grouped into distinct classes. If the classes do not have any natural ordering or ranking, the data are *nominal*. Examples of nominal data include binary outcomes such as gender or the presence or absence of disease, but also treatment group designation and such characteristics as hair color or country of residence. If the distinct classes have a predetermined or natural ordering, the data are *ordinal*. Some examples of ordinal data are classification of patients by disease severity, the commonly used

Likert scores for agreement, and plaque scores. Statistical methods have been developed specifically for the analysis of ordinal categorical data.[1] If statistical tests developed for nominal outcomes are used with ordinal data, the information contained in the ranking of the categories is lost. In contrast, use of the appropriate statistical methods for ordinal data would be expected to have greater statistical power.

Count data are also discrete but may often reasonably be analyzed using approaches developed for quantitative outcomes, particularly if they take on a wide range of values. For very restricted ranges, methods for ordinal data may be used. Special methods have also been developed for the evaluation of count data, such as Poisson and negative binomial modeling that will be covered later in this chapter.

Continuous data may assume any value on a continuous scale. Continuous data may be *interval* or *ratio* in scale. The scale of interval data is defined in terms of differences between observations, and the zero point is arbitrary. Temperature measured in degrees Fahrenheit or in degrees Celsius are examples, and the arbitrary nature of the zero value is obvious; other common examples are IQ scores and grade point averages. Notice that ratios of interval data are not readily interpretable. In contrast, the scaling of ratios is such that the ratio of two observations has real meaning: The income of one individual can be twice that of another. In ratio data, the zero point represents the total absence of the attribute being measured: One may indeed have no income.

An important distinction among statistical tests is whether the procedure is *parametric* or *nonparametric*. Parametric tests can be powerful approaches that yield readily interpretable results. However, it is important to emphasize that parametric tests make specific assumptions about the distribution of the outcome variable. For example, Student's t-tests and multiple linear regression assume that the underlying data are *normally distributed*. In a normal distribution, data are distributed such that most values cluster in the middle of a range of values and the remainder taper off symmetrically toward either extreme in a specific type of bell-shaped curve. This type of distribution is also called a *Gaussian distribution*. Other type of parametric tests, such as those used in survival analyses, assume that the data have other types of mathematical distributions. In some instances, *data transformations* such as logarithmic or square root transformation of the raw data can achieve conformance to assumptions of normality.

Many types of data are not normally distributed and, if parametric procedures assuming normality are inappropriately used, they can lead to incorrect conclusions. In contrast to parametric tests, nonparametric tests do not make specific distributional assumptions such as normality; rather, they make no or mild distributional assumptions, such as that the data are at least ordinal in terms of measurement scale. Many nonparametric tests are based on ranks and therefore are resistant to outliers. Nonparametric tests can be used in large samples, where large sample (asymptotic) methods are used to determine the significance probability. However, exact p-values are often easy to compute for small samples, and it is precisely in small samples that it is difficult to ascertain whether distributional assumptions like normality are valid. This is where the nonparametric approach can be especially helpful.

Nonparametric tests may be more difficult to interpret than parametric tests. *If* data actually meet the parametric test's distributional requirements, the nonparametric approach will have somewhat less power than the parametric one. This means that a slightly greater sample size is needed for nonparametric tests to achieve the same level of power as the analogous parametric test, again under

### • TABLE 13.3 Data Classification

| Type of Observation | Distinguishing Characteristics | Examples |
|---|---|---|
| **Categorical** | **Observations are grouped into distinct classes** | |
| A. Nominal group, | Distinct classes do not have any natural order or ranking | Sex, treatment presence or absence of disease |
| B. Ordinal | Distinct classes have a predetermined or natural ordering | Classification of patients by disease severity, scales for degree of agreement, plaque index |
| **Continuous** | **Observation may assume any value on a continuous scale** | |
| A. Interval | Scale is defined in terms of differences between observations; zero point is arbitrary | Temperature in degrees Fahrenheit or Celsius, IQ measurements, grade point average |
| B. Ratio | Scale differences represent real relationships in the items measured; zero point represents total absence of the attribute being measured | Height, weight, income, level of serum cholesterol, cytokine level |

## TABLE 13.4 Commonly Used Parametric Tests and Their Nonparametric Analogs

| Parametric Test | Nonparametric Test |
|---|---|
| **One-Sample T-Test** | **Wilcoxon Signed Rank Test** |
| $H_0$: $\mu = \mu_0$ [mean = fixed value] | (Sign Test is a less powerful competitor) |
| **Two-Sample T-Test** | **Wilcoxon Rank Sum Test** |
| $H_0$: $\mu_1 = \mu_2$ [equality of two means] | (also known as the Mann-Whitney U or Wilcoxon-Mann-Whitney test) |
| **Analysis of Variance** | **Kruskal-Wallis Test** |
| $H_0$: $\mu_1 = \mu_2 = \ldots = \mu_k$ [equality of several means] | |
| **Pearson (Product-Moment) Correlation** | **Spearman Rank Correlation** |
| $H_0$: $\rho = 0$ [no linear correlation] | |

the assumptions of the parametric model. It must be reiterated that if those assumptions are *not valid,* the performance of the nonparametric test may be far superior. Some examples of commonly used parametric tests and their nonparametric analogs are given in Table 13.4. The particular nonparametric tests shown have been selected because of their relatively high power.[13]

All statistical procedures are associated with specific assumptions and cannot be expected to produce valid inferences if the assumptions are not met. Good statistical practice makes sure that assumptions associated with a particular statistical model are satisfied. As noted, sample size may be a consideration in the choice of statistical test. Research design is another major factor that often dictates the statistical approach. Different designs require different analytic approaches; for example, statistical methods used to analyze data from two or more independent samples are quite different from those used for data from matched-pair designs or longitudinal studies. Specific approaches have been developed for specialized designs such as split-mouth and crossover designs. Careful consideration of research design is critical because use of an incorrect statistical test may lead to erroneous conclusions.

## Overview of Bivariate Analyses

When investigating clinical outcomes it is necessary to collect information about variables that may influence or be associated with the outcome. Examples include physical characteristics (height and weight), sociodemographic factors (income and household size), and behaviors (brushing, flossing, and regular dental cleanings). When trying to understand these relationships, it is often best to start with simple bivariate analyses. In these analyses, two variables are statistically examined for a relationship. This not only helps identify statistically significant patterns but also provides information that may be helpful in building statistical models.

Performing a bivariate analysis requires a careful matching of the variable types to the appropriate statistical methods. In the most general sense, there are three possibilities: two quantitative variables, two categorical variables, or one quantitative and one categorical variable. Some commonly used statistical tests follow.

### Two Quantitative Variables: Correlation and Simple Linear Regression

When examining two quantitative variables, X and Y, there are several ways to evaluate their relationship. Correlation coefficients are used to detect a linear trend (Pearson product-moment correlation) or a monotonic (increasing or decreasing) trend (Spearman rank correlation). Scatter plots use paired (X,Y) values to produce points along the X and Y axes. This plot is helpful for detecting outliers and visualizing the range of values actually observed in a data set. Moreover, if there is a straight-line function between the two variables, it can be formally tested using simple linear regression. This is an extension of the Pearson correlation analysis as it tries to predict the value of one variable from the other and specify that line defining the relationship. The Spearman approach may also be used when one or both of the variables are ordinal.

### Two Categorical Variables: Chi-Square/Fisher's Exact Test/Trend Tests

Cross-tabulation of variables is used to analyze two categorical variables in a *two-way contingency table.* Using these values, statistical procedures can test several kinds of hypotheses. The most common tests are Chi-square tests of association, which can test for independence of two categorical characteristics in a single population or assess the homogeneity of the distribution of a categorical outcome in independent samples from one or more populations. Such tests of association are asymptotic (large-sample) tests; in cases where counts are too sparse or certain categories too infrequent, the Fisher's exact test is used instead of the Chi-square test. When one of the categorical outcomes is ordinal, a test for trend such as the Cochran-Armitage test or a variant of the Cochran-Mantel-Haenszel test may be of use.[1] Associations between two ordinal variables can be assessed by a number of procedures, such as the Spearman rank and Kendall's tau-b. There are many other types of categorical data analyses for both nominal and ordinal categorical data.[1-3,19]

### One Quantitative and One Categorical Variable: Group Effects and Group Comparisons

Relationships between a quantitative and a categorical variable are generally explored by comparing the distribution of the quantitative variable among the groups defined by the categorical variable. One of the most common parametric approaches is the one-way *analysis of variance, or ANOVA.* This test is appropriate when the groups are approximately normally distributed and have similar variances. It provides an overall test as to whether the group means are the same. Provided that the sample sizes of the groups are approximately the same and that group variances are homogeneous, this procedure is quite robust with respect to the normality assumption. Determining the specifics of the mean differences will require follow-up testing that should involve suitable adjustment for multiple comparisons; for example, Tukey's method of adjusting for multiple testing is often used when performing all possible pairwise comparisons of group means. Note that the two-sample Student's t-test is a special case of one-way ANOVA.

In some cases, the data will not meet the distributional requirements for ANOVA. In these cases, nonparametric methods can be used. When comparing two groups, the Wilcoxon rank sum test is used. When comparing three or more groups, the Kruskal-Wallis test is used. These rank-based methods provide an overall test of whether the distributions of the quantitative variable are the same. Follow-up testing for the Kruskal-Wallis can be done using a modification of the Tukey procedure as described by Conover.[13] When sample sizes are small, follow-up testing for the Kruskal-Wallis test can be done using exact Wilcoxon rank sum tests in combination with the Bonferroni correction for multiple testing. Reporting the median and quantiles for the groups, with supplemental graphics, can assist in the interpretation of significant results for these methods.

When the particular outcome of interest is categorical, it may be suspected that membership in the categories may be associated with values of the quantitative variable. In this case, logistic regression can be used to formally test this hypothesis. Logistic regression will perform a significance test and provide an effect size for the strength of the association. Logistic models can be used for binary outcomes and when there are two or more groups, there are multinomial logistic regression approaches that are relevant to either nominal or ordinal outcomes.

The methods outlined above, applicable to a single random sample or several independent randomly sampled subpopulations, are by no means exhaustive. The statistical method must be suited to the design; for example, there are special analytic methods for paired designs, discussed in the section titled *"General Approaches to the Analysis of Correlated Data."*

## Statistical Modeling

### An Overview of Statistical Modeling

Under the appropriate circumstances, it is possible for relatively simple statistical procedures, such as bivariate testing, to definitively assess data and answer scientific questions. However, many phenomena of interest in dental public health, whether they represent disease processes or human behavior, are complex and affected by numerous factors. Statistical modeling provides a way to understand such complex phenomena. The basic idea of statistical modeling is to study the relationship between a response or outcome variable, often called the *dependent variable* and commonly denoted **Y**, and a set of predictor variables, also referred to as *explanatory* or *independent variables* (or as *covariates* or *covariables*), denoted $\mathbf{X_1}, \mathbf{X_2}, \ldots, \mathbf{X_p}$.

A model of the form below is generally used:

$$\mathbf{Y} = \mathbf{F}\left(\mathbf{X_1}, \mathbf{X_2}, \ldots, \mathbf{X_p}\right) \text{ where F is some mathematical function.}$$

Regression is commonly used in statistical modeling, with each model having its own mathematical function and associated assumptions. As a simple example, consider a continuous treatment response Y, which might be modeled using multiple linear regression. The independent (predictor or explanatory variables) might include data that describes demographic characteristics, treatment factors, or clinical status. The explanatory or independent variables of interest might also include quantitative variables such as age, body mass index, or blood pressure; categorical variables such as gender or treatment group; and/or count variables such as the number of concomitant conditions or cigarettes smoked per day. The model might include functions of the covariates to more fully capture relationships between the outcome and quantitative predictors or to explore statistical interaction (effect modification) involving predictors.

In addition to modeling continuous outcomes, binary outcomes and multilevel categorical responses can be modeled using methods such as multiple logistic regression. Time-to-event outcomes can be modeled using survival analysis, and there are specialized models for count data, such as the Poisson and negative binomial models, which are often used in the analysis of dental caries data. Statistical models have also been developed to address multivariate outcomes, where a set of responses is being modeled, as in the analysis of longitudinal data.

### Advantages of Modeling

Before considering specific models, it is important to understand some advantages of statistical modeling. Modeling does not require making arbitrary decisions when changing continuous variables to discrete variables or when categorizing patients into subgroups. For example, modeling avoids subgrouping patients by gender and age for separate subgroup analyses, which produces smaller groups, modest sample sizes, and less stable risk estimates. Modeling makes it possible to refine risk estimates because it permits full exploration of the relationship between the outcome and continuous explanatory variables such as age. It also makes it possible to consider many explanatory variables simultaneously and most importantly to assess the effect of each predictor variable on the response variable after adjusting for information from other covariates. Modeling makes it possible to assess the "independent" contribution of each variable in predicting or explaining the outcome variable. Modeling, therefore, permits researchers to assess the strength of the relationship between the dependent "Y" variable and a specific predictor "X" variable after adjusting for the effects of other predictors ($\mathbf{X_1}, \mathbf{X_2}, \ldots, \mathbf{X_p}$).

A particularly important advantage of modeling is that it allows the assessment of *confounding*, which can occur when an explanatory variable that is associated with an outcome is also associated with another covariate. In such a case, confounding can result in a spurious association between the second covariate and the outcome variable. For example, suppose exposures of both smoking and coffee consumption are recorded in a case-control study of cancer. Suppose further that smoking is indeed etiologically related to risk of this particular cancer, but coffee consumption is not. However, it is known that in many populations, smoking and coffee consumption are associated with each other. The relationship between the two exposures may lead to a spurious association between cancer and coffee consumption in a simple bivariate test of association. Modeling can evaluate whether the association between coffee consumption and cancer remains after the effect of smoking is taken into account. If the association is no longer significant after adjusting for the effect of smoking, it suggests that the simple bivariate association between cancer and coffee consumption was due to confounding; it simply reflected the correlation between smoking and coffee drinking. In this example, researchers would conclude that coffee consumption does not make an independent contribution to the model.

The ability to assess the independent contribution of a covariate after adjusting for other candidates is extremely valuable, since many of the putative risk factors in human studies are correlated. For example, positive (and negative) lifestyle factors often cluster in individuals. Modeling allows researchers to determine which correlated factors are most closely associated with the outcome of interest and which factors make independent contributions to the explanatory model. This property of modeling is also important in addressing imbalances in covariates between treatment groups, which sometimes occur despite the best attempts to achieve balanced samples through randomization. For example, one group of patients in a clinical trial may have more severe disease, fewer older or male subjects, more smokers, or more comorbidities. Each of these factors could affect the treatment response and perhaps even obscure important differences between treatments that are tested. Modeling makes it possible to assess the effect of treatment on the outcome of interest after adjusting for subject characteristics such as severity of condition, gender, age, lifestyle factors, and comorbid conditions. It permits researchers to determine whether there is a treatment effect after adjusting for other subject characteristics. This advantage of modeling also extends to observational studies that compare various conditions or diseases in populations.

Multivariable modeling also allows researchers to determine whether there is *statistical interaction* among predictor variables, that is, whether predictors appear to be related to the outcome variable in a nonadditive fashion. For example, the effects of a particular treatment may vary with age or gender, or a new treatment may be superior to a standard treatment but only in a subgroup of patients. An adjuvant treatment may prove to have value when used in conjunction with one medication but not another. Another example is gene–environment interaction, which may be present if a particular genotype predisposes to disease only if the individual is exposed to a particular environmental factor. Risk factors may interact such that each alone may have a negative (or beneficial) impact on an outcome, but together they have a synergistic effect that far outstrips what would be expected if the two effects were simply additive. Several of these features of statistical modeling will be illustrated in our consideration of multiple linear regression, but they can be used broadly in other types of modeling.

## Modeling Quantitative Outcomes: Multiple Linear Regression

### The Multiple Linear Regression Model

Multiple linear regression, also known simply as multiple regression, is used to model quantitative outcomes. In multiple regression, the model may be written in any of the following ways:

$$Y = \beta_0 + \beta_1 X_1 + \beta_2 X_2 + \cdots + \beta_p X_p + \varepsilon$$

$$E(Y) = \beta_0 + \beta_1 X_1 + \beta_2 X_2 + \cdots + \beta_p X_p$$

where E(Y) is the mean value of Y for a given set of **predictors ($X_1$, $X_2$, ..., $X_p$)**.

These equations convey that in the case of multiple regression, the model specifies that the mean value of a response variable Y for a given set of predictors is given by a linear function of the independent variables, $\beta_0 + \beta_1 X_1 + \beta_2 X_2 + \cdots + \beta_p X_p$, where the parameters $\beta_0$, $\beta_1$, $\beta_2$, ..., $\beta_p$ represent the model parameters to be estimated. The error term $\varepsilon$ acknowledges that individual outcomes will vary about that mean. The standard assumptions associated with multiple linear regression are that the error terms are normally distributed and homoscedastic, that is, the variance of the errors is the same across all levels of the independent variables. All of the observations must be independent, so this approach is not suitable for analyzing correlated data such as would be found in longitudinal studies or studies involving matched designs. Note that a particular regression coefficient represents the effects of its corresponding covariate adjusted for the effects of the other covariates in the model. Should the corresponding null hypothesis that the regression coefficient is zero be rejected, it would mean that there is evidence that the associated covariate made a significant contribution to the model after adjusting for the effect of the other covariates. In this way, we are able to assess the independent contribution of a particular covariate. See Box 13.4 for a detailed discussion of the interpretation of regression coefficients relevant to the results in Table 13.5.

### Specifying Multilevel Independent Variables

More generally, if the categorical covariate has $k$ levels, a series of (k-1) binary variables can be used to designate the adjustments of the other levels relative to the reference level. In this instance, the null hypothesis corresponds to the case where all (k-1) regression coefficients specifying that covariate are zero; this is the global test for the effect of that particular categorical covariate. This test assesses the significance of that particular multilevel (categorical) explanatory factor given that we have adjusted for all the other explanatory variables in the model. If this factor does contribute (is significant), then pairwise comparisons of the different levels may be of interest. An individual $\beta$ regression coefficient in this context will reflect a comparison with the reference group, but

---

**• BOX 13.4** | **Interpretation of Regression Coefficients: An Example**

To illustrate the interpretation of regression coefficients, consider a simple multiple regression model for a response variable **Y** to evaluate the effect of two explanatory factors, age (**$X_1$**) and sex (**$X_2$**). The model is

$$Y = \beta_0 + \beta_1 X_1 + \beta_2 X_2 + \varepsilon$$

Note that it specifies that there is a linear relationship between age and the response variable. The covariate **$X_1$** simply represents the age of the subject, but because sex is a dichotomous categorical variable, **$X_2$** is defined as a binary variable that takes on the value 0 if the subject is female and 1 if the subject is male.

To test the null hypothesis that age is not (linearly) related to the response Y is equivalent to testing that **$\beta_1 = 0$**. To assess whether the response differs with sex, we test the null hypothesis that **$\beta_2 = 0$**. Typically, the test of the intercept **$\beta_0$** is not of interest. As seen in the summary of regression results given in Table 13.5, the data provide evidence of an age effect ($P < .0001$) after adjustment for the effect of sex. The data also provide evidence that, after adjustment for age, the two sexes differ ($P = .0203$). In each instance, the test of that particular regression coefficient corresponds to the test of whether the corresponding explanatory variable makes a significant contribution to the model, given that other variable is in the model, that is, that we have adjusted for the effect of that other variable or controlled for that other variable.

As seen in Table 13.5, the estimated regression coefficient associated with age (**$\beta_1$**) is 2.05. This means that there is an average increase of 2.5 **Y** units for every increase of one year of age (Figure 13.3A). More generally, if **$X_i$** is a quantitative variable, then the coefficient **$\beta_i$** represents the average change in **Y** for each increase of one unit in **$X_i$**.

The estimate of the regression coefficient for sex (**$\beta_2$**) is 3.20. This implies that the response in males is, on average, 3.2 **Y** units greater than females (Figure 13.3A). If **$X_i$** is a binary variable used to denote the level of a categorical outcome, then the coefficient **$\beta_i$** represents an adjustment to the mean value of **Y** relative to a reference level. In this example, females represent the reference group.

Another way of looking at this is that the estimated regression equation for females (which corresponds to $X_2 = 0$) is Y = 19.01 + 2.05(Age), whereas the estimated regression equation for males (where $X_2 = 1$) is Y = 19.01 + 2.05(Age) + 3.20; the line for males is placed 3.20 units higher than that for females, as indicated in Figure 13.3A.

Note that a negative value of the regression coefficient for sex would have implied that males were, on average, lower than females in the outcome variable; if we had defined **$X_2$** differently, as 0 for males and 1 for females, then the value of the coefficient would have been −3.20, indicating that females were on average, 3.2 **Y** units less than males, the reference group.

| TABLE 13.5 Multiple Regression: One Quantitative and One Binary Predictor-Summary of Results | | | | |
|---|---|---|---|---|
| R-Square = 0.82 | | | | |
| P-Value for Overall F test: <.0001 | | | | |
| Parameter | Estimate | SE | t Value | Pr > \|t\|[a] |
| Intercept | 19.01 | 2.202 | 5.75 | 0.0004 |
| Age | 2.05 | 0.043 | 45.43 | <.0001 |
| Sex (0=F, 1=M) | 3.20 | 1.290 | 2.48 | 0.0203 |

[a]Note that in multiple regression, the test of a regression coefficient corresponds to the test of whether the corresponding explanatory variable makes a significant contribution to the model, given that the other variables are in the model.

other comparisons can be carried out as well. For example, suppose there were four treatment groups in the example above: It would probably be of interest to carry out all pairwise comparisons of treatments. In that context, it is appropriate to consider adjustment for multiple comparisons.

### Summarizing Regression Results

Typically, the summary table from a multiple regression analysis provides the estimated regression coefficients and their standard errors and the p-value associated with the test of the null hypothesis that the regression coefficient is equal to zero (i.e., that the corresponding predictor does not significantly contribute to the model). It may also include the test statistic associated with each test, like the t-statistics in Table 13.5. Sometimes a 95% confidence interval is given for the regression coefficient, which can be useful for the estimation of effect sizes.

When there is a categorical predictor with more than two levels (e.g., five levels of education), then a global test for the effect of that factor may also be presented.

Table 13.5 also provides a significance probability for the overall F test of the significance of the model with both age and gender specified as covariates ($P < .0001$) and an $R^2$ statistic, which gives the proportion of the variability in the response variable, which is explained by the stated relationship between the response variable and that particular set of predictors. In this instance, $R^2 = 0.82$, which implies that this particular model explains 82% of the variability in the response. $R^2$ is sometimes called the *coefficient of determination*. Note that large values of $R^2$ are needed ($R^2$ of 0.9 or greater are desirable) if the model is to be used for prediction.

Whenever we add a variable or group of variables to a model, the $R^2$ value will increase. We have noted that when we test whether a particular independent variable (or group of variables) is significant, we are testing whether the associated regression coefficient (s) = 0. This is actually equivalent to testing whether the value of $R^2$, that is, the explanatory capability of the model, was significantly increased by the addition of the new independent variable (s). Further discussion and examples from the dental literature are given by Petrie et al.[51]

### Beyond Simple Linear Relationships: Specifying More Complex Models

Multiple *linear* regression does not mean that the specification of relationships between the dependent variable Y and a quantitative independent variable X is limited to straight line relationships. It is possible to use additional predictor variables to specify other possible relationships. One example is *polynomial* regression, where the

terms represent the independent variable X used in a polynomial function of the form:

$$Y = \beta_0 + \beta_1 X + \beta_2 X^2 + \cdots + \beta_p X^p + \varepsilon$$

This form is used to express more complex, curvilinear relationships between the response Y and independent variable X. If appropriate, polynomial terms can be used to model nonlinear responses for several of the explanatory variables.

One or more predictor variables can also be used to define *interactions* between two or more independent variables. In our simple example, interaction between gender and age might look like this:

$$Y = \beta_0 + \beta_1 X_1 + \beta_2 X_2 + \beta_3 X_3 + \varepsilon \quad \text{where } X_3 = X_1 * X_2$$

This model essentially permits males and females to have separate lines with different slopes and intercepts (Figure 13.3B). In the original model, the effect of age was the same in males and females, as reflected in the parallel lines of Figure 13.3A; in this particular interaction model, the different slopes of the lines (Figure 13.3B) reflects a different relationship with age for males and females. It is the fourth term of the model, $\beta_3 X_3$, which permits the line for males to have a different slope than that for females. In the original model, gender and age had additive effects; it was possible to consider the effect of each independent variable on **Y** separately from the other. In the case of interaction, the difference between males and females depends on age, and the relationship with age is different for males and females, as illustrated in Figure 13.3B.

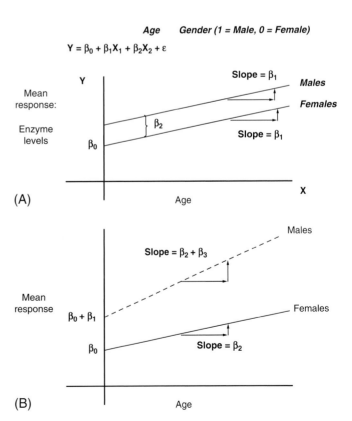

• **Figure 13.3** (A) One quantitative and one binary predictor. (B) Model with interaction of one quantitative and one binary predictor.

## Residual Analyses

As with any modeling endeavor, it is important to assess whether there is conformity to model assumptions. When fitting a multiple linear regression, it is important to perform *residual analyses* to assess the validity of the model. These include a series of diagnostic tests and graphics to assess such features as normality, variance homogeneity, and linearity and are detailed in any number of standard texts.[16,38]

## The Generalized Linear Model

Now that we are familiar with the details of multiple regression, we can now examine a more sophisticated technique whereby the linear model is extended to create the family of generalized linear models. You may already be familiar with some examples of a generalized linear model, such as a logistic regression model. Despite the variety seen among the generalized linear models, all models in this family are constructed such that the effect of the explanatory variables is modeled as a linear function:

$$\beta_0 + \beta_1 X_1 + \beta_2 X_2 + \cdots + \beta_p X_p.$$

This piece of the model is the same as was used in multiple regression. However, with generalized linear models we are moving beyond modeling only continuous, normally distributed response variables to modeling other types of response variables.

We accomplish this generalization through the use of a link function. It is through the link function that the effect of the explanatory variables is connected to the response variable. The specifics of the link function and the choice of which link function to use are all determined by the distribution of the response variable. In the case of logistic regression where the response variable is binary, a characteristic is present or not ($Y=1$ or $Y=0$), and we model the probability that the characteristic is present:

$$P\{Y=1\} = \exp\left\{\beta_0 + \beta_1 X_1 + \beta_2 X_2 + \cdots + \beta_p X_p\right\} / \left[1 + \exp\left\{\beta_0 + \beta_1 X_1 + \beta_2 X_2 + \cdots + \beta_p X_p\right\}\right].$$

In this case, the link function is the logit, also known as the log-odds, or the logarithm of the odds, defined as $P\{Y=1\}/[1-P\{Y=1\}]$.

The power of this approach stems from the fact that any outcome with a distribution that has a valid link function can be modeled in this way. This provides great flexibility through a unified approach to estimating the effects of covariates—but in the context of other model assumptions, and embedded in different modeling equations. Other examples include the Poisson and negative binomial regression models that are used with count data and are commonly used to model the number of decayed, missing, and filled teeth or surfaces.

From the nonstatistician's point of view, it is important to recognize that the *linear* designation refers to this specification of the way covariate effects are modeled—the model parameters (the regression coefficients $\beta_0$, $\beta_1$, $\beta_2$, ... , $\beta_p$) are part of a linear function. The basic interpretations are the same: If a particular $\beta$ coefficient is zero, then the associated independent variable drops out of the model and so makes no contribution to the model. Therefore, the key hypotheses tested are whether a particular regression coefficient (or set of coefficients) differs significantly from zero. If so, we have evidence that the corresponding predictors are associated with the outcome and contribute to the explanatory ability of the model.

There are other types of modeling, including nonlinear regression where the model function used is a nonlinear combination of the model parameters; other types of nonlinear modeling can even be nonparametric, such as kernel regression. However, the following discussion will be focused on linear modeling approaches.

## Modeling Categorical Outcomes: Logistic Regression

When the outcome of interest is categorical, we use a modeling method known as *multiple logistic regression*. If the response variable has two categories, we say that the outcome is *binary* or *dichotomous*. If the response variable has three or more categories, we say that the outcome is *polytomous* or *polychotomous*. Although the most common form of logistic regression is for binary outcomes, there are different implementations of logistic regression, and choosing among them depends on the number of categories in the outcome and elements of the study design.

*Binary logistic regression* is used when our outcome of interest has two possible outcomes. These may denote the presence or absence of some characteristic or may simply define two groups. One common example is when the two groups represent whether disease is present or not (e.g., cases and controls), but there are many other possibilities for binary outcomes, including whether or not an enamel defect, a microorganism, or clinical improvement is present. Other possibilities include whether or not a restoration is clinically acceptable or the assignment of a patient to one of two possible disease subclassifications.

### Binary Logistic Regression

When performing *binary logistic regression,* the response variable Y is a binary (0,1) outcome (e.g., $Y=0$ if disease is absent and 1 if it is present). Multiple logistic regression provides a method to assess the relationship between a group of independent variables $X_1$, $X_2$, ..., $X_p$ and the probability that an event occurs (or a characteristic is present). Logistic regression models the probability of an event happening, with the probability that $Y=1$ given by:

$$\exp\left\{\beta_0 + \beta_1 X_1 + \beta_2 X_2 + \cdots + \beta_p X_p\right\} / \left[1 + \exp\left\{\beta_0 + \beta_1 X_1 + \beta_2 X_2 + \cdots + \beta_p X_p\right\}\right].$$

If Y denotes the presence or absence of disease, then the independent variables may refer to any number of factors that may affect susceptibility to disease, including demographic factors, oral health habits, lifestyle factors, environmental exposures, or genetic status.

Examples of the functional form of the logistic function are seen in Figure 13.4A–B. In Figure 13.4A, we see that the risk of disease increases with age. The shape of the logistic function is *S*-shaped or *sigmoid*, and can take on values between 0 and 1. These properties are useful for modeling probabilities since they are restricted to the range of 0 to 1. In Figure 13.4B, we see an example of a logistic function where increasing age is again associated with increased risk of disease, but being male is also associated with greater disease risk.

The portion of the logistic function $\beta_0 + \beta_1 X_1 + \beta_2 X_2 + \cdots + \beta_p X_p$ is called the *logit*. The logit is the log-odds, or the logarithm of the odds $P\{Y=1\}/[1-P\{Y=1\}]$, which simplifies to the linear function $\beta_0 + \beta_1 X_1 + \beta_2 X_2 + \cdots + \beta_p X_p$.[28] The logistic model is a special case of the generalized linear model; the link function of the logistic model is established through the logit transformation. The effects of the independent variables are modeled as a linear function, the logit. The logit can be thought of as a kind of index of risk, with

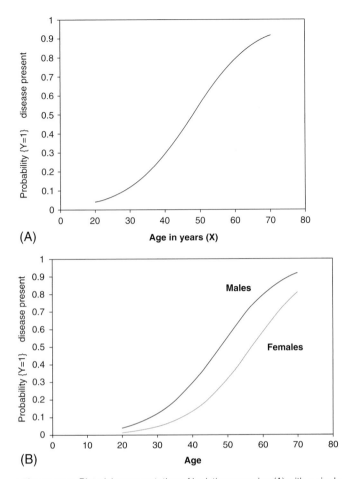

• **Figure 13.4** Pictorial representation of logistic regression (A) with a single continuous explanatory variable (age) and (B) with one continuous and one binary explanatory variable (age and sex).

weighting of the risk factors provided by the regression coefficients $\beta_1, \beta_2, ..., \beta_p$, which are estimated from the data. Individuals with many risk factors will tend to have high values of the logit and thus high risk of disease. Those with few risk factors or many protective factors will have lower logit values and correspondingly low risk of disease.

To assess whether a particular independent variable $X_i$ is related to the risk of disease, we test the null hypothesis that $\beta_i = 0$. This is a test for the significance of variable $X_i$ after having adjusted for all the other independent variables in the logistic regression model. As noted in the previous discussion of multiple linear regression, sometimes the impact of a factor is modeled by a series of regression coefficients; in those instances, the null hypothesis of interest is that all of the corresponding regression coefficients are equal to zero; that is, the factor makes no contribution to the logistic model.

### Odds Ratios in Logistic Regression

The *odds ratio* is the measure of association that is directly estimated by logistic regression. The odds ratio describes the strength of the association between the dependent variable and a particular independent variable, such as between disease status and a putative risk factor, and assists us in determining whether individuals with a particular characteristic are at greater (or lesser) risk of disease. If an odds ratio is greater than 1, the presence of the risk factor is associated with greater risk of disease; if it is less than 1, is it associated

with lesser risk of disease. An odds ratio of 1 corresponds to the null hypothesis, equivalent to a zero value of the associated regression coefficient. The estimated odds ratios are derived from the logistic regression using the regression coefficient(s) (the $\beta$s); associated confidence intervals are also routinely reported.

Under certain conditions, such as when the disease of interest is sufficiently rare,[21,47] the odds ratio will be *approximately* equal to another way of quantifying association between a putative risk factor and disease risk, the *relative risk* or *risk ratio*. For a particular exposure, the *risk ratio* is the ratio of the probability of disease for persons with the exposure to the probability of disease for persons without the exposure. However, in general, the odds ratio will be greater than the relative risk; it is only in certain circumstances that the approximation can be used. The odds ratio, however, is a valid descriptor of risk in its own right.[14]

Logistic regression can be usefully applied to case-control and cross-sectional studies as well as cohort studies, but there are important limitations to using logistic regression to analyze case-control and cross-sectional studies. In follow-up (e.g., cohort) studies, a fitted logistic model can be used to predict the risk for an individual with specific independent variables. However, although logistic modeling is applicable to case-control and cross-sectional studies, only estimates of odds ratios can be obtained for these studies. *The logistic model cannot be used to predict individual risk for these study types.*

### Other Types of Logistic Models

There are extensions to binary logistic regression that can be used when the outcome variable has more than two possible categorical outcomes. There are logistic regression methods for the modeling of either nominal or ordinal polytomous outcomes.[37,38] Another type of model, *conditional logistic regression,* can be used if the design specifies matched sets, as in studies of matched case-control pairs.[10] There are also extensions to logistic regression modeling that can be used to analyze correlated binary outcomes.[2,50] These are useful for modeling caries status for multiple surfaces within the same subject or periodontal status for multiple sites within the mouth.

## Modeling Count Data: Poisson and Negative Binomial Models

### Poisson Modeling

Count data feature prominently in many dental public health studies, such as caries investigations where the primary outcome is the number of decayed, missing, and filled teeth or surfaces (DMFT/DMFS). In studies of periodontal disease, counts of interest may include the number of teeth that meet criteria for periodontal disease and the number of teeth lost to periodontal disease. The *Poisson regression model*, a variant of the generalized linear model, is commonly used to model count data. It assumes that the response variable Y has a *Poisson distribution*. The Poisson distribution has a single parameter, $\lambda$, that is equal to both its mean and its variance. It describes the probability of the number of events, taking on the nonnegative integer values 0, 1, 2, ... . Figure 13.5 illustrates several examples of the Poisson distribution. It shows that as $\lambda$ increases, the corresponding Poisson distribution shifts to the right as the mean increases. In addition, as $\lambda$ increases, the distribution broadens with the increasing variance. As the Poisson parameter $\lambda$ increases, the distribution becomes less positively skewed and more symmetric.

Many natural phenomena conform to the Poisson distribution: stars in space, raisins in cakes, and the number of typing errors on a

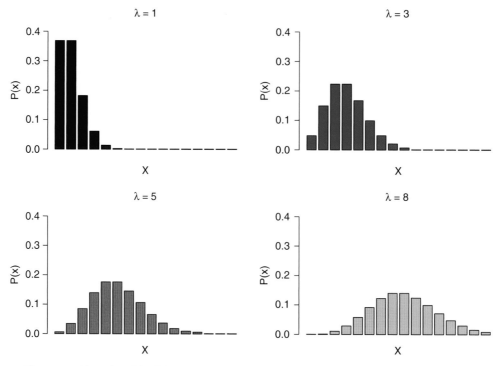

• **Figure 13.5** Examples of the Poisson distribution for differing values of the Poisson parameter λ, which is equal to the mean and the variance of the particular Poisson distribution.

page—all have been found to conform to the Poisson distribution. The classic Poisson example is Bortkiewicz's[7] distribution of the number of Prussian soldiers in a military corps killed by a kick from a horse in a 1-year period, which he modeled on observations from multiple corps over a 20-year period.

The Poisson distribution has applications in communications theory (number of signals or wrong numbers arriving at a receiver in a given period) and water testing (number of microorganisms in a given volume). It has been used to model rare events like accidents, adolescent suicides, and the occurrence of rare diseases like leukemia, in both epidemiologic and insurance contexts. In dentistry, it has found wide application in caries analysis.[43]

In Poisson regression, the logarithm of the mean is modeled as a linear combination: $\beta_0 + \beta_1 X_1 + \beta_2 X_2 + \cdots + \beta_p X_p$ of the independent variables; that is, the log serves as the link function. As before, the $X_1, X_2, \ldots, X_p$ represent the independent or explanatory variables, and the $\beta_0, \beta_1, \beta_2, \ldots, \beta_p$ are the regression coefficients to be estimated from the data. Poisson regression enables the investigator to assess and to incorporate the impact of the explanatory variables on the distribution of the outcome of interest—the count data. Essentially, the investigator is modeling the log of the Poisson parameter as a function of the covariates of interest.

Poisson regression can also be used to model rate data. This requires the original counts (the numerator of the rate) and the measure of time/area/volume (the denominator of the rate). Hujoel et al.[32] used Poisson regression to model caries incidence rates in a reanalysis of data from a xylitol trial, assessing their relationship to treatment, gender, age, and study period, as well as surface characteristics. In this instance, the accumulated posteruption surface time at risk served as the denominator of the rates, considered separately for molar pit-and-fissure surfaces versus all other surfaces.

In the Poisson distribution, the mean and variance are equal. When the observed variability is greater than that expected based on Poisson assumptions, this is known as *overdispersion*. Poisson models are often modified to address this by introducing a *scale parameter* into the Poisson model to deal with the overdispersion (the greater than expected variance); an example is found in the Hujoel et al.[32] analyses, which used an overdispersed Poisson model.

It is not uncommon for count data to have a greater probability of a zero response than would be indicated by a Poisson distribution. *Zero-inflated Poisson* (ZIP) models were developed to address such problems. The ZIP model allows for "excess zeros" in count models under the assumption that the population is a mixture. For example, imagine a population that is a mixture of two subpopulations, one where members always have zero counts (no carious lesions), and one where members may have either zero or positive counts, but where the counts follow a Poisson distribution. The specification of the first population accounts for the excess zero counts.

### Negative Binomial Modeling

The *negative binomial distribution* may also be used to model count data. This distribution has a variance that is larger than its mean. Negative binomial regression models therefore provide an alternative way to address overdispersion by broadening the Poisson restriction that the variance is equal to the mean response. There are also zero-inflated versions of negative binomial models (ZINB models).

In applications, the choice of model is typically empiric; it is a matter of which model best fits the data. Lewsey et al.[43] illustrate three approaches to caries analysis, using Poisson, negative binomial, and normal (Gaussian) assumptions. Given the shape of the Poisson distributions with large λ values in Figure 13.5, it is not surprising that the distribution of count data such as DMFS scores may be approximated by the normal distribution in some instances.

## Modeling Time-to-Event Outcomes: Survival Models

For time-to-event outcomes, the response variable is the time from entry into the study until the occurrence of the event of interest. Possible "events" include death, failure of an implant, onset of disease, or achievement of a developmental milestone, such as eruption of the complete primary dentition. The entry time will depend on the event of interest. It may be birth in studies of mortality, disease onset, or development, or it may reflect the time of diagnosis of disease or enrollment in the study.

Because the statistical methods for analyzing time-to-event data were initially used primarily to evaluate mortality, they are called *survival analysis*, although the term *time-to-event analysis* can be used interchangeably. These techniques are used to describe the survival (time-to-event) curve, to compare the survival experience of several groups, to assess whether particular variables are related to survival time, and to develop predictive models.

### Motivation

The problem of *censoring* was the underlying motivation for the development of survival methodology. Data are *censored* if follow-up ceases prior to the occurrence of the event of interest. Some individuals may be lost to follow-up, or the study may end before all units experience the outcome of interest. In such instances, the specialized methods of survival analysis are used to analyze the data in the presence of censoring. An illustration is provided in Box 13.5.

This type of censoring, where the subject does not experience the event of interest before the study ends, withdraws, or is otherwise lost to follow-up, is called *progressive censoring* or *right censoring*. In right censoring we know that survival time is more than a certain value, but it is unknown by how much. *Left censoring* is less commonly encountered; in this case, the subject has experienced the event prior to the time of study, but we do not know when it occurred. This problem is encountered in HIV research, where a subject may present with infection, but the time of infection is unknown. This discussion will be confined to right censoring methods.

If we have complete data, that is, each experimental or observational unit is followed until the event of interest occurs, many hypotheses can be tested using "conventional" techniques. For example, suppose all male and female children in a longitudinal study are followed from birth until primary first molars emerge. The time (age) of emergence could be compared for males and females using the Wilcoxon rank sum test. However, special methods must be used if the data are censored.

### Estimation and Comparison of the Survival Experience

The *survival function*, usually denoted $S(t)$, gives the probability that a subject survives longer than some specified time $t$, that is,

> ● BOX 13.5  **Illustration of Censoring in Survival Analysis**
>
> A study is conducted to compare the performance of two types of dental implants. The event of interest is implant failure. The two types of dental implants are placed and subjects are followed over time. Some subjects are lost to follow-up. They may move away, die from causes completely unrelated to the implant, or simply choose to withdraw from the study. In addition, at the end of the 5 years of funding (and follow-up!), as we are about to analyze the data, many of the implants are still functioning. The data are censored in all of these instances. We know that the implants were still functioning at the time of the censoring, after a known period of follow-up, but we do not know what happened afterward—when the implant failed.

the probability that the time to event exceeds the specified time $t$. This can also be interpreted as the proportion of the population still alive at time $t$. The *Kaplan-Meier (product-limit) estimator* is often used to estimate the survival function when individual survival times are available. It can be used with progressively censored observations and does not require any assumptions about the form of the survival function that is being estimated, that is, it is a nonparametric method. The Kaplan-Meier estimate provides a useful summary of the survival experience. It is generally used to give a pictorial representation of the observed survival experience. Median survival times and other percentile points may be estimated from the Kaplan-Meier survival curve, given sufficient information; a standard error can also be calculated for the estimated survival probability at a particular time $t$.

Figure 13.6A gives an example of an estimated survival function. At time zero, the value of the survival function is 1, reflecting the fact that all subjects are alive at the start. The survival function decreases over time, as more subjects die. In Figure 13.6A, the survival curve has a final value of zero: No subjects are alive at the end of the study, all have died or been censored. In Figure 13.6B, this is also true of the lower survival curve (solid line). In contrast, at the time that follow-up ended at 36 months, nearly half of the subjects being described by the upper curve (dashed line) were still alive. Clearly, for that subgroup, it would be possible to estimate the median (50th percentile point) but not the 25th percentile point.

In Figure 13.6B, the group corresponding to the lower curve (solid line) appears to have greater mortality, and a formal test of whether the survival curves differ for the two subgroups may be of interest. A number of alternative tests are available for comparing the survival experiences of two or more groups in the presence of censoring. This corresponds to the null hypothesis that the survival distributions of the groups under study are the same. Two commonly used procedures are the *log-rank test* and the *generalized Wilcoxon test*. The log-rank procedure tests whether the survival curves are equal by summarizing over the whole of the period studied. The test statistic can be interpreted in terms of the differences between the observed number of events in each group and the expected number under the null hypothesis of identical survival experiences for all the groups being considered. The log-rank test weights the difference scores comparing observed and expected numbers of events equally over all failure times over the entire period of observation.

Other tests directed at this same null hypothesis weight them differently. For example, the generalized Wilcoxon test differs from the log-rank statistic by a weighting factor that is based on the number of individuals "at risk" at a given time point. For this reason, the Wilcoxon test gives more weight to earlier survival times than to later ones. This would put more emphasis on the information at the beginning of the survival experience, where the number at risk is large, and less on failures in the later portion of the statistical curve, where the number at risk is smaller due to the attrition of earlier deaths. The Wilcoxon test therefore tends to be less sensitive than the log-rank procedure to differences occurring late in the period of observation. Each of the tests is more powerful than the other in certain specific instances, but neither has much power to detect group differences in situations where the survival curves cross, as in Figure 13.6C.

### The Hazard Function

The *hazard function* or *hazard rate* denotes the instantaneous potential per unit time for the event to occur, given that the individual has survived up to time $t$. In other words, given that the subject has lived to a particular time $t$, what is the probability that he

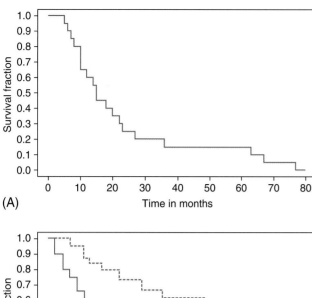

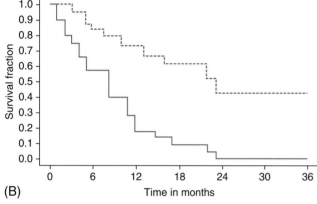

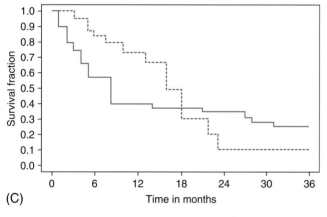

• **Figure 13.6** Examples of Survival Curves Estimated by the Kaplan-Meier Method. (A) For a single sample, (B) for two study subgroups: the lower curve (solid line) appears to have greater mortality, (C) example of survival curves that cross.

dies "in the next instant" of time? Other names for the hazard function are the conditional failure rate, the force of mortality, the instantaneous (relative) failure rate, the intensity rate, and the hazard rate. It is always nonnegative and has no upper bound. The hazard is mathematically related to the survival function and is usually what is modeled in survival analysis.

### The Cox Proportional Hazards Model

The *Cox proportional hazards model* is a frequently used approach that allows the investigator to study relationships between the time to event outcome Y and a set of explanatory variables $X_1, X_2, ..., X_p$. The Cox regression model is distribution free; no distributional

assumptions are required. In its original form, the Cox model assumes that the hazard rate of a person with one set of covariates is proportional to the hazard rate of a person with a different set of covariates—this is why the method is often referred to as the *proportional hazards model*, and this is the version we will consider first. If two survival distributions have *proportional hazards*, this means that one hazard differs from the other only by a multiplicative constant: $\mathbf{h_1(t) = c \cdot h_2(t)}$. Figure 13.6B is an example of estimated survival curves that appear reasonably consistent with the proportional hazards assumption; Figure 13.6C is not. The Cox proportional hazards model is a *robust* model; *provided* that the proportional hazards assumption is met, the results obtained using the Cox model typically will closely approximate the results for the correct parametric model (the model specifying the correct underlying distributional form of the survival function). This is why it is so widely used.

The Cox proportional hazards regression models the hazard rate, which is specified as:

$$\mathbf{h\left(t, X_1, X_2, ..., X_p\right) = h_0(t) \cdot exp\{\beta_0 + \beta_1 X_1 + \beta_2 X_2 + \cdots + \beta_k X_k\}}$$

The hazard function that is modeled by this approach has two parts – one is $\mathbf{h_0(t)}$—the "baseline hazard," and the other is the right-hand term: $\mathbf{exp\{\beta_0 + \beta_1 X_1 + \beta_2 X_2 + \cdots + \beta_p X_p\}}$—which is a function of the set of covariates $\underline{\mathbf{X}}$: $\mathbf{X_1, X_2, ..., X_p}$. The effect of the covariates on the hazard is modeled as a linear function in this equation (in the exponent of the transcendental number *e*). However, the distributional form of the baseline hazard, $h_0(t)$, does not need to be specified. This is why the Cox proportional hazards model is often called "semi-parametric." The Cox regression coefficients $\boldsymbol{\beta_1, \beta_2, ..., \beta_p}$ are estimated from the data. If any particular coefficient $\beta_i$ is zero, the implication is that the associated covariate $X_i$ is not related to survival, after adjustment is made for the other covariates in the model. To test whether a particular covariate is related to survival, we test the null hypothesis that the corresponding regression coefficient $\beta$ (or set of regression coefficients) is equal to zero. If the null hypothesis is rejected, then the data provide evidence that this particular covariate is associated with survival after adjustment for the other covariates in the model. Once the regression coefficients have been estimated, it is possible to produce estimated survival curves for persons with different constellations of covariate values. Such graphical representations can be extremely helpful in interpreting the results from Cox modeling.

Note that $h_0(t)$ does not involve the covariates, and note also that time is not part of the right-hand term where the covariate effects are specified. In considering the form of the hazard rate in the Cox proportional hazards model, we see that two individuals with different values of the covariates $\mathbf{X_1, X_2, ..., X_p}$ will have a different exponential portion (right-hand term) *but the same baseline hazard, $h_0(t)$*. This leads directly to the proportional hazards assumption that the hazard rate of a person with one set of covariates is *proportional* to the hazard rate of a person with a different set of covariates $\mathbf{X'_1, X'_2, ..., X'_p}$—that the hazards differ only by a multiplicative constant: $\mathbf{h_1(t) = c \cdot h_2(t)}$.

If we take the ratio of the hazard functions for two individuals, the first with the set of covariate values $(\mathbf{X_1, X_2, ..., X_p})$ and the second with covariate values $(\mathbf{X'_1, X'_2, ..., X'_p})$, the hazard ratio is:

$$\mathbf{HR = \frac{h_1(t, \underline{X}_1)}{h_2(t, \underline{X}_2)} = \frac{h_0(t) \cdot exp\{\beta_0 + \beta_1 X_1 + \beta_2 X_2 + \cdots + \beta_k X_k\}}{h_0(t) \cdot exp\{\beta_0 + \beta_1 X'_1 + \beta_2 X'_2 + \cdots + \beta_k X'_k\}} = c}$$

The two baseline hazards $h_0(t)$ are identical and cancel out. When the regression coefficients are estimated and the values for the covariates inserted, HR is just a constant value, $c$. Note that this implies that this relationship—and $c$—are time independent. The model assumes that the hazard ratio for these two individuals, each with his or her own set of covariates, does not change over time.

### Interpretation of the Hazard Ratio

Hazard ratios of interest are derived using the regression coefficient of the Cox model and can reflect comparison of two different sets of covariate values as shown previously or a single covariate. If, for example, the covariate $X_i$ is status for a particular risk factor (0 for risk factor absent, 1 for risk factor present), then the hazard ratio is obtained by the exponentiation of the estimated regression coefficient for $X_i$, that is, $\exp\{\beta_i\}$. Suppose this value is 3; this means the hazard for someone with the risk factor is three times as large as that for a subject without it, all other things being equal. A hazard ratio of 1 implies equal hazard in the two groups; if the hazard ratio is less than 1, it would mean that the hazard was less in persons with this putative risk factor—that its presence was protective. Spruance et al.[55] gives other examples and emphasizes that the hazard ratio alone is insufficient to convey the impact of covariates; survival curves and descriptors such as median survival times and other quantiles are helpful in describing the impact of the explanatory variables on survival. Other illustrations are given by Matthews and Farewell.[46] For further discussion of survival methodology, see Hosmer and Lemeshow[27] and Kleinbaum.[36]

As always, is important to assess the validity of the model assumptions. There are ways to assess the proportional hazards assumption of the Cox model, some involving graphical approaches and others using formal statistical testing. However, should the proportional hazards assumption prove to be untenable, there are ways to extend the Cox model so that the proportional hazards assumption is not required, such as models that provide for time-dependent covariates.

### Time-Dependent Covariates

There are alternative approaches to modeling the impact of covariates on time-to-event, including extensions to the Cox proportional hazards formulation that permit time-dependent covariates.[29,56] One situation where a model providing for time dependency is useful is when the impact of a covariate changes over time. Consider the potential impact of smoking in a study involving surgical intervention. If the effect on survival were mediated through impaired wound healing due to smoking, then smoking might exert its effect on survival only in the earlier postsurgical period and not in later parts of the period of follow-up. Another instance when allowing for time dependency is helpful is when the value of the covariate may change over time; for example, we may want to explore the effect on survival if the subject quits smoking.

### Interval-Censored Data

Special methods have been developed to address *interval censoring*. Interval censoring refers to situations where the outcome of interest is time-to-event, but the occurrence of the event of interest can only be recorded at specific intervals, such as at the time of periodic dental examinations. Such data arise when the time until the event of interest is not known precisely—only that it falls into a particular interval. This may be very relevant to certain dental outcomes, such as tooth eruption, development of caries, loss of a sealant, and colonization by *Streptococcus mutans*.[41] Statistical approaches have been developed for the analysis of interval-censored time-to-event data, including nonparametric approaches, extensions to the Cox model, and modeling approaches such as the accelerated failure time (AFT) model.[11]

### Other Approaches

Oral health research frequently involves the analysis of clustered (correlated) observations; such nonindependence arises when multiple sealants are placed in a single child as part of a sealant program or multiple implants are placed in a particular patient. Such applications require special methodology to address the correlated nature of the data. These can be addressed via extension of the Cox model, but there are other approaches, such as *frailty models*, that can be used for survival analysis of correlated outcomes, such as the clustered failure times observations in dental research.

### Parametric Survival Modeling

A variety of parametric methods and models have been used for survival analysis. Specialized survival distributions are frequently employed, such as exponential, Weibull, lognormal, gamma, or Gompertz. Distributional parameters can be expressed as functions of covariates. This again implies modeling the hazard function— the hazard function is different for persons (or other experimental units) with different sets of covariate values. Such parametric approaches have found particular use in dental materials research, where the outcome is not *time* to failure, but *force* to failure.

### Additional Considerations

The approaches discussed so far all assume that we have exact failure times for each individual experimental unit. There are other approaches for grouped data, such as traditional life-table analyses.

Planning for a time-to-event study can be very challenging. When considering sample size and power requirements, the investigator must consider not only the usual parameters, such as effect size and level of Type I error, but must also consider what the level and pattern of loss to follow-up is likely to be. The fact that most studies have rolling recruitment/accrual is a further complicating factor.

## Further Considerations Related to Statistical Modeling

### Overfitting

It is important to note that including too many explanatory (independent) variables relative to sample size can result in model *overfitting*. This is an important issue, because it has implications for the validity and reproducibility of the model. If too many explanatory variables are used relative to the available sample size, the resulting model will be of limited use for predicting the outcome of future observations. Moreover, overfitting statistical models by using too many explanatory variables may reveal idiosyncratic relationships among data in that particular sample rather than identifying reproducible ones. For these reasons, it is very important to validate predictive models by using data other than those used to develop the model. It is also important to emphasize that sample size considerations in statistical modeling are completely separate from the needed sample size to obtain sufficient statistical power. Although there are general guidelines for use of sufficient sample sizes to prevent model overfitting, they depend on the type of outcome being modeled and vary among experts and disciplines; for further discussion, see Harrell.[22]

### Evaluating Model Fit and Validity

All models are associated with specific assumptions; for example, the multiple regression model assumes normality and homoscedasticity (variance homogeneity), and the original time-independent formulation of the Cox model assumes proportional hazards. It is essential that the assumptions associated with the model are met to ensure that the interpretations and inferences made using the model will be valid. Both statistical tests and graphical methods have been developed for evaluating model assumptions.

Tests are also available to test the goodness of fit of a particular model; one example is the Hosmer-Lemeshow goodness of fit test used in logistic regression modeling. More generally, there are multiple *information criteria* that can be used in comparing different models. Two commonly used approaches are the Akaike information criterion (AIC) and the Bayesian information criterion (BIC). The BIC is also known as the Schwarz information criterion (abbreviated SBC or SBIC). Such criteria are intended to assist in choosing between competing models and can be used in a wide variety of situations.

When fitting models, it is possible to increase the goodness of fit by adding explanatory variables and so more model parameters but with the cost of added complexity and possible overfitting. *Information criteria* are measures that have been developed to try to address the trade-off between the goodness of fit of the model and the complexity of the model by introducing a penalty for the number of parameters. Different information criteria apply more or less stringent penalties, for example, the penalty term is larger in the BIC approach than in the AIC. A particular use of such criteria is in evaluating competing models. By way of example, suppose one effect under consideration is the impact of the number of treatments, with one to four applications of the treatment being studied. One might model the effect of the number of treatments with only one explanatory variable as a linear trend. Alternatively, one might model its impact using a four level categorical variable, using three binary covariates to estimate separate effects for one, two, three, or four courses of treatment. Obviously, the model with more parameters will fit better—but at the cost of added complexity. Is linear fit reasonable? Is the gain in fit worth those extra parameters? Information criteria can assist with such decisions.

Finally, we emphasize that it is important to validate the usefulness of models that will be used for prediction using data other than those used to develop the model. There are various approaches to model validation. A simple method—often called data splitting, simple validation, or the holdout method—involves splitting the sample into training (model development) and test (model validation) samples. More complex methods that are improvements on data splitting include resampling approaches, such as bootstrapping and jackknifing, and cross-validation methods to estimate model prediction performance.[22]

### Model Selection Procedures

Modeling, like the practice of dentistry, is something of an art form. Various approaches are used to select the explanatory variables to be included in statistical models. Some rely heavily on hypothesis testing, others on guidance based on a theoretical model or biological considerations, often combined with more statistical approaches. Some approaches are wholly data driven, such as the use of algorithms for automatic variable selection (e.g., forward, backward, and stepwise selection methods). Other approaches rely on

considerations of fit. For example, information criteria such the BIC or AIC and its variants may be used in the process of model selection.

Since candidate covariates in human studies are frequently correlated, it is not surprising that different approaches to model selection—or different modelers—may develop alternative models that are very similar in terms of predictive ability. This underlying correlation among explanatory variables has actually been of help to scientific investigation, since key factors in the biological process being modeled may not even be in our set of candidate explanatory variables. However, the associations identified often point toward potential involvement of a particular pathway or system, generating new hypotheses and opening up new avenues of investigation.

### Multicollinearity

The fact that some explanatory variables may be very highly correlated can cause serious problems in model fitting. Multicollinearity, or simply collinearity, occurs when two or more independent explanatory variables in a model are determined by a linear combination of other covariates in the model or are very highly correlated. For example, consider three candidate covariates: current subject age, subject age at onset of disease, and duration of disease. Clearly, any one of these covariates can be derived based on knowledge of the other two. Another example of collinearity between explanatory variables would be the age of dentists and number of years of practice; these two covariates are likely to be strongly related.

If some of the explanatory variables are very highly correlated, it may be difficult or even impossible to fit the model, as when there is perfect collinearity. Serious computation problems may also occur because the variables are conveying essentially the same information, as in the case of dentist age and years in practice. Moderate multicollinearity is not uncommon, and it may or may not cause problems in the predictive model. When severe multicollinearity occurs, the standard errors of the regression coefficients tend to become inflated, and the associated significance tests lose power. In some instances, estimates of the regression coefficients become unstable and unreliable, making it difficult to ascertain the effect of any single explanatory variable. Two commonly used measures of multicollinearity are the variance inflation factor, which is an indicator of the extent to which standard errors could be inflated due to multicollinearity, and the tolerance measure, which is simply its inverse. Regardless of the type of model being fit—multiple regression, logistic, survival, or Poisson—it is essential to evaluate potential multicollinearity among the predictor variables. Further examples and discussion of multicollinearity may be found in the dental literature.[6,15]

### Categorization of Quantitative Measures

Quantitative measures are rich in information. When a continuous measure is categorized, a portion of the information is lost along with the statistical power it implies. For those who have had the privilege of experiencing middle age, it is clear that 20 years of age is not 30, 30 is not 40, and 40 most assuredly is not 50. Nevertheless, it is not unusual to see dichotomizations of age, such as less than 40 versus 40 plus years, used in modeling. In addition to reducing power, the true relationship between outcome and the quantitative predictor is lost, and estimates of risk will be made with less precision. It is entirely possible that an arbitrary choice of cutpoint for the dichotomization will be unfortunate, and an existing relationship between the outcome and predictor will go undetected. Perhaps worse, repeated selection and evaluation of a series of cutpoints may lead to declarations of spurious associations. Finally, the ability to detect relationships with other covariates such as statistical interaction (effect modification) is likely to be impaired. This is not to say that categorization of quantitative measures can never be useful. Categorized intervals of some quantitative measures can have real implications. Consider developmental epochs in children and adolescents, the completion of a specific stage of the educational process, or specifications of intervals for clinical use. However, categorization should not automatically be the first approach taken in modeling.

### Final Words of Caution

The investigator must always be ready to explore new models as new information becomes available. A key consideration is the recognition that models are only tools that are used in an attempt to shed light on the phenomenon of interest; at best, models are approximations that may help gain insight on how reality functions. This was frequently emphasized by the noted statistician George E. P. Box[8,9] who stated that "Essentially, all models are wrong, but some are useful."

## Statistical Approaches to the Complexity of Oral Health Data

### Special Considerations for Oral Health Research

Oral health data are complex by their very nature. The analysis of observations involving teeth is complicated by the natural developmental processes of eruption of the primary teeth, the eventual shedding of the primary teeth, and the gradual emergence of the permanent dentition. Teeth may be lost to trauma or disease. These factors add to the usual missing data issues and lead to complications in the handling of missing data and other aspects of analysis. Moreover, oral health research includes many examples of correlated or clustered data. When multiple teeth, surfaces, or implants are evaluated within the same subject, it must be recognized that such observations would be expected to be correlated. Dental public health investigations often focus on classrooms, nursing homes, clinics, or dental practices. It is similarly reasonable to think that there may be similarities with respect to subjects within one of these units, and so the observed outcomes for those subjects would be expected to be correlated. In other instances, research paradigms such as split-mouth and crossover designs lead to the generation of correlated data, because they involve repeated measures on the same experimental unit. The approach to the statistical analysis of such data must take into account the correlated nature of such data; analyzing such data as if they were independent constitutes a serious error. We will now consider how such complexities can be addressed analytically.

### Missing Data

When data are missing, we are concerned primarily for two reasons: the associated loss of power and potential bias. The difficulty caused by missing data is clearly seen in matched designs—the loss of data for one member of the pair results in the loss of the entire pair. Missing data also have considerable potential impact on multivariable modeling; in certain approaches, missing data for one explanatory variable causes the subject to be eliminated from contributing to the model (known as *listwise deletion*). Further, certain subgroups of subjects may be more likely to have missing data, giving rise to the potential for bias in the results. For example, the sickest patients may not return for clinical follow-up; or conversely, the patient with an implant who is experiencing no problems may not see the need to return for a follow-up visit. Respondents to a questionnaire may be quite different from those who chose not to respond.

In considering possible remedies to the problem of missing data, it is important to consider the nature of the missing data and how they came about. Data may be missing due to loss, as when there is a recording error, or loss or mishandling of a physical sample. They may be missing due to refusal on the part of the subject to provide data, either because of the rigor associated with the testing or the sensitivity of the information. In time-to-event studies, the key outcome is unknown when there is censoring, that is, when follow-up ceases prior to occurrence of the event of interest. Particularly concerning are instances when there is a relationship between the outcome and an important covariate, such as when a subject fails to come to recall because of factors such as severity of illness or economic hardship.

The best way to address missing data is by efforts at the planning stage—prevention is best! Concerted efforts at retention or recontacting nonrespondents to secure key data items by telephone can help ameliorate missing data problems. Care in construction of questionnaires, such as providing ranges for sensitive items such as income, may also help lower rates of non response.

There are also analytic approaches, which include comparison of subjects with and without missing data. In this way, a profile can be created of those who fail to complete follow-up or have a particular item missing. In some instances, there may be analytic solutions, such as the survival methodology developed specifically to deal with the problem of censoring, or types of longitudinal data analyses that are able to deal with missing data. Sensitivity analyses may be carried out to explore the potential impact of missing data. Other solutions use some form of data imputation. One of the most widely used is multiple imputation, a method by which missing data are replaced by multiple simulated versions. Each of the simulated data sets are analyzed, and their results are combined, typically to obtain estimates, standard errors and confidence errors.[45,54,57]

These analytic solutions may be partial, may be analytically complex, and may rely on assumptions about the nature of the "missingness." There are different classifications of "missingness." One example is "missing completely at random," which assumes that the probability a data point is missing is independent of all responses. Another is "missing at random," which implies that the likelihood a data point is missing is related to at least some of the observed data but not to the missing data. Most analytic approaches to addressing the problem of missing data make some assumption, implicit or otherwise, about the nature of missing data, at least with respect to the inferences drawn from the analysis.

### Special Analytic Considerations for Interventional Studies

Both observational and interventional studies may involve prolonged periods of follow-up, and missing data due to attrition represent a serious concern. Active retention efforts are therefore critically important to both types of studies. However, there are special analytic issues that are primarily relevant to intervention studies. One is the standard of using *intention to treat (ITT)* analysis—also called "as randomized" or "method effectiveness" analysis—in the context of a randomized trial. The ITT principle requires that any comparison of treatments be based on comparison of outcomes of all subjects in the treatment groups to which they were originally assigned via the randomization. For treatment comparisons to be valid, they must be accomplished via analyses consistent with the design used to generate the data. The protection against bias afforded by randomization is thwarted if the analysis is biased. In the case of the RCT, this means analysis should be carried out according to the ITT principle, which preserves the benefits of randomization.

Analyses based on treatment administered or requirements such as strict adherence to treatment protocol (*per protocol* analyses) may be performed, but these should represent supplementary analyses. In no instance should they supplant the ITT analyses as the primary analyses. *Per protocol* analyses, as well as analyses comparing groups defined by factors other than the randomization schedule, can be associated with considerable potential for bias. This is especially true when the groups are defined by factors influenced by treatment. For example, if the comparison is with only patients who actually fully complied with the prescribed treatments, then observed differences might be due not to treatment but to factors associated with compliance; there are many other possibilities.

Another fairly common analytic aspect of interventional studies is the use of sequential testing.[20] They provide for several planned interim analyses of the data and specify stopping criteria for each of the planned interim analyses. It may be desirable to stop an interventional study early if there is convincing evidence that one treatment is superior to the others, that there is no difference between treatments, or if there is evidence of harm associated with one or more treatments. Group sequential testing methods have been developed for dental clinical trials with longitudinal data on multiple outcomes.[39] However, in many situations, more flexible methods of monitoring trials—usually administered via a data safety monitoring board—are felt to be appropriate.

Approaches using propensity scores may be useful in instances where estimation of treatment effects are of interest. Broadly speaking, a propensity score is the probability that a subject (or other experimental unit) is assigned to a particular group given a set of covariates associated with that subject; typically, the group represents a treatment assignment. In the absence of randomization, as is used in a randomized control trial, it is often likely that the characteristics of an individual make it more or less likely that he or she will receive a certain treatment. For this reason, there is a clear risk of bias in observational studies or nonrandomized trials due to this "confounding by indication." Individuals directed toward a particular treatment may differ from those not receiving that particular treatment by factors that are strongly related to prognosis, such as the presence of concomitant conditions or the severity of the disease. Statistical techniques using propensity scores attempt to reduce bias in the estimation of the effect of an intervention by taking account of the covariates that predict receiving that treatment. The propensity score represents a summary of the information from the explanatory covariates and may be used in several possible analytic approaches. In one approach, a subject receiving the treatment of interest is matched with an individual who did not receive the treatment on the basis of propensity score. In stratified approaches, subgroups are defined by propensity score. In other approaches, the propensity score is used for adjustment in the context of a regression analysis. Further discussion is given by Williamson and Forbes.[59] Although such approaches are typically used in the analysis of data from observational studies or nonrandomized trials, they have also found utility in addressing imbalances in subject characteristics in randomized trials. As discussed by Nicholas and Gulliford,[49] they may have particular value in cluster randomized trials, where such imbalances may be more likely to occur, either because only a limited number of clusters is being randomized or because the covariate profiles of subjects may differ from cluster to cluster.

## Analysis of Correlated/Clustered Data

Appropriate analysis is a matter of critical importance in oral health research, where the following are commonplace:

- Multiple evaluations of the same outcome over time
- Study of multiple teeth, sealants, implants, or restorations in a single subject
- Study of multiple surfaces on the same tooth
- Evaluation by multiple raters of a set of experimental units
- Study of an experimental unit under several different conditions
- Clustered designs that evaluate subjects within groups such as classrooms, nursing home, dental practices and so forth; examples are cluster randomized trials where the groups of subjects are randomized rather than having randomization carried out on the level of the individual subject. Such designs induce dependency: The observations of individuals within a cluster would be expected to be correlated.

All of these represent instances where outcome data are likely to be correlated and where statistical approaches that can appropriately address that lack of independence must be applied. Although the terms "multivariable" and "multivariate" may be used interchangeably in other contexts, statisticians reserve the term "multivariate analysis" for instances where there are many outcome variables, such as those just outlined. Multivariate analysis is indicated when more than one response variable is analyzed simultaneously. The term "multivariable" is more generic, indicating only that multiple variables are involved. For example, a multivariable logistic regression model has more than one explanatory variable. One way this can occur is when multiple response characteristics are measured on each subject. Examples include the caries status of multiple teeth or surfaces within the same subject; attachment level measurements for a set of sites in the same subject; a set of cephalometric measures; microbial profiles; or outcomes for multiple implants, sealants, or restorations within the same subject. Multivariate analysis is also used when a single response variable is measured under different conditions or at different times, as in longitudinal studies. Of course, one can also look at multivariate profiles over time, combining these two possibilities. Multivariate approaches will take into account the correlation among multivariate responses. Analyzing correlated measures with univariate methods, which assume all observations are mutually independent, is a common mistake that can have grave consequences in terms of improper inference and erroneous conclusions.

### *General Approaches to the Analysis of Correlated Data*

In the simplest situations associated with correlated data, arising from before-and-after or matched pair designs, well-known statistical procedures such as the paired t-test, the Wilcoxon signed rank test, and McNemar's test are commonly used. A few procedures for analyzing more complex correlated data have already been mentioned, some quite specialized, such as extensions to logistic regression for analyzing correlated binary outcomes,[4,50] and methods relevant to correlated time-to-event outcomes,[29,56] but there are many others, including specifically dental applications.[5,48,53,60]

Among the general analytic approaches that have been found to be useful in analyzing the correlated observations frequently encountered in dental public health and oral health research in general, one of the simplest employs *summary measures* on the level of the subject. The multivariate data are combined into a single index for analysis, sidestepping the issue of their correlation; a common example is the DMFS (number of decayed, missing or filled surfaces) commonly used in caries research. Such summary measures are quite data reductive and may obscure details; for example, the simple DMFS measure does not facilitate consideration of differences in caries susceptibility among the various tooth types or between pit-and-fissure versus smooth surfaces.

Repeated measures analysis of variance (repeated measures ANOVA) has some utility in the analysis of correlated data, but more recently developed statistical models have broader applicability. These approaches are generalizations of the linear model for clustered data, such as random effects models, which can accommodate both quantitative and categorical outcomes, and varying cluster sizes, and can allow for general correlation structure. For measurements in the oral cavity, the ability to specify different correlation structures is an important consideration, since observations of some teeth or surfaces may be more highly correlated than others. In longitudinal studies, observations that are further apart in time may be less highly correlated than those measured in closer time proximity.

One form of the generalized linear model for correlated data is the *random effects model*. The term *mixed model* often is used to denote a model including both random and fixed effects. Random effects are generally used to model individual variation, whereas fixed effects are intended to elucidate the impact of covariates such as treatment group and patient characteristics. A second generalized linear model approach for correlated data is the *generalized estimating equation (GEE) model* first proposed by Liang and Zeger.[44] These two approaches, contrasted and illustrated by Begg[5] and Hujoel et al.,[32] used general estimating equation approaches to estimate and assess model parameters while taking account of the clustering of caries outcomes for multiple surfaces within a subject. A variety of specialized methods are available for the analysis of longitudinal data.[18] All of these approaches are able to address nonindependence among observations and provide ways to address more complicated data structures when repeated measures are made on the same subject.

### Analysis of Split-Mouth and Crossover and Split-Mouth Designs

Crossover and split-mouth designs are two designs involving correlated data that are frequently used in oral health research. Data from these designs must be analyzed using methods that take into account the fact that the observations include repeated measures on the same individual. There are also key assumptions that must be met for these analyses to be valid. In theory, efficiency will be increased for these matched designs because each subject "serves as his own control"—the matched design is intended to control for sources of error due to individual differences and eliminate confounding. If that is the case, fewer subjects are needed to obtain equivalent power.

In the simplest form of crossover design (Figure 13.7), there are two treatments, A and B, and each subject receives both treatments. Subjects are randomized to one of two treatment sequences: Half of the participants begin with one treatment and then switch to the second treatment; the other half of the subjects have the opposite sequence: A-B or B-A. There is typically a *washout period* between treatments. The key assumption that must be fulfilled for results from crossover studies to be valid is that after the washout period, the subject is returned to the identical state the subject was in before the first treatment was applied. *This is critical—and is a very strong assumption.* It is not always clear what the washout period should be or if this key assumption can be met. The potential for *carryover effects* from one treatment to another (i.e., when

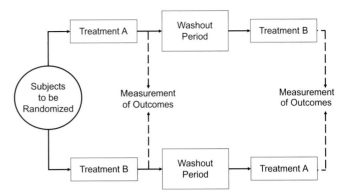

A "Simple" Cross-Over Design

• **Figure 13.7** Schematic for the conduct of a simple cross-over design.

this key assumption is violated) represents a serious disadvantage. If carryover is present, results of statistical tests may not be valid and the estimates of treatment effects incorrect. The seriousness of this potential problem cannot be overstated.

The design adds to the complexity of the data analysis—the analysis must take account of the paired design. One approach is to use a general linear mixed model to estimate the effects of treatment and the two carryover effects (i.e., a separate carryover effect for each treatment sequence); it is then possible to assess whether there are significant carryover effects and whether they differ.[23] When more treatments are added, things become even more complicated. If such experiments are not properly planned and balanced, treatment effects cannot be properly estimated. The handling of dropouts, protocol infractions, and errors in treatment assignment or dosage can be quite problematic. A disadvantage of the crossover design is that it tends to lengthen the duration of the study.

In split-mouth designs, the oral cavity of an individual is divided into two or more subunits, and treatments are randomly assigned to the subunits rather than to the entire mouth of a given subject, as in a parallel design. This design has been applied to implant studies, studies of pain associated with injection, and in trials of periodontal and orthodontic treatment; its first use in dentistry was reported by Ramfjord et al.[52] Potentially, this design can reduce the time to conduct a trial and/or the number of patients needed to conduct the trial, in comparison to parallel or crossover designs, and under certain conditions, split-mouth designs can offer significant gains in efficiency as compared with whole mouth designs.[30,31,33,42] However, in practice, *carry-across effects* may represent a significant problem.[40] This design is only appropriate if no treatment affects the outcomes of any of the other treatments. In instances where there is physical contamination or systemic effects of any treatment, this key assumption will not be met. In the presence of carry-across effects, validity of statistical tests is questionable, and treatment effects are confounded with carry-across effects. In the absence of carry-across effects, statistical approaches similar to those used in crossover studies are typically applied.

There are some other potential disadvantages of the split-mouth approach. Asymmetry of disease severity within the mouth may be a problem, and it may be difficult to recruit appropriately symmetric subjects. When there are more treatments than experimental units (sites) within blocks (subjects), then the design will be some form of incomplete block structure. If these are not properly balanced, treatment effects cannot be properly estimated. Further, not all treatment comparisons will be estimated with the same precision, so this must be considered carefully at the design stage. It follows that the handling of dropouts may be problematic.

## Effective Consultation With Statisticians

Clinicians work in the language of disease, diagnosis, treatment, and outcomes. Biostatisticians work in the language of hypothesis testing, statistical power, sample size, data analysis, and probability. Early and respectful collaboration between clinicians and biostatisticians is the most effective way of designing and planning a productive and mutually satisfying research project.

Biostatisticians often have a familiarity with clinical and scientific terminology and procedures, especially within the research areas they have previously supported. This has developed as a necessity for clear communication with researchers. However, this does not make the biostatistician a content expert nor should he or she be expected to function as one. Therefore, the researchers consulting with the statistician should expect to provide all expert decisions, such as determining a clinically meaningful difference, assessing the quality or appropriateness of clinical methods used in research, and reviewing the primary literature for the clinical state of the art.

To help focus the collaboration and before consulting with a biostatistician, it is very helpful if clinical researchers prepare a brief written background statement of the problem to be addressed and questions to be answered in the proposed study. Clearly defining the primary and secondary research questions in writing is the first issue that needs to be resolved in designing any research study. Doing so saves valuable time and effort in developing the research hypothesis and design of the proposed study. In this regard, the biostatistician and clinical researcher will need to work together to answer the proposed questions that will include the type of study to be conducted (i.e., observational or interventional) and other important details about the study. These details include such things as calculating appropriate sample size and statistical power, selection of appropriate test or control subjects, clearly defining the magnitude or effect size of the clinically meaningful primary and secondary outcomes that will achieve a clinical impact, deciding the specific measurements and covariates that need to be collected, and the various analytical approaches that will be used (the statistical analysis plan).

Successful collaborations will continue this give-and-take into the analytic phase, where time invested in reciprocal education will enable the refinement of models and enhance their interpretation. An evolving understanding and discussion can lead to new questions, supplemental analyses, and ideas for future work. Navigating this process can be subject to setbacks, difficulties in communicating clearly, and external pressure to perform. However, as in any collaboration, the best results are achieved when there is mutual respect and understanding of the interdisciplinary nature of those involved in the work.

For the best outcome, design and analysis must go hand in hand. It is essential that the statistician be part of the investigative team from the beginning of study planning. Just as it is frequently impossible to retrieve a key data item overlooked in the development of a study, it is typically impossible for the statistician to amend a significant design flaw through statistical manipulation.

As Sir Ronald Aylmer Fisher warned in his presidential address to the first Indian Statistical Congress[17]: "To consult the statistician after an experiment is finished is often merely to ask him to conduct a post mortem examination. He can perhaps say what the experiment died of."

## References

1. Agresti A. *Analysis of Ordinal Categorical Data.* 2nd ed. New York: Wiley; 2010.
2. Agresti A. *Categorical Data Analysis.* 3rd ed. New York: Wiley; 2013.
3. Agresti A. *An Introduction to Categorical Data Analysis.* New York: Wiley; 2007.
4. Ananth CV, Kantor ML. Modeling multivariate binary responses with multiple levels of nesting based on alternating logistic regressions: an application to caries aggregation. *J Dent Res.* 2004 Oct;83 (10):776–781.
5. Begg MD. Analysis or correlated responses. In: Lesaffre E, Feine J, Leroux B, et al. eds. *Statistical and Methodological Aspects of Oral Health Research,* eds. New York: Wiley; 2009:221–240.
6. Binkley CJ, Beacham A, et al. Genetic variations in the melanocortin-1 receptor (MC1R) gene associated with red hair color and fear of dental pain, anxiety regarding dental care and avoidance of dental care. *J Am Dent Assoc.* 2009;140(7):896–905.
7. Bortkiewicz L. *Das Gesetz der kleinen Zahlen.* Leipzig: B.G. Teubner; 1898.
8. Box GEP. Science and statistics. *J Amer Stat Assoc.* 1976;71:791–799.
9. Box GEP, Draper NR. Empirical Model Building and Response Surfaces. *New York: Wiley.* 1987;424.
10. Breslow NE, Day NE. *Statistical Methods in Cancer Research Volume 1: The Analysis of Case-Control Studies.* International Agency for Research on Cancer; Lyon; 1980.
11. Chen D-G, Sun J, Peace KE. *Interval-Censored Time-to-Event Data: Methods and Applications.* London, England: Chapman & Hall; 2013.
12. Cohen J. *Statistical Power Analysis for the Behavioral Sciences.* Mahwah, NJ: Lawrence Erlbaum Associates; 1988.
13. Conover WJ. *Practical Nonparametric Statistics.* 3rd ed. New York: Wiley; 1999.
14. Cook TD. Advanced statistics: up with odds ratios! A case for odds ratios when outcomes are common. *Acad Emerg Med.* 2002;9: 1430–1434.
15. Dawson DV. Variants in the melanocortin-1 receptor (MC1R) gene appear to be associated with increased dental care-related anxiety, increased fear of dental pain, and greater likelihood of dental care avoidance. *J Evid Based Dent Pract.* 2010;10:169–171.
16. Draper NR, Smith H. *Applied Regression Analysis.* 3rd ed. New York: Wiley; 1998.
17. Fisher RA. Presidential address. *Sankhya Ser B.* 1938;4(1):14–17.
18. Fitzmaurice GM, Laird NM, Ware JH. *Applied Longitudinal Analysis.* 2nd ed. New York: Wiley; 2011.
19. Fleiss JL, Levin B, Paik MC. *Statistical Methods for Rates and Proportions.* 3rd ed. New York: Wiley; 2003.
20. Friedman LM, Furberg CD, DeMets DL, Reboussin DM, Granger CB. *Fundamentals of Clinical Trials.* 5th ed. New York: Springer; 2015.
21. Gordis L. *Epidemiology.* 5th ed. New York: Elsevier; 2013.
22. Harrell FE. *Regression Modeling Strategies: With Applications to Linear Models, Logistic Regression, and Survival Analysis,* 2nd ed. New York: Springer.
23. Hedayat A, Afsarinejad K. Repeated measurements designs, II. *Ann Stat.* 1978;6:619–628.
24. Hochberg Y, Benjamini Y. More powerful procedures for multiple significance testing. *Stat Med.* 1990;9:811–818.
25. Hochbeg Y, Tamhane AC. *Multiple Comparisons Procedures.* New York: Wiley; 2009.
26. Holm S. A simple sequentially rejective multiple test procedure. *Scand J Statist.* 1979;6:65–70.
27. Hosmer DW Jr, Lemeshow S. *Applied Survival Analysis: Regression Modeling of Time to Event Data.* New York: Wiley; 1999.

28. Hosmer DW, Lemeshow S, Sturdivant RX. *Applied Logistic Regression*. 3rd ed. New York: Wiley; 2013.
29. Hougaard P. *The Statistical Analysis of Failure Time Data*. 2nd ed. New York: Wiley; 2000.
30. Hujoel PP. Design and analysis issues in split mouth clinical trials. *Community Dent Oral Epidemiol*. 1998;26:85–86.
31. Hujoel PP, DeRouen TA. Validity issues in split-mouth trials. *J Clin Periodontol*. 1992;19:625–627.
32. Hujoel PP, Isokangas PJ, Tiekso J, Davis S, Lamont RJ, DeRouen TA, Makinen KK. A re-analysis of caries rates in a preventive trial using Poisson regression models. *J Dent Res*. 1994;73: 573–579.
33. Hujoel PP, Loeschle WJ. Efficiency of split-mouth designs. *J Clin Periodontol*. 1990;17:722–728.
34. Imrey PB1, Chilton NW, Pihlstrom BL, et al. Proposed guidelines for American Dental Association acceptance of products for professional, non-surgical treatment of adult periodontitis. Task Force on Design and Analysis in Dental and Oral Research. *J Periodontal Res*. 1994;29:348–60.
35. Ioannidis JPA. The proposal to lower p value thresholds to .005. *JAMA*. 2018;319:1429–1430.
36. Kleinbaum DG. *Survival Analysis: A Self-Learning Text*. New York: Springer; 1996.
37. Kleinbaum DG, Klein M. *Logistic Regression: A Self-Learning Text*. 3rd ed. New York: Springer; 2010.
38. Kleinbaum DG, Kupper LL, Nizam A, et al. Applied Regression Analysis, 5th ed. Boston: Cengage. *Learning*. 2014.
39. Leroux BG, Mancl LA, DeRouen TA. Group sequential testing in dental clinical trials with longitudinal data on multiple outcome variables. *Stat Meth Med Res*. 2005;14:591–602.
40. Lerous B, Lesaffre E. Design and analysis of randomized clinical trials in oral health. In: Lesaffre E, Feine J, Leroux B, eds. *Statistical and Methodological Aspects of Oral Health Research*. New York: Wiley; 2009:221–240.
41. Lesaffre E, Komárek A. An overview of methods for interval-censored data with an emphasis on applications in dentistry. *Stat Methods Med Res*. 2005;14:539–552.
42. Lesaffre E, Pihlstrom B, Needleman I, Worthington H. The design and analysis of split-mouth studies: What statisticians and clinicians should know. *Stat in Med*. 2009;28:3470–3482.
43. Lewsey JD, Gilthorpe MS, Bulman JS. Bedi R. Is modelling dental caries a "normal" thing to do? *Community Dent Health*. 2000;17:212–217.
44. Liang KY, Zeger S. Longitudinal data analysis using generalized linear models. *Biometrics*. 1986;73:13–22.
45. Little RJA, Rubin DB. *Statistical Analysis with Missing Data*. 2nd ed. New York: Wiley; 2002.
46. Matthew DE, Farewell VT. *Using and Understanding Medical Statistics*. 5th ed. Basel, Switzerland: Karger; 2015.
47. McNutt LA, Wu C, Hafner JP. Estimating the relative risk in cohort studies and clinical trials of common outcomes. *Am J Epidemiol*. 2003;157:940–943.
48. Mutsvari T, Bandyopadhyay D, Declerck D, Lesaffre E. A multilevel model for spatially correlated binary data in the presence of misclassification: an application in oral health research. *Stat Med*. 2013;32:5241–5259.
49. Nicholas J, Gulliford MC. Commentary: what is a propensity score? *Br J Gen Prac*. 2008;58:687.
50. Perin J, Preisser JS. Alternating logistic regressions with improved finite sample properties. *Biometrics*. 2017;73:696–705.
51. Petrie A, Bulman JS. Osborn. Further statistics in dentistry. Part 6: Multiple linear regression. *Br Dent J*. 2002;193:675–682.
52. Ramfjord SP, Nissle RR, Shick RA, Cooper H Jr. Subgingival curettage versus surgical elimination of periodontal pockets. *J Periodontol*. 1968;39:167–175.
53. Reich BJ, Bandyopadhyay D, Bondell HD. A nonparametric spatial model for periodontal data with non-random missingness. *J Am Stat Assoc*. 2013;108:820–831.
54. Schafer J. Multiple imputation: a primer. *Stat Methods Med Res*. 1999;8:3–15.
55. Spruance SL, Reid JE, Grace M, Samore M. Hazard ratio in clinical trials. *Antimicrob Agents Chemother*. 2004;48:2787–2792.
56. Therneau TM, Grambsch P. *Modeling Survival Data: Extending the Cox Model*. New York: Springer-Verlag; 2000.
57. van Buuren S. *Flexible Imputation of Missing Data. London*. Chapman & Hall: England; 2012.
58. Wasserstein RL, Lazar NA. The ASA's statement on P-values: context, process, and purpose. *Am Stat*. 2016;70:129–133.
59. Williamson EJ, Forbes A. Introduction to propensity scores. *Respirology*. 2014;19:625–635.
60. Zhang Y, Todem D, Kim K, Lesaffre E. Bayesian latent variable models for spatially correlated tooth-level binary data in caries research. *Stat Modelling*. 2011;11:25–47.

## Further Reading

Brunette DM, Hornby K, Oakley C. *Critical Thinking: Understanding and Evaluating Dental Research*. Chicago: Quintessence Publishing; 2007.
Giannobile WV, Burt BA, Genco RJ. *Clinical Research in Oral Health*. Wiley-Blackwell: Ames, IA; 2010.
Lesaffre E, Feine J, Leroux B, Declerk D, eds. *Statistical and Methodological Aspects of Oral Health Research*. Chichester, UK: Wiley; 2009.

# 14

# Measurement and Distribution of Dental Caries

MARISOL TELLEZ MERCHAN, BDS, MPH, PhD

AMID I. ISMAIL, BDS, MPH, MBA, DrPH

## CHAPTER OUTLINE

## Description and Etiology of Dental Caries

Dental caries is a chronic disease that is caused by the interaction of the intraoral microbial biofilm (microbiome) accumulated on tooth surfaces with fermentable sugars in an environment where salivary buffering and remineralization systems are weakened or cannot counteract the continuous cycles of demineralization. Additionally, dental caries is an ecologic and behavioral disease facilitated by multiple risk factors—direct or indirect, causal or not—that interplay to lead to shifts in the balance of the normal noncariogenic oral microbiota driven by a change in the oral environment and lifestyle.[66]

Our basic understanding of the caries process dates back over 125 years to W.D. Miller's chemo-parasitic theory, and to a large extent we are still managing dental caries using similar late-19th century surgical approaches intended to control the disease process.[67] Today, dental caries is understood as a dynamic process with rapidly alternating periods of tooth demineralization and remineralization. If net demineralization can occur over a sufficient time, this results in the initiation of a carious lesion at certain anatomic plaque-stagnation areas on tooth surfaces.[66] Dental caries can also develop on nonplaque stagnation areas when the challenge of demineralization is overwhelming and is not counteracted by natural remineralization of tooth structure (enamel and dentin). Although dental caries is a disease that can occur throughout one's lifetime, the most susceptible period of caries initiation is when a tooth erupts until full eruption and mineralization of the outer tooth enamel is complete.

The multilevel interactions between caries risk factors and the chronic nature of the disease process presents a challenge for assessing caries risk, which has been shown to have low predictive validity.[28] The number of predicative indicators, pathologic and protective, that may directly or indirectly influence caries risk is extensive, especially in young children,[2] and includes clinical/biological factors (e.g., caries experience of child and caregiver, plaque/microbiology, gingivitis, saliva, tooth developmental defects, medical factors, genetics), environmental factors (e.g., exposure to fluoride, antibiotic usage, exposure to lead), and behavioral/psychosocial/sociodemographic factors (e.g., diet, oral hygiene habits, age, parenting styles, child temperament, beliefs, caregiver's education level, socioeconomic status, insurance status, and access to dental care).[29] Some of these risk factors not only influence dental caries but also play a role in the development of major non-communicable diseases.[70] For example, diet is a shared common risk factor not only for dental caries, but also for obesity, diabetes, heart disease, stroke, and some cancers.

## Measurement of Dental Caries

### Models Used in the 20th Century

The clinical detection of caries is traditionally made by detailed visual inspection of clean teeth by trained examiners. Although sharply pointed dental probes (or explorers) are still often used, they provide little additional diagnostic benefit and can do some damage.[25,26] Dental radiographs or other supportive diagnostic methods are also needed in clinical practice to detect lesions that are hidden to visual assessment, particularly those situated on the approximal tooth surfaces.[43] It has been recognized since the late 19th century that detection and classification of dental caries are not easy tasks. The problems of misdiagnosis of caries lesions and "hidden caries" are not new phenomena.[50] Conversely, misdiagnosing sound tooth surfaces as carious (false positive) may have greater consequences by leading to unnecessary restorative care.

The concept that dental caries is a process rather than a binary disease with "cavitated" and "not cavitated" states was reported over 100 years ago.[53] Indeed, G.V. Black advocated for the study and detection of early caries lesions. Nevertheless, as the focus on surgical repair of damaged tooth structure (euphemistically referred to as "drilling and filling") and the misunderstanding that early lesions could not be reliably measured became central to dental practice, the development of early dental caries criteria systems inaccurately reflected the contemporary understanding of dental caries epidemiology, prevention, and management.[43] This began to change based on some early work by European researchers dating to the 1960s, where they had included early signs of dental caries in their criteria systems. By contrast, criteria developed in the United States remained focused on measuring cavitation only using explorers. This led to a dichotomy where the sensibility of the European criteria systems favored the disease process, while the sensibility of the US systems favored reliability and comparability.[43] However, in the past 20 years, there have been renewed attempts globally to expand the methodology to detect and diagnose caries lesions.

The range of criteria employed in the last half of the 20th century to assess for dental caries varied substantially and was reported in review describing the content validity of caries detection criteria reported in the literature between January 1, 1966, and May 1, 2000.[43] Analysis was based on evaluation of the disease process, exclusion of noncaries lesions, subjectivity, use of explorers, and drying of teeth prior to examination. This review included 29 unique criteria systems. Of those, 13 originated from the United Kingdom, three from the United States, four from Denmark, and others from the World Health Organization (WHO), Sweden, Switzerland, Norway, the Netherlands, and Canada. Thirteen of the criteria systems either measured active and inactive early and cavitated lesions or defined separate criteria for smooth and occlusal tooth surfaces. Nine systems measured early and cavitated stages of the caries process, and seven measured cavitation only. Eleven of the criteria systems provided explicit descriptions of the disease process measured or information on how to exclude noncaries from caries lesions. The use of explorers varied widely as did other procedures and examination conditions (Table 14.1).[43]

The WHO criteria are the most widely used in oral health surveys globally. The case definition for caries as proposed by the WHO is "Caries is recorded as present when a lesion in a pit or fissure, or on a smooth tooth surface, has an unmistakable cavity,

## • TABLE 14.1  Selected Criteria for Detection of Dental Caries (20th Century)

| Diagnostic System | Year/Country | Tooth Surface | Description |
|---|---|---|---|
| Backer-Dirks et al. | 1961, Netherlands | Crown | For approximal caries, the clinical examination by mirror and explorer was completely abandoned, because of poor accuracy, which makes it almost impossible to standardize diagnosis. Pits and fissures were cleaned with a new sharp explorer and dried with compressed air. The diagnosis was made with a small hand light of high intensity. Incident and transmitted light was used. Caries was estimated in four different grades. Caries I signifies a minute black line at the bottom of the fissure. In caries II, there is also a white zone along the margins of the fissure. Caries III denotes the smallest perceptible break in the continuity of the enamel (cavity) with or without undermined margins. Caries IV is a large cavity more than 3 mm wide. |
| Radike | 1968, USA | Crown | (I) Frank lesions—The detection of these lesions on the basis of gross cavitation usually does not present a problem in diagnosis. When cavitation is present, the diagnosis is positive.<br>(A) Cavitation in this context can be defined as a discontinuity of the enamel surface caused by loss of tooth surfaces.<br>(B) Cavitation that is the result of the caries process must be distinguished from fractures and smooth lesions or erosion and abrasion.<br>(II) Lesions not showing cavitation—The most difficult part of the examiner's task is the detection of lesions without frank cavitation. These are lesions close to the decision point between carious and sound. The criteria for detection of these lesions are summarized in three categories, each presenting its special problems.<br>(A) Detection of pit and fissure lesions of the occlusal, facial, and lingual surfaces.<br>(1) Area is carious when the explorer "catches" or resists removal after insertion into a pit or fissure with moderate to firm pressure and when accompanied by one or more of the following signs of caries:<br>(a) a softness at the base of the area<br>(b) opacity adjacent to the pit or fissure as evidence of undermining or demineralization<br>(c) softened enamel adjacent to the pit or fissure that may be scraped away with the explorer<br>(2) Area is carious if there is loss of the normal translucency of the enamel, adjacent to a pit, which is in contrast to the surrounding tooth structure. This condition is considered reliable evidence of undermining. In some of these cases, the explorer may not catch or penetrate the pit.<br>(B) Detection of lesions on smooth area[s] of facial and lingual surfaces<br>(1) Area is carious if surface is etched or if there is a white spot as evidence of subsurface demineralization and if the area is found to be soft by:<br>(a) penetration with explorer<br>(b) enamel can be scraped away with explorer<br>(2) Area is sound when there is apparent evidence of demineralization (etching or white spots) but no evidence of softness.<br>(C) Detection of lesions on proximal surfaces: It was not possible to attain agreement on a single set of criteria, since procedures used for diagnosis of proximal surfaces varied considerably. Some examiners depended largely upon visual-tactile methods, some depended largely on radiographs |

(Continued)

**• TABLE 14.1  Selected Criteria for Detection of Dental Caries (20th Century)—Cont'd**

| Diagnostic System | Year/Country | Tooth Surface | Description |
|---|---|---|---|
| | | | and transillumination, while others used a combination of these procedures. The following is intended to be a composite of the best elements from all procedures: <br>(1) For area exposed to direct visual and tactile examination, these are diagnosed as under "B" above for smooth areas. <br>(2) For hidden areas not exposed to direct visual-tactile examinations: <br>  (a) (visual examination) If the marginal ridge shows an opacity as evidence of undermined enamel, the proximal surface is carious. <br>  (b) (tactile examination) Any discontinuity of the enamel in which an explorer will enter is carious if it also shows other evidence of decay, such as softness, shadow by transillumination, or loss of translucency. <br>  (c) (radiography) Any definite radiolucency indicating a break in the continuity of the enamel surface is carious. <br>  (d) (transillumination; use mostly for anterior teeth) A loss of translucency producing a characteristic shadow in a calculus-free and stain-free proximal surface is adequate evidence of caries. |
| NIDCR | 1987, USA | Crown and root | Coronal caries: Frank lesions are detected as gross cavitation. Incipient lesions may be subdivided into three categories according to location, each with special diagnostic considerations. These categories are: <br>(I) Pits and fissures on occlusal, buccal, and lingual surfaces. These areas are diagnosed as carious when the explorer catches after insertion with moderate to firm pressure and when the catch is accompanied by one or more of the following signs of decay: <br>  (A) softness at the base of the area <br>  (B) opacity adjacent to the area, providing evidence of undermining or demineralization <br>  (C) softened enamel adjacent to the area that may be scraped away with the explorer. (Care should be taken to avoid removal of enamel that could be remineralized.) <br>(II) Smooth areas on buccal (labial) or lingual surfaces These areas are carious if they are decalcified or if there is a white spot as evidence of subsurface demineralization and if the area is found to be soft by: <br>  (A) penetration with the explorer, or <br>  (B) scraping away the enamel with the explorer. These areas should be diagnosed as sound when there is only visual evidence of demineralization but no evidence of softness. <br>(III) Proximal surfaces: For areas exposed to direct visual and tactile examination, as when there is no adjacent tooth, the criteria are the same as those for smooth areas on facial or lingual surfaces. For areas not available to direct visual-tactile examination, the following criterion applies: A discontinuity of the enamel in which the explorer will catch is carious if there is softness. Visual evidence of undermining under a marginal ridge is not acceptable evidence of a proximal lesion unless a surface break can be entered with the explorer. <br>Root caries: Active caries lesions in root surfaces are yellow/orange, tan, or light brown. Lesions in remission tend to be darker, sometimes almost black. When root caries is covered by small amounts of plaque, the discoloration of the lesions usually shows through. The tactile criterion of softness to an explorer tip must be met for a definite diagnosis of root caries. |
| WHO | 1987, World | Crown | Caries is recorded as present when a lesion in a pit or fissure or on a smooth tooth surface has a detectably softened floor, undermined enamel, or softened wall. A tooth with a temporary filling should also be included in this category. On approximal surfaces, the examiner must be certain that the explorer has entered a lesion. When any doubt exists, caries should not be recorded as present. |
| WHO | 1997, World | Crown | Caries is recorded as present when a lesion in a pit or fissure or on a smooth tooth surface has an unmistakable cavity, undermined enamel, or a detectably softened floor or wall. A tooth with a temporary filling or one that is sealed but also decayed should also be included in this category. In cases where the crown has been destroyed by caries and only the tooth is left, the caries is judged to have originated on the crown and therefore is scored as crown caries only. The CPI probe should be used to confirm visual evidence of caries on the occlusal, buccal, and lingual surfaces. Where any doubt exists, caries should not be recorded as present. |

undermined enamel, or a detectably softened floor or wall."[75] The WHO criteria are based on the assumption that measuring earlier stages that can be controlled through preventive therapy is not feasible in epidemiologic surveys, and it further assumes that clinical decision making is irrelevant to the measurement of caries. The linkage between epidemiologic data and clinical decisions should be seamless and help practitioners and policy makers design programs to control, treat caries, and preserve oral health. The data generated by the WHO criteria have so far only been used to show the overall burden of what is referred to by the WHO as an irreversible chronic condition at the cavitation level. Hence, health planners and providers of care are restricted to the end stage of caries rather than the earlier stages where they can prevent, arrest, or reverse the caries process.

Outside of operative dentistry, in the research and epidemiology domains, details of the classification of the disease into various stages of severity have been widely known and used. When referring to diagnostic thresholds, the D3 caries threshold has been used for decades.[68] D3 refers to large lesions with open cavities extending into the dental pulp together with more moderate lesions with open cavities extending only into the dentin. If caries were measured at this threshold, then only these two stages of lesion severity were counted, and all other lesions were called "sound," along with truly sound tooth surfaces. If, however, the classification used also recognized clinically detectable cavities in enamel (where the enamel surface was broken but dentin was not visually involved) and clinically detectable lesions in enamel with macroscopically intact surfaces (the so-called white-spot lesions), then many more lesions were properly regarded as caries and the estimates of caries present in an individual or a population increased. This was known as the D1 threshold, which is the D3 threshold value with enamel lesions added.[65,68]

## The DMF Index

The traditional global index used to measure caries prevalence in epidemiologic studies—but not in clinical practice—is the DMF (decayed, missing, and filled) index, which is a numerical count of affected teeth per individual collected at either the tooth (DMFT) or tooth surface level (DMFS).[49] The count of DMFT for an individual or group records their caries experience (i.e., the total of both current and past caries). The index can be used at different diagnostic thresholds, which affect both the mean DMFT and the proportion of individuals affected.

The DMF index has been used since 1938 and is expressed as the total number of permanent teeth or surfaces that are decayed (D), missing (M), or filled (F) in an individual. The DMFT scores per individual can range from 0 to 28 or 32, depending on whether the third molars are included in the scoring of teeth. When the index is applied only to tooth surfaces (five per posterior tooth and four per anterior tooth), it is called the DMFS and scores per individual can range from 0 to 128 or 148, depending on whether the third molars are included in the scoring.

When written in lowercase letters, the def index is a variation that is applied to the primary dentition. The caries experience for a child is expressed as the total number of teeth or surfaces that are decayed (d), indicated for extraction (e), or filled (f). The deft index expresses the number of affected teeth in the primary dentition, with scores ranging from 0 to 20 for children. The defs index expresses the number of affected surfaces in primary dentition (five per posterior tooth and four per anterior tooth), with a score range of 0 to 88 surfaces. Because of the difficulty in distinguishing between primary teeth extracted due to caries and those that have naturally exfoliated, missing teeth may be ignored according to some protocols. In this case, it is called the df index.

While DMF indices can provide useful data and perspectives on the burden of dental caries, they also have some limitations. For one, researchers have noted a significant amount of interobserver bias and variability in each component of the index. For example, in developed countries where the F (filled) component is higher than the other components, measuring caries can be influenced substantially by the wide variation in dentists' professional experience who are generally not trained or calibrated to use either consistent criteria or definitions. Similarly, the (M) missing component may be influenced by dentists' and patients' decisions that were not related to dental caries exposure for that particular

tooth. In addition, the absence of a denominator requires that DMF values are always presented in an age-related form to have much meaning. Other criticisms include that the values do not provide any indication as to the number of teeth at risk or data that are useful in estimating treatment needs; that the indices give equal weight to missing, untreated decayed, or repeatedly restored teeth; that the indices do not account for teeth lost for reasons other than decay (such as periodontal disease); and that they do not account for sealed teeth because sealants and other cosmetic restorations did not exist in the 1930s when this method was devised.

### Health and the DMF Index

Although the DMF/dmf indices are measures of dental caries experience, the component missing from the measurement is the number of sound (S) teeth or tooth surfaces that are not affected by caries. Counting the number of sound teeth or tooth surfaces may represent another important measure of oral health. For example, with the DMFT/dft index, the increasing number of surfaces restored due to recurrent decay on the same tooth are not adequately captured. This can be accounted for by counting the number of sound tooth surfaces, which could provide an important assessment of health maintenance.

### "Caries-Free"

When the DMF/dmf equals zero, this does not mean that a patient is "caries free" because this status depends on the definition of caries used (noncavitated vs. cavitated) and the use of radiographs or other diagnostic aids. Hence, all statistics on the prevalence of caries-free individuals are biased by the type of study protocols implemented to assess for and define dental caries during the examinations. To provide greater transparency, we recommend defining the caries stages and diagnostic tools used whenever caries-free statistics are presented or compared with over time rather than simply using the designation of DMFT/dmft equals to zero.

## Emergence of New Models (21st Century)

More recent diagnostic systems of dental caries have placed substantial emphasis on early noncavitated carious lesions as studies have shown that early lesions are more prevalent than cavitated lesions in economically developed countries,[1,42] are more likely to be restored compared with sound tooth surfaces,[39,42] may serve as indicators of caries activity,[31,37] and may provide a better understanding of the mechanism of action of fluoride, sealants, and other preventive agents.[42]

Among more recent detection systems for caries, there are three systems that have gone through histologic and clinical validation (Table 14.2). First, the *Nyvad criteria* define caries as a progression that ranges from surface demineralization to deep cavitation.[61] The criteria differentiate between active and nonactive lesions as well as noncavitated and cavitated lesions.[61] The criteria have been validated in a clinical trial that found that the criteria clearly demonstrated difference in caries progression or arrestment based on the stage of the caries process at baseline.[61] The differentiation among the stages of caries progression is conducted using visual and tactile examination. Radiographs are not considered in the classification, but additional data from radiographs can be added.

A second system developed and adopted by practitioners around the world is the International Caries Detection and Assessment System (ICDAS). ICDAS was developed to integrate information from several caries criteria systems that were published over

**• TABLE 14.2 Selected Criteria for Detection of Dental Caries (21st Century)**

| Diagnostic System | Year/Country | Tooth Surface | Description |
|---|---|---|---|
| Nyvad et al. | 1998, Denmark | Crown | (I) Active caries (intact surface): Surface of enamel is whitish/yellowish opaque with loss of luster; feels rough when the tip of the probe is moved gently across the surface; generally covered with plaque. No clinically detectable loss of substance. Smooth surface: Caries lesion is typically located close to gingival margin. Fissure/pit: intact fissure morphology; lesion extending along the walls of the fissure (II) Active caries (surface discontinuity): Same criteria as score 1. Localized surface defect (microcavity) in enamel only. No undermined enamel or softened floor detectable with the explorer. (III) Active caries (cavity): Enamel/dentin cavity easily visible with the naked eye; surface of cavity feels soft or leathery on gentle probing. There may or may not be pulpal involvement. (IV) Inactive caries (intact surface): Surface of enamel is whitish, brownish, or black. Enamel may be shiny and feels hard and smooth when the tip of the probe is moved gently across the surface. No clinically detectable loss of substance. Smooth surface: Caries lesion is typically located some distance from gingival margin. Fissure/pit: Intact fissure morphology; lesion extending along the walls of the fissure. (V) Inactive caries (surface discontinuity): Same criteria as score 4. Localized surface defect (microcavity) in enamel only. No undermined enamel or softened floor detectable with explorer. (VI) Inactive caries (cavity): Enamel/dentin cavity easily visible with the naked eye; surface of cavity may be shiny and feels hard when probed with gentle pressure. No pulpal involvement. |
| ICDAS | 2007, World | Pits and fissures | Sound tooth surface-0: • There should be no change in enamel translucency after 5 seconds air drying. • First visual change in enamel-1: • When seen wet there is no evidence of any change in color but after 5 seconds air drying a carious opacity or discoloration is visible that is not consistent with the clinical appearance of sound enamel and is limited to the confines of the pit and fissure area. • Distinct visual change in enamel-2: • When wet there is a carious opacity and/or brown carious discoloration that is wider than fissure (the lesion is still visible when dry) • Localized enamel breakdown due to caries with no visible dentin or underlying shadow-3: • When wet there is a carious opacity and/or brown carious discoloration that is wider than fissure. • Once dried for approximately 5 seconds there is carious loss of tooth structure at the entrance to or within the pit or fissure/fossa, but dentin is not visible in the walls or base of the discontinuity. • Underlying dark shadow from dentin with or without enamel breakdown-4: • This lesion appears as a shadow of discolored dentin visible through an apparently intact enamel surface that may or may not show signs of localized breakdown. • The darkened area may appear as gray, blue, or brown and is seen more easily when the tooth is wet • Distinct cavity with visible dentin-5: • Cavitation in opaque or discolored enamel exposing the dentin beneath. • Extensive distinct cavity with visible dentin-6: • The cavity is deep and wide and dentin is clearly visible |
| | | Smooth Surface | Sound tooth surface-0: • There should be no change in enamel translucency after 5 seconds air drying. • First visual change in enamel-1: • When seen wet there is no evidence of any change in color but after air drying a carious opacity is visible that is not consistent with the clinical appearance of sound enamel and is seen from the buccal or lingual surface. • Distinct visual change in enamel-2: • When wet there is a carious opacity and/or brown carious discoloration and the lesion is still visible when dry. Lesion may be seen when viewed from the buccal or lingual direction. • When viewed from the occlusal direction, this opacity may be seen as a shadow confined to enamel, seen through the marginal ridge. • Initial enamel breakdown due to caries with no visible dentin-3 • Once dried for approximately 5 seconds there is distinct loss of enamel integrity viewed from the buccal or lingual direction. • Underlying dark shadow from dentin with or without enamel breakdown-4 • This lesion appears as a shadow of discolored dentin visible through an apparently intact marginal ridge, buccal, or lingual walls of enamel. • This shadow may appear as gray, blue, or brown and is often seen more easily when tooth is wet. • Distinct cavity with visible dentin-5: • Cavitation in opaque or discolored enamel with exposed dentin. • Extensive distinct cavity with visible dentin-6: • Obvious loss of tooth structure, extensive cavity may be deep or wide and dentin is clearly visible on both walls and at the base. The marginal ridge may or may not be present. |
| | | CARS | Sound tooth surface with restoration or sealant-0: • A sound tooth surface adjacent to a restoration/sealant margin. There should be no evidence of caries • First visual change in enamel-1: • When wet there is no evidence of any change in color but after air drying a carious opacity or discoloration is visible that is not consistent with the clinical appearance of sound enamel. • Distinct visual change in enamel/dentin adjacent to a restoration/sealant margin-2: • If the restoration margin is placed on enamel, tooth must be viewed wet. When wet there is an opacity consistent with demineralization that is not consistent with the clinical appearance of sound enamel. The lesion is still visible when dry. • If the restoration margin is placed on dentin, discoloration can be seen that is not consistent with the clinical appearance of sound dentin. • Caries defect of 0.5 mm in width. • Distinct cavity adjacent to restoration/sealant-6: • With visible dentin in interfacial space with signs of caries as described in code 4, in addition to a gap >0.5 mm. |

the last several decades.[41] The premise of ICDAS is that caries is a process that should be measured at different stages of progression from the early changes in enamel translucency, which can be detected by visually examining clean and dried tooth surfaces, to extensive cavitation causing the destruction of more than half of a tooth surface. The stages of ICDAS are meticulous and have been validated through extensive in vitro and in vivo evaluations.

ICDAS was designed as a system for caries classification, but not diagnosis, that could be applied in research, public health, education, and clinical practice. The evolution of ICDAS led to the development of the International Caries Classification and Management System (ICCMS),[64] which is the only system so far with a detailed clinical and radiographic protocol for caries detection, diagnosis, risk assessment, and plans to manage caries using risk-adjusted preventive strategies, control of noncavitated lesions, surgical or restorative care for cavitated or deep dentinal lesions, recall and review of behavioral change targets and lesions' progression, and assessment of outcomes. ICCMS can also be used in epidemiologic research and surveys and can be applied without the use of radiographs.

Unlike the Nyvad criteria and ICDAS, the Caries Assessment Spectrum and Treatment (CAST) defines caries demineralization at the histologic penetration of enamel or dentin with or without cavitation.[16] This system does not require cleaning or drying the teeth and does not include radiographs. The CAST model for caries classification was developed for epidemiologic studies with no consideration of outcomes of care and public health planning.

## New Challenges in Dental Caries Measurement

### Early Childhood Caries

The term early childhood caries (ECC) appeared from a workshop held at the Centers for Disease Control and Prevention that characterized dental caries in young children as having a progressive pattern of tooth decay.[46] This was based on the current understanding of the etiology of caries and its unique relationship with inappropriate infant feeding practices. Regarding the measurement of ECC, this term and a classification system were proposed in the late 1990s to facilitate epidemiologic research of dental caries in young children.[17]

A review conducted in 2015 that aimed to assess the impact of those early childhood caries recommendations on the prevalence and measurement of caries in preschool children found that diagnostic criteria varied greatly.[18] This review found that most studies used some element of Klein's dental caries index based on summing the dmft or dmfs. A few studies used a modified dmft version proposed by Gruebbel where the missing component was specified as extracted because of dental caries (deft). Nevertheless, the most frequently used index was dmft/deft. When the study provided prevalence of the primary outcome measure, such as ECC, it typically was based on calculating the dmft/deft using information from all 20 primary teeth, while others calculated prevalence using only primary maxillary anterior teeth, and a final group reported some estimate of prevalence using both.[18]

### Root Caries

The early detection of root caries is critical for the implementation of appropriate preventive therapeutic regimes. While much research activity has been seen in the detection and monitoring of enamel caries, this has not been seen in root caries—despite the possibilities for shorter clinical trials due to the more rapid remineralization and arrest of such lesions.[12] Surveys describing the clinical appearance of root caries began to appear in the

literature in the early 1970s, and many studies on root caries were reported over the next two decades. These clinical studies primarily used diagnostic criteria proposed by several investigators.[6,47] A systematic review conducted in 2001 concluded that there was insufficient evidence on the validity of clinical diagnostic systems for root caries.[5]

Generally root caries lesions have been described as having a distinct outline and presenting with a discolored appearance in relation to the surrounding noncarious root. Many root caries lesions are cavitated, although this is not necessarily the case with early lesions. The base of the cavitated area can be soft, leathery, or hard to probing. Probing of root caries lesions with a sharp explorer using controlled, modest pressure, however, may create surface defects that prevent complete remineralization of the lesion.[38] Therefore, for detection and classification of root caries utilizing ICDAS criteria, examiners are directed to use a Community Periodontal Index (CPI) probe.

The ICDAS Committee recommends that the following clinical criteria be used for the detection and classification of root caries: (1) color (light/dark brown, black); (2) texture (smooth, rough); (3) appearance (shiny or glossy, matte or nonglossy); (4) perception on gentle probing (soft, leathery, hard); and (5) cavitation (loss of anatomical contour). Additionally, the outline of the lesion and its location on the root surface are useful in detecting root caries lesions. Root caries appears as a distinct, clearly demarcated circular or linear discoloration at the cemento-enamel junction (CEJ) or wholly on the root surface.[38]

### Caries Around Restorations and Sealants

Dental caries around or under restorations and sealants is very common, especially when the caries risk factors are not controlled. Restoration or sealant margins, regardless of how good they are, trap bacteria. There has been debate on whether secondary caries (in Europe) or recurrent caries (United States) is primary caries that remained after the cavity was prepared when the original restoration was placed. It is hard to determine whether recurrent or secondary caries was a residual form of caries or not.[55] Thus ICDAS has adopted the term "caries around restorations and sealants."

The sealing of pits and fissures is highly recommended as a primary and a secondary preventive measure. The use of opaque sealant material is recommended to ease detection but not widely used because of aesthetics. Most often clear sealants are used. Clear sealants are difficult to detect in epidemiologic or clinical examinations. Examiners can differentiate between sealed and unsealed surfaces by running an explorer or a probe to feel the tooth surface (glassy when sealed) and an optical finding of the probe or explorer not touching the base of the pit or fissure. Moreover, the presence of a cavity outline may indicate that the material is actually a restoration rather than a sealant. Sealants are usually grouped with sound tooth surfaces unless there is recurrent caries at the margin; then they should be grouped with untreated decay or restorations with recurrent caries.

### Special Populations: Institutionalized Elderly and People With Developmental Disabilities

Most of what we know about dental caries is based on data collected from coronal tooth surfaces. As the number of old and very old individuals increases rapidly over the next decades, the problem of root caries will become more evident. There is a dearth of data on the epidemiology of this form of caries, and there have been no clear or agreed-upon criteria for measurement. While the caries process is the same on root caries as it was described for coronal caries, the lack of protective enamel and the quick removal of less remineralized cementum when the roots are exposed present significant challenges in measurement. The stages of root caries include noncavitated and cavitated, which can be active or inactive. Active noncavitated root caries looks like a normal root surface but the dentin is usually leathery or soft. Hence, the use of ball-ended explorers is recommended.

Another challenge is the measurement of caries in homebound elderly and individuals with disabilities. Measurement of caries in these populations is difficult, and data are not available. The use of disposable mouth mirrors, headlamps, and gauze or cotton is recommended. These population groups may benefit highly from preventive programs that stop or control the disease process. Thus careful assessment of early signs of dental caries is necessary.

## Risk Factors and Indicators for Dental Caries

A few high-quality, prospective studies or systematic reviews have looked at risk assessment.[29] The scientific evidence relating standardized caries risk assessment (CRA) models is still limited.[10,73] CRA is not widely used in clinical practice or public health settings. Generally, caries risk assessment is more effective in the selection of patients at low risk than those with high caries risk.[73] Furthermore, the prediction models have not been validated in independent populations, weakening the external validity of their results as model sensitivity may vary considerably. Regardless of the lack of evidence, past caries experience is far from ideal but the most important single risk component for more caries at all ages, so any clinical sign of likely active demineralization on any surface should be taken as a signal for the implementation of tailored preventive and management measures.[73]

There are numerous risk factors/indicators for dental caries, and those that are most frequently reported in the literature are presented here.

*Past caries experience.* It is an indicator of the complex interaction among ecologic, behavioral, and genetic factors that result in the development and progression of caries. It summarizes the cumulative effect of all risk factors and protective factors to which an individual has been exposed over a lifetime. Children with previous caries experience are at increased risk of future caries (evidence grade equals 2++).[70] This factor has also been identified as a strong predictor when used by nondental personnel such as primary care pediatricians when examining toddlers.[63] However, past caries experience is the effect and not the cause of disease, so its predictive ability is questionable.[73] It represents all factors measured or not measured, known or unknown, that cause tooth demineralization. Past caries experience is also influenced by access to care and the variation in restorative decision making among dentists.

*Microbiological risk factors.* The oral microbiota grows on surfaces as functionally organized communities of interrelating species, termed dental plaque. Dental plaque is an example of a biofilm,[66] which now is referred to as microbiome because endogenous or natural flora exists in the human body that is necessary for health and disease. The presence of *Streptococcus mutans* or lactobacilli in saliva or plaque as a sole predictor for caries in the primary dentition has shown low accuracy because caries is caused by a community of bacteria that is part of the normal microbiome of the oral cavity.[59] However, caries in young children historically has been associated with high oral levels of *Streptococcus mutans* (evidence grade equals 2++).[70] As more epidemiologic studies have been performed, caries is observed in the apparent absence of these bacteria, whereas these organisms could persist on other surfaces that remained sound. More recently, studies using molecular approaches have found associations between caries and other groups of acid-producing and acid-tolerating bacteria such as *Actinomyces* spp. and *Propionibacterium* spp., among others.[66]

*Saliva.* Saliva plays an important role in the health of soft and hard tissues in the oral cavity. Salivary pH and buffering capacity can contribute to the ion exchanges during remineralization and demineralization of enamel, with supersaturation of calcium and phosphate, and in the presence of fluoride.[27] Hence there is biological plausibility for changes in salivary characteristics to contribute to the development of dental caries. Despite this, salivary markers have generally proved unhelpful in the formal assessment of caries risk in children (evidence grade equals 4).[70] Another piece of evidence for the potential biological plausibility of saliva on dental caries is studies conducted in people who have chronic salivary disturbances, which typically have higher rates of dental caries.[72] Nevertheless, the effect of saliva on dental caries in people without pathologic conditions is less well understood. Evidence from epidemiologic studies is scarce and of low quality. A recent study conducted by the Northwest PRECEDENT (Practice-based REsearch Collaborative in Evidence-based DENTistry) that collected data pertaining to the 2-year cumulative incidence of dental caries and salivary characteristics in a random sample of 1763 patients visiting 63 general dental practices reported that salivary characteristics were associated weakly with previous dental caries experience. No consistent trends among different age groups were identified.[14]

*Dietary risk factors.* Both the amount of sugars and the frequency with which they are consumed are risk factors for the development of dental caries as shown in early animal studies.[32,51] Some human epidemiologic studies show that frequency of intake of sugars is an important causative factor for caries development,[33,35] but only studies that measure both variables simultaneously can conclude on the relative importance of amount and frequency. Few studies have measured the daily amount and frequency of free sugars from all sources and related this to dental caries. Some studies have found amount only or both to be important.[9]

WHO has issued guidelines that recommend intake of free sugars should provide 10% or less of energy intake and suggest further reductions to less than 5% of energy to protect dental health throughout life. WHO concluded that both amount and frequency of sugars consumed are important.[76] As intake of free sugars has been associated with obesity risk and an increased risk of cardiovascular disease mortality,[56,57] it is imperative that the dental community be mindful of the importance of educating patients on limiting frequency and amount of intake of free sugars.

*Sociodemographic risk factors.* Sociodemographic conditions have been included in several multivariate models tested to assess caries risk in preschool children, with immigrant status and parents' education/beliefs being significant in several studies. As reviewed recently by Scottish Intercollegiate Guidelines Network (SIGN), children from families with low socioeconomic status or who live in high-deprivation areas have significantly higher caries severity and prevalence than those from high socioeconomic areas (evidence grade equals 2++).[70] Among US adults, people of lower socioeconomic position have a higher burden of oral diseases compared with those who are socioeconomically better off, and these disparities also apply to issues of access to oral health services. A study among US adults reported that people living in poverty and those with the least education had fewer dentist visits compared with more affluent and educated individuals.[44] Disparities by age and race and Hispanic origin for dental caries have also been observed with data from the National Health and Nutrition Examination Survey (NHANES).[21] In 2011 and

2012, for adults ages 20 to 64, dental caries was lower for Hispanic, non-Hispanic black, and non-Hispanic Asian adults compared with non-Hispanic white adults, whereas untreated tooth decay was more prevalent among Hispanic and non-Hispanic black adults compared with non-Hispanic white and Asian adults. Also caries experience was more prevalent among adults ages 35 to 64 than among younger adults. In contrast, a little more than one-quarter of adults ages 20 to 64 (27%) had untreated tooth decay, and the prevalence of untreated caries did not vary as adults aged.[21] Hence, socioeconomic position, race/ethnicity, and age seem to be risk indicators that remain across the life span.

## Distribution of Dental Caries

### Prevalence of Dental Caries in the 20th Century Throughout the Life Cycle

#### Global

Worldwide data on caries prevalence are limited both in quantity and reliability. WHO has collected data for the indicator group of 12-year-olds in the WHO's Oral Health Country/Area Profile Program (CAPP) database.[73] Comparison among countries, however, is difficult because of differences in methodology and data collection periods. Caries severity is often reported in the form of the DMFT or DMFS value of the population. As caries can be scored at various diagnostic thresholds or levels of severity ranging from early noncavitated carious lesions to extensive cavitation, the D may be noted with a suffix indicating at which level of severity caries is reported. $D_1$ includes all severity levels, while $D_3$ only includes moderate to frank cavitation.[75]

From data collected before 1990, a significant proportion of countries in the region of the Americas reached the WHO objective of a mean DMFT less than 3, and many countries showed trends toward low prevalence in the 1990s.[7] The largest decline was seen in the high- and middle-income countries. Still, there are countries such as China, Nepal, and Thailand, among others, in which the decline was less explicit (Table 14.3). The decline was first observed in the United States and western and Nordic European countries as fluoride toothpaste became widely available in the mid-1970s.[52] In eastern Europe, the decline only started after the fall of the Iron Curtain, when the market was opened for sale of reputable brands of fluoride toothpaste. This partially explains current caries differences between eastern and western European countries. Analyses performed in each of the six WHO regions—the Americas (AMRO), Africa (AFRO), South East Asia (SEARO), Europe (EURO), Eastern Mediterranean (EMRO), and Western Pacific (WPRO)—revealed that while the Americas and South East Asia have traditionally been the areas more affected by dental caries, the Western Pacific and Africa are the regions with the lowest DMFT scores respectively[15] (Figure 14.1).

#### United States

##### Children and Adolescents

The prevalence of dental caries in the primary dentition in the United States developed with some important changes before the 1990s, particularly related to operational definitions used across NHANES periods (all primary teeth contributing to the denominator vs. only maxillary anterior teeth).[18] In general, approximately one in five preschoolers had untreated dental caries from the 1970s to the late 20th century. In the early 1990s, the distribution of dfs shifted from majority untreated (ds) to majority restored (fs) when all primary dentition was assessed,[19,20] and little

| Country | DMFT 1980s | DMFT 1990s | DMFT 2000s |
|---|---|---|---|
| **High Income** | | | |
| Australia | 3 | 0.8 | 1.1 |
| Austria | 3.8 | 1.7 | 1.4 |
| Czech Republic | 3.3 | 3.4 | 2.1 |
| Denmark | 2.2 | 1.2 | 0.4 |
| France | 4.2 | 1.9 | 1.2 |
| Greece | 2.4 | 2.7 | 1.4 |
| Iceland | 6.6 | 1.5 | 1.4 |
| Italy | 4.9 | 2.1 | 1.2 |
| Japan | 4.9 | 2.4 | 1.4 |
| Korea | 2.8 | 3.1 | 1.8 |
| Norway | 2.6 | 1.5 | 1.7 |
| Spain | 4.2 | 2.3 | 1.1 |
| Sweden | 2.2 | 0.9 | 0.8 |
| Switzerland | 2 | 0.9 | 0.9 |
| UK | 3.1 | 1.1 | 0.8 |
| USA | 2.6 | 1.3 | 1.2 |
| **Middle Income** | | | |
| Bangladesh | 1.5 | 1.4 | 1 |
| Brazil | 6.7 | 4.9 | 2.1 |
| China | 0.8 | 1 | 0.9 |
| Colombia | 4.8 | 2.3 | 1.7 |
| Cuba | 6 | 2.9 | 1.5 |
| Indonesia | 2.3 | 2.7 | 3.2 |
| Malaysia | 2.4 | 1.6 | 1.1 |
| Mexico | 4.4 | 2.5 | 1.1 |
| Russia | 3.2 | 2.9 | 2.5 |
| Thailand | 1.5 | 1.6 | 1.3 |
| Ukraine | 3.7 | 4.4 | 2.8 |
| **Low Income** | | | |
| Jordan | 3.2 | 3.3 | 1.1 |
| Nepal | 2.1 | 0.8 | 2.3 |

**TABLE 14.3** Mean DMFT Scores in 12-Year Olds, in Selected High-, Medium-, and Low-Income[a] Countries Since the 1980s

[a]As defined by the World Bank in World Bank Group, Data and statistics, Country groups. Available from: https://datahelpdesk.worldbank.org/knowledgebase/articles/906519-world-bank-country-and-lending-groups.
*DMFT,* Decayed, missing, and filled teeth.

differences were observed in the prevalence of caries by surface group (smooth, interproximal, and occlusal).[18]

Likewise, the prevalence of dental caries in permanent teeth in children and adolescents remained relatively unchanged since the 1980s.[18] Approximately one in two children ages 6 to 11 had

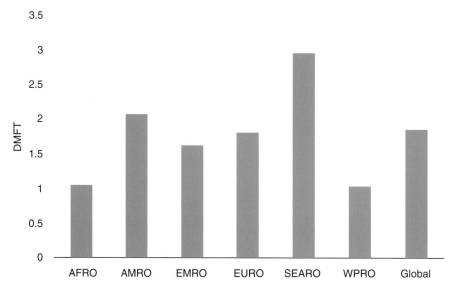

• **Figure 14.1** WHO region-specific* weighted mean DMFT among 12-year-olds. *AFRO = African region; AMRO = American region; EMRO = Eastern Mediterranean region; EURO = European region; SEARO = South-East Asia region; WPRO = Western Pacific region.

dental caries experience in permanent teeth in the early 1970s, decreasing to one in four since the late 1980s.[48] A similar decline was observed between the 1970s and 1980s regarding untreated dental caries, where one in four children used to have untreated disease, compared later to one in 10.[20,48] When it came to adolescents, 90% of them had experienced dental caries, and 50% had untreated disease. After the mid-1980s, three in five adolescents had caries experience, and one in five had untreated disease.[20]

### Adults (20–64 Years Old)

Overall, adult oral health did improve between the late 1980s and 1990s. Although untreated dental caries remained unchanged for most adults ages 35 to 44 years, untreated caries significantly decreased for non-Hispanic black people, but increased for near-poor and nonpoor Mexican American adults.[22]

The prevalence of adult coronal caries slightly declined from approximately 95% in 1988 to 1994, to 92% from 1999 to 2004. Untreated caries remained unchanged for most adults ages 35 to 44 years. There was a statistically significant decline (2.21 percentage points overall) in mean DMFT scores for all adults between the two NHANES periods.[20] Compared with coronal caries in adults, the prevalence of root caries in this group was relatively low at 14% in 1999 to 2004, which represented a decrease from 19% in 1988 to 1994.[20]

### Adults 65 Years or Older

Untreated coronal caries significantly declined, from approximately 28% to 18% between 1988 and 1994 and 1999 and 2004 for this age group. During the same period, there was a statistically significant decline in DMFT scores for all dentate seniors (19.11 vs. 17.96), and the contribution of the number of decayed coronal surfaces to the overall DFS declined (13% vs. 8%). Moreover, root caries experience improved among dentate seniors (46% vs. 36%) with the largest decrease observed for seniors living below 100% the federal poverty level (FPL) (16%).[20]

## Prevalence of Dental Caries in the 21st Century Throughout the Life Cycle

### Global

Dental caries has historically been considered the most important global oral health burden.[63] As revealed by the Global Burden of Diseases, Injuries, and Risk Factors Study (GBD),[54] untreated caries in permanent teeth was the most prevalent of all 291 conditions evaluated for the entire GBD 2010 study (global prevalence of 35% for all ages combined), and untreated caries in primary teeth was the 10th most prevalent condition, affecting 9% of the global population.[54]

At present the distribution and severity of dental caries vary in different parts of the world and within the same region or country. Studies in industrialized countries over recent decades have shown a decline in dental caries, and the number of caries-free individuals and of restorations has increased. The incidence and effects of dental caries in children and adolescents have been thoroughly investigated, but caries experience among adults has received less attention. More studies on the total number of decayed teeth per person in a population and the proportion of adults with untreated caries are needed, along with caries etiologic studies among elderly populations.[45] Recent analyses as presented in the next sections demonstrate the significant variations across world areas.

### Americas (Latin America and the Caribbean)

Dental caries experience is still relatively high in the Americas compared with European and African countries.[62] A recent systematic review and metaanalysis of 75 studies evaluating the prevalence of caries in Latin American and Caribbean countries reported significant differences in pooled prevalence between Brazilian surveys and those performed in other Latin American and Caribbean countries.[30] In particular, it was found that the metaanalysis including only Brazilian surveys in primary teeth showed approximately 20% lower pooled prevalence than other studied countries.[30]

For the permanent dentition, analyses were based on 86,358 patients who participated in 63 different studies. The metaanalysis showed an overall caries prevalence close to 60%. Although there was no statistical difference in pooled prevalence between region subgroups for permanent teeth ($P = .42$), a significant decreasing trend in caries prevalence was observed only in Brazil. The caries prevalence in permanent teeth in Brazil decreased on average 3% per year after 2000. It is important to recognize that caries is still a problem in Brazil and in Latin America and the Caribbean. Results indicate that a significant proportion of children and adolescents have cavitated carious lesions, even considering improvement in socioeconomic conditions, availability of preventive measurements, access to fluorides, or new initiatives in oral health education.[30]

### Australia and New Zealand

The prevalence of dental caries in 5- to 11-year-old Australian children in 2003 and 2004 ranged from 43.9% to 66.2%. A study examining 30-year trends for caries experience in the primary dentition of 6-year-old children and the permanent dentition of 12-year-old children enrolled in the school dental service (SDS) found that the reduction of caries experience in school children from 1977 up to now in Australia represents a significant achievement in oral health.[4] Public health programs such as water fluoridation in some jurisdictions, extended fluoridated toothpaste use, and the existence of the SDSs are key factors contributing to that success. However, since 1997 there has been a clear increasing trend for caries in the primary dentition of Australian children attending SDSs.[4] More importantly, rural Aboriginal children are generally at a disadvantage compared with their urban counterparts. Aboriginal children have an approximately twofold higher caries experience score. The 2000 to 2003 national estimates for caries experience showed that Aboriginal 6-year-olds had a dmft score that was 2.38 times higher than non-Aboriginal children (3.68 vs. 1.54). For 12-year-olds, the magnitude of disparity was not as marked, though the direction was similar.[13]

Regarding the indicators of dental caries experience of the Australian adult population for the period 2004 to 2006, untreated tooth decay was experienced by one in four Australians. The percentage of people with untreated disease did not differ notably between generations. However, the average number of decayed tooth surfaces was lower among the older generations.[3] Females had less evidence of untreated disease, on average, than males. As seen with children, indigenous Australians were more likely to have untreated decay.

### United Kingdom

The first national survey of children's dental health in England and Wales was carried out in 1973, and subsequent surveys in 1983, 1993, and 2003 involved all four United Kingdom health departments. A total of 69,318 children, ages 5 to 15 years, were involved from 1973 to 2013. Caries prevalence has been reduced from 72% to 41% in 5-year-olds and from 97% to 46% in 15-year-olds in 40 years.[58] The addition of enamel caries added an extra dimension in 2013 and allowed an indication of the extent of caries activity that extended beyond children with lesions into dentin. In both 5- and 15-year-olds the addition of early lesions meant that there was an increase in the proportion of children with signs of caries activity; a 16 percentage point increase in 5-year-olds and a 27 percentage point increase were seen in 15-year-olds. The 2013 survey reported that 42% of 15-year-olds had obvious decay experience.

The downward trend in dentin caries in permanent teeth was most obvious between 1973 and 1983; however, the rate of decline has continued but slowed between 2003 and 2013.[58]

### Sweden

Studies conducted in Sweden and other industrialized countries over recent decades have shown a decline in dental caries' severity as measured by the DMFT index, and the number of individuals without caries or restorations has increased.[23,60] A recent study that investigated the prevalence of dental caries in an adult population (20–85 years) using four different cross-sectional studies over a 30-year period in the county of Dalarna, Sweden, demonstrated that the proportion of individuals with at least one decayed surface (DS) was 58% in 1983 and significantly lower, 34% in 2008 ($P < .05$) and 33% in 2013. The mean number of DS was 2.0 in 1983 and 1.1 in 2013 in the age group 35 to 75 ($P < .05$).[24] However, in the age group 78 to 85, the mean number of DS was 1.2 in 2008 and 2.4 in 2013, indicating a possible beginning of an increase. This finding was also corroborated by another large study evaluating age, period, and cohort trends of permanent teeth in four developed countries including Sweden. This study found that despite marked recent declines in caries among children, caries levels increase with age and remain problematic in adults.[8]

### United States

National estimates demonstrate profound improvements in most dental caries indicators over the 21st century. Caries severity in permanent dentition has decreased to historically low levels, and progress is being made in addressing long-standing inequalities in untreated disease. This downward trend in caries prevalence and severity is carrying over into adulthood as cohorts born since the beginning of the "fluoride era" continue to be exposed to effective caries prevention strategies as they age. Dental caries is now characterized as a slowly progressive chronic disease affecting people throughout life rather than a rapidly progressing disease of childhood.[69]

#### Children and Adolescents

Except for a small increase in caries prevalence (or severity or both) in the primary dentition of young children in the late 1990s, the prevalence of pediatric caries in the United States has remained consistent for the past three decades.[19] Among children ages 2 to 5 years, caries experience was lower comparing the two periods (1999 thorough 2004 and 2011 thorough 2014; 28% vs. 24%, respectively), although this difference was not significant.[19] The same pattern was observed for untreated caries for preschool-age children (20% vs. 11%) (Figure 14.2). Among children ages 6 to 8 years, approximately one-half had experienced dental caries in their primary teeth, and there was no change in this result between the same two periods. Among children ages 2 to 8 years, untreated dental caries in the primary dentition significantly decreased ($P < .05$) from approximately 24% to 14% between the two periods, and it was significantly lower regardless of sex or poverty status. Severe untreated caries in primary teeth (having three or more dental surfaces with caries) also significantly decreased ($P < .05$) from 10% to 6%.

Untreated caries was substantially lower among children ages 2 to 5 years from families with high income compared with families with income less than 100% of Federal Poverty Guidelines (FPG) (31% vs. 18%) (Figure 14.3). Overall, severe untreated caries in

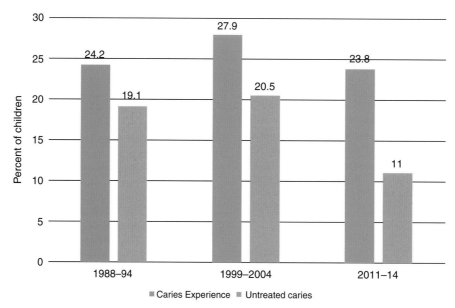

• **Figure 14.2** Prevalence of dental caries in primary dentition among preschool-age children: United States, 1988–2014.

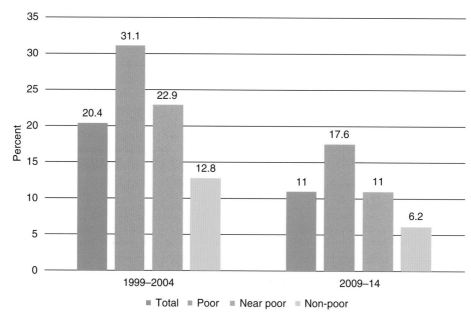

• **Figure 14.3** Prevalence of untreated caries in primary dentition (dt > 0) among children ages 2 to 5 years by poverty status: United States, 1999–2014.

primary teeth significantly decreased ($P < .05$) for children regardless of gender, race, or ethnicity. Among preschool children ages 2 to 5 years, the prevalence of severe untreated caries decreased by approximately one-half, and in families with incomes less than 100% of FPG, the decrease was greater than 50%, declining from 16% to 7%.[19] In other words, the disparity in the prevalence of caries between children in families with lower incomes and children in families with higher incomes was reduced, resulting in an extensive decline in caries experience in young children in families classified as "poor."

Overall, there were no substantial changes in dental caries for adolescents ages 12 to 19 years for the same two periods. Approximately 58% of all adolescents had dental caries from 2011 through 2014 (Figure 14.4), with adolescents in families with incomes less than 100% of FPG having a higher prevalence (66%) than adolescents in families with incomes greater than or equal to 200% of FPG (50%).[19] (Figure 14.5, Tables 14.4 and 14.5).[19]

In conclusion, for primary tooth surfaces in preschool-age children, there were significant reductions in untreated caries and significant increases in restored tooth surfaces, an important

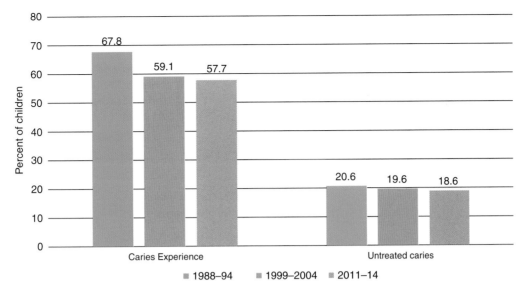

• **Figure 14.4** Prevalence of dental caries in permanent dentition among adolescents ages 12 to 19 years: United States, 1988–2014.

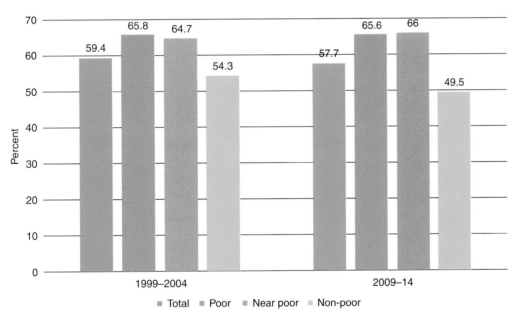

• **Figure 14.5** Prevalence of dental caries in permanent dentition among adolescents ages 12 to 19 by poverty status: United States, 1999–2014.

change in the proportional distribution of the number of tooth surfaces with caries—from most of them being untreated to most of them being restored. Poverty status did not affect this change, which suggests that activities to improve access to care have been effective for many preschool-age children in the United States.[21]

### Adults (20–64 Years Old)

Approximately 91% of US adults ages 20 to 64 had dental caries in permanent teeth in 2011 and 2012. Dental caries among adults ages 35 to 64 was higher (94%–97%) compared with adults ages 20 to 34 (82%). The prevalence of caries among adults ages 20 to 64 was lower for Hispanic (85%), non-Hispanic black (86%), and non-Hispanic Asian (85%) adults compared with non-Hispanic white adults (94%). During 2011 and 2012, about 27% of adults ages 20 to 64 had untreated tooth decay in permanent teeth. Little difference was seen in the prevalence of untreated dental caries between the age groups examined. The prevalence of untreated dental caries was nearly twice as high for non-Hispanic black adults (42%) compared with non-Hispanic white (22%) and Asian (17%) adults (Table 14.6 and 14.7).[21]

• TABLE 14.4    **Mean DMFT and DT Scores by Race, Ethnicity, and Poverty Status Among 6- to 11-Year-Old Children and 12- to 19-Year-Old Adolescents in Three National Surveys in the United States, 1988–94, 1999–2004, and 2011–14**

| Variable | 1988–94 DMFT | DT | 1999–2004 DMFT | DT | 2011–14 DMFT | DT |
|---|---|---|---|---|---|---|
| **Ages 6–11 Years** | | | | | | |
| **Race and Ethnicity** | | | | | | |
| White, non-Hispanic | 0.53 | 0.12 | 0.38 | 0.08 | 0.4 | 0.11 |
| Black, non-Hispanic | 0.52 | 0.2 | 0.43 | 0.14 | 0.52 | 0.13 |
| Mexican American | 0.62 | 0.2 | 0.7 | 0.22 | 0.62 | 0.17 |
| **Poverty status** | | | | | | |
| <100% FPL | 0.61 | 0.23 | 0.63 | 0.18 | 0.58 | 0.16 |
| 100%–199% FPL | 0.72 | 0.2 | 0.55 | 0.21 | 0.54 | 0.14 |
| ≥200% FPL | 0.47 | 0.08 | 0.32 | 0.05 | 0.32 | 0.09 |
| **Ages 12–19 Years** | | | | | | |
| **Race and Ethnicity** | | | | | | |
| White, non-Hispanic | 3.01 | 0.37 | 2.54 | 0.42 | 2.44 | 0.45 |
| Black, non-Hispanic | 2.8 | 0.84 | 2.2 | 0.56 | 2.67 | 0.59 |
| Mexican American | 3.06 | 0.78 | 2.82 | 0.63 | 3.19 | 0.72 |
| **Poverty Status** | | | | | | |
| <100% FPL | 3.25 | 0.74 | 2.88 | 0.62 | 3.19 | 0.73 |
| 100%–199% FPL | 3.6 | 0.83 | 2.81 | 0.7 | 3.08 | 0.63 |
| ≥200% FPL | 2.89 | 0.27 | 2.28 | 0.3 | 2.02 | 0.29 |

*DMFT,* Decayed, missing, and filled teeth; *DT,* decayed teeth; *FPL,* federal poverty level.

• TABLE 14.5    **Prevalence of Dental Caries in Permanent Teeth (DMFT > 0) by Race, Ethnicity and Poverty Status Among 6- to 11-Year-Old Children and 12- to 19-Year-Old Adolescents in Three National Surveys in the United States, 1988–94, 1999–2004, and 2011–14**

| Variable | 1988–94 % | 1999–2004 % | 2011–14 % |
|---|---|---|---|
| **Ages 6–11 Years** | | | |
| **Race and Ethnicity** | | | |
| White, non-Hispanic | 23.69 | 18.59 | 15.2 |
| Black, non-Hispanic | 23.38 | 19.03 | 22.3 |
| Mexican American | 27.56 | 30.76 | 22.7 |
| **Poverty Status** | | | |
| <100% FPL | 28 | 28.28 | 23.7 |
| 100%–199% FPL | 29.89 | 24.09 | 20.4 |
| ≥200% FPL | 22.28 | 16.31 | 13.4 |
| Overall | 25.49 | 21.06 | 18.2 |
| **Ages 12–19 Years** | | | |
| **Race and Ethnicity** | | | |
| White, non-Hispanic | 68.15 | 58.08 | 55.6 |
| Black, non-Hispanic | 62.93 | 54.36 | 57.8 |
| Mexican American | 68.53 | 64.49 | 64.5 |
| **Poverty Status** | | | |
| <100% FPL | 72.29 | 65.55 | 65.6 |
| 100%–199% FPL | 69.16 | 64.4 | 66.0 |
| ≥200% FPL | 65.58 | 54 | 49.5 |
| Overall | 67.8 | 59.11 | 57.7 |

*DMFT,* Decayed, missing, and filled teeth; *FPL,* federal poverty level.

## Adults 65 Years or Older

In 2011 and 2012, nearly all US adults ages 65 and over (96%) with any permanent teeth had dental caries, and about one in five adults ages 65 and over had untreated tooth decay. The prevalence of dental caries was similar among those ages 65 to 74 and those ages 75 and over (Figure 14.6). Caries prevalence was lower among non-Hispanic black adults (91%) and Hispanic adults (86%) compared with non-Hispanic white adults (98%)[21] (Tables 14.8 and 14.9).

## Population Disparities of Dental Caries

The prevalence of untreated caries in people of all ages is strongly influenced by social determinants.[11,34,36] Due to improvements in access to care and promotion of good health, the differences in income-related untreated caries in children appear to have narrowed over the last decade.[69] For example, the percentage of 13- to 15-year-old poor children with any untreated caries in their permanent teeth declined from 27.9% in 1999 to 2004 to 18.2% in 2011 and 2012. However, another recent study analyzed data from the NHANES conducted in 1988 to 1994, 1999 to 2004, and 2011 to 2014 and generated absolute and relative measures of inequality comparing caries experience in families below the poverty level with families where income was at least three times the poverty threshold. It found that substantial income-related disparities in dental caries among US children and adolescents persisted over those NHANES periods.[71] Countries such as Australia have been able to demonstrate fewer socioeconomic inequalities in children's dental caries particularly among those exposed to community water fluoridation when compared to nonfluoridated areas.[72]

The income disparity in untreated caries prevalence among working-age adults remained about the same between 1999 and 2004 and 2011 and 2014 but worsened among those 65 years of age or older, reaching an absolute disparity of 32.3 percentage

**TABLE 14.6** Mean DMFT and DT Scores by Race, Ethnicity, and Poverty Status Among Adults Ages 20 to 64 Years in Three National Surveys in the United States, 1988–94, 1999–2004, and 2011–12

| Variable | 1988–94 DMFT | 1988–94 DT | 1999–2004 DMFT | 1999–2004 DT | 2011–12 DMFT | 2011–12 DT |
|---|---|---|---|---|---|---|
| **Race and Ethnicity** | | | | | | |
| White, non-Hispanic | 13.04 | 0.66 | 10.67 | 0.68 | 9.93 | 1.05 |
| Black, non-Hispanic | 11.61 | 1.46 | 9.78 | 1.12 | 9.19 | 1.75 |
| Mexican American | 9.03 | 1.14 | 8.07 | 0.99 | 8.12 | 1.49 |
| **Poverty Status** | | | | | | |
| <100% FPL | 11.67 | 1.76 | 10.22 | 1.51 | 9.28 | 2.21 |
| 100%–199% FPL | 12.3 | 1.32 | 10.55 | 1.24 | 9.71 | 1.78 |
| ≥200% FPL | 12.75 | 0.47 | 10.3 | 0.48 | 9.45 | 0.65 |

*DMFT, Decayed, missing, and filled teeth; DT, decayed teeth; FPL, federal poverty level.*

**TABLE 14.7** Prevalence of Dental Caries (DMFT) Scores by Race, Ethnicity, and Poverty Status Among Adults Ages 20 to 64 Years in Three National Surveys in the United States, 1988–94, 1999–2004, and 2011–12.

| Variable | 1988–94 % | 1999–2004 % | 2011–12 % |
|---|---|---|---|
| **Race and Ethnicity** | | | |
| White, non-Hispanic | 96.42 | 93.49 | 93.8 |
| Black, non-Hispanic | 89.75 | 87.51 | 85.6 |
| Mexican American | 87 | 82.97 | 85.4 |
| **Poverty Status** | | | |
| <100% FPL | 88.05 | 88.69 | - |
| 100%–199% FPL | 92.57 | 88.91 | - |
| ≥200% FPL | 96.28 | 93.05 | - |
| Overall | 94.6 | 91.63 | - |

*DMFT, Decayed, missing, and filled teeth; FPL, federal poverty level.*

points between the lowest and highest income categories.[69] In 2011 to 2014, the prevalence of untreated caries was 42.2% among adults 65 years of age and older in the 100% or under FPL income category and 9.9% in the 400% or over FPL category (Tables 14.8 and 14.9).

# Dental Caries and Public Health

## Perspectives on Measurement and Health Outcomes

Dental caries epidemiology is important and should ideally provide all stakeholders (governments, health professions and their associations, the public and patients) with timely, accurate, and understandable indications for key age groups across the life course of the following: amount of disease present (prevalence), rate of progress of disease (incidence), and disease trends over time to help planning. In addition, information on variations in disease levels between and within countries and trends in inequalities and health gradients are now actively sought by many.[67] The field of public health should focus on disease measurement that leads to implementing primary and secondary preventive programs at all levels of intervention in communities. Hence, measurement of dental caries should be designed based on the type of intervention and goals of programs. Whenever feasible it is advisable that both noncavitated and cavitated stages of caries are measured.

## Pathways for Caries Management and Measurement of Caries in Clinical and Public Health Practice

The primary goal of a contemporary caries management system, in the wellness and health promotion era of the 21st century, is to "preserve dental tissues [through prevention, control, and minimal restorative techniques] and restore [conservatively] only when indicated."[40] This focused goal requires that dentists or other dental or health providers should assess the presence of early or noncavitated stages of the caries process that can be managed through secondary (or medical) preventive therapies. Dentists should also evaluate the extent and size of the stages that are advanced beyond the caries control phase. These caries stages should be managed surgically and conservatively to preserve tooth structure. They also should assess the caries risk status of a tooth, and of the patient, so that preventive therapies can be risk based and account for future caries development.

The traditional restorative-only approach is not a therapy for caries that will prevent future disease development; instead the aim of restorative care is to replace lost tooth structure, restore function, and remove decayed and infected hard tissues. Any cavity preparation made to place a restoration has the potential side effect of weakening the tooth structure and increasing the probability of developing new caries at the margins of contact between the restoration and the abutting tooth. In this century, caries management should consider these four modalities of care:[40]

1. Prevention of caries development on sound tooth surfaces.
2. Control (medical care) of noncavitated caries lesions that do not extend into dentin (the cutoff point when these lesions should be restored varies among different countries and practitioners). (It is recommended that these lesions have no clinical cavitation and can extend radiographically to the outer one-third of dentin.)
3. Preservative surgical or restorative therapy to remove the decayed structure and replace it with a restorative material. This therapy may require, in some cases, pulpal therapy when the tissue is infected or necrotic.
4. Tooth extraction of nonrestorable teeth.

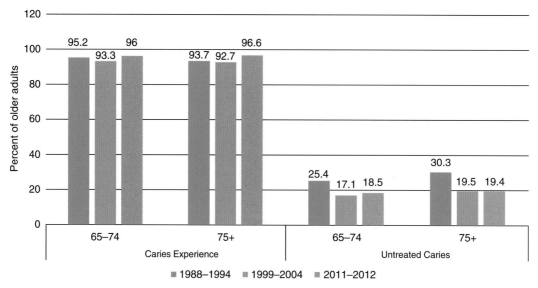

• **Figure 14.6** Prevalence of dental caries in permanent dentition among adults ages 65 and older: United States, 1988–2012.

• TABLE 14.8 **Mean DMFT and DT Scores by Race, Ethnicity, and Poverty Status Among Adults Age 65 Years and Above in Three National Surveys in the United States, 1988–94, 1999–2004, and 2011–12**

| Variable | 1988–94 DMFT | DT | 1999–2004 DMFT | DT | 2011–12 DMFT | DT |
|---|---|---|---|---|---|---|
| **Race and Ethnicity** | | | | | | |
| White, non-Hispanic | 19.47 | 0.54 | 18.23 | 0.36 | 17.3 | 0.51 |
| Black, non-Hispanic | 16.74 | 1.71 | 16.9 | 1.04 | 16.84 | 1.25 |
| Mexican American | 15.69 | 1.64 | 15.11 | 1.1 | 15.6 | 2.11 |
| **Poverty Status** | | | | | | |
| <100% FPL | 18.49 | 1.62 | 17.3 | 1.01 | 17.96 | 1.8 |
| 100–199% FPL | 18.72 | 0.97 | 18.21 | 0.58 | 17.99 | 1.24 |
| ≥200% FPL | 19.32 | 0.38 | 18.15 | 0.29 | 17.03 | 0.31 |

*DMFT,* Decayed, missing, and filled teeth; *DT,* decayed teeth; *FPL,* federal poverty level.

• TABLE 14.9 **Prevalence of Dental Caries (DMFT > 0) by Race, Ethnicity, and Poverty Status Among Adults Age 65 Years and Above in Three National Surveys in the United States, 1988–94, 1999–2004, and 2011–12**

| Variable | 1988–94 % | 1999–2004 % | 2011–12 % |
|---|---|---|---|
| **Race and Ethnicity** | | | |
| White, non-Hispanic | 95.89 | 94.86 | 97.8 |
| Black, non-Hispanic | 82.65 | 80.2 | 90.5 |
| Mexican American | 87.37 | 83.82 | 86.1 |
| **Poverty Status** | | | |
| <100% FPL | 84.1 | 83.47 | - |
| 100–199% FPL | 93.36 | 90.92 | - |
| ≥200% FPL | 96.63 | 95.53 | - |
| Overall | 94.54 | 93 | - |

*DMFT,* Decayed, missing, and filled teeth; *FPL,* federal poverty level.

# References

1. Amarante E, Raadal M, Espelid I. Impact of diagnostic criteria on the prevalence of dental caries in Norwegian children aged 5, 12 and 18 years. *Community Dent Oral Epidemiol.* 1998;26:87–94.
2. American Academy of Pediatric Dentistry. Guideline on caries risk assessment and management for infants, children, and adolescents. Reference Manual 2013–2014. *Pediatr Dent.* 2013;35:13–14. Available from: http://www.aapd.org/media/Policies_Guidelines/G_CariesRiskAssessment.pdf.
3. Australian Research Centre For Population Oral Health. Dental caries experience in the Australian adult population. *Aust Dent J.* 2007;52(3):249–251.
4. Australian Research Centre For Population Oral Health. Dental caries trends in Australian school children. *Aust Dent J.* 2011;56(2):227–230.
5. Bader JD, Shugars DA, Bonito AJ. Systematic review of selected dental caries diagnostic and management methods. *J Dent Educ.* 2001;65:960–968.
6. Banting DW. The diagnosis of root caries. *J Dent Educ.* 2001;65:991–996.
7. Beltrán-Aguilar ED, Estupiñán-Day S, Báez R. Analysis of prevalence and trends of dental caries in the Americas between the 1970s and 1990s. *Int Dent J.* 1999;49(6):322–329.
8. Bernabé E, Sheiham A. Age, period and cohort trends in caries of permanent teeth in four developed countries. *Am J Public Health.* 2014;104(7):e115–e121.

9. Burt BA, Eklund SA, Morgan KJ, et al. The effects of sugars intake and frequency of ingestion on dental caries increment in a three-year longitudinal study. *J Dent Res.* 1988;67:1422–1429.

10. Cagetti MG, Bontà G, Cocco F, et al. Are standardized caries risk assessment models effective in assessing actual caries status and future caries increment? A systematic review. *BMC Oral Health.* 2018;18:123.

11. Capurro DA, Iafolla T, Kingman A, et al. Trends in income-related inequality in untreated caries among children in the United States: findings from NHANES I, NHANES III, and HNHANES 1999–2004. *Community Dent Oral Epidemiol.* 2015;43(6):500–510.

12. MRO Carrilho. *Root Caries: From Prevalence to Therapy.* Monographs in Oral Science; vol 26. Basel, Switzerland: Karger; 2017.

13. Christian B. Blinkhorn AS. A review of dental caries in Australian aboriginal children: the health inequalities perspective. *Rural Remote Health.* 2012;12:1–11.

14. Cunha-Cruz J, Scott J, Rothen M, et al. Salivary characteristics and dental caries: Evidence from general dental practices. *J Am Dent Assoc.* 2013 May;144(5):e31–e40.

15. Da Silveira MR. In: Virdi M, ed. *Epidemiology of Dental Caries in the World, Oral Health Care—Pediatric, Research, Epidemiology and Clinical Practices.* Available from: http://www.intechopen.com/books/oral-health-care-pediatric-research-epidemiology-andclinical-practices/epidemiology-of-dental-caries-in-the-world; 2012. Accessed January 22, 2018.

16. De Souza AL, Leal SC, Chaves SB, et al. The caries assessment spectrum and treatment (CAST) instrument: construct validation. *Eur J Oral Sci.* 2014;122:149–153.

17. Drury TF, Am Horowitz, Ismail AI, et al. Diagnosing and reporting early childhood caries for research purposes: a report of a workshop sponsored by the National Institute of Dental and Craniofacial Research, the Health Resources and Services Administration, and the Health Care Financing Administration. *J Public Health Dent.* 1999;59:192–197.

18. Dye BA, Hsu K-LC, Afful J. Prevalence and Measurement of Dental Caries in Young Children. *Pediatr Dent.* 2015;37(3):200–216.

19. Dye BA, Mitnik GL, Lafolla TJ. Trends in dental caries in children and adolescents according to poverty status in the United States from 1999 through 2004 and from 2011 through 2014. *J Am Dent Assoc.* 2017;148(8):550–565e7.

20. Dye BA, Tan S, Smith V, et al. Trends in oral health status—United States, 1988–1994 and 1999–2004. *Vital Health Stat 11.* 2007;248. Available from: http://www.cdc.govchs/data/series/sr_11/sr11_248.pdf.

21. Dye BA, Thornton-Evans G, Lafolla TJ. Dental caries and tooth loss in adults in the United States, 2011-2012. *NCHS Data Brief.* 2015;197:1–7.

22. Dye BA, Thornton-Evans G. Trends in oral health by poverty status as measured by Healthy People 2010 objectives. *Public Health Rep.* 2010 Nov-Dec;125(6):817–830.

23. Edman K, Ohrn K, Holmlund A, et al. Comparison of oral status in an adult population 35–75 year of age in the county of Dalarna, Sweden in 1983 and 2008. *Swed Dent J.* 2012;36:61–70.

24. Edman K, Öhrn K, Nordström B, et al. Prevalence of dental caries and influencing factors, time trends over a 30-year period in an adult population. Epidemiological studies between 1983 and 2013 in the county of Dalarna, Sweden. *Acta Odontol Scand.* 2016;74(5):385–392.

25. Ekstrand K, Qvist V, Thylstrup A. Light microscope study of the effect of probing in occlusal surfaces. *Caries Res.* 1987;21:368–374.

26. Ekstrand KR, Ricketts DN, Kidd EA. Occlusal caries: pathology, diagnosis and logical management. *Dent Update.* 2001;28:380–387.

27. Featherstone JD. The caries balance: the basis for caries management by risk assessment. *Oral Health Prev Dent.* 2004;2(suppl 1):259–264.

28. Fisher-Owens SA, Gansky SA, Platt LJ, et al. Influences on children's oral health: a conceptual model. *Pediatrics.* 2007 Sep;120(3):e510–e520.

29. Fontana M. The clinical, environmental, and behavioral factors that foster early childhood caries: evidence for caries risk assessment. *Pediatr Dent.* 2015;37(3):217–225.

30. Gimenez T, Bispo B, Souza D, et al. Does the decline in caries prevalence of Latin American and Caribbean children continue in the new century? Evidence from systematic review with meta-analysis. *PLoS One.* 2016;11(10):1–14. e0164903.

31. Grindefjord M, Dahlöf G, Modéer T. Caries development in children from 2.5 to 3.5 years of age: a longitudinal study. *Caries Res.* 1995;29:449–454.

32. Guggenheim B, König KG, Herzog E, et al. The cariogenicity of different dietary carbohydrates tested on rats in relative gnotobiosis with a Streptococcus producing extracellular polysaccharide. *Helv Odontol Acta.* 1966;10:101–113.

33. Gustafsson BE, Quensel CE, Lanke LS, et al. The Vipeholm dental caries study; the effect of different levels of carbohydrate intake on caries activity in 436 individuals observed for five years. *Acta Odontol Scand.* 1954;11:232–264.

34. Health Policy Institute, American Dental Association. *Untreated Caries Rates Falling Among Children, Rising Among Low-Income Adults and Seniors.* Available from: https://www.ada.org/en/publications/ada-news/2016-archive/september/hpi-unmet-dental-needs-falling-for-children-rising-for-lowincome-adults-seniors?nav=news; 2016. Accessed January 24, 2018.

35. Holt RD, Joels D, Winter GB. Caries in preschool children: the Camden study. *Br Dent J.* 1982;153:107–109.

36. Hybels CF, Wu B, Landerman LR, et al. Trends in decayed teeth among middle-aged and older adults in the United States: socioeconomic disparities persist over time. *J Public Health Dent.* 2016 Sep;76(4):287–294.

37. Imfeld TN, Steiner M, Menghini GD, et al. Prediction of future caries increments for children in a school dental service, and in private practice. *J Dent Educ.* 1995;59:941–944.

38. *International Caries Detection and Assessment System Coordinating Committee Rationale and Evidence for the International Caries Detection and Assessment System (ICDAS II).* Available from: https://pdfs.semanticscholar.org/0478/3d0cfe0a96ffb865c358f780f5227b9baca9.pdf; 2011. Accessed January 22, 2018.

39. Ismail AI, Gagnon P. A longitudinal evaluation of fissure sealants applied in dental practices. *J Dent Res.* 1995;74:1583–1590.

40. Ismail AI, Pitts NB, Tellez M, et al. The International Caries Classification and Management System (ICCMS™): an example of a caries management pathway. *BMC Oral Health.* 2015;15(suppl 1):S9.

41. Ismail AI, Sohn W, Tellez M, et al. The International Caries Detection and Assessment System (ICDAS): an integrated system for measuring dental caries. *Community Dent Oral Epidemiol.* 2008;36:55–68.

42. Ismail AI. Clinical diagnosis of precavitated carious lesions. *Community Dent Oral Epidemiol.* 1997;25:13–23.

43. Ismail AI. Visual and visuo-tactile detection of dental caries. *J Dent Res.* 2004;83. Spec No C:C56-66.

44. Kailembo A, Quiñonez C, Lopez Mitnik GV, et al. Income and wealth as correlates of socioeconomic disparity in dentist visits among adults aged 20 years and over in the United States, 2011–2014. *BMC Oral Health.* 2018;18:147.

45. Kassebaum NJ, Bernabé E, Dahiya M, et al. Global burden of untreated caries: a systematic review and metaregression. *J Dent Res.* 2015 May;94(5):650–658.

46. Kaste LM, Gift HC. Inappropriate infant bottle feeding status of the Healthy People 2000 objective. *Arch Pediatr Adolesc Med.* 1995;149:786–791.

47. Katz RV. Development of an index for the prevalence of root caries. *J Dent Res.* 1984;63:814–818.

48. Kelly JE, Scanlon JV. Decayed, missing, and filled teeth among children, United States. *Vital Health Stat.* 1974;11(106):1–53.

49. Klein H, Palmer CE, Knutson JW. Studies on dental caries: I. Dental status and dental needs of elementary school children. *Public Health Rep.* 1938;53:751–765.

50. Knapp J. Hidden dental caries. *Am Dent Assoc Trans.* 1868;8:108–112.

51. König KG, Schmid P, Schmid R. An apparatus for frequency-controlled feeding of small rodents and its use in dental caries experiments. *Arch Oral Biol.* 1968;13:13–26.

52. Lagerweij M, van Loveren C. Declining caries trends: are we satisfied? *Curr Oral Health Rep.* 2015;2(4):212–217.

53. Magitot E. Therapeutic indications in dental caries. *Br J Dent Sci.* 1886;29:405–410.

54. Marcenes W, Kassebaum N, Bernabé E, et al. Global burden of oral conditions in 1990-2010. *J Dent Res.* 2013;92(7):592–597.

55. Mjör IA, Toffenetti F. Secondary caries: a literature review with case reports. *Quintessence Int.* 2000;31(3):165–179.

56. Moynihan P. Sugars and dental caries: evidence for setting a recommended threshold for intake. *Adv Nutr.* 2016 Jan;7(1):149–156.

57. Moynihan PJ, Kelly SA. Effect on caries of restricting sugars intake: systematic review to inform WHO guidelines. *J Dent Res.* 2014;93:8–18.

58. Murray J, Vernazza C, Holmes R. Forty years of national surveys: An overview of children's dental health from 1973-2013. *Br Dent J.* 2015;219(6):281–285.

59. National Institute of Health. Diagnosis and Management of Dental Caries Throughout Life. *NIH Consensus Statement.* 2001 March 26–28;18(1):1–30. Available from: https://consensus.nih.gov/2001/2001DentalCaries115PDF.pdf. Accessed January 30 2018.

60. Norderyd O, Koch G, Papias A, et al. Oral health of individuals aged 3-80 years in Jonkoping, Sweden during 40 years (1973–2013). II. Review of clinical and radiographic findings. *Swed Dent J.* 2015;39:69–86.

61. Nyvad B, Machiulskiene V, Baelum V. Construct and predictive validity of clinical caries diagnostic criteria assessing lesion activity. *J Dent Res.* 2003;82:117–122.

62. Petersen P, Bourgeois D, Ogawa H, et al. The global burden of oral diseases and risk to oral health. *Bull World Health Organ.* 2005;83(9):661–669.

63. Pierce KM, Rozier RG, Vann WF Jr. Accuracy of pediatric primary care providers' screening and referral for early childhood caries. *Pediatrics.* 2002;109(5):1–7. E82.

64. Pitts NB, Ekstrand KR. International Caries Detection and Assessment System (ICDAS) and its International Caries Classification and Management System (ICCMS)—methods for staging of the caries process and enabling dentists to manage caries. *Community Dent Oral Epidemiol.* 2013;41:e41–e52.

65. Pitts NB, Fyffe HE. The effect of varying diagnostic thresholds upon clinical caries data for a low prevalence group. *J Dent Res.* 1988;67:592–596.

66. Pitts NB, Zero DT, Marsh PD, et al. Dental caries. *Nat Rev Dis Primers.* 2017 May 25;3(17030):67.

67. Pitts NB, Zero DT. White Paper on Dental Caries Prevention and Management. A summary of the current evidence and the key issues in controlling this preventable disease. Available from: https://www.fdiworlddental.org/sites/default/files/media/documents/2016-fdi_cpp-white_paper.pdf.

68. Poulsen S, Horowitz H. An evaluation of a hierarchical method of describing the pattern of dental caries attack. *Community Dent Oral Epidemiol.* 1974;2:7–11.

69. Rozier RG, White BA, Slade GD. Trends in oral diseases in the U.S. population. *J Dent Educ.* 2017;81(8):eS97–eS109.

70. Scottish Intercollegiate Guidelines Network (SIGN). *Dental Interventions to Prevent Caries in Children. SIGN Publication No. 138. A National Clinical Guideline.* March 2014. Edinburgh, UK: SIGN; 2104. Available from: http://www.sign.ac.uk/assets/sign138.pdf.

71. Slade GD, Sanders AE. Two decades of persisting income-disparities in dental caries among U.S. children and adolescents. *J Public Health Dent.* 2017 Dec 15. https://doi.org/10.1111/jphd.12261. [Epub ahead of print].

72. Slade GD, Spencer AJ, Davies MJ, Stewart JF. Influence of exposure to fluoridated water on socioeconomic inequalities in children's caries experience. *Community Dent Oral Epidemiol.* 1996 Apr;24(2):89–100.

73. Tellez M, Gomez J, Pretty I, Ellwood R, Ismail AI. Evidence on existing caries risk assessment systems: are they predictive of future caries? *Community Dent Oral Epidemiol.* 2013;41(1):67–78.

74. World Health Organization. *WHO's Oral Health Country/Area Profile Programme (CAPP) Database.* Available from: http://www.mah.se/CAPP/Country-Oral-Health-Profiles/; 2013. Accessed January 22, 2018.

75. World Health Organization. *Oral Health Surveys: Basic Methods—5th Edition.* Available from: http://www.who.int/oral_health/publications/9789241548649/en/; 2015. Accessed January 22, 2018.

76. World Health Organization. Diet, nutrition and the prevention of chronic diseases. *World Health Organ Tech Rep Ser* 2003;916:i–viii, 1–149, backcover.

# 15

# Measurement and Distribution of Periodontal Diseases

PAUL I. EKE, PhD, MPH, PhD

WENCHE S. BORGNAKKE, DDS, MPH, PhD

JASIM M. ALBANDAR, DDS, DMD, PhD

## Description and Etiology of Periodontal Diseases

"Periodontal diseases" is a generic term for a group of related but distinctly different diseases that affect the soft and hard tissues that surround and support the teeth. The most common of these are gingivitis and periodontitis, which are inflammatory diseases of only the soft gingival tissue or of both the soft and hard tissues around the teeth, respectively. These two diseases are the focus of this chapter. The plural form "periodontal diseases" connotes situations referring collectively to involvement of either one or both diseases or other diseases and conditions affecting the periodontium.

In addition to a novel classification of periodontal health, the 2017 World Workshop on the Classification of Periodontitis and Peri-Implant Disease and Conditions reclassified various forms of gingival diseases and periodontitis using a staging and grading system.[17,20,72,86] The Workshop also proposed a new classification of non-plaque–induced gingival diseases.[46]

## Periodontal Health

The 2017 World Workshop classification suggested four levels of periodontal health: (1) pristine periodontal health, defined as total absence of clinical inflammation and physiologic immune response affecting the periodontium with no attachment or bone loss; (2) well-maintained clinical periodontal health, presenting as a structurally and clinically intact periodontium; (3) periodontal disease stability, presenting as a reduced periodontium in a stable periodontitis patient; and (4) periodontal disease remission/control with a reduced periodontium.[17]

## Gingival Diseases

In the 2017 World Workshop classification, gingival diseases/conditions are categorized into (1) dental biofilm-induced gingivitis and (2) non-dental biofilm induced gingival diseases (see Box 15.1).[17] Biofilm-induced gingivitis occurs as a gingival inflammatory response to plaque biofilm accumulation at the gingival margin, in which the junctional epithelium—although altered by the disease—still remains attached to the tooth at or about its original level. Also, gingivitis may be mediated by systemic and local risk factors, hormonal level, and medication-influenced gingival enlargements. Other non-dental biofilm-induced gingival diseases are recognized with a wide spectrum of other etiologies. Typically, gingivitis manifests clinically as visual signs of inflammation (edema, redness, gingival enlargement) of the gingiva that bleeds either spontaneously or only on probing, and where the gingival sulcus/pocket is still less than 3 mm deep and there is no clinical attachment loss (CAL).

## Periodontitis

The 2017 World Workshop classification made significant changes to the 1989[4] and 1999[5] classifications of periodontitis.

• **BOX 15.1** Periodontal Health, Gingival Diseases/Conditions[17]

1. Periodontal health and gingival health
   a. Clinical gingival health on an intact periodontium
   b. Clinical gingival health on a reduced periodontium
      i. Stable periodontitis patient
      ii. Non-periodontitis patient
2. Gingivitis—dental biofilm-induced
   a. Associated with dental biofilm alone
   b. Mediated by systemic or local risk factors
   c. Drug-influenced gingival enlargement
3. Gingival diseases—non-dental biofilm induced
   a. Genetic/developmental disorders
   b. Specific infections
   c. Inflammatory and immune conditions
   d. Reactive processes
   e. Neoplasms
   f. Endocrine, nutritional, and metabolic diseases
   g. Traumatic lesions
   h. Gingival pigmentation

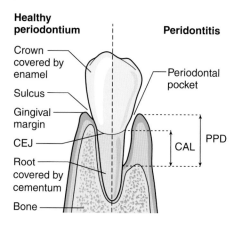

• **Figure 15.1** Terminology for measuring periodontal tissues in health *(left)* and periodontitis *(right)*. CAL: attachment loss. PDD: periodontal probing depth.

It defines three distinct forms of periodontitis: (1) periodontitis (formerly "chronic" or "aggressive" periodontitis), (2) necrotizing periodontitis, and (3) periodontitis as a manifestation of systemic diseases (Box 15.2).[17,72,86] This new classification is based on emerging scientific evidence and current knowledge of the pathophysiology of periodontitis. It recognizes that several systemic diseases and conditions, such as Papillon–Lefèvre syndrome, affect periodontal health, whereas several common systemic diseases, such as uncontrolled diabetes mellitus, have variable effects that modify the course of periodontitis.[2]

Periodontitis develops as an extension of gingivitis in especially susceptible individuals, but only a portion of gingivitis sites make this transition. Although gingivitis is reversible to a state of health, the sequela of periodontitis remain for life even after successful therapy. Loss of periodontal tissues due to periodontitis is irreversible, and the lost tissue cannot be restored to its original structure. An understanding that periodontitis can only be controlled, not healed, is important for patients and dental care providers alike. In periodontitis, the local inflammatory process leads to chronic destruction of periodontal tissues manifested as apical migration of the epithelial attachment, CAL of the periodontal ligament, loss of alveolar bone, and eventually tooth mobility and possibly loss of the tooth (Figure 15.1).

## Dental Plaque (Biofilm)

The vast majority of periodontal diseases are dental plaque biofilm induced. Biofilms are structurally and functionally organized viable microbial communities enclosed in an extracellular polymeric substance matrix and found on natural and artificial oral surfaces. The oral cavity has two types of surfaces for biofilm colonization: shedding surfaces (mucosa) and solid surfaces (teeth and various artificial materials in fixed and removable oral appliances). At gingival sites around teeth, dental biofilm can grow, develop, and accumulate into a complex supragingival and subgingival dental plaque, both of which can mineralize into dental calculus.

Dental plaque biofilms can be diverse and complex, consisting of variable combinations of the oral flora. About 700 different bacterial species have been identified in the human oral cavity as of early 2019,[83] but estimates suggest that the number may be as high as 1200.[22] Only about one-half of the microorganisms detected in the mouth are officially named, and only about three-quarters of those are indisputably oral commensals. The rest may represent transient colonization, but some may turn out to inhabit the mouth on a regular basis and consequently are found in oral biofilms.[12] Biofilm ecology may provide the organisms within biofilms with collective virulence properties that include resistance to host immune system clearance, reduced susceptibility to antimicrobial agents, and the ability to project a greater concentration of collective virulence factors produced by the microbes, such as the production of endotoxins by Gram-negative organisms in the biofilm community.

## Dental Biofilm-Induced Periodontal Diseases: Pathogenesis

Overall, there is compelling evidence that gingivitis, the reversible inflammation of the gingiva (soft tissue), is primarily a nonspecific inflammatory response to dental biofilms. At some sites and in some subjects, when the host response is inadequate or dysregulated, gingivitis could progress over time to the onset and progression of irreversible chronic destruction of soft and hard periodontal tissues, resulting in periodontitis. Depending on underlying host

• **BOX 15.2** Forms of Periodontitis[17,72,86]

1. Necrotizing Periodontal Diseases
   a. Necrotizing gingivitis
   b. Necrotizing periodontitis
   c. Necrotizing stomatitis
2. Periodontitis as Manifestation of Systemic Disease
3. Periodontitis
   a. **Stages**: based on severity and complexity of management
      i. Stage 1: initial periodontitis
      ii. Stage 2: moderate periodontitis
      iii. Severe periodontitis with potential for additional tooth loss
      iv. Severe periodontitis with potential for loss of the dentition
   b. **Extent and Distribution**: localized; generalized; molar-incisor distribution
   c. **Grades**: evidence or risk of rapid progression, anticipated treatment response
      i. Grade A: slow rate of progression
      ii. Grade B: moderate rate of progression
      iii. Grade C: rapid rate of progression

factors and other risk factors (e.g., genetic, acquired, or environmental), periodontitis may be localized to certain teeth or sites or progress to a generalized disease affecting the entire dentition and could lead to tooth loss.

Overall, the pathogenesis of dental biofilm-induced periodontal diseases is a complex interplay of dental biofilm and host inflammatory immune responses locally at the periodontal tissues that mutually and adversely affect each other in a vicious cycle. Hence, the breakdown of periodontal tissues occurs mainly as a result of the host inflammatory responses to the assault by the dental biofilm community of bacteria, which causes a microbial imbalance (dysbiosis).

Due to the shift from a symbiotic relationship to a dysbiotic state, the collective effect of pathogenic levels of biofilm communities is to initiate and exacerbate periodontitis, which results in dysbiosis. A more recent proposed model called polymicrobial synergy and dysbiosis requires only the presence of low abundance of "community activators," so-called keystone pathogens (e.g., *Porphyromonas gingivalis*), and the increased virulence of their synergy with other organisms to cause dysbiosis.[43] Keystone pathogens are able to act synergistically with other nonpathogens to elevate and project the virulence of the dental biofilm community.

Bartold and Van Dyke proposed an additional paradigm assuming that periodontal bacteria cause the deepened periodontal pockets, instead of resulting from them.[8] They suggest that the initial enlargement of the marginal gingiva due to inflammation may be sufficient to lead to changes in the gingival microenvironment for the microbiome in the plaque in the healthy sulcus. As bacteria that require less oxygen (facultative anaerobes or anaerobes) thrive in the bottom of the healthy sulcus, they multiply into a disproportionate overgrowth, which results in an imbalance in the finely balanced composition of the healthy microbiome. Eventually this process may continue in especially susceptible individuals whose immune responses will be the main determinants of the progress and the extent of this destruction of supportive tissue around the teeth. As the process advances and the pockets become more oxygen deprived, the composition of the microbiome in the pocket changes to a composition dominated by anaerobic bacteria and spirochetes. In this model, inflammation plays a role in the initiation and progression that may be more important than the actual abundance and composition of the bacteria in the plaque.

An important 2019 systematic review by Bartold and van Dyke supported the notion that there are no specific periodontal bacteria that always are present and lead to periodontitis and therefore could be labeled "periodontal pathogens."[6] In periodontitis, there is a disproportionate overgrowth of nonspecific members of the commensal microbiome that also are present in periodontal health. Thus it can be disputed that gingivitis and periodontitis actually represent infections, a notion that usually pertains to invasion of microbes external to the infected site.

Several factors, such as genetics, sex, age, and some underlying systemic conditions, moderate the inflammatory interactions between the host and dental plaque and will be described in the risk factor section of this chapter.

## Nondental Biofilm-Induced Periodontal Diseases: Etiology-Based Classification

Because some gingival diseases are not induced by dental plaque, the 2017 World Workshop updated a review by the 1999 International Workshop for a Classification of Periodontal Diseases and Conditions[47] and proposed a classification based on the etiology of the lesions that is shown in Box 15.3.[48]

## Measurement of Periodontal Diseases

### Dental Plaque and Calculus

Control of dental plaque remains a primary prevention strategy for gingivitis and periodontitis. Dental plaque biofilm accumulates on the surface of teeth and can be visible in the oral cavity (supragingival plaque) or extends apical to the gingival margin (subgingival plaque). When the plaque is not removed, it may become mineralized and is then called dental calculus, often referred to as tartar in lay language. Calculus cannot be removed by the patient and thus needs to be removed by a dental professional. The accumulation of dental plaque biofilm alone or in combination with calculus is associated with the development of gingivitis.

Plaque and calculus are still measured in terms of quantity rather than quality, so most indexes are variations of this theme. Silness and Löe developed the Plaque Index (Pl) to be used along with the Gingival Index Score (Box 15.4).[81] The same surfaces of the same teeth are scored as in the GI using a 0 to 3 ordinal scale. The World Health Organization no longer recommends that assessment of presence of calculus be included in the Community Periodontal Index (CPI).[73] As always, however, the index chosen depends on the purpose of the given survey and the way the data are to be used.

The Volpe-Manhold Index (VMI) has been used widely in the United States in trials to test agents for plaque control and calculus inhibition.[93] It is intended to score new deposits of supragingival calculus, following a prophylaxis to remove all calculus, in clinical trials. The VMI scores the height of calculus on the lingual, distal, and mesial planes of the lingual surfaces of each of the lower six anterior teeth. A probe is used to measure the linear extent of calculus in each plane in increments of 0.5 mm up to 5 mm. The tooth score is the sum of the scores in the three planes; patient total score is the sum of the tooth scores, and a person can have a maximum score of 90.

### Gingivitis

Bleeding on probing (BOP) is the primary parameter to set the threshold for gingivitis and is recorded using the gingival index score (GI) by Silness and Löe (Box 15.5).[81]

The healthy gingiva is pink (unless pigmented in dark-skinned persons), firm, and free of swelling and redness due to inflammation. It does not bleed when a periodontal probe is passed along the gingival crevice or while brushing or flossing gently. Healthy gingiva has less than 3 mm crevice with no bone loss on radiographs. In gingivitis, the gum becomes red and the margin enlarges due to inflammation and bleeds when brushed or probed, or it may even bleed spontaneously. Teeth surfaces are scored for gingivitis on a 0 to 3 scale or for BOP on a 0 to 1 ordinal scale. The World Health Organization modified the CPI in 2013 to assess gingival bleeding and periodontal probing depth (PPD) at all teeth present and CAL at six index teeth in adults only (all first molars [second molars as substitutes], the upper right central incisor, and the lower left central incisor) (Box 15.6)[73] using the special CPI periodontal probe.

### Periodontitis

Periodontitis is most often determined by clinical measures of pocket depth (PD), also called periodontal probing depth (PPD), and/or attachment loss (AL), also called clinical attachment loss (CAL), both of which are the consequence of recent or past accumulation of periodontal destruction. The main reason that

---

**• BOX 15.3** **Classification of Non-Plaque–Induced Gingival Diseases and Conditions[48]**

1 Genetic/Developmental Disorders
  1.1 Hereditary gingival fibromatosis (HGF)
2 Specific Infections
  2.1 Bacterial Origin
    Necrotizing periodontal diseases (*Treponema* spp., *Selenomonas* spp.,
      *Fusobacterium* spp., *Prevotella intermedia,* and others)
    *Neisseria gonorrhoeae* (gonorrhea)
    *Treponema pallidum* (syphilis)
    *Mycobacterium tuberculosis* (tuberculosis)
    Streptococcal gingivitis (strains of streptococcus)
  2.2 Viral Origin
    Coxsackie virus (hand–foot–and–mouth disease)
    Herpes simplex 1/2 (primary or recurrent)
    Varicella-zoster virus (chicken pox or shingles affecting V nerve)
    Molluscum contagiosum virus
    Human papilloma virus (squamous cell papilloma, condyloma)
  2.3 Fungal
    Candidosis
    Other mycoses (e.g., histoplasmosis, aspergillosis)
3 Inflammatory and Immune Conditions and Lesions
  3.1 Hypersensitivity Reactions
    Contact allergy
    Plasma cell gingivitis
    Erythema multiforme
  3.2 Autoimmune Diseases of Skin and Mucous Membranes
    Pemphigus vulgaris
    Pemphigoid
    Lichen planus
    Lupus erythematosus
  3.3 Granulomatous Inflammatory Conditions (Orofacial Granulomatosis)
    Crohn's disease
    Sarcoidosis
4 Reactive Processes
  4.1 Epulides
    Fibrous epulis

    Calcifying fibroblastic granuloma
    Pyogenic granuloma (vascular epulis)
    Peripheral giant cell granuloma (or central)
5 Neoplasms
  5.1 Premalignant
    Leukoplakia
    Erythroplakia
  5.2 Malignant
    Squamous cell carcinoma
    Leukemia
    Lymphoma
6 Endocrine, Nutritional, and Metabolic Diseases
  6.1 Vitamin Deficiencies
    Vitamin C deficiency (scurvy)
7 Traumatic Lesions
  7.1 Physical/Mechanical Insults
    Frictional keratosis
    Toothbrushing-induced gingival ulceration
    Factitious injury (self-harm)
  7.2 Chemical (Toxic) Insults
    Etching
    Chlorhexidine
    Acetylsalicylic acid
    Cocaine
    Hydrogen peroxide
    Dentifrice detergents
    Paraformaldehyde or calcium hydroxide
  7.3 Thermal Insults
    Burns of mucosa
8 Gingival Pigmentation
    Gingival pigmentation/melanoplakia
    Smoker's melanosis
    Drug-induced pigmentation (antimalarials; minocycline)
    Amalgam tattoo

---

**• BOX 15.4** **Scores and Criteria for the Silness and Löe Plaque Index (PI)[81]**

0: No plaque
1: A film of plaque adhering to the free gingival margin and adjacent area of the tooth; the plaque may be seen in situ only after application of disclosing solution or by using the probe on the tooth surface
2: Moderate accumulation of soft deposits within the gingival pocket or on the tooth and gingival margin that can be seen by the naked eye
3: Abundance of soft matter within the gingival pocket and/or on the tooth and gingival margin

---

**• BOX 15.5** **Scores and Criteria for Löe and Silness Gingival Index (GI) System[64]**

0: Absence of inflammation
1: Mild inflammation—slight change in color and little change in texture
2: Moderate inflammation—moderate glazing, redness, edema, and hypertrophy; bleeding on pressure
3: Severe inflammation—marked redness and hypertrophy, tendency to spontaneous bleeding, ulceration

---

using the PPD expression is preferable over PD is that this refers to both the healthy sulcus and the pathologic pocket. Another reason is the risk of confusing the two meanings of the acronym PD often used, namely probing depth and periodontal disease.

When the gum becomes separated from the tooth as a result of inflammation, a periodontal pocket develops. Pocket depth is measured using a periodontal probe as the distance in millimeters from the free gingival margin (FGM), also called the gumline, to the bottom of the pocket formed between the gingiva and the tooth. Gingival recession develops when the gumline recedes

• BOX 15.6  Codes and Criteria for Community Periodontal Index (CPI) modified in 2013 by
the World Health Organization[73]

**Gingival Bleeding (All Teeth Present)**

0: Absence of condition
1: Presence of condition
9: Tooth excluded
X: Tooth not present

**Periodontal Pocket (All Teeth Present)**

0: Absence of condition
1: Pocket 4–5 mm
2: Pocket $\geq$6 mm
9: Tooth excluded
X: Tooth not present

**Loss of Attachment (6 Index Teeth)**

0: 0–3 mm
1: 4–5 mm (CEJ within black band)
2: 6–8 mm (CEJ between upper limit of black band and 8.5 mm ring)
3: 9–11 mm (CEJ between 8.5 and 11.5 mm ring)
$\geq$12 mm (CEJ beyond 11.5 mm ring)
X: Excluded

*CEJ*, cemento-enamel junction.

apically, and it is measured as the distance in millimeters from the FGM to the cemento-enamel junction (CEJ). The CEJ is the border between the smooth enamel of the tooth crown and the tooth root's rough-textured cover called cementum (Figure 15.2).

Because the level of the attachment of the soft tissue to the root of the tooth initially is at the CEJ, the terms *level* and *loss* are used interchangeably. Hence, loss of attachment (LOA) is the same as

attachment loss (AL) and clinical attachment loss (CAL), which again is the same as clinical attachment level, namely clinical detachment of the gum from the tooth root and loss of other supporting tissues, such as the jawbone and the periodontal ligament that consists of connective tissue fibers that hold the tooth in place in its alveolus (socket in the jawbone). It is a measure of the difference between the gingival recession and pocket depth and is calculated by subtracting the gingival recession from the pocket depth. If the FGM has receded apically to the CEJ onto the tooth root, gingival recession (the distance from the FGM to the CEJ) will be a negative number. Attachment loss due to disease, if present, is usually greater at the four interproximal sites than at the midfacial and midlingual sites (see Figure 15.2). Oral hygiene measures are usually more easily executed on the two latter that are easily accessible, but overzealous brushing may push the gingival margin to recede apically even if no periodontal disease is present.

Measurements are obtained from a maximum of six sites per tooth. The three probing sites on the surface of the tooth closest to the face or lip are called facial or buccal sites, and the three on the surface of the tooth closest to the tongue are called the lingual sites. On each side of the tooth, measurements are taken by probing at one site closer to the front or centerline of the mouth (mesial, mesio-), another site toward the back of the mouth (distal, disto-), and a final site about halfway between the mesial and distal sites (mid-). The six probing sites are called the mesiofacial, midfacial, distofacial, mesiolingual, midlingual and distolingual sites. The mesial and distal sites are also called interproximal (interdental) sites because they are located near the space between two adjacent teeth.

The **severity** of periodontitis is determined by the greatest CAL measurement, namely the most severely diseased site, which usually occurs at an interproximal site. The **extent** of periodontitis is expressed by the proportion of probed sites (or teeth) that are affected. Some classifications call the periodontitis localized if a

**A)** Gingiva coronally to cemento-enamel junction

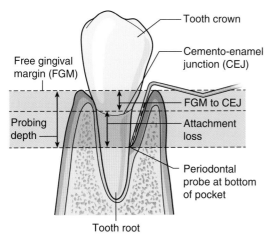

**B)** Gingiva apically to cemento-enamel junction

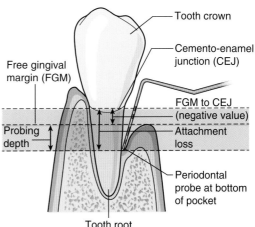

**Attachment loss = (Probing depth) - (FGM to CEJ)**

• **Figure 15.2**  Terminology for measuring periodontal probing depth (PPD) and distance from the free gingival margin (FGM) to the cemento-enamel junction (CEJ) to calculate clinical attachment loss (CAL) when the FGM is located coronally and apically the CEJ, respectively. Note the distance "FGM to CEJ" is positive in the left figure and negative in the right figure. Clinical attachment loss = periodontal probing depth minus the distance "FGM to CEJ." That is: CAL = PPD - (FGM to CEJ).

CAL of at least a specified threshold is found at less than 30% of the sites (or teeth), and generalized if present at 30% or more of the sites (or teeth). An often-used threshold for determining the presence of periodontitis is 3 mm CAL, a value often used to define a pathologic pocket in contrast to a healthy sulcus of less than 3 mm. The thresholds used for severity and extent of periodontitis vary considerably between studies and investigators.

Historically, several national probability surveys have assessed the periodontal status of the US adult population. The earliest of these surveys, namely the 1960–62 Health Examination Survey (HES) and the 1971–74 National Health and Nutrition Examination Survey (NHANES), assessed periodontal status visually, whereas subsequent surveys, such as the National Institute of Dental Research (NIDR) Survey of Employed Adults and Seniors 1985–86, NHANES III (1988–94), and NHANES 1999–2004, have used probing measurements to assess PPD and CEJ. These assessments were made using various partial mouth periodontal examinations (PMPE) protocols.[16,24] The PMPE protocols used by NHANES have evolved from collecting measurements from two randomly selected quadrants of the mouth assessing PPD and CAL at two sites per tooth (midbuccal and mesiobuccal sites) in NHANES III and NHANES 1999–2000 to assessing three sites (midbuccal, mesiobuccal, and distobuccal sites) in NHANES 2001–04.

Because periodontitis is site specific, and hence not evenly distributed in the mouth, prevalence estimates from surveys using PMPE protocols underestimate disease in the population, and this underestimation can be significant in NHANES.[30] The NHANES 2009–14 used for the first time a full-mouth periodontal examination protocol, obtaining measurements from six sites around all teeth, except third molars.[26,27,31]

## Measurements From Partial-Mouth Versus Full-Mouth Periodontal Examination

Full-mouth periodontal examinations can be time consuming and resource intensive, and measuring and recording gingival bleeding and probing measurements—possibly also including calculus scoring—can present substantial discomfort and time consumption to the patient. Thus, full-mouth periodontal examination is not commonly used in large-scale periodontal studies. Investigators have tried using various indexes on a subset of teeth to save time and thereby costs. The expectation is that the selected subset of teeth will act as a representative sample of all teeth in the mouth, yielding information that can be applied to the whole mouth while requiring much less examination time. This partial-mouth recording approach was pioneered in 1959 by Ramfjord using the so-called Ramfjord teeth subset.[75] There is agreement that partial-mouth recording is valid for assessing plaque formation and gingivitis, both of which usually are generalized conditions. However, partial-mouth recording is less accurate for the site-specific conditions of CAL and pocketing, for which measures systematic underreporting occurs with partial-mouth examination methods. Partial-mouth recording is adequate for surveys in which a degree of underestimation is an acceptable trade-off for lower costs, but it is not recommended for use in clinical trials or in any other situation that demands a high degree of precision.

A study that assessed the accuracy of periodontitis prevalence determined from a full-mouth periodontal examination *versus* a partial-mouth periodontal examination protocols used in the NHANES determined that both PMPE protocols used in

NHANES substantially underestimated the true prevalence of periodontitis by as much as 50% or more, depending on the periodontitis case definition used.[30] Overall, PMPE protocols performed below threshold levels for moderate to high levels of validity for surveillance. Prevalence varied widely by case definition. These findings suggest low validity for previous national prevalence estimates for periodontitis using NHANES PMPE protocols. Consequently, during the 6 years from 2009 to 2014, NHANES implemented a full-mouth periodontal examination (FMPE) protocol to collect PPD and CEJ probing measurements from six sites per tooth around all teeth, except third molars, as described by Eke and coauthors.[23,26-29,31,32,71]

## Case Definitions for Periodontitis

A major obstacle to comparing and pooling findings regarding the presence and prevalence of periodontitis in clinical and epidemiologic studies among different groups or populations and countries is the lack of standard case definitions for periodontitis. Many different classifications of periodontal diseases for use in the clinic and in clinical studies have been proposed and applied, and their evolution is well documented in the various world workshops held over the years. These workshops are gatherings of international experts to review the state of knowledge in the periodontal field and were held in 1966, 1977, 1989, 1996 (reported in the first issue of *Annals of Periodontology*), 1999, and 2001. The most recent workshop was held in 2017 to update clinical periodontal disease classifications and produced a new classification of periodontal diseases (see Box 15.1)[17] and forms of periodontal diseases that for the first time were based on staging and grading (see Box 15.2).[17,72,86]

Overall, the case definition, severity, and extent of periodontitis are determined by the values of clinical attachment loss and periodontal probing depth and numbers or proportions of affected sites or teeth. In general, larger values of attachment loss and pocket depth, at greater numbers of teeth with affected sites, indicate more severe periodontal disease. However, many different measurement thresholds have been used to classify periodontitis.

Examples of case definitions of "serious" periodontitis that have been used in epidemiologic studies are shown in Box 15.7.[9,63,66] Two of these definitions use CAL plus the presence of pockets, whereas the third is based on a cutoff point in a statistical distribution. There is moderate agreement in the literature that CAL of 6 mm or more is a reasonable cutoff point to differentiate severe from moderate periodontitis; the latter term is usually applied to CAL of 4 to 5 mm or less. Moderate periodontitis could mean periodontitis in which pocketing, CAL, or even some bone loss can be clinically or radiographically demonstrated, but the condition is not yet sufficiently severe to threaten the loss of teeth.

---

| • BOX **15.7** | Some Definitions of "Serious" Periodontitis Used in Periodontal Studies |
| --- | --- |

- $\geq$4 sites with CAL $\geq$5 mm, with PPD $\geq$4 mm at $\geq$1 of these sites[9]
- $\geq$2 teeth with CAL $\geq$6 mm, plus $\geq$1 site(s) with PPD $\geq$5 mm[66]
- Mean CAL in the top 20th percentile of the distribution[63]

*CAL*, clinical attachment loss; *PPD*, periodontal probing depth.

## Standard Measurements and Periodontitis Case Definitions for Surveillance

An international workgroup was convened in 2005 by the Centers for Disease Control and Prevention (CDC) and the American Academy of Periodontology (AAP) in response to the historic need for a global, standard periodontitis case definition to use for surveillance of population groups to compare the prevalence of periodontitis in different population groups worldwide or in similar population groups over time.[28]

### CDC/AAP Periodontitis Case Definitions for Surveillance

This CDC/AAP workgroup suggested case definitions of no/mild, moderate, and severe periodontitis for use in surveillance.[71] Separate categories for no and mild periodontitis were suggested in 2012.[29] The case definition for severe periodontitis was stringent to ensure that cases identified by the definition do have disease. Only measurements from interproximal sites are used in contrast to buccal and lingual sites because the disease usually begins at and is most severe at interproximal sites. In addition, CAL at midbuccal and midlingual sites could be caused by vigorous toothbrushing and thus may not represent disease. Furthermore, the effect of gingival recession on the accuracy of the probing depth measurements is minimized. Both CAL and PPD were used in this classification but could not occur on the same tooth. Although CAL is considered a more valid measure of periodontitis than PPD, and CAL is accepted as the gold standard for disease severity and progression, use of CAL alone could mistakenly include some periodontally healthy sites because attachment loss can accompany noninflammatory gingival recession.

This case definition requirements of at least one site with PPD 5 mm or greater was partly aimed to exclude cases that have been treated successfully but still have CAL or have CAL not resulting from periodontitis. It's important to note that these case definitions are intended for use in surveillance of populations, not for clinical practice. Periodontitis was classified as displayed in Box 15.8.[29]

Studies have validated these classifications and report strong correlations between periodontal inflamed surface area and case definition based on this classification.[61] These case definitions are increasingly used as the global standard and reference in population

> ### • BOX 15.8 Periodontitis Case Definitions for Population-Based Surveillance[29]*
>
> - *Severe* periodontitis: ≥2 interproximal sites with CAL ≥6 mm (not on the same tooth) **and** ≥1 interproximal site with PPD ≥5 mm
> - *Moderate* periodontitis: ≥2 interproximal sites with CAL ≥4 mm (not on the same tooth) **or** ≥2 interproximal sites with PPD ≥5 mm (not on the same tooth)
> - *Mild* periodontitis: ≥2 interproximal sites with CAL ≥3 mm **and** ≥2 interproximal sites with PPD ≥4 mm (not on the same tooth) **or** ≥1 site with PPD ≥5 mm
> - *No* periodontitis: no evidence of mild, moderate, or severe periodontitis
> Two additional categorizations were subsequently constructed, namely:
> - "*Total* periodontitis" (*any* periodontitis) is the presence of severe, moderate, or mild periodontitis.
> - Moderate/severe periodontitis is defined as presence of either moderate or severe periodontitis.
>
> *These four mutually exclusive categories of periodontitis are now commonly referred to as the "CDC/AAP case definitions for surveillance of periodontitis" and are used worldwide.
> CAL, clinical attachment loss; PPD, periodontal probing depth.

> ### • BOX 15.9 European Workshop in Periodontology Definition Risk Factor Research[85]
>
> Two mutually exclusive groups, incipient or severe cases of periodontitis were defined:
> - *Severe* periodontitis was defined as having >30% teeth with CAL ≥5 mm
> - *Incipient* cases, among those who were not classified as having severe periodontitis, with CAL >3 mm on two non-adjacent teeth
> Additionally, *any* (or *total*) periodontitis was defined as presence of either incipient or severe periodontitis
>
> CAL, clinical attachment loss.

> ### • BOX 15.10 A Current Model of Periodontal Diseases
>
> - Mild gingivitis is common, nearly ubiquitous.
> - Gingivitis precedes periodontitis, but only some sites with gingivitis develop periodontitis.
> - Only a small proportion of persons (5%–15%) exhibit severe periodontitis.
> - The vast majority of gingivitis and periodontitis are associated with dental plaque biofilms that are complex microbial communities colonizing the tooth and gingiva.
> - Plaque-induced gingivitis manifests as gingival inflammation without clinical attachment loss (CAL) and is reversible.
> - Periodontitis manifests as inflammation accompanied by CAL and alveolar bone loss and is irreversible.
> - Untreated periodontitis may progress and will eventually lead to tooth mobility and ultimately the loss of the tooth.
> - Periodontitis is the leading cause of tooth loss and edentulism in adult populations.
> - Both gingivitis and periodontitis are mediated by local risk factors and underlying systemic diseases or conditions.
> - Periodontitis is not a natural consequence of aging; it is usually related to age in cross-sectional studies, but this is partly due to its chronic, irreversible, cumulative nature and to the higher prevalence of systemic diseases and other factors in older subjects.
> - Periodontitis is a site-specific condition that is asymmetrically distributed in the dentition.
> - Progression of periodontitis occurs in bursts of destructive activity with intermittent quiescent periods.
> - Presence and severity of periodontitis is associated with hyperglycemia in poorly or uncontrolled diabetes, not in well-controlled diabetes.

studies, and epidemiologic findings of periodontitis prevalence from different studies around the world can now be compared.

The periodontitis case definitions proposed in 2005 by the European Workshop in Periodontology are displayed in Box 15.9,[85] and a current model for periodontal diseases summarizing the most common features of gingivitis and periodontitis is shown in Box 15.10.

## Risk Factors/Indicators for Periodontitis

### Nonmodifiable Risk Factors

#### Age

Increasing age is traditionally cited as the most important determinant of periodontitis with greater prevalence with advancing age, "but not necessarily due to age *per se*."[84] The greater prevalence of greater CAL at various thresholds found in older people in cross-sectional surveys are mostly due to the cumulative nature of the irreversible lesions over time. Importantly, the 2009–14 NHANES revealed that neither mild nor severe periodontitis increased a lot with age; the observed greater prevalence was driven by the moderate type of periodontitis.[26,27,31]

Several explanations have been proposed regarding the relationship with age. Notably, the effectiveness of the inflammatory responses do decrease with increasing age, with altered immunoactivation, immunosenescence, and a changing balance between pro- and antiinflammatory processes in favor of a chronic, macrophage-centered, low-grade inflammation in senescence, a phenomenon known as inflammaging.[25,35]

### Sex

Surveys of periodontal conditions have historically shown that men have poorer periodontal health than women. Sex-specific differences in periodontitis prevalence may not only be due to different gender-based health behaviors, as previously believed.[40] Women usually exhibit better oral hygiene, resulting in less plaque accumulation, which could explain the differences seen in gingivitis prevalence. The prevalence of periodontitis is consistently greater in males of all ages in all countries and subgroups. Especially noteworthy is the strength of sex as a risk factor. For example, in NHANES 2009–14 only 4.3% of dentate women 30 years and older *versus* 11.5% of the men had severe periodontitis.[31] Conversely, almost two-thirds (65.4%) of the females *versus* half (49.8%) of males had no periodontitis.

### Race/Ethnicity

There is little evidence to suggest different susceptibility to periodontitis among different races or ethnic groups. This should not come as a surprise when taking into account that race and ethnicity are largely social constructs, not based on any inherent traits. Any observed differences between racial/ethnic groups are likely due to differences in other risk factors, such as socioeconomic status (SES) and smoking habits. Nonetheless, some types of periodontitis, for instance that formerly known as aggressive periodontitis, may be more prevalent among African subjects or those of African descent.[82]

### Socioeconomic Status

Socioeconomic status (SES) is a multifaceted, complex measure of social standing that can include cultural, societal, and geographical factors in addition to the educational, occupational, and financial components. Generally, those who are better educated, wealthier, and live in more affluent circumstances enjoy better health status, including periodontal health, than the less educated and poorer segments of society. This association might be explained by factors associated with low SES status, such as smoking, stress, depression, anxiety, poor coping skills, and allostatic load (the latter is discussed in more detail in subsequent text). A study in a Norwegian population found that SES and smoking are the main predictors of periodontitis, whereas the likelihood of periodontitis was not reduced by regular dental visits,[46] a finding further demonstrated by a systematic review.[87]

### Genetic Factors

Genetic factors play an important role in the development and progression of periodontal tissue[91] with studies in twins suggesting that approximately half of the variance in a population may be attributed to genetic variance.[67] Likely, many gene variants, not a single trait, are implicated while also being impacted by environmental factors. This may merely suggest a potentially increased predisposition to periodontitis—or even susceptibility to any infection-/inflammation-related disease or condition—rather than inevitable occurrence of the disease. Nonetheless, familial aggregation of periodontitis, particularly the aggressive forms of the disease, has been documented.[91] At present, significant association of periodontitis with three genes has been validated through genome-wide association studies, namely glycosyltransferase 6 domain containing 1 (GLT6D1),[79] defensin α1 and α3 (DEFA1A3),[68] and sialic acid–binding Ig-like lectin 5 (SIGLEC5).[68] Other genes that also may have clinical significance include vitamin D receptor (VDR), Fc gamma receptor IIA (Fc-γRIIA), interleukin 10 (IL10),[18,70] and cyclooxygenase 2 (COX2) genes.[98] No genetic variant is identified for gingivitis.

### Family/Individual History of Disease

History of periodontitis in a family member or a member of one's household is not generally recognized as a risk factor, except for any inherited genetic predisposition to susceptibility to infection/inflammation, coupled with the shared household environment and behavioral norms.

## Modifiable Risk Factors

The modifiable risk factors are all due to lifestyle and hence should in theory be modifiable or preventable.

### Plaque, Microbiota, and Oral Hygiene

As described earlier, microbes in dental plaque initiate the local inflammatory responses, whereas it is mostly the host response to often prolonged exposure to such plaque that determines the degree to which the periodontal tissues will be affected.[7,54] More specifically, the dysbiotic microbiome as a community is responsible for this initial insult, not any particular individual bacterium or bacteria.[6-8]

A logical consequence of this understanding of the pathogenesis of periodontal diseases is that although there is a clear relationship between poor oral hygiene and gingivitis, the relationship between oral hygiene status and periodontitis is less straightforward. Good oral hygiene can favorably influence the ecology of the subgingival microbial flora of already treated (shallow) pockets, but it does not affect flora in untreated patients.

### Hyposalivation

The term "dry mouth" refers to both xerostomia (subjective feeling of mouth dryness) and hyposalivation (diminished saliva secretion). Notably, the two conditions do not necessarily occur simultaneously, as a substantial proportion of people complaining of xerostomia actually do not have decreased salivary output and *vice versa*.[10] Decreased amounts of saliva leads to poorer efficiency in plaque removal with resulting accumulation, which in turn predisposes to gingivitis. It is a common misconception that older people secrete significantly less saliva than their younger counterparts. Rather, hyposalivation is caused by diseases of the salivary glands and by several systemic diseases—and by the medications taken to treat them, as all major groups of pharmaceuticals are capable of leading to hyposalivation. Because older individuals tend to suffer from more diseases and take more medication than younger people, they often suffer from hyposalivation but not due to age *per se*. Disease or radiation of the salivary glands and diabetic neuropathy can also lead to hyposalivation.[10]

## Orthodontic Appliances

Fixed orthodontic appliances cause changes in the bacterial composition of dental plaque and can lead to gingivitis. Also, both fixed and removable space retainers are shown to cause an increase in the abundance of both bacteria and yeast (mostly *Candida*) colonization. However, these changes seem to revert back to normal several months after removal of the appliances and not lead to periodontitis.[42]

## Dentures

Prosthodontic appliances can function as a microbial reservoir and increase the load of bacteria and fungi. In a 10-year study of older Japanese aged 70 years at baseline, those with either fixed or removable partial dentures were more likely to experience progression of periodontitis.[45]

## Tobacco Use

The evidence is clear that tobacco smoking is a major causal factor of periodontal tissue loss. The first line of treatment for periodontitis should always be to encourage patients who smoke to quit.[10]

### Current Cigarette Smokers

Cigarette smoking is the strongest independent risk factor for periodontitis. Several reports on the health effects of smoking were published by the Surgeon General starting in 1964.[88] The 2004 version added periodontitis as being causally linked to smoking.[89] The analyses of data from NHANES 1971–74 by Ismail, Burt, and Eklund at the University of Michigan first reported a clear association between smoking and periodontal disease—independent of oral hygiene, age, or any other factor—in a large population-based epidemiologic study representative of US adults.[49]

Both human and microbial cells are affected by nicotine.[94] The pathogenicity of oral microorganisms is increased by nicotine, which leads to the formation of greater abundance of biofilm or to increased expression of virulence factors. A 2018 systematic review and meta-analysis concluded that smokers were 85% more likely to have periodontitis.[62] Analysis of data from the 2009–12 NHANES estimated cigarette smoking to cause about 20% (16.0 million) of all periodontitis cases in dentate US adults age 30 years or older.[92] Of these cases, 9.7 million were current, active cigarette smokers, and another 5.7 million cases were nonsmokers (i.e., never or former smokers) who currently were exposed to environmental tobacco exposure (ETS), formerly known as secondhand cigarette smoke.

### Former Cigarette Smokers

Former cigarette smokers consistently have higher rates of (especially severe) periodontitis than never smokers, but longer time since quitting smoking is associated with a lower likelihood of periodontitis.[3]

### Tobacco Use Other Than Cigarette Smoking

A small proportion of the population smoke a pipe, cigars, little cigars, and cigarillos, and there is evidence that such vehicles have detrimental effects on periodontal health similar to cigarette smoking.[1]

### Environmental Tobacco Exposure

The prevalence of periodontitis is also elevated in individuals who do not themselves smoke but are exposed to ETS, also known as secondhand smoke exposure, with up to twice the odds of periodontitis compared to those unexposed.[77,92]

## E-Cigarette Smoking/Vaping

Regardless of nicotine content, e-cigarette vapor may damage oral tissues due to sugars and other ingredients. The evidence for periodontal consequences is emerging.

## Nutrition, Minerals, and Vitamins

Growing interest has focused on the role of nutrition for a healthy periodontium. Even though a 2014 systematic review found insufficient evidence to support the link between nutritional status and periodontal inflammation,[58] calcium and minerals that play antioxidant roles in the immune responses might be important.[90] Moreover, diets rich in saturated fat and meat are pro-inflammatory and are associated with missing more teeth.[56]

### Sugar

Sugar is traditionally associated with caries, but partly due to its pro-inflammatory effects, it has become evident that it is also a risk driver in periodontal diseases. High-frequency consumption of added sugars was found to be independently associated with the extent of BOP and periodontal probing depth of 3 mm or more among 18- to 25-year-olds participating in NHANES III.[65]

### Alcohol

A 2016 meta-analysis of 18 observational studies concluded that alcohol consumption is significantly associated with increased periodontitis risk in both sexes.[95] Women are especially susceptible, having more than twice the risk for periodontitis *versus* a 25% increased risk for men. A linear dose-response relationship was found, in which the risk of periodontitis significantly increases by 0.4% for each 1 g/day increment in alcohol consumption.[95] Evidence for adverse effects on periodontal health of vaping alcohol-containing liquids is emerging.

## Other Modifiable Factors

### Obesity

Obesity is a metabolic disorder found to be associated with increased prevalence of periodontal diseases. It is estimated that obese individuals have a 35% increased risk of developing periodontitis compared to normal weight individuals.[69] Notably, not all obese individuals have a high risk of periodontitis, although persons affected with adipose tissue dysfunction may be at particularly higher risk. However, a recent study with NHANES data shows that obesity is not a risk indicator for periodontitis after controlling for all sociodemographic factors and known risk factors.[33]

### Pregnancy

Pregnancy is another transient condition known to significantly increase gingival inflammation without an accompanying increase in levels of dental plaque throughout pregnancy.[97] This increased inflammatory response is most pronounced during the second and third trimesters and reverses postpartum.

### Sleep Disturbances

There is a novel, strong association between obstructive sleep apnea (OSA) and periodontitis, especially with moderate/severe periodontitis, and nonapnea sleep disorders can also increase the risk for periodontitis. In NHANES 2009–12 (N=3740), an unadjusted association between subjects sleeping less than 7 hours and periodontitis was reported,[90] and disordered breathing during sleep was independently associated with severe periodontitis among US Hispanics.[76]

### Stress, Depression, Anxiety, Poor Coping Skills, Allostatic Load

A cross-sectional study by Genco and coauthors found stress, depression, and inadequate coping behaviors to be risk indicators of periodontitits.[41] Self-reported depression and clinically assessed periodontitis were associated, in a dose-response manner, with periodontitis severity.

The term *allostasis* is the process of adaptation to the social and physical environments in which we live. The concept "allostatic load" refers to physiologic consequences of neural, neuroendocrine, and immune reactions ("wear and tear" on the body) by chronic or repeated exposure to stress and has been linked to poorer periodontal health in minorities.[15]

### Low Health Literacy

A 2017 systematic review concluded that a reduced number of teeth and greater CAL were associated with lower levels of oral health literacy.[34]

## Systemic Diseases

The loss of periodontal supporting tissues can be potentiated, sometimes profoundly, by certain systemic diseases and conditions.[2] Diseases that compromise the host responses to infections may lead to significant loss of periodontal attachment and alveolar bone, and the tissue loss is usually proportional to the degree of deficiency of the host response. Thus patients with immunologic disorders show severe periodontitis and a high rate of disease progression, and these clinical manifestations often occur at a young age. Examples of these disorders include leukocyte adhesion deficiency syndromes—primary immunodeficiency diseases, Papillon-Lefèvre syndrome, Haim-Munk syndrome, Chediak-Higashi syndrome, Kostmann syndrome, and Cohen syndrome.[2,51]

Dental professionals should be cognizant of important associations between periodontal diseases and systemic diseases, both in designing preventive and intervention measures for managing oral diseases and in detecting undiagnosed underlying systemic diseases in the dental office.

### Diabetes

Of the chronic, common, endocrine, metabolic, and inflammation-based diseases; systemic diseases; and conditions that affect the health of the periodontium, the strongest scientific evidence for the strongest effect pertains to hyperglycemia/diabetes, as per extensive literature reviews.[13,14,19,55,59,78] It is often stated that diabetes is a risk factor for periodontitis. However, it is not a diabetes diagnosis *per se* that is the deciding factor. Rather, the degree of hyperglycemia dictates the magnitude of effect on the periodontium, as expressed by Genco in 1996: "Risk factors which we know today as important include diabetes mellitus, especially in individuals in whom metabolic control is poor."[39] Nonetheless, only rather recently has this important qualifier been acknowledged and reported.[36] This dose–response effect was illustrated by a population study among 3086 Germans that demonstrated that although poorly controlled type 2 diabetes was associated with periodontitis, well-controlled diabetes and prediabetes were not.[57] Another study reported worse periodontal parameters in participants with prediabetes compared to normoglycemia.[50] A rare study of the effect of controlling glycemia on the peridontium found that improving glycemic control in type 2 diabetes with no accompanying periodontal treatment significantly lowered the BOP especially in those with higher baseline bleeding levels.[53] In contrast, periodontal pocket depths did not improve.

### Effect of Nonsurgical Periodontal Treatment on Blood Glucose Level

A large number of clinical trials report that nonsurgical periodontal treatment (scaling and root planing) can lead to decreased glycated hemoglobin level (improved glucose control) of clinical importance in type 2 diabetes.[21,44]

However, other studies did not find any statistically significant decrease in levels of glycated hemoglobin or fasting blood glucose. Hence, this is still a hotly debated topic. Nonetheless, nonsurgical periodontal treatment is safe and effective in improving both periodontal health and quality of life also for people with type 2 diabetes. However, the evidence is scant among people with the insulin-requiring type 1 diabetes.

### Other Systemic Diseases and Conditions

Greater prevalence, extent, and severity of periodontitis are reported in people with a metabolic syndrome; allergies and asthma; hypertension, atherosclerosis, and a history of myocardial infarction; ischemic stroke and intracranial hemorrhage; rheumatoid arthritis, Sjögren's syndrome, Crohn's disease, and other autoimmune diseases; cognitive decline, Alzheimer's disease; adverse pregnancy outcomes (preterm delivery, small for gestational age delivery, preeclampsia); cancer (oral, digestive system); and possibly osteoporosis or osteopenia.

## Prevalence/Distribution of Periodontal Diseases in US Adults

### Gingivitis

Gingivitis is nearly ubiquitous, with up to 90% in any population worldwide affected.[74] The 2017 World Workshop proposed case definitions for gingival health and for gingivitis for use in individual patients (clinical practice) and for surveillance.[20] Nonetheless, because BOP was not included in the protocol for 2009–14 NHANES to examine for gingivitis, no further description will be provided regarding the prevalence of this reversible disease.

### Periodontitis

The three 2-year NHANES cycles (2009–10, 2011–12, and 2013–14) referred to as NHANES 2009–14 used for the first time the full mouth (except third molars) gold standard periodontal examination protocol for consenting dentate adults aged 30 to 79 years ("≥30 years"). Because of its extent, magnitude, and representativeness, this survey has generated data that represent the most stable, accurate, and reliable estimates of the prevalence of periodontitis in US adults currently in existence. The following description is based on these data with the CDC/AAP periodontitis case definitions applied. Some estimates are generated specifically for this chapter, whereas others are published earlier[26,27,31] and will be cited instead of repeated.

Overall, 42% of US dentate adults 30 years and older had *total* periodontitis, consisting of 7.8% with severe periodontitis and 34.4% with nonsevere (mild or moderate) periodontitis (Table 15.1).[31]

Further analyses of the NHANES 2009–14 data estimated the prevalence of *total* periodontitis (mild, moderate, or severe) to be 62.4% in current smokers (16.9% severe periodontitis and 45.4% nonsevere [mild or moderate]), 45.8% in former smokers (8.0% severe plus 37.7% nonsevere), and 34.4% in nonsmokers (4.9% severe and 29.5% nonsevere).[31] No other demographic or health behavior group of characteristics (potential confounders) showed

**● TABLE 15.1**  Prevalence of *Severe* and *Nonsevere* (*Mild* or *Moderate*) Periodontitis Classified by the CDC/AAP Case Definitions[29] Among Dentate Adults 30 Years and Older by Demographic and Health Related Subgroups—National Health and Examination Survey 2009–14 (N = 10,683)[31]

| | PERIODONTITIS | | |
|---|---|---|---|
| Characteristic [%(SE)] | Severe %(SE) | Nonsevere (Mild/Moderate) %(SE) | Total %(SE) |
| Total | 7.8(0.5) | 34.4(1.2) | 42.2(1.4) |
| **Age** | | | |
| 30–44 years | 4.1(0.3) | 25.3(1.4) | 29.5(1.5) |
| 45–64 years | 10.4(0.8)*** | 35.6(1.4)*** | 46.0(1.6)*** |
| ≥65 years | 9.0(1.0)*** | 50.7(1.9)*** | 59.8(2.1)*** |
| **Sex** | | | |
| Male | 11.5(0.8)*** | 38.8(1.2)*** | 50.2(1.4)*** |
| Female | 4.3(0.4) | 30.2(1.4) | 34.6(1.5) |
| **Race/Ethnicity** | | | |
| Mexican Americans | 13.4(1.4)*** | 46.4(1.5)*** | 59.7(1.7)*** |
| Other Hispanics | 7.8(0.9) | 40.7(1.5)*** | 48.5(1.6)*** |
| Non-Hispanic whites | 5.9(0.6) | 31.1(1.5) | 37.0(1.7) |
| Non-Hispanic blacks | 14.7(1.1)*** | 42.0(1.3)*** | 56.6(2.0)*** |
| Other race, incl. multiracial | 9.3(1.4)* | 36.9(2.3)* | 46.2(2.6)** |
| **Smoking Status** | | | |
| Nonsmokers | 4.9(0.5) | 29.5(1.2) | 34.4(1.4) |
| Former smokers | 8.0(0.7)* | 37.7(1.8)*** | 45.8(1.8)*** |
| Current smokers | 16.9(1.3)*** | 45.4(1.7)*** | 62.4(1.7)*** |
| **Socioeconomic Level** | | | |
| **Income Categories A)[a]** | | | |
| <100% FPL | 13.9(1.0)*** | 46.5(1.5)*** | 60.4(1.7)*** |
| 100%–199% FPL | 12.1(1.1)*** | 41.5(1.9)*** | 53.6(2.0)*** |
| 200–399% FPL | 7.2(0.8)*** | 37.4(1.8)*** | 44.6(2.0)*** |
| ≥400% FPL | 4.0(0.6) | 24.6(1.2) | 28.6(1.4) |
| **Income Categories B)[a]** | | | |
| Low ≤130% | 13.8(1.0)*** | 45.2(1.4)*** | 59.0(1.7)*** |
| Middle 131%–350% | 8.6(0.7)*** | 40.0(1.7)*** | 48.5(1.8)*** |
| High ≥351% | 4.5(0.6) | 25.3(1.2) | 29.7(1.4) |
| **Body Mass Index (BMI)[b]** | | | |
| <25 kg/m² | 7.6(0.6) | 31.6(1.6) | 39.2(1.8) |
| 25–30 kg/m² | 8.1(0.7) | 34.0(1.3) | 42.1(1.4) |
| >30 kg/m² | 7.7(0.7) | 36.7(1.5)** | 44.4(1.5)* |
| **Diabetes Mellitus** | | | |
| Yes | 10.8(1.3)* | 49.0(2.5)*** | 59.9(2.2)*** |
| No | 7.5(0.5) | 32.8(1.2) | 40.4(1.4) |
| **Use of Dental Floss in Past 7 Days** | | | |
| Yes | 5.8(0.5) | 32.1(1.2) | 37.9(1.3) |
| No | 12.8(1.0)*** | 40.3(1.6)*** | 53.1(1.8)*** |

*(Continued)*

| • TABLE 15.1 | Prevalence of *Severe* and *Nonsevere* (*Mild* or *Moderate*) Periodontitis Classified by the CDC/AAP Case Definitions[29] Among Dentate Adults 30 Years and Older by Demographic and Health Related Subgroups—National Health and Examination Survey 2009–14 (N = 10,683)[31]—Cont'd |
|---|---|

| | PERIODONTITIS | | |
|---|---|---|---|
| Characteristic [%(SE)] | Severe %(SE) | Nonsevere (Mild/Moderate) %(SE) | Total %(SE) |
| Total | 7.8(0.5) | 34.4(1.2) | 42.2(1.4) |
| **Last Dental Visit[c]** | | | |
| ≤6 months | 3.9(0.6) | 26.4(1.6) | 30.3(1.7) |
| >6–12 months | 6.3(1.0)* | 31.6(2.2)* | 37.9(2.4)** |
| >12 months/never | 13.3(1.1)*** | 41.5(1.7)*** | 54.8(1.8)*** |
| **# Teeth Missing** | | | |
| 0 teeth missing | 2.6(0.5) | 20.9(1.2) | 23.5(1.4) |
| 1–5 teeth missing | 7.0(0.7)*** | 36.0(1.2)*** | 43.0(1.3)*** |
| 6–27 teeth missing | 17.1(1.2)*** | 51.5(1.7)*** | 68.6(1.5)*** |

[a]n = 895 respondents were missing values on income.
[b]n = 64 respondents were missing values for Body Mass Index.
[c]Based on data from National Health and Examination Survey 2011–14 only.
*P < =.05, **P < 0.01, ***P < 0.001.
#, number; *FPL*, federal poverty limit; *SE*, standard error.
3rd molars excluded
Wald Chi-square test was used for testing significance of proportion difference in each group

such a high prevalence of periodontitis as in current smokers, supporting that cigarette smoking is regarded as the strongest risk factor for periodontitis. In only one subgroup—those with 6 to 27 teeth missing—was the prevalence of total periodontitis greater, namely 68.6%.[31] This is likely due to many of the missing teeth having been lost due to periodontitis and the remaining teeth still suffering from that disease.

The *severity* of CAL and PPD is reported in Table 15.2 for the years 2009–12. For all six years (2009–14), the population mean CAL was 1.7 mm and increased with age (not shown).[31] About 89% of all adults had ≥1 site with CAL ≥3 mm with an average of 19.0% of sites per person and an average of 37.1% of teeth per person affected (not shown).[31]

The *extent* of periodontitis is displayed by various cut points for CAL and PPD in Table 15.2.[27] An estimated 58.2% of adults had ≥3 mm CAL in ≥5% of sites. Overall, the mean proportion of sites with ≥3 mm CAL was 19.3%. At the tooth level, 80.1% of adults had CAL ≥3 mm at ≥5% of their teeth, whereas 47.4% (almost half) had ≥30% of their teeth affected by CAL ≥3 mm. The mean proportion of teeth with ≥3 mm CAL was 37.4%. An estimated 17.0% of adults had PPD ≥4 mm at ≥5% of all sites and 3.1% at ≥30% of all sites. Overall, the mean proportion of sites with PPD ≥4 mm was 3.8%. At the tooth level, 32.8% of adults had PPD ≥4 mm at ≥5% of their teeth, whereas 12.5% had ≥30% of their teeth affected by PPD ≥4 mm. The overall mean proportion of teeth with PDD ≥4 mm was about 1 in 10 (10.6%).

Importantly, the recent 2009–14 NHANES data suggest that the prevalence of *severe* and *mild* periodontitis, respectively, remains ≤15% and ≤10% of adults in all age groups between the ages of 30 and 79 years (Figure 15.3). The prevalence of *moderate* and *total* periodontitis increases with age from about 20% or less at age 30 to more than 50% at age 75 and older. The important

conclusion is that it is the *moderate* type that drives this increase with age, not the *severe* form.[31]

There is substantial disparity in the distribution of severe periodontitis by sex, race/ethnicity, and income status (Figure 15.4). Men are more than twice as likely as women age 45 to 64 to have severe periodontitis (15% *vs.* 6%). A similar pattern is seen for Mexican Americans and non-Hispanic blacks compared to non-Hispanic whites, and the prevalence of severe periodontitis is three times greater among low-income adults compared to high-income adults (20% *vs.* 6%). Among adults in the United States, severe periodontitis continues to be three to four times more prevalent in current smokers compared to nonsmokers.

Figure 15.5 shows the prevalence of increasing severity of CAL as adults age. By age 65, more than half of older adults have at least one periodontal site with CAL ≥5 mm, and nearly 20% have CAL ≥7 mm. Among all adults age 30 and older, 38% have at least one periodontal site with CAL ≥5 mm (Figure 15.6). In the United States, older adults, males, Mexican Americans and non-Hispanic blacks, low-income adults, and smokers have a higher prevalence of CAL ≥5 mm.

The prevalence of increasing severity of PPD as adults age is shown in Figure 15.7. By age 50, the prevalence of adults with at least one periodontal site with PPD ≥4 mm fluctuates around 40%, ranging from as high as 50% to as low as 30%. Unlike the increasing severity of CAL with increasing age (see Figure 15.5), increasing severity of PPD remains relatively consistent across the age span (see Figure 15.7). Although 38% of adults age 30 and older have at least one periodontal site with PPD ≥4 mm (Figure 15.8), similar to CAL ≥5 mm, the distribution of PPD ≥4 mm by key risk indicators is not as pronounced for age compared to CAL. The prevalence of PPD ≥4 mm is higher among males, Mexican Americans and non-Hispanic blacks, low-income adults, and current smokers in the United States.

**• TABLE 15.2** Site- and Tooth-Specific Prevalence and Extent of Periodontal Probing Depth and Clinical Attachment Loss Among Adults 30 Years and Older by Severity—NHANES 2009–12[27]

| | | SEVERITY | | | | | | | | | |
| | | ≥3 mm | | ≥4 mm | | ≥5 mm | | ≥6 mm | | ≥7 mm | |
| | Extent | % | SE | % | SE | % | SE | % | SE | % | SE |
| Site-Specific: | % | | | | | | | | | | |
|---|---|---|---|---|---|---|---|---|---|---|---|
| PPD: | ≥5% sites | 44.9 | 22 | 17.0 | 0.9 | 6.3 | 0.6 | 2.4 | 0.3 | 0.6 | 0.09 |
| | ≥10% sites | 31.2 | 18 | 10.6 | 0.6 | 3.1 | 0.4 | 1.2 | 0.2 | 0.2 | 0.05 |
| | ≥30% sites | 12.8 | 10 | 3.1 | 0.4 | 0.8 | 0.1 | 0.2 | 0.04 | 0.02 | 0.01 |
| Mean % sites | | 11.9 | 07 | 3.8 | 0.2 | 1.2 | 0.1 | 0.5 | 0.05 | 0.1 | 0.01 |
| CAL: | ≥5% sites | 58.2 | 16 | 31.8 | 1.4 | 17.3 | 0.8 | 9.7 | 0.5 | 5.3 | 0.4 |
| | ≥10% sites | 43.8 | 16 | 21.9 | 1.0 | 11.7 | 0.6 | 6.4 | 0.4 | 3.6 | 0.3 |
| | ≥30% sites | 21.3 | 10 | 10.0 | 0.7 | 5.0 | 0.4 | 2.9 | 0.3 | 1.6 | 0.2 |
| Mean % sites | | 19.3 | 08 | 9.8 | 0.5 | 5.2 | 0.3 | 2.9 | 0.2 | 1.5 | 0.1 |
| Tooth-specific: | | | | | | | | | | | |
| PPD: | ≥5% teeth | 70.6 | 16 | 32.8 | 1.2 | 14.6 | 0.8 | 7.1 | 0.7 | 2.5 | 0.3 |
| | ≥10% teeth | 61.4 | 19 | 25.7 | 0.9 | 10.4 | 0.7 | 4.6 | 0.5 | 1.5 | 0.2 |
| | ≥30% teeth | 35.5 | 20 | 12.5 | 0.7 | 3.9 | 0.4 | 1.5 | 0.2 | 0.3 | 0.05 |
| Mean % teeth | | 28.4 | 13 | 10.6 | 0.5 | 3.7 | 0.3 | 1.6 | 0.2 | 0.5 | 0.05 |
| CAL: | ≥5% teeth | 80.1 | 11 | 49.5 | 1.7 | 31.5 | 1.2 | 18.0 | 0.8 | 10.7 | 0.5 |
| | ≥10% teeth | 73.2 | 14 | 42.4 | 1.5 | 24.7 | 0.9 | 13.4 | 0.6 | 7.9 | 0.5 |
| | ≥30% teeth | 47.4 | 17 | 23.4 | 1.0 | 12.0 | 0.7 | 6.4 | 0.4 | 3.5 | 0.3 |
| Mean % teeth | | 37.4 | 11 | 19.2 | 0.8 | 10.6 | 0.5 | 5.9 | 0.3 | 3.2 | 0.2 |

*CAL,* clinical attachment loss; *PPD,* periodontal probing depth; *SE,* standard error.

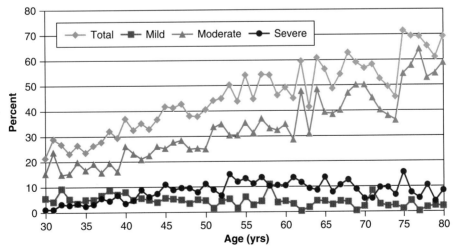

**• Figure 15.3** Prevalence of periodontitis classified by the CDC/AAP case definitions[29] (mild, moderate, and severe periodontitis, respectively) and *total* periodontitis (mild, moderate, or severe) by age among dentate adults 30 years or older, NHANES 2009–14 (N = 10,683).[31]

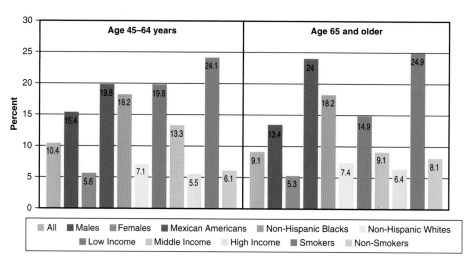

• **Figure 15.4** Prevalence of *severe* periodontitis classified by the CDC/AAP case definitions[29,71] by age groups 45–64 years and 65 years and older for select characteristics among dentate adults, NHANES 2009–14.[31]

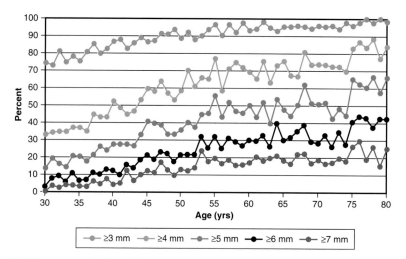

• **Figure 15.5** Prevalence of periodontitis by severity categorized by minimum clinical attachment loss (CAL) by age among dentate adults 30 years or older, NHANES 2009–14 (N = 10,683).[31]

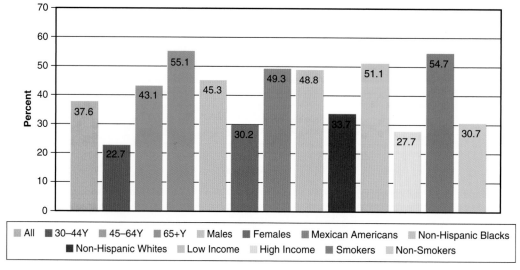

• **Figure 15.6** Prevalence of CAL => 5 mm for dentate adults 30 years or older according to selected characteristics. National Health and Nutrition Examination Survey 2009–14.[31]

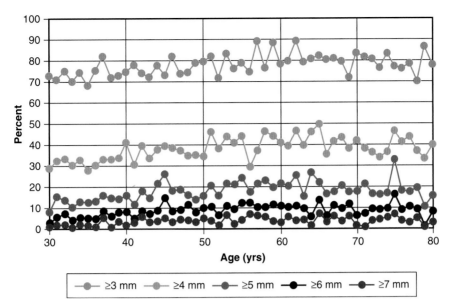

• **Figure 15.7** Prevalence of periodontitis by severity categorized by minimum periodontal probing depth (PPD) by age among dentate adults 30 years or older, NHANES 2009–14.[31]

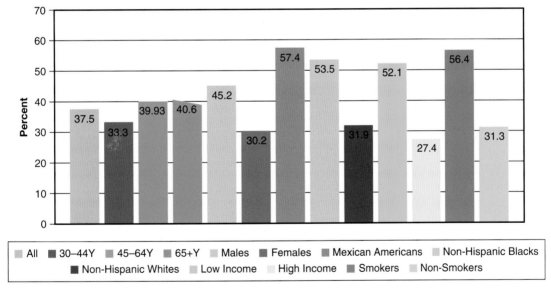

• **Figure 15.8** Prevalence of periodontal probing depth (PPD) ≥4 mm for dentate adults 30 years or older according to selected characteristics, National Health and Nutrition Examination Survey, 2009–14.[31]

## Public Health Importance of Periodontal Diseases

Several factors contribute to the public health significance of periodontal diseases. First, when the integrity of the gingival epithelium is compromised by periodontal disease, virulent subgingival bacteria can gain direct access to the systemic blood circulation and may directly invade tissues located remotely from the oral cavity.[12] The resulting bacteremia together with the bacterial virulence factors provoke the release of responding host inflammatory mediators, hence increasing the level of systemic inflammation. This mechanism has been proposed as the biologically plausible main mechanism underlying the link between periodontitis and systemic diseases and conditions, notably type 2 diabetes mellitus, atherosclerotic cardiovascular disease, rheumatoid arthritis, and adverse pregnancy outcomes.

It is important to note that periodontitis shares several risk factors with other systemic chronic diseases.[10,11,80] Common modifiable risk factors for periodontitis and noncommunicable diseases include tobacco use, alcohol use, poor diet and nutrition, and psychosocial factors. The importance of hyperglycemia/diabetes as a risk factor for periodontal disease is also attributed to its high prevalence worldwide, particularly in older age groups.

The potential process by which periodontitis can result in bacteremia and increased levels of systemic inflammation—together with its shared unhealthy lifestyle (e.g., smoking) and metabolic and dietary risk factors with other chronic noncommunicable disease—presents an opportunity for joint interventions targeting local etiologic factors and systemic factors. This common risk factor approach[80] and accompanying targeted health promotion and education will be useful in persons at high risk for periodontitis. Moreover, with the risk factors for periodontitis being similar, if not identical, to those of other chronic diseases, it should be possible to identify subpopulations at increased risk for periodontitis, which could facilitate the institution of preventive and intervention measures. Consequently, a patient-centered, interprofessional collaboration would be warranted for the improvement of both oral and general health.

There are important potential consequences of periodontal diseases, notably pain and discomfort, gingival bleeding, tooth displacement and mobility, and eventually tooth loss. Increased tooth mobility and tooth loss may contribute to decreased masticatory function, which in turn may lead to difficulty consuming a proper diet and to poor nutrition when one must resort to soft food items that often contain high levels of fat and sugar. Bacteria that are usually located in the periodontal pockets also travel everywhere in the body and thereby cause bacteremia and more importantly induce potentially strong antiinflammatory responses that also are risk factors for cardiovascular disease and events.

Furthermore, periodontitis can have a significant impact on patients' quality of life and self-esteem, through social, functional, and aesthetic impairment. Periodontitis also affects general health, with the potential to severely affect a person's overall health and well-being, and hence may negatively affect quality of life. Quality of life and oral function can be severely diminished by periodontitis-related problems, such as pain, foul taste and smell (halitosis), not eating in public, not daring to smile, poor self-esteem, and having trouble getting a job. Several studies have reported strong correlations between health-related quality of life and periodontitis.

There are inequalities in the prevalence of periodontitis, with great disparities by social determinants and race/ethnicity. About 60% of the oldest adults, the poorest, lowest socioeconomic ethnic groups, those with uncontrolled diabetes, and current smokers are disproportionately affected. Other populations disproportionally affected include socially disadvantaged, disabled, and chronically ill persons.

Finally, the significance of periodontitis can be appreciated by its burden in populations. Periodontal disease is the most important oral disease contributing to the global burden of chronic diseases. The Global Burden of Disease collaborators reported periodontal disease to be the 11th most common chronic disease in the world in 2015, affecting 537.5 million people of all ages.[37,38] There was a 25.4% increase in the number of persons affected by periodontitis from 2005 to 2015, mostly due to the aging of the world's population, as the age-standardized rate increase was only 1.2%.[37] Periodontitis is widespread, as it affects more than 4 in 10 adults with natural teeth.[31] Importantly, *severe* periodontitis was found to be the sixth most prevalent condition in the world, affecting 11% of

adults age 15 years and older in 37 countries.[52] The latter global estimate is consistent with the burden of severe periodontitis in the United States.[31]

Successful population-based interventions for periodontitis are currently rare and need further evaluation. The surveillance, prevention, treatment, and management of periodontitis are important public health issues that require extensive attention from all stakeholders for the benefit of the public's oral and general health. There is no total health without oral health.

# References

1. Albandar JM, Streckfus CF, Adesanya MR, et al. Cigar, pipe, and cigarette smoking as risk factors for periodontal disease and tooth loss. *J Periodontol*. 2000;71:1874–1881.
2. Albandar JM, Susin C, Hughes FJ. Manifestations of systemic diseases and conditions that affect the periodontal attachment apparatus: Case definitions and diagnostic considerations. *J Clin Periodontol*. 2018;45(suppl 20):S171–S189.
3. ALHarthi SSY, Natto ZS, Midle JB, et al. Association between time since quitting smoking and periodontitis in former smokers in the national health and nutrition examination surveys (NHANES) 2009 to 2012. *J Periodontol*. 2019;90(1):16–25.
4. American Academy of Periodontology. *Proceedings of the World Workshop in Clinical Periodontics*. Chicago, IL: American Academy of Periodontology; 1989.
5. Armitage GC. Development of a classification system for periodontal diseases and conditions. *Ann Periodontol*. 1999;4(1):1–6.
6. Bartold PM, Van Dyke TE. An appraisal of the role of specific bacteria in the initial pathogenesis of periodontitis. *J Clin Periodontol*. 2019;0(ja).
7. Bartold PM, Van Dyke TE. Host modulation: controlling the inflammation to control the infection. *Periodontol 2000*. 2017;75(1):317–329.
8. Bartold PM, Van Dyke TE. Periodontitis: a host-mediated disruption of microbial homeostasis. Unlearning learned concepts. *Periodontol 2000*. 2013;62(1):203–217.
9. Beck JD, Koch GG, Rozier RG, et al. Prevalence and risk indicators for periodontal attachment loss in a population of older community-dwelling blacks and whites. *J Periodontol*. 1990;61(8):521–528.
10. Borgnakke WS. Modifiable risk factors for periodontitis and diabetes. *Curr Oral Health Rep*. 2016;3(3):254–269.
11. Borgnakke WS. "Non-modifiable" risk factors for periodontitis and diabetes. *Curr Oral Health Rep*. 2016;3(3):270–281.
12. Borgnakke WS. Ch3. The traveling oral microbiome. In: Glick M, ed. *The Oral-Systemic Health Connection: A Guide to Patient Care*. Pp 38–85. Chicago, IL: Quintessence; 2019. 384 pp.
13. Borgnakke WS, Genco RJ. Ch6. Associations between periodontal disease and hyperglycemia/diabetes. In: Glick M, ed. *The Oral-Systemic Health Connection: A Guide to Patient Care*. Chicago, IL: Quintessence; 2019:384 pp. 135–163.
14. Borgnakke WS, Genco RJ, Eke PI, et al. Ch31. Oral health and diabetes. In: Cowie CC, Casagrande SS, Menke A, et al, eds. *Diabetes in America*. 3rd ed. Bethesda, MD: National Institutes of Health/National Institute of Diabetes and Digestive and Kidney Diseases (NIH/NIDDK); 2018:31.01–31.51. NIH Pub No. 17-1468. Available from: https://www.niddk.nih.gov/about-niddk/strategic-plans-reports/diabetes-in-america-1463rd-edition
15. Borrell LN, Crawford ND. Social disparities in periodontitis among US adults: the effect of allostatic load. *J Epidemiol Community Health*. 2011;65(2):144–149.
16. Brown LJ, Brunelle JA, Kingman A. Periodontal status in the United States, 1988–1991: prevalence, extent, and demographic variation. *J Dent Res*. 1996;75:672–683.
17. Caton JG, Armitage G, Berglundh T, et al. A new classification scheme for periodontal and peri-implant diseases and conditions -

introduction and key changes from the 1999 classification. *J Clin Periodontol.* 2018;45(suppl 20):S1–S8.

18. Chapple IL, Bouchard P, Cagetti MG, et al. Interaction of lifestyle, behaviour or systemic diseases with dental caries and periodontal diseases: Consensus report of group 2 of the joint EFP/ORCA workshop on the boundaries between caries and periodontal diseases. *J Clin Periodontol.* 2017;44(suppl 18):S39–S51.

19. Chapple IL, Genco R. Working group 2 of joint EFP/AAP workshop. Diabetes and periodontal diseases: Consensus report of the joint EFP/AAP workshop on periodontitis and systemic diseases. *J Clin Periodontol.* 2013;40(suppl 14):S106–S112.

20. Chapple ILC, Mealey BL, Van Dyke TE, et al. Periodontal health and gingival diseases and conditions on an intact and a reduced periodontium: Consensus report of workgroup 1 of the 2017 world workshop on the classification of periodontal and peri-implant diseases and conditions. *J Clin Periodontol.* 2018;45(suppl 20): S68–S77.

21. D'Aiuto F, Gkranias N, Bhowruth D, et al. Systemic effects of periodontitis treatment in patients with type 2 diabetes: A 12 month, single-centre, investigator-masked, randomised trial. *Lancet Diabetes Endocrinol.* 2018;6(12):954–965.

22. Dewhirst FE, Chen T, Izard J, et al. The human oral microbiome. *J Bacteriol.* 2010;192(19):5002–5017.

23. Dye BA, Li X, Lewis BG, et al. Overview and quality assurance for the oral health component of the National Health and Nutrition Examination Survey (NHANES), 2009–2010. *J Public Health Dent.* 2014;74(3):248–256.

24. Dye BA, Thornton-Evans G. A brief history of national surveillance efforts for periodontal disease in the united states. *J Periodontol.* 2007;78(suppl 7):1373–1379.

25. Ebersole JL, Dawson DA, Emecen Huja P, et al. Age and periodontal health—immunological view. *Curr Oral Health Rep.* 2018;5(4): 229–241.

26. Eke PI, Dye BA, Wei L, et al. Prevalence of periodontitis in adults in the United States: 2009 and 2010. *J Dent Res.* 2012;91(10): 914–920.

27. Eke PI, Dye BA, Wei L, et al. Update on prevalence of periodontitis in adults in the United States: NHANES 2009 to 2012. *J Periodontol.* 2015;86(5):611–622.

28. Eke PI, Genco RJ. CDC periodontal disease surveillance project: background, objectives, and progress report. *J Periodontol.* 2007;78(suppl 7):1366–1371.

29. Eke PI, Page RC, Wei L, et al. Update of the case definitions for population-based surveillance of periodontitis. *J Periodontol.* 2012;83(12):1449–1454.

30. Eke PI, Thornton-Evans GO, Wei L, et al. Accuracy of NHANES periodontal examination protocols. *J Dent Res.* 2010;89(11): 1208–1213.

31. Eke PI, Thornton-Evans GO, Wei L, et al. Periodontitis in US adults: National Health and Nutrition Examination Survey 2009–2014. *J Am Dent Assoc.* 2018;149(7):576–588; 588.e1–588.e6.

32. Eke PI, Wei L, Borgnakke WS, et al. Periodontitis prevalence in adults ≥65 years of age, in the USA. *Periodontol 2000.* 2016;72(1): 76–95.

33. Eke PI, Wei L, Thornton-Evans GO, et al. Risk indicators for periodontitis in US adults: NHANES 2009 to 2012. *J Periodontol.* 2016;87(10):1174–1185.

34. Firmino RT, Ferreira FM, Paiva SM, et al. Oral health literacy and associated oral conditions: A systematic review. *J Am Dent Assoc.* 2017;148(8):604–613.

35. Franceschi C, Garagnani P, Vitale G, et al. Inflammaging and 'garb-aging'. *Trends Endocrinol Metab.* 2017;28(3):199–212.

36. Garcia D, Tarima S, Okunseri C. Periodontitis and glycemic control in diabetes: NHANES 2009 to 2012. *J Periodontol.* 2015;86(4): 499–506.

37. GBD 2015 DALYs and HALE Collaborators (610 collaborators). Global, regional, and national disability-adjusted life-years (DALYS) for 315 diseases and injuries and healthy life expectancy (HALE),

1990–2015: A systematic analysis for the global burden of disease study 2015. *Lancet.* 2016;388(10053):1603–1658.

38. GBD 2015 Disease and Injury Incidence and Prevalence Collaborators. Global, regional, and national incidence, prevalence, and years lived with disability for 310 diseases and injuries, 1990–2015: a systematic analysis for the global burden of disease study 2015. *Lancet.* 2016;388(10053):1545–1602.

39. Genco RJ. Current view of risk factors for periodontal diseases. *J Periodontol.* 1996;67(suppl 10):1041–1049.

40. Genco RJ, Borgnakke WS. Risk factors for periodontal disease. *Periodontol 2000.* 2013;62(1):59–94.

41. Genco RJ, Ho AW, Grossi SG, et al. Relationship of stress, distress and inadequate coping behaviors to periodontal disease. *J Periodontol.* 1999;70(7):711–723.

42. Guo R, Lin Y, Zheng Y, et al. The microbial changes in subgingival plaques of orthodontic patients: a systematic review and meta-analysis of clinical trials. *BMC Oral Health.* 2017;17(1):90.

43. Hajishengallis G, Darveau RP, Curtis MA. The keystone-pathogen hypothesis. *Nat Rev Microbiol.* 2012;10(10):717–725.

44. Hasuike A, Iguchi S, Suzuki D, et al. Systematic review and assessment of systematic reviews examining the effect of periodontal treatment on glycemic control in patients with diabetes. *Med Oral Patol Oral Cir Bucal.* 2017;22(2):e167–e176.

45. Hirotomi T, Yoshihara A, Ogawa H, et al. Tooth-related risk factors for periodontal disease in community-dwelling elderly people. *J Clin Periodontol.* 2010;37(6):494–500.

46. Holde GE, Baker SR, Jonsson B. Periodontitis and quality of life: What is the role of socioeconomic status, sense of coherence, dental service use and oral health practices? An exploratory theory-guided analysis on a Norwegian population. *J Clin Periodontol.* 2018;45 (7): 768–779.

47. Holmstrup P. Non-plaque-induced gingival lesions. *Ann Periodontol.* 1999;4(1):20–31.

48. Holmstrup P, Plemons J, Meyle J. Non-plaque-induced gingival diseases. *J Clin Periodontol.* 2018;45(suppl 20):S28–S43.

49. Ismail AI, Burt BA, Eklund SA. Epidemiologic patterns of smoking and periodontal disease in the united states. *J Am Dent Assoc.* 1983;106(5):617–621.

50. Javed F, Thafeed Alghamdi AS, Mikami T, et al. Effect of glycemic control on self-perceived oral health, periodontal parameters, and alveolar bone loss among patients with prediabetes. *J Periodontol.* 2014;85(2):234–241.

51. Jepsen S, Caton JG, Albandar JM, et al. Periodontal manifestations of systemic diseases and developmental and acquired conditions: consensus report of workgroup 3 of the 2017 World Workshop on the Classification of Periodontal and Peri-Implant Diseases and Conditions. *J Clin Periodontol.* 2018;45(suppl 20): S219–S229.

52. Kassebaum NJ, Bernabe E, Dahiya M, et al. Global burden of severe periodontitis in 1990–2010: A systematic review and meta-regression. *J Dent Res.* 2014;93(11):1045–1053.

53. Katagiri S, Nitta H, Nagasawa T, et al. Effect of glycemic control on periodontitis in type 2 diabetic patients with periodontal disease. *J Diabetes Investig.* 2013;4(3):320–325.

54. Kinane DF, Stathopoulou PG, Papapanou PN. Periodontal diseases. *Nat Rev Dis Primers.* 2017;3:17038.

55. Kocher T, König J, Borgnakke WS, et al. Periodontal complications of hyperglycemia/diabetes mellitus: Epidemiologic complexity and clinical challenge. *Periodontol 2000.* 2018;78(1):59–97.

56. Kotsakis GA, Chrepa V, Shivappa N, et al. Diet-borne systemic inflammation is associated with prevalent tooth loss. *Clin Nutr.* 2017.

57. Kowall B, Holtfreter B, Volzke H, et al. Pre-diabetes and well-controlled diabetes are not associated with periodontal disease: the ship trend study. *J Clin Periodontol.* 2015;42(5):422–430.

58. Kulkarni V, Bhatavadekar NB, Uttamani JR. The effect of nutrition on periodontal disease: a systematic review. *J Calif Dent Assoc.* 2014;42(5):302–311.

59. Lalla E, Papapanou PN. Diabetes mellitus and periodontitis: a tale of two common interrelated diseases. *Nat Rev Endocrinol.* 2011;7(12):738–748.

60. Lamont RJ, Hajishengallis G. Polymicrobial synergy and dysbiosis in inflammatory disease. *Trends Mol Med.* 2015;21(3):172–183.

61. Leira Y, Martin-Lancharro P, Blanco J. Periodontal inflamed surface area and periodontal case definition classification. *Acta Odontol Scand.* 2018;76(3):195–198.

62. Leite FRM, Nascimento GG, Scheutz F, et al. Effect of smoking on periodontitis: a systematic review and meta-regression. *Am J Prev Med.* 2018;54(6):831–841.

63. Locker D, Leake JL. Risk indicators and risk markers for periodontal disease experience in older adults living independently in Ontario, Canada. *J Dent Res.* 1993;72(1):9–17.

64. Löe H, Silness J. Periodontal disease in pregnancy. I. Prevalence and severity. *Acta Odontologica Scandinavica.* 1963;21(6):533–551.

65. Lula EC, Ribeiro CC, Hugo FN, et al. Added sugars and periodontal disease in young adults: an analysis of NHANES III data. *Am J Clin Nutr.* 2014;100(4):1182–1187.

66. Machtei EE, Christersson LA, Grossi SG, et al. Clinical criteria for the definition of "established periodontitis." *J Periodontol.* 1992;63(3):206–214.

67. Michalowicz BS, Diehl SR, Gunsolley JC, et al. Evidence of a substantial genetic basis for risk of adult periodontitis. *J Periodontol.* 2000;71(11):1699–1707.

68. Munz M, Willenborg C, Richter GM, et al. A genome-wide association study identifies nucleotide variants at SIGLEC5 and DEFA1A3 as risk loci for periodontitis. *Hum Mol Genet.* 2017;26(13):2577–2588.

69. Nascimento GG, Peres MA, Mittinty MN, et al. Diet-induced overweight and obesity and periodontitis risk: an application of the parametric g-formula in the 1982 Pelotas birth cohort. *Am J Epidemiol.* 2017;185(6):1–10.

70. Nibali L, Di Iorio A, Tu YK, et al. Host genetics role in the pathogenesis of periodontal disease and caries. *J Clin Periodontol.* 2017;44(suppl 18):S52–S78.

71. Page RC, Eke PI. Case definitions for use in population-based surveillance of periodontitis. *J Periodontol.* 2007;78(suppl 7):1387–1399.

72. Papapanou PN, Sanz M, Buduneli N, et al. Periodontitis: Consensus report of workgroup 2 of the 2017 World Workshop on the Classification of Periodontal and Peri-Implant Diseases and Conditions. *J Clin Periodontol.* 2018;45(suppl 20):S162–S170.

73. Petersen PE, Baez RJ. World Health Organization (WHO). In: *Oral Health Surveys: Basic Methods*: 5th ed. 2013. Available from: http://www.who.int/oral_health/publications/9789241548649/en.

74. Pihlstrom BL, Michalowicz BS, Johnson NW. Periodontal diseases. *Lancet.* 2005;366(9499):1809–1820.

75. Ramfjord SP. Indices for prevalence and incidence of periodontal disease. *J Periodontol.* 1959;30(1):51–59.

76. Sanders AE, Essick GK, Beck JD, et al. Periodontitis and sleep disordered breathing in the Hispanic community health study/study of Latinos (seecomment by billings2015). *Sleep.* 2015;38(8): 1195–1203.

77. Sanders AE, Slade G. State cigarette excise tax, secondhand smoke exposure, and periodontitis in us nonsmokers. *Am J Public Health.* 2013;103(4):740–746.

78. Sanz M, Ceriello A, Buysschaert M, et al. Scientific evidence on the links between periodontal diseases and diabetes: consensus report and guidelines of the Joint Workshop on Periodontal Diseases and Diabetes by the International Diabetes Federation and the European Federation of Periodontology. *J Clin Periodontol.* 2018;45(2):138–149.

79. Schaefer AS, Richter GM, Nothnagel M, et al. A genome-wide association study identifies GLT6D1 as a susceptibility locus for periodontitis. *Hum Mol Genet.* 2010;19(3):553–562.

80. Sheiham A, Watt RG. The common risk factor approach: a rational basis for promoting oral health. *Community Dent Oral Epidemiol.* 2000;28(6):399–406.

81. Silness J, Löe H. Periodontal disease in pregnancy. II. Correlation between oral hygiene and periodontal condition. *Acta Odontol Scand.* 1964;22:121–135.

82. Susin C, Haas AN, Albandar JM. Epidemiology and demographics of aggressive periodontitis. *Periodontol 2000.* 2014;65(1):27–45.

83. The Forsyth Institute. *Expanded Human Oral Microbiome Database (eHOMD).* Available from: http://www.homd.org/#expanded; 2019.

84. Tonetti MS, Bottenberg P, Conrads G, et al. Dental caries and periodontal diseases in the ageing population: call to action to protect and enhance oral health and well-being as an essential component of healthy ageing—consensus report of group 4 of the joint EFP/ORCA workshop on the boundaries between caries and periodontal diseases. *J Clin Periodontol.* 2017;44(suppl 18):S135–S144.

85. Tonetti MS, Claffey N. Advances in the progression of periodontitis and proposal of definitions of a periodontitis case and disease progression for use in risk factor research. Group C consensus report of the 5th European workshop in periodontology. *J Clin Periodontol.* 2005;32(suppl 6):210–213.

86. Tonetti MS, Greenwell H, Kornman KS. Staging and grading of periodontitis: framework and proposal of a new classification and case definition. *J Clin Periodontol.* 2018;45(suppl 20):S149–S161.

87. Trombelli L, Franceschetti G, Farina R. Effect of professional mechanical plaque removal performed on a long-term, routine basis in the secondary prevention of periodontitis: a systematic review. *J Clin Periodontol.* 2015;42(suppl 16):S221-236.

88. U. S. Department of Health and Human *Services. Smoking and health; report of the Advisory Committee to the Surgeon General of the Public Health Service.* 386 pp. 1964. Available from: https://www.govinfo.gov/app/details/GPO-SMOKINGANDHEALTH/context

89. US Department of Health and Human Services. Office of the Surgeon General. *The Health Consequences of Smoking: A Report of the Surgeon General.* 2004; Atlanta GA. Available from: https://www.cdc.gov/tobacco/data_statistics/sgr/2004/complete_report/index.htm.

90. Varela-Lopez A, Giampieri F, Bullon P, et al. A systematic review on the implication of minerals in the onset, severity and treatment of periodontal disease. *Molecules.* 2016;21(9):1183.

91. Vieira AR, Albandar JM. Role of genetic factors in the pathogenesis of aggressive periodontitis. *Periodontol 2000.* 2014;65(1):92–106.

92. Vogtmann E, Graubard B, Loftfield E, et al. Contemporary impact of tobacco use on periodontal disease in the USA. *Tob Control.* 2017;26(2):237–238.

93. Volpe AR, Manhold JH, Hazen SP. *In vivo* calculus assessment. I. A method and its examiner reproducibility. *J Periodontol.* 1965;36:292–298.

94. Wagenknecht DR, BalHaddad AA, Gregory RL. Effects of nicotine on oral microorganisms, human tissues, and the interactions between them. *Curr Oral Health Rep.* 2018;5(1):78–87.

95. Wang J, Lv J, Wang W, et al. Alcohol consumption and risk of periodontitis: a meta-analysis. *J Clin Periodontol.* 2016;43(7):572–583.

96. Wiener RC. Relationship of routine inadequate sleep duration and periodontitis in a nationally representative sample. *Sleep Disord.* 2016;2016(NoIss):9158195.

97. Wu M, Chen SW, Jiang SY. Relationship between gingival inflammation and pregnancy. *Mediators Inflamm.* 2015;2015. 623427.

98. Xie CJ, Xiao LM, Fan WH, et al. Common single nucleotide polymorphisms in cyclooxygenase-2 and risk of severe chronic periodontitis in a chinese population. *J Clin Periodontol.* 2009;36(3):198–203.

# 16

# Measurement and Distribution of Oral Cancer

ATHANASIOS I. ZAVRAS, DMD, DDS, MS, DrMedSc

JAYAPRIYAA R. SHANMUGHAM, BDS, MPH, DrPH

## Description and Classification of Oral Cancer

The general term "oral cancer" is used to describe a malignancy of epithelial origin that is found in the oral cavity, lip, nasopharynx, oropharynx, and/or pharynx. These malignancies are classified by the International Classification of Diseases (ICD) coding system as C00–C06 (for malignant neoplasms of the lip, tongue, gums, floor of mouth, palate, and other parts of the mouth); C09–13 (tonsils, oropharynx, nasopharynx, and other pharyngeal sites); and C14 (other unspecified areas in the lip, oral cavity, and pharynx). Cancers of the salivary glands, coded as C07 and C08, are excluded from the traditional definition of epithelial oral cancer and are not discussed in this chapter.[68]

The ICD was originally developed by the World Health Organization (WHO) as a global reference classification system. An updated ICD-10 released in October 2018 is the current version of the coding system that is in use globally. In the United States, the National Center for Health Statistics (NCHS) adapted the coding system to develop the ICD-10 Clinical Modification, comparable to WHO's original version, to be used primarily by healthcare providers to classify and code health conditions. While the ICD-10 classification scheme is broadly used, alternative nomenclature may include head and neck cancer (HNC), head and neck squamous cell carcinoma (HNSCC), oral squamous cell carcinoma (OSCC), oropharyngeal carcinoma (OPC), and oral cavity cancers (OCC).

Oral cancers can also be classified based on histologic characteristics.[71] The mucosal epithelial lining of the oral cavity is made of stratified squamous epithelial cells, which line the inside of the oral cavity, nose, pharynx, larynx, and throat. Neoplasms derived from this layer are referred to as oral squamous cell carcinoma (OSCC). OSCC is the most common type of oral cancer, and more than 90% of diagnosed oral cancers are OSCCs.[64] Subtypes of OSCCs include papillary, anaplastic, keratinizing, and nonkeratinizing squamous cell carcinoma. In addition to the stratified squamous epithelium, several other tissues in the head and neck, such as salivary glands (major and minor), bone and lymphatic tissues, and melanin-producing melanocytes, may develop malignancies as well.

## Measurement of Oral Cancer

Measures used to describe the overall burden of oral cancer include rates such as incidence, mortality and survival, and proportions such as prevalence. Age-adjusted or age-standardized incidence rates are weighted averages of age-specific rates and are particularly helpful statistics as they allow comparisons across different populations with different age distributions. Lifetime risk for oral cancer portrays the cumulative probability of oral cancer incidence or mortality, whereas prevalence proportions are useful in describing existing cases as a reflection of past incidence and survival. Survival rates, specifically 5-year survival rates, are important measures that describe the proportion of patients surviving 5 years or more following the diagnosis of oral cancer.[58] The Surveillance, Epidemiology and End Results program (SEER) in the United States (US), supported by the National Cancer Institute (NCI), is the nation's leading source of information on the distribution of malignancies based on data from population-based cancer registries from 19 geographic areas scattered across the United States and represents approximately 34% of the population. SEER cancer distribution and survival results are usually presented stratified in the following categories: localized (cancer that is localized to its original site); regional (cancer that has spread to regional lymph nodes); distant (cancer that has metastasized to distant tissues); and unknown stage.

The staging of cancer is a vital process that is used not only for statistical purposes and surveillance but also to assist clinicians in planning treatment and patient management. The tumor, node, and metastasis (TNM) staging system is the most commonly used staging system for cancers.[14] It was developed and is currently maintained and published in the *Cancer Staging Manual* (CSM) by the American Joint Committee on Cancer (AJCC). TNM describes the tumor's location, the extent of cancer, the presence of regional lymph node involvement, and distant metastasis. The AJCC first published the CSM in 1977 with the most recent (eighth) edition released in 2018.[33] Updates in the latest edition include the subgrouping of oropharyngeal cancers based on the presence or absence of human papilloma virus (HPV), a risk factor for oral cancer, and updated tumor and nodal staging of cancers of oral cavity and nasopharynx.

Finally, in addition to measures of occurrence, survival and staging, qualitative measures, such as quality of life (QoL), have been developed in the last decade to track and report important patient outcomes, such as various functional dimensions during or after treatment and patient satisfaction.[48]

# Risk Factors and Risk Indicators for Oral cancer

In the United States, tobacco use is an important risk factor for oral cancer and is used in various forms, such as cigarette, cigar or pipe smoking, and smokeless tobacco use (chewing tobacco or snuff). Other established risk factors include excessive alcohol intake and oral oncogenic HPV infection, followed by secondary factors, such as genetic susceptibility, diet, and marijuana use.[17] Existence of Potentially Malignant Disorders (PMDs) or premalignant oral lesions such as leukoplakia, erythroplakia, etc may also be viewed as a risk factor, and it is discussed later.

## Cigarette Smoking

Cigarette smoking continues to be an important risk factor for oral cancer globally, with about 25% of oral cancer cases developing among smokers.[25] According to the Global Health Observatory (GHO), more than 1.1 billion people around the world smoke tobacco.[45] Smoking is an important risk factor in the United States and a leading cause for significant morbidity and mortality. Although dramatic reductions in smoking prevalence have been reported since the dawn of the 21st century, an estimated 40 million US adults and 4.7 million middle school and high school students currently smoke some form of tobacco.[27,54] Smoking is more prevalent among men (17.5%) when compared to women (13.5%), adults 45 to 64 years of age (18%), and among American Indians/Alaska Natives (31.8%) followed by whites (16.6%) and blacks (16.5%).[27] Smoking is most prevalent in the Midwest (18.5%) followed by the South (16.9%) and more prevalent among individuals of lower income and educational levels.[27]

The International Agency for Research on Cancer (IARC) has established that tobacco smoking is causally associated with oral cancer.[49] A dose response has been established. For current smokers, those who smoke more cigarettes have a higher risk compared to those smoking fewer cigarettes. For past smokers, those who smoked for longer durations and those who began smoking at younger ages are at a higher risk for oral cancer. With regards to gender differences, women tend to smoke less than men in the developed world but at equal rates in developing nations.[64] The effects of smoking tend to be more severe among women than among men. Previous studies have reported that the risk for oral cancer measured in pack-years (number of cigarette packs smoked per day over the total number of years smoked) is four times higher among women who smoked more than 18 pack-years, whereas among men the risk was comparatively lower for those who smoked for more than 30 pack-years.[34,74]

## Smokeless Tobacco

Smokeless tobacco is less popular than cigarette smoking in the United States. In 2014, 3% of adults 18 years and older and 6% of high school students used some form of smokeless tobacco.[57] Men were more likely to use smokeless tobacco compared to women (6.7% vs. 0.3% respectively), and this habit is more common among non-Hispanic American Indians/Alaska Natives (7.1%). Smokeless tobacco use was highest in Wyoming, West Virginia, Montana, and Mississippi. Forms of smokeless tobacco include snuff (dry or wet), chewing tobacco, and tobacco strips or sticks.[3] Epidemiologic evidence reports that among those who use moist snuff or chew tobacco, the relative risk (RR) for oral cancer ranges from 0.6 to 1.7, whereas among dry snuff users, the risk of oral cancer is 4 to 13 times higher.[11] The primary carcinogenic agent in smokeless tobacco associated with the development of oral cancer is tobacco specific nitrosamines (TCNS).[17] Although smokeless tobacco is often promoted as a tool to control or quit cigarette smoking—and sometimes even promoted by manufacturers as a "risk reduction" strategy to reduce the probability of lung cancer—evidence suggests that various forms of smokeless tobacco are associated with an increased risk of oral cancer.[57] Smokeless tobacco is increasingly prevalent worldwide, particularly in Asian countries, where it is often combined with betel quid chewing. Betel quid chewing, a mixture of the areca nut, with tobacco and lime, is highly carcinogenic and more common in Southeast Asian countries with prevalence rates ranging between 25% to as high as 80%.[22] Interestingly, betel quid chewing is more common among women than men, and in highly prevalent regions, 90% of oral cancer cases among women are among betel quid users.

## Alcohol Consumption

Alcohol consumption has been increasingly prevalent globally, with the highest consumption in European countries, ranging from 13.5 to 17.5 liters per capita per year, which is about 25% of the total alcohol consumed worldwide.[45] High levels of alcohol drinking have been associated with increased risk of various types of cancer, particularly cancers of the liver, digestive tract, and oral cavity. Overall, 7% to 19% of oral cancer cases are attributable to alcohol consumption, and those who consume four to five drinks per day are at two to three times higher risk for oral cancer.[45] Evidence from various studies report relative risks ranging from 3.2 to 9.2 for those consuming more than 60 g/day (equivalent to approximately four drinks per day) when adjusting for tobacco smoking.[19] In fact, heavy consumption of alcohol has been found to be an independent risk factor of oral cancer, causing up to 19% of oral cancer cases among nonsmokers.[24] In the United States, oral cancer incidence is higher among men who consume more than two drinks per day and women who consume more than one drink per day. However, it is the joint use of smoking and alcohol drinking that causes the highest risk. Those exposed to high amounts of tobacco and alcohol experience more than 15 times higher oral cancer risk.[25]

What exactly causes such a disproportionately high risk among those who are heavy users of tobacco and alcohol has been the subject of multiple studies, but the methodologic limitations of those studies pose interpretation challenges. Most epidemiologic studies in oral cancer involve men, especially smokers. Collinearity between smoking and alcohol drinking is one example of a methodologic challenge when trying to disentangle causative pathways. Another challenge is the small samples of female participants in the studies of nonsmokers.[24]

Like tobacco use, gender differences seem to exist when comparing the risk for oral cancer among alcohol drinkers based on intensity and duration. Previous evidence reports oral cancer risks up to three times higher at very high alcohol intake (>60 g/day) among men, whereas recent evidence suggests that among women even with moderate drinking the risk starts to increase.[69] For example, the increase in risk for oral cancer for every 10 g of alcohol intake is higher among women (relative risk [RR]: 1.18; 95% CI: 1.04 to 1.33) when compared to men (RR: 1.15; 95% CI: 1.10 to 1.20) in one cohort study,[65] and in another study,[15] at one to three drinks per day, the risk increases almost three times higher among women (RR: 1.74; 0.95 to 3.20) than among men (RR: 1.22; 0.85 to 1.76). One limitation is that these cohort studies included small samples of female drinkers. Overall the role and extent of alcohol as a risk factor of oral cancer among women is based on mostly case-control studies.[4,24] A large multicenter pooled analysis of 15 case-control studies from North America, Europe, and South America showed that overall the odds ratio (OR) for three or more drinks/day versus no drinking was two times higher (OR: 2.04; 95% CI: 1.29 to 3.21) among never-users of tobacco, and this increased to almost three times higher for those consuming more than five drinks per day (OR: 2.8; 95% CI: 1.49 to 5.27).[24] The observed gender differences in oral cancer risk may be due to varying levels of susceptibility to alcohol-induced carcinogenesis and differences in gastric metabolism, which in turn may affect the bioavailability of acetaldehyde in the oral epithelial tissue.[5] Studies on cancer of the liver have shown that liver damage is higher among females when compared to men at lower intake of alcohol and shorter duration of intake.

In studies designed to look at the role of diet in oral cancer, low serum folate levels have been reported among head and neck cancer patients.[16] One example of a high-quality prospective study that looked at diet and oral cancer is the Nurses' Health Study (NHS), a cohort of 87,621 female registered nurses who were followed for 26 years.[50] In this study, women who consumed over 30 g of alcohol per day were at almost two times higher risk for oral cancer when compared to nondrinkers. The investigators in this study also reported a significant interaction between folate intake and alcohol consumption. Those who consumed more than 30 g/day and reported low folate intake (<350 μg/day) had a significantly higher risk for oral cancer (RR: 3.36; 95% CI: 1.57 to 7.20). In another large prospective analysis of approximately 84,000 registered female nurses (NHS data) age 34 to 59 years over a period of 16 years, those who consumed high amounts of alcohol (>30 g/day) and low total folate (<180 μg/day) reported the highest risk for major

chronic disease, which included alcohol-related cancers as a group.[28] Observational studies report similar findings on the role of folate in protecting against oral cancer risk. Interestingly, the mechanism related to the role of folate on the relationship between alcohol and oral cancer has been studied in recent years. Folate is important for DNA synthesis, methylation, and repair.[23] Cleavage of folate can occur in the microenvironment of the oral cavity, deterring the positive effects of folate, where the metabolism of acetaldehyde from ethanol can also occur. Thus, alcohol may impair folate status and metabolism, which in turn can disrupt DNA synthesis, methylation, and repair of the oral squamous epithelial cells leading to carcinogenesis.

## Human Papilloma Virus (HPV)

Human papilloma virus (HPV) is another important factor that has been identified to increase the risk of specific types of oral cancer. Since the late 20th century, there has been a decline in the rates of oral cancers that is associated with smoking and drinking, particularly in developed countries.[10] However, a rise in oropharyngeal cancer incidence has been reported among younger adults and among those with nontraditional risk profiles. This change in trend may be attributed to the prevalence of high-risk oncogenic HPV in intraoral infections. HPV is a nonencapsulated double-stranded DNA virus that infects the basal epithelial layer of the squamous epithelium through microabrasions, penetration, and vegetative replication.[9] HPV infection has been reported to be a necessary cause for cervical cancer, which is the fourth most common cancer among women globally.[70] Among more than 100 strains of HPV reported globally, HPV 16 and 18 are considered the most common high-risk strains and have been reported in more than 70% of cervical cancers. HPV was first identified as a potential carcinogenic virus in the risk for oral cancer in the late 20th century. Epidemiologic evidence suggests that more than 20% of oral cancers and 60% to 80% of oropharyngeal cancers are caused by HPV globally, with a population attributable risk of 26%.[13] Prevalence is higher among developed countries in Europe (Sweden) and in the United States and among younger individuals and males. In the United States, between 1999 and 2015, HPV-related oropharyngeal SCCs increased among men (2.7% per year) and women (0.8% per year). Notably, a decrease of 1.6% per year was observed in HPV-related cervical cancers.[61] Currently oropharyngeal SCCs are the most common HPV-related cancers in the United States, with 18,917 cases reported in 2015, 82% among men and 18% among women.

The comparison between HPV-related oropharyngeal cancer with other types of oral cancer is important for public health reasons. While oropharyngeal cancers have increased significantly over the last decade, with the national age-adjusted incidence rates being 2.4/100,000, non-HPV–related oral cavity cancers show higher incidence rates nationally (11.3/100,000) and are caused primarily by smoking and alcohol drinking.[41]

NCHS data from 2011 to 2015 show that 63% and 51% of all oropharyngeal SCCs among men and women, respectively, are related to HPV strains 16 or 18.[62] The prevalence of HPV-related oral SCCs is highest among whites (1.9%) followed by blacks (1.3%) and are more prevalent in the Midwest and Southern regions (1.9% in both regions). Epidemiologic evidence suggests that the increase in oral HPV infections may be due to a recent increase in oral sexual activity among young adults.[2] Prophylactic vaccination against a limited set of high-risk HPV strains is currently in place to prevent cervical cancers. Immunity against the vaccinated strains HPV 16 and 18 would protect against oropharyngeal cancers. However, because of the long duration of oral carcinogenesis, there is currently limited evidence regarding the effectiveness of vaccination in the prevention of oral HPV infection and HPV-related oral cancers.[29] Other viruses, such as the Epstein Barr virus (EBV) and hepatitis C virus (HCV), have also been explored as potential risk factors, but limited evidence is available on the level of risk and pathogenesis of OSCC.[35]

## Dietary Factors

Dietary factors, particularly the protective effects of fruit and vegetable intake, play a role in the epidemiology of oral cancer. In industrialized countries, dietary factors account for approximately 30% of cancers overall and 10% to 15% of oral cancers.[45,72] According to the WHO, poor nutrition has a higher toll on oral cancer statistics in developing countries, where 60% of cancers of the oral cavity, pharynx, and esophagus are attributed to a low intake of fruits and vegetables.[72] Fruits and vegetables are rich in anticarcinogenic compounds, including antioxidants, carotenoids, fiber, folate, flavonoids, plant sterols, phenolic acids, and vitamin C, which play a role in reducing the risk for oral cancer.[55] There is some evidence that the anticarcinogenic effect of a diet rich in fruits can possibly offset the cancerous effect of tobacco smoking. In the late 20th century, reports from the World Cancer Research Fund (WCRF) and American Institute for Cancer Research (AICR) suggested that the effect of total fruits and vegetables on decreasing the risk for cancer of the mouth, pharynx, larynx, esophagus, stomach, and lung as "probable."[18] Prospective studies in the United States have evaluated the inverse association of fruits and vegetables and the risk for oral cancer, confirming strong inverse associations with increased intake of fruits (RR range: 0.65–0.87) and vegetables (RR range: 0.53–0.65).[16,37] In Europe, the European Prospective Investigation into Cancer and Nutrition study (EPIC) documented a strong protective association related to the intake of fruits but not for vegetables.[6] Meta-analysis of several case-controls studies also reported a significant decrease of about 40% to 60% in oral cancer risk among those with a high intake of fruits and vegetables.[43] Other evidence suggests that vegetable intake was protective for oral cancer but not fruit intake.[47] A matched case-control study from Greece on the relationship between overall diet and oral cancer reported a significantly lower risk for oral cancer among those with a higher intake of cereals and lipids, such as olive oil.[44] This study also reported a lower risk among those with a higher intake of micronutrients, such as riboflavin, magnesium, and iron. The protective effect from consuming plant-based foods may be due to the vitamin and mineral content of fruits and vegetables. Vitamin D deficiency is reported to be higher among those with oral cancer, but the association is weak and needs further corroboration.[20] Stronger evidence is reported for the antioxidant effect of vitamin E in the prevention of oral cancer and in decreasing the risk of malignant transformation of precancerous lesions.[36]

## Potentially Malignant Disorders

Oral premalignant lesions—or more appropriately, potentially malignant disorders (PMD)—are a group of oral lesions that exhibit increased probability for malignant transformation if left undiagnosed and untreated.[40,73] The most common oral PMDs include leukoplakia, erythroplakia, and submucous fibrosis. Other oral PMDs include lichen planus, discoid lupus erythematosus, and abnormal palatal lesions in reverse smokers. Common risk factors for oral PMDs include tobacco smoking, alcohol, diet, and more recently, HPV infections.

**Malignant Transformation of PMD:** In oral PMD, it is believed that malignant transformation is a multistate process and occurs as a result of progressive changes and cellular alterations in populations of cells that are already "initiated." Genetic and epigenetic factors seem to play a role in such transformation, as the epithelium responds to environmental insults and the tissue moves from its normal state to a dysplastic state to malignancy. While PMDs are diagnosed clinically, histologically the tissue exhibits certain unique characteristics, all described under the term oral epithelial dysplasia (OED).[59] Dysplastic regions are characterized by increasing numbers of atypical and immature cells and decreasing numbers of mature cells. According to a recent WHO workshop, OED is stratified as mild, moderate, and severe dysplasia and carcinoma in situ. In a more recent pilot study, a binary grading system for predicting malignant transformation has been developed to classify OED as low risk or high risk for malignant transformation and was found to be 82% accurate with sensitivity and specificity of 85% and 80%, respectively.[31] Malignant transformation rate (MTR) is a useful measure to evaluate the rate of disease progression in oral PMDs. A meta-analysis of 16 cohort studies using data from different geographic regions calculated the average MTR by comparing the incidence rate of malignant cases developing among those with mild, moderate, or severe dysplasia.[51] The pooled MTR for confirmed OED patients was reported to be 10.5% and varies by severity of dysplasia (Table 16.1). The rate of malignant transformation varies by each type of PMD as reported later and therefore becomes a valuable tool in aiming for early diagnosis and setting up individualized monitoring plans for patients.

**Types of PMD: Leukoplakia** is the most common oral PMD. It was first identified in the late 1800s and is defined clinically as a white patch or plaque that cannot be scraped off and that cannot be characterized as any other disease.[40] There are various types of leukoplakia, including homogenous, speckled, verrucous, and proliferative verrucous leukoplakia. Leukoplakia can occur at any age, including among young adults and most commonly among males. The average worldwide prevalence of leukoplakia is around 2%, with prevalence proportions ranging from 1.1% to 11.7% globally.[46] Based on data from a pooled analysis, the oral cancer rate attributable to leukoplakia was reported to be between 6.2 and 29.1 per 100,000. Tobacco smokers are more likely to develop leukoplakia than nonsmokers.[60] A dose-response relationship has been reported between tobacco smoking and leukoplakia, with a significant regression following the cessation of smoking. Alcohol is another risk factor for leukoplakia and plays a role in accelerating malignant transformation.[38,53] Leukoplakia that develops on the floor of the mouth, the lateral surface of tongue and on the lower lip show higher rates of malignant transformation. For example, buccal lesions have a lower MTR (3.53%), whereas cancers of the tongue have much higher transformation rates (24.22%).[1] Factors that contribute to malignant transformation include larger lesions with longer duration, increased epithelial dysplasia, and presence of candida infection.[59] Based on epidemiologic data from 24 studies between 1960 and 2013, the overall mean MTR for leukoplakia was reported to be 14.9%, with a range of 0.13% to 34%.[63] Among the various types of leukoplakia, speckled leukoplakia and erosive leukoplakia are at higher risk for transforming into carcinoma.[59]

• **TABLE 16.1** Malignant Transformation Rates for Mild, Moderate and Severe Oral Epithelial Dysplasia[51] .

| First Author | Year | ORAL EPITHELIAL DYSPLASIA | | | | MALIGNANT TRANSFORMATION | | | | | | | |
|---|---|---|---|---|---|---|---|---|---|---|---|---|---|
| | | Total | Mild | Mod | Sev | Total | Mild | Mod | Sev | Total | Mild | Mod | Sev |
| Bánóczy (13) | 1976 | 68 | 13 | 43 | 12 | 9 | 1 | 3 | 5 | 13.2% | 7.7% | 7.0% | 41.7% |
| Mincer (17) | 1972 | 45 | NA | 32 | 13 | 5 | NA | 2 | 3 | 11.1% | NA | 6.3% | 23.1% |
| Gupta (7) | 1980 | 90 | NA | NA | NA | 6 | NA | NA | NA | 6.7% | NA | NA | NA |
| Lumerman (18) | 1995 | 43 | 19 | 18 | 6 | 7 | 3 | 3 | 1 | 16.3% | 15.8% | 16.7% | 16.7% |
| Cowan (12) | 2001 | 165 | NA | NA | NA | 24 | NA | NA | NA | 14.6% | NA | NA | NA |
| Holmstrup (11) | 2006 | 82 | 42 | 26 | 14 | 8 | 5 | 2 | 1 | 9.8% | 11.9% | 7.7% | 7.1% |
| Hsue (8) | 2007 | 166 | NA | NA | NA | 8 | NA | NA | NA | 4.8% | NA | NA | NA |
| Ho (9) | 2009 | 33 | NA | NA | NA | 8 | NA | NA | NA | 24.2% | NA | NA | NA |
| Arduino (16) | 2009 | 207 | 135 | 50 | 22 | 15 | 4 | 2 | 9 | 7.3% | 3.0% | 4.0% | 43.0% |
| Bradley (21) | 2010 | 1434 | 959 | 326 | 149 | 139 | 47 | 43 | 49 | 9.7% | 4.9% | 13.2% | 32.9% |
| Liu (10) | 2011 | 138 | 92 | NA | 46 | 37 | 17 | NA | 20 | 26.8% | 18.5% | NA | 43.5% |
| Warnakulasuriya (15) | 2011 | 204 | 104 | 70 | 30 | 24 | 5 | 11 | 8 | 11.8% | 4.8% | 15.7% | 26.7% |
| Ho (14) | 2012 | 91 | 40 | 31 | 20 | 23 | 8 | 11 | 11 | 25.3% | 20.0% | 35.5% | 55.0% |
| Zhang (22) | 2012 | 296 | 127 | 135 | 34 | 41 | 16 | 19 | 6 | 13.9% | 12.6% | 14.1% | 17.7% |
| Sperandio (19) | 2013 | 201 | 103 | 69 | 29 | 17 | 4 | 7 | 6 | 8.5% | 3.9% | 10.1% | 20.7% |
| Dost (20) | 2014 | 368 | 221 | 85 | 55 | 26 | 9 | 6 | 1 | 7.1% | 4.1% | 7.1% | 1.8% |

NA: Not available

**Erythroplakia** is defined as a red velvety patch or plaque that cannot be characterized as any other definable disease. It occurs mostly in the floor of the mouth, lateral side of the tongue, retromolar pad, and soft palate region.[60] Types of erythroplakia include homogenous erythroplakia, erythroleukoplakia (erythroplakia speckled with white patches), and speckled erythroplakia. Erythroplakia is less common than leukoplakia, with worldwide prevalence ranging from 0.02% to 0.83%. It is more common among 60- to 70-year-olds and among males.[60] Tobacco smoking and alcohol are the most common risk factors. Although the prevalence is much lower for erythroplakia, the malignant transformation rates are highest in erythroplakia, ranging from 20% to 68% when compared to all other premalignant lesions.[60]

**Oral submucous fibrosis** (OSF) is a chronic and debilitating premalignant disorder that is characterized by inflammation and fibrosis of the mucosal lining, most commonly in the buccal region but sometimes in the oropharyngeal region as well.[39] OSF is most prevalent in the Asian subcontinent, with a prevalence of 0.2% to 1.2%. Although smoking and alcohol are potential risk factors, areca nut, an ingredient in betel quid chewing, is the primary risk factor for OSF.[26] Overall the MTR varies between 2% and 8% but can increase to 30% in the Asian subcontinent where the prevalence of OSF and betel quid chewing is higher.

Oral lichen planus (OLP) has the lowest prevalence compared to other oral PMDs, with a global prevalence of approximately 1% and risk factors that are similar to other PMDs.[59] Over the years, inconsistent results have been reported on the malignant potential of OLP, as there is some suggestion that oral lichenoid lesions (OLL), which appear similar to OLP, may have higher malignant potential.[52] The MTR for OLP is reported to be less than 1%, but this is based on limited evidence, and more evaluation is needed.

## Distribution of Oral Cancer

### Incidence of Oral Cancer

In the United States, the estimated number of new oral cancer cases in 2018 was 51,540, with 10,030 deaths.[58] The median age at diagnosis is 63 years with the highest incidence between 55 to 75 years of age. In 1975, the overall age-adjusted incidence rate of cancers of the oral cavity and pharynx was 13.2 per 100,000, whereas this declined to 11.8 per 100,000 in 2015.[41] In the period of 2011 to 2015, the age-adjusted oral cancer incidence among adults under 65 years was 6.7 per 100,000, whereas among older individuals (>65 years) the incidence increased to 42.9 per 100,000. Over the years, a steady increase in incidence is evident among adults 50 years and older (Figure 16.1A). A decline in incidence rates has been reported among blacks since the beginning of the 21st century, whereas incidence rates have been increasing among whites, particularly non-Hispanic whites (Figure 16.1B). When comparing trends by gender, the incidence has been increasing among males since the earlier part of the 21st century (Figure 16.1C). This recent increase in incidence in males could be due to higher incidence of HPV-related oropharyngeal cancers particularly among white males.[41] In 2015 SEER data the cancer incidence among white males was 18.5 per 100,000, whereas the incidence among black males was 13.6 per 100,000.[41] When compared to black females (5.3 per 100,000), the incidence was also higher among white females (6.9 per 100,000).[41]

Worldwide, oral cancer is among the top 20 cancers worldwide among both men and women.[7,67] A report released in 2018 from the WHO IARC highlighted that the overall cancer burden has increased. For oral cancer, 354,864 new cases were estimated for 2018 (oral cavity and lip combined) with age standardized rate (ASR) of incidence at 4 in 100,000 cases.[67] Similar to the findings from the United States, globally the incidence rate increases with age, and it triples between the middle and the older age groups. The incidence ranges between 6.4 per 100,000 at 45 to 49 years of age to 20.8 per 100,000 for those older than 70 years of age. Regions with highest human development report higher ASR of incidence (4.3 per 100,000) when compared to less developed regions (ASR 1.9 per 100,000). Among males the incidence is higher (ASR 5.8 per 100,000) when compared to females (2.3 per 100,000).

## Mortality

In the United States, the first 17 years of the 21st century brought about declines in the mortality rates when compared to the 20th century.[41] In 1975, the overall age-adjusted mortality rate was 4.3 per 100,000. In 2015, the mortality rate decreased to 2.5 per 100,000.[41] Similar to the trends observed in incidence, the mortality rates also increase with increasing age. Overall, the oral cancer mortality rate is 1.1 per 100,000 among those younger than 65 and climbs to 12 per 100,000 for older Americans. Males have a higher mortality rate (3.9 per 100,000) than females (1.3 per 100,000). With regards to racial disparities, overall, higher mortality rates were reported in 2011 to 2015 among black males (4.8 per 100,000) in comparison to white males (3.8 per 100,000).[41] Minor differences in mortality rates were reported between white and black females, with more recent trends showing a slight increase in rates among white females.

Globally, the number of estimated deaths from oral cancer was 177,384 in 2018 (ASR of mortality 2/100,000).[67] In contrast to the trends in incidence rates, the mortality rates are higher in less developed regions. Mortality trends also vary by WHO region (Figure 16.2). Mortality rates are highest in the Southeast Asian region (ASR 4.6 per 100,000) and lowest in the Americas (ASR 0.9 per 100,000).[67] Worldwide, higher mortality is reported among older individuals and males.

## Prevalence of Oral Cancer

Prevalence estimates are useful because they provide information on the total number of existing (live) cases. Based on 2015 SEER data, the overall prevalence in the United States was reported to be 359,718 cases.[41] Higher prevalence was observed among males when compared to females, a finding that is related to the higher incidence in males.

Globally, geographic patterns in oral cancer are based on local variations in exposure to lifestyle risk factors.[21,45] In 2018, the overall 3-year prevalence for cancer of the oral cavity and lip was 620,445 (8.1 per 100,000).[67] The highest prevalence proportions for oral cancer were reported in the Southeast Asia region followed by the European region, but this trend is currently reversing. High prevalence of oral and pharyngeal cancers was also reported in France and Hungary, increasing prevalence of oral and oropharyngeal cancers was reported in the United States whereas high prevalence of lip cancer was reported in Australia and Brazil.[21,67]

## Survival and Patient Outcomes

Based on data reported by SEER, the overall 5-year relative survival rate for oral cancer was lower in the mid-70s (52.5%) between

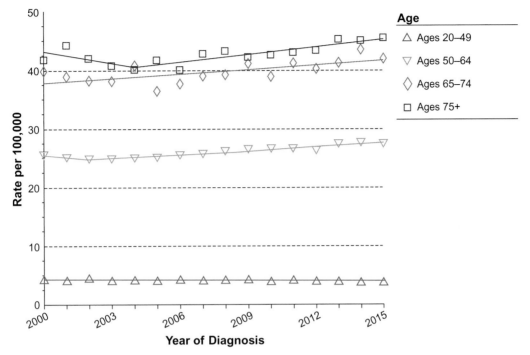

Oral Cavity and Pharynx Cancer
Recent Trends in SEER Incidence Rates, 2000–2015
By Age
Both Sexes, All Races (includes Hispanic), Observed Rates

SEER 18 areas [http://seer.cancer.gov/registries/terms.html] (San Francisco, Connecticut, Detroit, Hawaii, Iowa, New Mexico, Seattle, Utah, Atlanta, San Jose-Monterey, Los Angeles, Alaska Native Registry, Rural Georgia, California excluding SF/SJM/LA, Kentucky, Louisiana, New Jersey and Georgia excluding ATL/RG).
Rates are per 100,000 and are age-adjusted to the 2000 US Std Population (19 age groups - Census P25-1130).
Cancer Incidence Rates Adjusted for Reporting Delay. [https://surveillance.cancer.gov/delay/]
The Annual Percent Change (APC) estimates were calculated from the underlying rates using the Joinpoint Trend Analysis Software [http://surveillance.cancer.gov/joinpoint], Version 4.6, February 2018, National Cancer Institute.
The APC's direction is "rising" when the entire 95% confidence interval (C.I.) is above 0, "falling" when the entire 95% C.I. is lower than 0, otherwise, the trend is considered stable.
Rates for American Indians/Alaska Natives only include cases that are in a Contract Health Service Delivery Area (CHSDA). See SEER Race Recode Documentation for American Indian/Alaskan Native Statistics [http://seer.cancer.gov/seerstat/variables/seer/race_ethnicity/#ai-an].
Hispanics and non-Hispanics are not mutually exclusive from whites, blacks, Asian/Pacific Islanders, and American Indians/Alaska Natives. Incidence data for Hispanics and non-Hispanics are based on the NAACCR Hispanic Latino Identification Algorithm (NHIA) and exclude cases from the Alaska Native Registry. See SEER Race Recode Documentation for Spanish-Hispanic-Latino Ethnicity [http://seer.cancer.gov/seerstat/variables/seer/race_ethnicity/#hispanic].
Cancer sites are defined using the SEER Site Recode ICD-O-3/WHO 2008 Definition [https://seer.cancer.gov/siterecode/icdo3_dwhoheme/index.html].
Created by seer.cancer.gov/explorer/application.php on 02/27/2019 10:58 pm.

(A)

• **Figure 16.1** SEER age-adjusted incidence rates for cancer of the oral cavity and pharynx in the United States by (A) age, (B) race/ethnicity, and (C) sex—SEER 18 2000–2015.[41]

*(Continued)*

1975 and 1977. The relative survival has significantly improved since the 1970s ($P < 0.05$) and is currently 67.9% based on data available from 2008 to 2014.[41] Females have higher survival rates (69.7%) when compared to males (67.1%). Survival is better among younger adults, for example, survival rate among those diagnosed before the age of 45 years was 80%. This decreases as age at diagnosis increases, with survival rates decreasing to as low as 56.5% for those diagnosed at or after 65 years.[41] Survival rates are higher among whites when compared to blacks, and this has not changed over the years since the 20th century. Between 2008 and 2014, the overall survival rates for whites was 69.7%, whereas among blacks it was 49.6%. The survival rates decrease to 39% for cases diagnosed in the distant stage where the cancer has

metastasized. These SEER data also report that 20% of oral cancer cases are diagnosed in the distant stage (Figure 16.3). Location of cancer also determines survival, with higher survival rates for cancer of the tongue (65%) and lower survival when the cancer reaches the oropharynx (40%).

## Quality of Life

Developing a malignancy in the oral cavity or pharynx can have a dramatic and severe impact on the patient's overall health, quality of life (QoL) and survival, due to the location of the tumors and the invasiveness of the treatments.[48] The oral cavity is critical for several functions of everyday life, such as mastication, swallowing,

**Oral Cavity and Pharynx Cancer**
**Recent Trends in SEER Incidence Rates, 2000–2015**
**By Race/Ethnicity**
**Both Sexes, All Ages, Observed Rates**

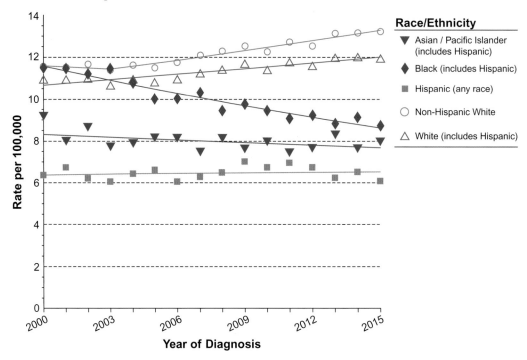

SEER 18 areas [http://seer.cancer.gov/registries/terms.html] (San Francisco, Connecticut, Detroit, Hawaii, Iowa, New Mexico, Seattle, Utah, Atlanta, San Jose-Monterey, Los Angeles, Alaska Native Registry, Rural Georgia, California excluding SF/SJM/LA, Kentucky, Louisiana, New Jersey and Georgia excluding ATL/RG).
Rates are per 100,000 and are age-adjusted to the 2000 US Std Population (19 age groups - Census P25-1130).
Cancer Incidence Rates Adjusted for Reporting Delay. [https://surveillance.cancer.gov/delay/]
The Annual Percent Change (APC) estimates were calculated from the underlying rates using the Joinpoint Trend Analysis Software [http://surveillance.cancer.gov/joinpoint], Version 4.6, February 2018, National Cancer Institute.
The APC's direction is "rising" when the entire 95% confidence interval (C.I.) is above 0, "falling" when the entire 95% C.I. is lower than 0, otherwise, the trend is considered stable.
Rates for American Indians/Alaska Natives only include cases that are in a Contract Health Service Delivery Area (CHSDA). See SEER Race Recode Documentation for American Indian/Alaskan Native Statistics [http://seer.cancer.gov/seerstat/variables/seer/race_ethnicity/#ai-an].
Hispanics and non-Hispanics are not mutually exclusive from whites, blacks, Asian/Pacific Islanders, and American Indians/Alaska Natives. Incidence data for Hispanics and non-Hispanics are based on the NAACCR Hispanic Latino Identification Algorithm (NHIA) and exclude cases from the Alaska Native Registry. See SEER Race Recode Documentation for Spanish-Hispanic-Latino Ethnicity [http://seer.cancer.gov/seerstat/variables/seer/race_ethnicity/#hispanic].
Cancer sites are defined using the SEER Site Recode ICD-O-3/WHO 2008 Definition [https://seer.cancer.gov/siterecode/icdo3_dwhoheme/index.html].
Created by seer.cancer.gov/explorer/application.php on 02/27/2019 11:02 pm.

(B)

• **Figure 16.1,** cont'd

taste, speech, and salivation.[56] Patients may be affected on the emotional, psychologic, and social levels due to the pain, discomfort, and sometimes loss of function caused by the disease or the resulting treatment. Several studies have been conducted to evaluate QoL in oral cancer patients, including randomized clinical trials, and evaluate the effect of symptoms, disease, and treatment factors. Overall QoL scores are lower in the initial period but tend to slowly rise in the years that follow treatment. QoL scores are better among older patients in the first year after treatment, with no difference in scores between males and females. Lower scores are reported among patients with cancers of the posterior aspect of the tongue and oropharynx, which affect basic functions, and with cancers diagnosed in later stages. Facial appearance and

disfigurement are major concerns among oral cancer patients undergoing treatment. Emotional stress, an increased level of anxiety, and depression are common among head and neck cancer patients.

## Oral Cancer and Public Health

### Impact of Oral Cancer Trends

Historically, epidemiologic evidence over the years has clearly demonstrated that cigarette smoking and alcohol drinking are the two major causes of oral cancer[45] both globally and in the United States, as described in this chapter. This trend continues in the current decade, and causal associations between smoking and oral

Oral Cavity and Pharynx Cancer
Recent Trends in SEER Incidence Rates, 2000–2015
By Sex
All Races (includes Hispanic), All Ages, Observed Rates

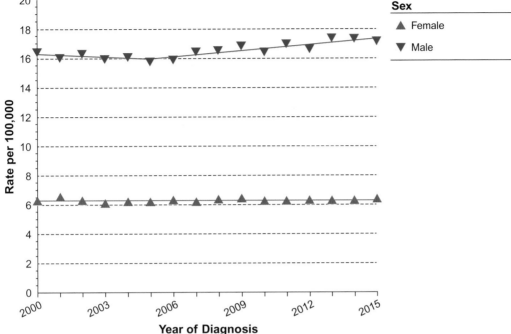

SEER 18 areas [http://seer.cancer.gov/registries/terms.html] (San Francisco, Connecticut, Detroit, Hawaii, Iowa, New Mexico, Seattle, Utah, Atlanta, San Jose-Monterey, Los Angeles, Alaska Native Registry, Rural Georgia, California excluding SF/SJM/LA, Kentucky, Louisiana, New Jersey and Georgia excluding ATL/RG).
Rates are per 100,000 and are age-adjusted to the 2000 US Std Population (19 age groups - Census P25-1130).
Cancer Incidence Rates Adjusted for Reporting Delay. [https://surveillance.cancer.gov/delay/]
The Annual Percent Change (APC) estimates were calculated from the underlying rates using the Joinpoint Trend Analysis Software [http://surveillance.cancer.gov/joinpoint], Version 4.6, February 2018, National Cancer Institute.
The APC's direction is "rising" when the entire 95% confidence interval (C.I.) is above 0, "falling" when the entire 95% C.I. is lower than 0, otherwise, the trend is considered stable.
Rates for American Indians/Alaska Natives only include cases that are in a Contract Health Service Delivery Area (CHSDA). See SEER Race Recode Documentation for American Indian/Alaskan Native Statistics [http://seer.cancer.gov/seerstat/variables/seer/race_ethnicity/#ai-an].
Hispanics and non-Hispanics are not mutually exclusive from whites, blacks, Asian/Pacific Islanders, and American Indians/Alaska Natives. Incidence data for Hispanics and non-Hispanics are based on the NAACCR Hispanic Latino Identification Algorithm (NHIA) and exclude cases from the Alaska Native Registry. See SEER Race Recode Documentation for Spanish-Hispanic-Latino Ethnicity [http://seer.cancer.gov/seerstat/variables/seer/race_ethnicity/#hispanic].
Cancer sites are defined using the SEER Site Recode ICD-O-3/WHO 2008 Definition [https://seer.cancer.gov/siterecode/icdo3_dwhoheme/index.html].
Created by seer.cancer.gov/explorer/application.php on 02/27/2019 11:00 pm.

(C)

• Figure 16.1, cont'd

cancer, and alcohol intake and oral cancer have been established by evidence reported by the World Cancer Research Fund (WCRF), AICR, and the IARC.[69] Dental health professionals have a unique role in screening for oral cancer risk factors and for early signs of malignancy, and can actively work toward increasing knowledge and awareness among patients on the harmful risks of smoking and alcohol drinking.

The late 20th century and early 21st century witnessed a new trend, with increasing numbers of HPV-related oropharyngeal SCCs. As mentioned previously, the burden of disease from HPV-related oropharyngeal cancer now exceeds that of HPV-related cervical cancers,[61] yet the public remains relatively uninformed. Although oropharyngeal cancers are just a subset of oral cancer, oropharyngeal cancers pose a significant public health concern (see previous section on HPV). Dental health professionals can play a significant role in preventive efforts to avoid intraoral HPV

infections through patient education, as well as in screening for the oral presence of high-risk HPV. Given the proven effectiveness of HPV vaccinations in reducing cervical and other cancers, dental professionals are also considering their role in vaccinating boys and girls against high-risk HPV. Expanding dentists' scope of practice to vaccinate against high-risk HPV may allow for an increased number of vaccinated children. By participating in such public health efforts, dental health professionals may play a vital role in decreasing the morbidity and mortality of oropharyngeal cancers.

## Economic Impact

Oral cancer is a complex disease requiring a multidisciplinary approach to treatment and management, leading to costs that have a severe economic impact on public health. The costs involved in the management of oral cancer depend on various factors, such as

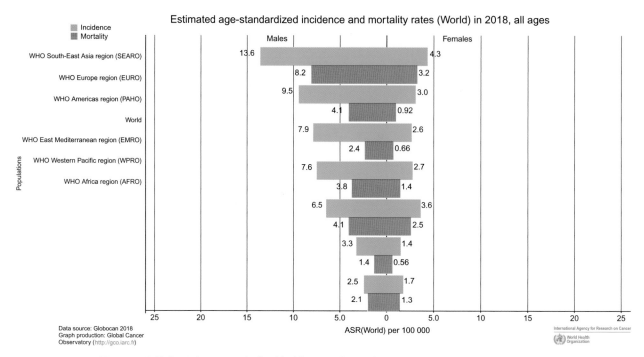

• **Figure 16.2** Estimated age-standardized incidence and mortality rates worldwide for cancer of the oral cavity and lip—age-standardized rates (ASR) per 100,000 among males and females, 2018.[67]

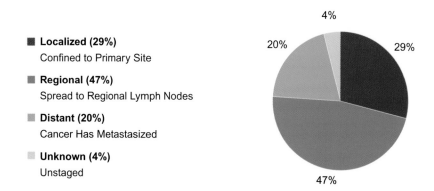

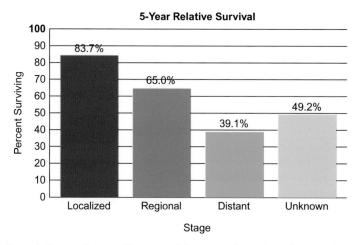

• **Figure 16.3** Percent of cases diagnosed by stage of disease at diagnosis and 5-year relative survival by stage of diagnosis – SEER 18 2008-2014.[41]

stage, severity, site of cancer, and patient factors, such as demographics, comorbidities, and access to care.[66] In the United States between 2007 and 2013, only 30% of the cases were diagnosed when the disease was localized. The majority of the cases were diagnosed when the disease had spread.[58] In a review of 77 studies between 2003 to 2013, investigators reported that patients with early stage head and neck cancer may require only one treatment modality, whereas patients diagnosed with oral cancer that has localized to lymph nodes require a combination of treatments.[66] This review, which included mostly studies from the United States, also reported that the majority of the expense was due to systemic therapies rather than surgery or radiotherapy. However, due to price controls of drugs in Europe, costs tend to be higher for surgical procedures in European studies.

In an analysis of excess direct medical costs among patients with head and neck cancer using SEER Medicare data, investigators reported $369 million excess cost in 2010 when compared to those without head and neck cancer.[51] Using data between 1995 and 2005, investigators also reported $11,450 more in costs among blacks when compared to whites. Another pooled analysis reported annual expenditures of $3.18 billion in 2008 dollars as attributable costs for patients with head and neck cancer.[12]

In a recent analysis of economic burden of head and neck cancers conducted by the authors, data from the Centers for Medicaid and Medicare (CMS) and wage data from the World Bank Group were abstracted and evaluated. In this analysis, patients were categorized based on stage of disease and by single or combination treatment modalities. Mean costs of treatment in the first 3 months were calculated along with costs for the 5-year follow-up period. The study included dental rehabilitation costs for the 5-year postoperative period and loss of pay and expenses related to hospital stay. In this analysis, the total economic loss annually for new cases of head and neck cancer in 2018 was reported to be $4.4 billion, which included treatment costs, rehabilitation, and loss of wages (Table 16.2). The cost per patient and total costs were higher for patients with advanced stage of head and neck cancer and for those who received more than one treatment, such as surgery and radiotherapy or surgery and chemotherapy. This analysis concurs with previous evidence that the economic burden can be significantly decreased for oral cancer–related costs when the cancer is diagnosed in the earlier stages.

## Screening and Early Detection

Although the benefits of diagnosing oral cancer early are significant, the US Preventive Services Task Force (USPSTF) has found insufficient evidence to support population screening by primary care physicians for the early detection of oral cancer.[42] Opposition to population screening of asymptomatic adults by their primary care physicians is mainly due to the low prevalence of the condition and the high risk of false positives and false negatives.[8] However, recent comprehensive reviews have concluded that while overall there is insufficient evidence for such screening of asymptomatic individuals, there is evidence that screening may be effective in decreasing mortality among high-risk individuals such as smokers and/or alcohol drinkers.[8,42] Because the majority of oral cancer cases are preceded by premalignant lesions or PMDS, an opportunity exists to identify these lesions early and to monitor them aggressively for signs of malignant transformation.[59] This aggressive monitoring should be performed by dentists and other healthcare professionals with appropriate training and should take into consideration the rate of disease progression based on the type and severity of PMD and the types and severity of exposure to risk factors.

**• TABLE 16.2**  **Total Medical Costs for Initial 3 Months of Treatment and 5-Year Follow-up. Data Stratified by Stage and Payor Type (Private vs. Government), using data from 2012.**

| Private Payors | Surgery | S + RT | S + CRT | CRT | Cost per Patient | No. of Patients | Total Cost |
|---|---|---|---|---|---|---|---|
| Stage 1 | $48,665 | $0 | $0 | $0 | $48,665 | 9,031 | $439,504,905 |
| Stage 2 | $24,333 | $0 | $0 | $128,886 | $153,218 | 2,852 | $436,972,833 |
| Stage 3 | $10,323 | $29,342 | $60,440 | $62,490 | $162,595 | 3,327 | $541,000,685 |
| Stage 4 | $2,704 | $43,035 | $69,254 | $57,282 | $172,275 | 8,556 | $1,473,968,837 |
| | | | | | Total cost for 2012 (all stages combined) | | $2,891,447,260[a] |

| Government Payor | Surgery | S + RT | S + CRT | CRT | Cost per Patient | No. of Patients | Total Cost |
|---|---|---|---|---|---|---|---|
| Stage 1 | $20,363 | $0 | $0 | $0 | $20,363 | 7,096 | $144,495,196 |
| Stage 2 | $10,182 | $0 | $0 | $37,329 | $47,511 | 2,241 | $106,463,049 |
| Stage 3 | $4,319 | $13,529 | $16,780 | $18,099 | $52,728 | 2,614 | $137,846,467 |
| Stage 4 | $1,131 | $19,843 | $19,228 | $16,591 | $56,792 | 6,722 | $381,784,740 |
| | | | | | Total cost for 2012 (all stages combined) | | $770,589,452[b] |

Abbreviations – CRT, Chemoradiation therapy; RT, radiation therapy; S, surgery.

[a,b]Original calculations performed in 2012.

[a]Assuming a 2.62% annual medical inflation rate between 2012 and 2018, total private payer expenses for 2018 in US dollars: $3,377,760,568

[b]Assuming a 2.62% annual medical inflation rate between 2012 and 2018, total public payer expenses for 2018 in US Dollars: $999,216,563

Total direct medical costs for oral cancer in US dollars taking into consideration the annual medical inflation rate between 2012 – 2018 is 4,376,977,131

Risk-based screening is defined as targeted screening of individuals with easily identifiable risk factors. Risk-based screening has gained acceptance in dentistry, especially in the management of dental caries. However, risk-based screening for oral cancer, the most lethal disease of the oral cavity, is not yet broadly accepted by the medical community. Advances in cellular genetic and epigenetic analysis will soon allow risk-based screening to become more efficient by further stratifying high-risk individuals to narrower, better defined strata of risk. As highlighted in previous sections, the benefits of screening for oral cancer include reductions in mortality, morbidity and economic savings.[30] In a recent cost-effectiveness analysis of risk-based screening of a theoretical US population of approximately 10 million high-risk individuals between the ages of 40 and 80 years, with estimated screening costs of $200 per person, the total screening costs were calculated at $2 billion. This excess cost for screening has the potential to reduce significantly the much higher annual treatment-related cost of $4.3 billion (see Table 16.2) via early detection and early treatment, while improving health outcomes.

Risk-based screening and monitoring for oral cancer should become part of a national wellness strategy that mobilizes the organized efforts of dental health professionals. Allocating the time to use simple visual inspection during provision of standard clinical care can be vital in detecting early lesions. In addition, appropriate training can be provided to dental health personnel in conducting visual inspection and identification of lesions, which can minimize inaccuracies and improve accuracy of detection, thus allowing more efficient screening. While various technologies such as toluidine blue, oral cytology, brush biopsy, DNA- and RNA-based genetic arrays, and various light-based detection methods are available, these methods need further investigation to evaluate their efficacy in diagnosing early lesions.[32]

Oral cancer is a debilitating disease that affects the patients' quality of life and leads to high morbidity and avoidable mortality. A national evidence- and risk-based screening approach should become part of a coherent national strategy to control the burden of this dreadful disease.

# References

1. Anderson A, Ishak N. Marked variation in malignant transformation rates of oral leukoplakia. *Evid Based Dent.* 2015;16(4):102–103.
2. Bajos N, Bozon M, Beltzer N, et al. Changes in sexual behaviours: from secular trends to public health policies. *AIDS.* 2010;24(8):1185–1191.
3. Bassiony M, Ail A, Khalili M, et al. Tobacco consumption and oral, pharyngeal and lung cancers. *Open Cancer J.* 2015;8:1–11. https://benthamopen.com/contents/pdf/TOCJ/TOCJ-8-1.pdf.
4. Blot WJ, McLaughlin JK, Winn DM, et al. Smoking and drinking in relation to oral and pharyngeal cancer. *Cancer Res.* 1988;48(11):3282–3287.
5. Blume SB. Women and alcohol. A review. *JAMA.* 1986;256(11):1467–1470.
6. Boeing H, Dietrich T, Hoffmann K, et al. Intake of fruits and vegetables and risk of cancer of the upper aero-digestive tract: the prospective EPIC-study. *CCC.* 2006;17(7):957–969.
7. Bray F, Ferlay J, Soerjomataram I, et al. Global cancer statistics 2018: GLOBOCAN estimates of incidence and mortality worldwide for 36 cancers in 185 countries. *CA Cancer J Clin.* 2018;68:394–424.
8. Brocklehurst P, Kujan O, O'Malley LA, et al. Screening programmes for the early detection and prevention of oral cancer. *Cochrane Database Syst Rev.* 2013;(11). CD004150.
9. Campisi G, Panzarella V, Giuliani M, et al. Human papillomavirus: its identity and controversial role in oral oncogenesis, premalignant and malignant lesions (review). *Int J Oncol.* 2007;30(4):813–823.
10. Chaturvedi AK, Engels EA, Pfeiffer RM, et al. Human papillomavirus and rising oropharyngeal cancer incidence in the United States. *J Clin Oncol.* 2011;29(32):4294–4301.
11. Chi AC, Day TA, Neville BW. Oral cavity and oropharyngeal squamous cell carcinoma—an update. *CA Cancer J Clin.* 2015;65(5):401–421.
12. Coughlan D, Frick KD. PCN150 Direct medical costs of head and neck cancer in the United States: an analysis using pooled Medical Expenditure Panel Survey (MEPS) data. *Value Health.* 2012;15(4):A235.
13. de Martel C, Ferlay J, Franceschi S, et al. Global burden of cancers attributable to infections in 2008: a review and synthetic analysis. *Lancet Oncol.* 2012;13(6):607–615.
14. Edge S, Byrd D, Compton C, et al. *Head and Neck Cancer Staging.* 7th ed. Chicago, IL: Springer; 2010.
15. Freedman N, Absent C, Leitzmann M, et al. A prospective study of tobacco, alcohol, and the risk of esophageal and gastric cancer subtypes. *Am J Epidemiol.* 2007;165:1424–1433.
16. Freedman ND, Park Y, Subar AF, et al. Fruit and vegetable intake and head and neck cancer risk in a large United States prospective cohort study. *Int J Cancer.* 2008;122(10):2330–2336.
17. Gillison ML. Current topics in the epidemiology of oral cavity and oropharyngeal cancers. *Head Neck.* 2007;29(8):779–792.
18. Glade MJ. Food, nutrition, and the prevention of cancer: a global perspective. American Institute for Cancer Research/World Cancer Research Fund, American Institute for Cancer Research, 1997. *Nutrition.* 1999;15(6):523–526.
19. Goldstein BY, Chang SC, Hashibe M, et al. Alcohol consumption and cancers of the oral cavity and pharynx from 1988 to 2009: an update. *Eur J Cancer Prev.* 2010;19(6):431–465.
20. Grimm M, Cetindis M, Biegner T, et al. Serum vitamin D levels of patients with oral squamous cell carcinoma (OSCC) and expression of vitamin D receptor in oral precancerous lesions and OSCC. *Med Oral Patol Oral Cir Bucal.* 2015;20(2):e188–e195.
21. Gupta N, Gupta R, Acharya AK, et al. Changing trends in oral cancer - a global scenario. *Nepal J Epidemiol.* 2016;6(4):613–619.
22. Gupta PC, Ray CS. Epidemiology of betel quid usage. *Ann Acad Med Singapore.* 2004;33(suppl 4):31–36.
23. Hamid A, Wani NA, Kaur J. New perspectives on folate transport in relation to alcoholism-induced folate malabsorption—association with epigenome stability and cancer development. *FEBS J.* 2009;276(8):2175–2191.
24. Hashibe M, Brennan P, Benhamou S, et al. Alcohol drinking in never users of tobacco, cigarette smoking in never drinkers, and the risk of head and neck cancer: pooled analysis in the International Head and Neck Cancer Epidemiology Consortium. *J Natl Cancer Inst.* 2007;99(10):777–789.
25. Hashibe M, Brennan P, Chuang SC, et al. Interaction between tobacco and alcohol use and the risk of head and neck cancer: pooled analysis in the International Head and Neck Cancer Epidemiology Consortium. *Cancer Epidemiol Biomarkers Prev.* 2009;18(2):541–550.
26. Ho PS, Yang YH, Shieh TY, et al. Consumption of areca quid, cigarettes, and alcohol related to the comorbidity of oral submucous fibrosis and oral cancer. *Oral Surg Oral Med Oral Pathol Oral Radiol Endod.* 2007;104(5):647–652.
27. Jamal A, Phillips E, Gentzke AS, et al. Current cigarette smoking among adults—United States, 2016. *MMWR Morb Mortal Wkly Rep.* 2018;67(2):53–59.
28. Jiang R, Hu FB, Giovannucci EL, et al. Joint association of alcohol and folate intake with risk of major chronic disease in women. *Am J Epidemiol.* 2003;158(8):760–771.
29. Kim HJ. Current status and future prospects for human papillomavirus vaccines. *Arch Pharm Res.* 2017;40(9):1050–1063.
30. Kujan O, Glenny AM, Oliver RJ, et al. Screening programmes for the early detection and prevention of oral cancer. *Cochrane Database Syst Rev.* 2006;(3). CD004150.
31. Kujan O, Oliver RJ, Khattab A, et al. Evaluation of a new binary system of grading oral epithelial dysplasia for prediction of malignant transformation. *Oral Oncol.* 2006;42(10):987–993.

32. Lingen MW, Kalmar JR, Karrison T, et al. Critical evaluation of diagnostic aids for the detection of oral cancer. *Oral Oncol.* 2008;44(1):10–22.

33. Lydiatt W, Patel S, O'Sullivan B, et al. Head and neck cancers-major changes in the American Joint Committee on cancer eighth edition cancer staging manual. *CA Cancer J Clin.* 2017;67(2):122–137.

34. Macfarlane GJ, Zheng T, Marshall JR, et al. Alcohol, tobacco, diet and the risk of oral cancer: a pooled analysis of three case-control studies. *Eur J Cancer B Oral Oncol.* 1995;31b(3):181–187.

35. Marcopoulos AK. Current aspects on oral squamous cell carcinoma. *Open Dent J.* 2012;6:126–130.

36. Maserejian NN, Giovannucci E, Rosner B, et al. Prospective study of vitamins C, E, and A and carotenoids and risk of oral premalignant lesions in men. *Int J Cancer.* 2007;120(5):970–977.

37. Maserejian NN, Giovannucci E, Rosner B, et al. Prospective study of fruits and vegetables and risk of oral premalignant lesions in men. *Am J Epidemiol.* 2006;164(6):556–566.

38. Maserejian NN, Joshipura KJ, Rosner BA, et al. Prospective study of alcohol consumption and risk of oral premalignant lesions in men. *Cancer Epidemiol Biomarkers Prev.* 2006;15(4):774–781.

39. Messadi DV. Diagnostic aids for detection of oral precancerous conditions. *Int J Oral Sci.* 2013;5(2):59–65.

40. Nair DR, Pruthy R, Pawar U, et al. Oral cancer: Premalignant conditions and screening—an update. *J Cancer Res Ther.* 2012;8(suppl 1).S57–S66.

41. Noone A, Howlader N, Krapcho M, et al. *SEER Cancer Statistics Review, 1975–2015*, National Cancer Institute, based on November 2017 SEER data submission, posted to the SEER web site April 2018. Available from https://seer.cancer.gov/csr/1975_2015.

42. Olson CM, Burda BU, Beil T, et al. *U.S. Preventive Services Task Force Evidence Syntheses, formerly Systematic Evidence Reviews. Screening for Oral Cancer: A Targeted Evidence Update for the US Preventive Services Task Force.* Rockville, MD: Agency for Healthcare Research and Quality; 2013.

43. Pavia M, Pileggi C, Nobile CG, et al. Association between fruit and vegetable consumption and oral cancer: a meta-analysis of observational studies. *Am J Clin Nutr.* 2006;83(5):1126–1134.

44. Petridou E, Zavras AI, Lefatzis D, et al. The role of diet and specific micronutrients in the etiology of oral carcinoma. *Cancer.* 2002;94(11):2981–2988.

45. Petti S. Lifestyle risk factors for oral cancer. *Oral Oncol.* 2009;45(4-5):340–350.

46. Petti S. Pooled estimate of world leukoplakia prevalence: a systematic review. *Oral Oncol.* 2003;39(8):770–780.

47. Riboli E, Norat T. Epidemiologic evidence of the protective effect of fruit and vegetables on cancer risk. *Am J Clin Nutr.* 2003;78(3 Suppl):559s–569s.

48. Rogers SN, Ahad SA, Murphy AP. A structured review and theme analysis of papers published on 'quality of life' in head and neck cancer: 2000–2005. *Oral Oncol.* 2007;43(9):843–868.

49. Sadri G, Mahjub H. Tobacco smoking and oral cancer: a meta-analysis. *J Res Health Sci.* 2007;7(1):18–23.

50. Shanmugham J, Zavras A, Rosner B, et al. Alcohol-folate interactions in women's oral cancer risk: a prospective cohort study. *Cancer Epidemiol Biomarkers Prev.* 2010;19(10):2516–2524.

51. Shariff J, Zavras A. Malignant transformation rate in patients presenting oral epithelial dysplasia: systemic review and meta-analysis. *J Oral Dis.* 2015;1–10.

52. Shirasuna K. Oral lichen planes: Malignant potential and diagnosis. *Oral Science International.* 2014;11(1):1–7.

53. Shiu MN, Chen TH. Impact of betel quid, tobacco and alcohol on three-stage disease natural history of oral leukoplakia and cancer: implication for prevention of oral cancer. *Eur J Cancer Prev.* 2004;13(1):39–45.

54. Singh T, Arrazola RA, Corey CG, et al. Tobacco Use Among Middle and High School Students–United States, 2011–2015. *MMWR Morb Mortal Wkly Rep.* 2016;65(14):361–367.

55. Taghavi N, Yazdi I. Type of food and risk of oral cancer. *Arch Iran Med.* 2007;10(2):227–232.

56. Torres-Carranza E, Infante-Cossio P, Hernandez-Guisado JM, et al. Assessment of quality of life in oral cancer. *Med Oral Patol Oral Cir Bucal.* 2008;13(11). E735-41.

57. US Public Health Service, Centers for Disease Control and Prevention (CDC). A clinical practice guideline for treating tobacco use and dependence: a report, 2008 update. *Am J Prev Med.* 2008;35(2):158–176.

58. US Public Health Service, National Cancer Institute (NCI). SEER Cancer Surveillance 2018. *Oral Cavity and Pharynx Cancer.* Available from: http://seer.cancer.gov/statfacts/html/oralcav.html.

59. van der Waal I. Oral potentially malignant disorders: is malignant transformation predictable and preventable? *Med Oral Patol Oral Cir Bucal.* 2014;19(4):e386–e390.

60. van der Waal I. Potentially malignant disorders of the oral and oropharyngeal Article ID: 854636:1-10. mucosa; terminology, classification and present concepts of management. *Oral Oncol.* 2009;45(4-5):317–323.

61. Van Dyne E, Henley S, Saraiya M, et al. Trends in human papillomavirus–associated cancers—United States, 1999–2015. *MMWR Morb Mortal Wkly Rep.* 2018;67:918–924.

62. Viens LJ, Henley SJ, Watson M, et al. Human papillomavirus-associated cancers—United States, 2008–2012. *MMWR Morb Mortal Wkly Rep.* 2016;65(26):661–666.

63. Warnakulasuriya S, Ariyawardana A. Malignant transformation of oral leukoplakia: a systematic review of observational studies. *J Oral Pathol Med.* 2016;45(3):155–166.

64. Warnakulasuriya S. Global epidemiology of oral and oropharyngeal cancer. *Oral Oncol.* 2009;45:309–316.

65. Weikert C, Dietrich T, Boeing H, et al. Lifetime and baseline alcohol intake and risk of cancer of the upper aero-digestive tract in the European Prospective Investigation into Cancer and Nutrition (EPIC) study. *Int J Cancer.* 2009;125:406–412.

66. Wissinger E, Griebsch I, Lungershausen J, et al. The economic burden of head and neck cancer: a systematic literature review. *Pharmacoeconomics.* 2014;32(9):865–882.

67. World Health Organization (WHO), International Agency for Research on Cancer (IARC). Globocan. In: *Cancer Incidence, Mortality and Prevalence Worldwide, 2018.* IARC; 2018. Available from: http://gco.iarc.fr.

68. World Health Organization (WHO) Library Cataloguing-in-Publication Data. *WHO International Statistical Classification of Diseases and Related Health Problems (ICD),* 2016.

69. World Health Organization (WHO), International Agency for Research on Cancer (IARC) working group on the evaluation of carcinogenic risk to humans. *Part E: Personal Habits and Indoor Combustions. Consumption of Alcoholic Beverages.* France: Lyon; 2012. Available from: https://www.ncbi.nlm.nih.gov/books/NBK304390.

70. World Health Organization (WHO), International Agency for Research on Cancer (IARC). Biological agents. A review of human carcinogens. *IARC Monogr.* 2012;100(Pt B):1–441.

71. World Health Organization (WHO), International Agency for Research on Cancer (IARC). *Histological Classification of Tumours.* 4th ed. IARC; 2017.

72. World Health Organization (WHO). Diet, nutrition and the prevention of chronic diseases. *WHO Tech Rep Ser.* 2003;916:1–149, i–viii.

73. Yardimci G, Kutlubay Z, Engin B, et al. Precancerous lesions of oral mucosa. *World J Clin Cases.* 2014;2(12):866–872.

74. Zavras AI, Douglass CW, Joshipura K, et al. Smoking and alcohol in the etiology of oral cancer: gender-specific risk profiles in the south of Greece. *Oral Oncol.* 2001;37(1):28–35.

# 17

# Measurement and Distribution of Edentulism and Tooth Retention

**VINODH BHOOPATHI, BDS, MPH, DScD**

**HIROKO IIDA, DDS, MPH**

## CHAPTER OUTLINE

Description and Etiology of Tooth Loss
Measurement of Tooth Loss
Risk Factors and Risk Indicators for Tooth Loss
Distribution of Tooth Loss
    Edentulism
    Tooth Retention
Tooth Loss and Public Health

## Description and Etiology of Tooth Loss

Tooth loss, especially edentulism or complete tooth loss, is considered "the dental equivalent of mortality."[3,65] The primary reason that teeth are lost is that they are extracted by dentists most commonly due to consequences of dental diseases, such as dental caries or periodontitis.[52] However, not all carious or periodontally affected teeth are lost during the lifetime, and there are various factors that may contribute to tooth loss in different subgroups. Tooth loss can lead to morbid oral health and psychologic health consequences.[8,51] An individual with complete or partial tooth loss may experience difficulty in chewing and speaking and also may have low self-esteem, which altogether can affect his or her oral health–related quality of life.[51] Tooth loss and tooth retention are, therefore, important oral health indicators measured in many national and worldwide surveys to determine the oral health status and well-being of an individual and the community.

## Measurement of Tooth Loss

Unlike other dental diseases and conditions, measurement of tooth loss does not require complex indices. Tooth loss is measured by counting the number of missing teeth. The challenge, especially in surveillance, is to validate the etiology of tooth loss—separating tooth loss occurring due to disease compared to other reasons, such as extraction for orthodontic treatment—by investigating past events. Complete tooth loss or edentulism is defined as having all natural teeth missing, including third molars.[9-11] Partial tooth loss is loss of some teeth due to caries or periodontal disease. Complete tooth retention is defined as having all 28 natural permanent teeth present, excluding third molars.[10,11] A "functional dentition" is another measure of tooth retention, derived from the concept that an individual must have a minimal set of natural teeth to have adequate dental function without needing prosthetic replacements.[16,40] The presence of 21 or more natural teeth is the definition of functional dentition that is often used.[16,40]

## Risk Factors and Risk Indicators for Tooth Loss

It was once believed that caries was the main reason for tooth loss before age 35 and periodontal disease the main reason after age 35.[3] This thought process, however, has changed considerably. Many studies show demographic characteristics, health behaviors, environment, and systemic conditions as possible risk factors/indicators linked to tooth loss.

Demographic factors, such as race/ethnicity and socioeconomic status (SES) indicators measured by education and income, are associated with tooth loss.[19,32,63] The National Health and Nutritional Health Survey (NHANES) data indicate that those with fewer years of education and those with lower incomes are more likely to have a greater number of missing teeth or be edentulous.[32,63] The influences of socioeconomic factors on tooth loss are not consistent across race/ethnicity.[29,43] Jimenez and colleagues found that the associations between SES and tooth loss were weaker for African American and Mexican American adults (18 years and older) than for Whites.[29] Naorungroj et al. reported that education was inversely associated with the incidence of tooth loss in African Americans ages 53 to 74 years, while lower income was a predictor of tooth loss among Whites.[43] SES also influences having dental insurance and use of dental care[36] and therefore consequently may affect oral health outcomes, such as tooth loss. Data from the Florida Dental Care Study showed that subjects (45 years and older) of lower SES and African Americans had worse oral health status (having fewer teeth and oral symptoms) at baseline and were more likely to have lost teeth and continue to have oral symptoms 48 months later than their counterparts.[20] Being an African American was also associated with getting care at busier dental practices and practices that performed a greater number of dental extractions each month after controlling for dental disease factors.[20]

Among the lifestyle factors, smoking is most frequently associated with tooth loss.[1,6,7,33,42] While the association between poor diet and tooth loss is less clear, it is known that the number and distribution of teeth lost influences masticatory ability and efficiency and therefore can influence an individual's food preferences or choices.[30,55] Studies have reported that being edentulous is associated with lower consumption of dietary fiber, fresh fruits, vegetables, and proteins and increased consumptions of soft processed foods.[26,27,30,44,55,62]

Certain systemic diseases and conditions are associated with tooth loss. Diabetes has a bidirectional relationship with tooth loss.[34] For example, type 2 diabetes increases the risk for periodontitis, and periodontitis is associated with reduced glycemic control in those with diabetes.[5,54] While no study has determined causality or elucidated biological mechanisms, tooth loss is also reportedly linked to diabetes mellitus,[5,47,54] cardiovascular diseases,[14,15,45,56] cancer,[35,39] and other conditions, such as obesity, rheumatoid arthritis, and respiratory/pulmonary diseases.[17]

Eklund and Burt reported the importance of early tooth loss as a determinant of edentulism.[13] Their findings may imply the importance of examining early life influences on the risk of tooth loss as well as the historical or cumulative effect of risk factors across the life stages. Associations between tooth loss and depression,[46,53,60] social isolation,[21,38] and rural residency[24,53] indicate that etiology of tooth loss is complex and definitely entails more than individual biological influences. Acculturation has also been strongly associated with edentulism among Hispanic immigrants.[58] All these associations further substantiate the fact that tooth loss at different life stages is influenced by various factors that present across social, economic, educational, cultural, psychologic/emotional, environmental, biological, and medical domains.[18]

## Distribution of Tooth Loss

### Edentulism

Over several decades, the prevalence of edentulism has declined substantially in the United States.[8,9,12,51,52,57] In continuation of a trend previously seen, among older adults (65+ years of age), the overall prevalence of edentulism declined from 26.5% in 1999 to 2004 to 17.6% in 2009 to 2014.[12] Although dental care use by gender is relatively unchanged today,[41] gender differences in edentulism prevalence have disappeared since the NHANES III,[3] and the prevalence continues to decline in both genders. The edentulism prevalence in male and female older adults declined from 23.7% to 17.1% and 28.5% to 17.8%, respectively, between 1999 and 2004 and 2009 and 2014.[12] The absolute decline in edentulism prevalence between these two time periods was large in Hispanics (17.3%) and non-Hispanic Whites (9%) but not in non-Hispanic Black adults (3.4%).[12] Previous national level data showed interesting tooth loss patterns in different Hispanic subgroups. The Hispanic Health and Nutrition Examination Survey (HHANES) indicated that Cuban American adults (14.4%) had higher edentulism prevalence compared to Mexican Americans (12.9%),[28] and the NHANES III data showed a significantly lower prevalence in Mexican American adults (5%) compared to Whites (18%).[29]

A current disparity in edentulism prevalence by poverty status is evident with a higher proportion (33.5%) of poor older adults experiencing edentulism compared to near-poor (26%) and non-poor adults (11.1%) (Figure 17.1). When race/ethnicity is taken into account, larger differences are seen by poverty status among non-Hispanic Whites than among Hispanic people.[12] Geographically across the United States as seen in Figure 17.2, variations in age-adjusted prevalence are evident, with the highest in West Virginia (31.5%) and the lowest in Hawaii (5.8%).[4]

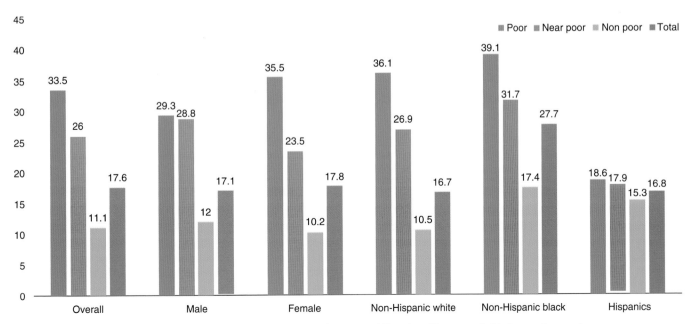

• **Figure 17.1** Prevalence percentage of edentulism among US seniors 65 years and older by gender, race/ethnicity, and poverty: 2009–14 NHANES data.[9]

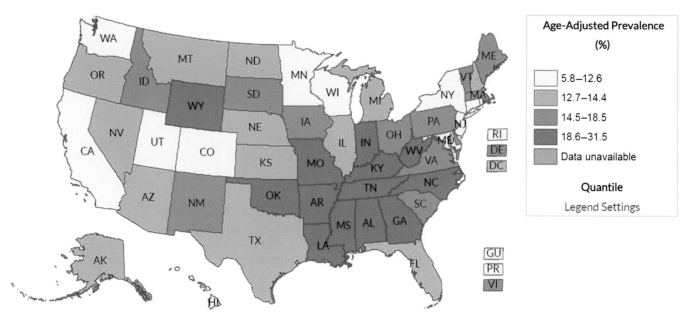

• **Figure 17.2** Age-adjusted prevalence percentage of edentulism in the United States by individual states: 2016 BRFSS data.[4]

The Healthy People (HP) initiative that provides 10-year national objectives for improving the health of all Americans used decreasing edentulism as an objective and assessed progress in meeting the objective for the years 2000, 2010, and 2020.[22,23] The most recent 2009 to 2014 NHANES data suggest that reducing the prevalence of edentulism among adults ages 65 to 74 to 21.6% was met (13% prevalence in 2009 to 2014) for the overall US population in this age group but not for the subgroups living in poverty (29%) or near poverty (23%).[23] Further, all but six states (Oklahoma [21.8%], Tennessee [22.1%], Kentucky [22.5%], Arkansas [23.4%], Mississippi [27.0%], and West Virginia [31.5%]) did not meet the objective and reported an age-adjusted edentulism prevalence of greater than 21.6% in 2016.[4] It does need to be pointed out that there were still 4 to 6 years left to 2020.

Globally, the prevalence of complete and partial tooth loss varies across different regions and countries. In 2003, the World Health Organization (WHO) recommended that countries set their own standards or monitor the oral health progress in their population for the year 2020.[25,48] One recommended goal was for each participating country to reduce the number of edentulous persons ages 35 to 44 and 65 to 74 years by a set percentage.[48] Edentulism prevalence varied substantially between the WHO regions and by gross national income (set by World Health Bank criteria).[49,50] The 2006 World Health Survey (WHS) study, in which 72 countries from different WHO regions participated, showed that older adults ages 65 to 74 years in African (AFRO) and South East Asia Region (SEARO) countries had a lower prevalence (<20%) of edentulism compared to countries in East Mediterranean (EMRO), American (AMRO), and Western Pacific (WPRO) regions, with the highest (>30%) in the European (EURO) region.[49] When countries were categorized by national income, the prevalence was as high as 35% in upper-middle–income countries compared to only 10% in low-income countries.[49] More recent data (2015) also shows that the global

prevalence of edentulism is higher in high sociodemographic index (SDI) countries compared to low SDI countries.[8] When disability-adjusted life years (DALYs) are considered instead of prevalence, edentulism is now responsible for a significant proportion of disease burden worldwide compared to other oral diseases.[8] This burden is more extensive in high SDI countries compared to low SDI countries.[8]

In a study using data from the 2013 Survey of Health, Ageing and Retirement in Europe (SHARE) of adults 50 to 90 years of age, representing 14 European countries and Israel, an overall prevalence of edentulism among older adults (65 to 74 years) was estimated at 13.8% (95% CI: 12.7, 14.9) (Table 17.1).[59] This study set edentulism prevalence of 15% or less as an oral health goal[2,64] and determined that this goal was only met by five of the 14 countries (Sweden, Switzerland, Denmark, France, and Germany) in 2013.[59] Further, in most of the countries studied, almost 50% of the population under the age of 90 and 25% under the age of 80 were edentulous. In the 2015 Global Burden of Disease (GBD) study, which used data from 195 countries and territories, the authors estimated that the global age-standardized rate for edentulism was 4.1% (95% uncertainty interval [UI]: 3.9 to 4.3).[31]

## Tooth Retention

From 1988 to 1994, 30.1% of adults 35 to 44 years of age had completely retained all of their teeth compared to 38.3% during the period from 1999 to 2004, indicating a sizable improvement within just a decade.[9] A continued increasing trend was seen in prevalence of complete tooth retention from 14.1% to 20.9% among those ages 50 and older between 1999 to 2004 and 2009 to 2014, respectively.[12] The prevalence of complete tooth retention increased between these two survey periods across all racial/ethnic groups and income levels, except the poor subgroup.[12] The greatest increase was observed among the nonpoor, and non-Hispanic White

| TABLE 17.1 | Prevalence Percentage of Edentulism in 65- to 74-Year-Olds and Number of Natural Teeth Retained in 50- to 90-Year-Olds in 14 European Countries and Israel in 2013[59] |

| Country | ESTIMATED EDENTULISM PREVALENCE[a] Percentage % (95% CI) | NUMBER OF NATURAL TEETH RETAINED[b] Mean (95% CI) | Median (95% CI) |
|---|---|---|---|
| Austria | 21.3 (18.9, 23.8) | 17.1 (16.7, 17.4) | 21.1 (20.5, 21.8) |
| Belgium | 18.2 (15.5, 21.0) | 16.7 (16.3, 17.1) | 20.4 (19.6, 21.2) |
| Czech Republic | 18.7 (16.4, 21.1) | 16.9 (16.5, 17.3) | 20.5 (19.8, 21.2) |
| Denmark | 6.8 (5.3, 8.4) | 22.4 (22.1, 22.7) | 26.0 (25.8, 26.2) |
| Estonia | 18.1 (16.2, 20.0) | 14.3 (14.0, 14.6) | 15.0 (14.1, 15.9) |
| France | 9.1 (6.9, 11.4) | 19.4 (19.0, 19.8) | 22.5 (22.1, 22.9) |
| Germany | 10.7 (9.0, 12.4) | 18.2 (17.9, 18.5) | 21.8 (21.3, 22.3) |
| Israel | 17.7 (13.9, 21.5) | 18.6 (18.0, 19.3) | 24.0 (23.4, 24.7) |
| Italy | 16.9 (13.2, 20.7) | 18.7 (18.3, 19.2) | 22.1 (21.7, 22.6) |
| Luxembourg | 17.7 (13.9, 21.5) | 18.0 (17.5, 18.6) | 22.0 (21.5, 22.5) |
| The Netherlands | 27.6 (24.7, 30.4) | 17.5 (17.1, 17.9) | 23.0 (22.4, 23.6) |
| Slovenia | 19.2 (15.5, 22.9) | 14.9 (14.3, 15.4) | 15.5 (13.8, 17.1) |
| Spain | 16.7 (12.9, 20.5) | 18.1 (17.6, 18.6) | 21.9 (21.1, 22.6) |
| Sweden | 2.7 (1.9, 3.5) | 24.5 (24.3, 24.7) | 27.0 (26.9, 27.2) |
| Switzerland | 6.7 (5.0, 8.4) | 22.2 (21.9, 22.6) | 25.9 (25.6, 26.3) |
| Overall | 13.8 (12.7, 14.9) | 18.7 (18.5, 18.8) | 22.3 (22.2, 22.5) |

[a]Estimated in older adults ages 65 to 74 only for complete edentulism prevalence.
[b]Estimated in adults ages 50 to 90, standardized to European population.
*CI*, Confidence interval.

group.[12] In both time periods, disparity was evident with a higher proportion of non-Hispanic Whites retaining all teeth compared to non-Hispanic Blacks and Hispanics.[12]

An individual's functional dentition is also an important indicator of oral health–related quality of life. Lack of a minimum set of natural teeth can result in compromised oral function with eating problems and selective food avoidance.[16] Similar to trends in edentulism and tooth retention, the prevalence of functional dentition (21 or more teeth in the mouth) among US adults ages 50 and older was 55% from 1999–2004 and increased to 67% from 2009–2014.[12] This trend of increase was seen (Figure 17.3) across all racial/ethnic groups and poverty levels, including the subgroups living in poverty.[12] In both time periods, disparity was evident with a higher prevalence in non-Hispanic whites compared to non-Hispanic blacks and Hispanics. The nonpoor group across all racial/ethnic groups had a higher prevalence of functional dentition compared to near-poor and poor groups in both periods.

Global perspectives of tooth retention were also estimated using the 2013 SHARE data (see Table 17.1).[59] The mean and median tooth retention estimates for all 15 countries in Table 17.1 clearly illustrate substantial variation by countries, with means ranging from 14.3 (Estonia) to 24.5 (Sweden), and similarly for medians.[59] These 2013 data also suggest that many European countries are struggling to reach the 1992 goal set by WHO of retaining at least 20 teeth by age 80.[61]

## Tooth Loss and Public Health

Tooth loss is an ultimate end point of the oral disease process that is influenced by various factors. While extraction of teeth with advanced disease and infection is sometimes the only solution to relieve pain and discomfort, loss of teeth impairs an individual's ability to chew, speak, and smile, as well as their quality of life.[51]

Despite the aging of our society, it is expected that tooth retention will continue to increase in the coming decades. It is therefore important that surveillance systems monitor the distribution of tooth loss and tooth retention using case definitions that are comparable to monitor the progress toward oral health goals and determine the impact on the population's oral health and well-being.

In the United States, the news is mixed, as edentulism has almost disappeared from some groups (higher income) but is now concentrated in the lower income subpopulation, and thus disparity in tooth loss has exacerbated over the last several decades. Non-Hispanic black adults still experience a relatively higher prevalence of edentulism and a lower prevalence of having complete and/or functional dentition compared to non-Hispanic white adults. More policies at the state and federal levels in favor of these disadvantaged groups are necessary to improve their access to dental care to further decrease dental diseases leading to tooth loss and to promote oral health behaviors at the appropriate time. Globally, severe tooth loss is a major public health issue and is one of the most commonly observed conditions.[37] Individual countries

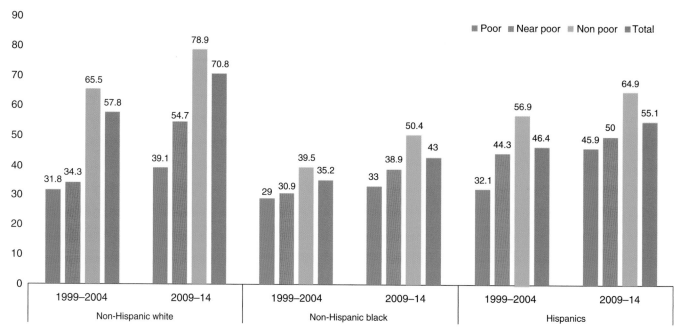

• **Figure 17.3** Prevalence percentage of functional dentition among US adults 50 years and older by race/ethnicity and poverty status.[9]

and/or WHO should develop strategies, policies, and programs to address this issue, especially in low-income and middle-income countries.

Further improvements in our understanding of the socio-behavioral factors associated with tooth loss in different racial/ethnic subgroups throughout the life stages would help better prevent and manage the direct and indirect causes of tooth loss. As socioeconomic inequity and demographic diversity widen, the effort of promoting tooth retention must incorporate public health and a collaborative approach to effectively address social determinants and risk factors for tooth loss in the most disadvantaged subgroups. Because etiology of tooth loss is complex, researchers, public health specialists, and policy makers should take into consideration various social, economic, educational, cultural, psychologic/emotional, environmental, and medical domains.

## References

1. Arora M, Schwarz E, Sivaneswaran S. Cigarette smoking and tooth loss in a cohort of older Australians: the 45 and up study. *J Am Dent Assoc.* 2010;141(10):1242–1249.
2. Bravo M, Cortes J, Casals E, Llena C, Almerich-Silla JM, Cuenca E. Basic oral health goals for Spain 2015/2020. *Int Dent J.* 2009; 59:78–82.
3. Burt BA, Eklund SA. Chapter 19. In: *Tooth Loss. Dentistry, Dental Practice, and the Community.* 6th ed. St. Louis, MO: Elsevier Saunders; 2005.
4. Centers for Disease Control and Prevention. Chronic Disease Indicators (CDI) Data. Available from: https://nccd.cdc.gov/cdi; 2016. Accessed May 20, 2019.
5. Corbella S, Francetti L, Taschieri S, et al. Effect of periodontal treatment on glycemic control of patients with diabetes: A systematic review and meta-analysis. *J Diabetes Investig.* 2013;4(5):502–509.
6. Dietrich T, Maserejian NN, Joshipura KJ, et al. Tobacco use and incidence of tooth loss among US male health professionals. *J Dent Res.* 2007;86(4):373–377.
7. Dietrich T, Walter C, Oluwagbemigun K, et al. Smoking, smoking cessation, and risk of tooth loss: the EPIC-Potsdam study. *J Dent Res.* 2015;94(10):1369–1375.
8. Dye BA. The global burden of oral disease: research and public health significance. *J Dent Res.* 2017;96(4):361–363.
9. Dye BA, Tan S, Smith V, et al. Trends in oral health status: United States, 1988–1994 and 1999–2004. *Vital Health Stat 11.* 2007; (248).
10. Dye BA, Li X, Beltrán-Aguilar ED. *Selected Oral Health Indicators in the United States, 2005–2008.* NCHS Data Brief, no 96. Hyattsville, MD: National Center for Health Statistics; 2012.
11. Dye BA, Thornton-Evans G, Li X, Iafolla TJ. *Dental Caries and Tooth Loss in Adults in the United States, 2011–2012.* NCHS Data Brief, No 197. Hyattsville, MD: National Center for Health Statistics; 2015.
12. Dye BA, Weatherspoon DJ, Mitnik GL. Tooth Loss Among Older Adults by Poverty Status in the United States from 1999–2004 to 2009–2014. *J Am Dent Assoc.* 2019;150(1):9–23.
13. Eklund SA, Burt BA. Risk factors for total tooth loss in the United States: longitudinal analysis of national data. *J Public Health Dent.* 1994;54(1):5–14.
14. Elter JR, Offenbacher S, Toole JF, et al. Relationship of periodontal disease and edentulism to stroke/TIA. *J Dent Res.* 2003;82(12): 998–1001.
15. Elter JR, Champagne CM, Offenbacher S, et al. Relationship of periodontal disease and tooth loss to prevalence of coronary heart disease. *J Periodontol.* 2004;75(6):782–790.
16. Evin RB, Dye BA. The effect of functional dentition on Healthy Eating Index scores and nutrient intakes in a nationally representative sample of older adults. *J Public Health Dent.* 2009;69(4):207–216.
17. Felton DA. Complete edentulism and comorbid diseases: an update. *J Prosthodont.* 2016;25(1):5–20.
18. Friedman PK, Lamster IB. Tooth loss as a predictor of shortened longevity: exploring the hypothesis. *Periodontol 2000.* 2016;72(1): 142–152.
19. Gilbert GH, Duncan RP, Shelton BJ. Social determinants of tooth loss. *Health Serv Res.* 2003;38(6):1843–1862.
20. Gilbert GH, Shewchuck RM, Litaker MS. Effect of dental practice characteristics on racial disparities in patient-specific tooth loss. *Med Care.* 2006;44(5):414–420.

21. Hanson BS, Liedberg B, Owall B. Social network, social support and dental status in elderly Swedish men. *Community Dent Oral Epidemiol.* 1994;22:331–337.
22. Healthy People. *Oral Health-Chapter 21.* Washington, DC: US Department of Health and Human Services, Office of Disease Prevention and Health Promotion; 2010. https://www.cdc.gov/nchs/data/hpdata2010/hp2010_final_review_focus_area_21.pdf. Accessed May 20, 2019.
23. Healthy People. *Oral Health of Adults (OH-4).* Washington, DC: US Department of Health and Human Services, Office of Disease Prevention and Health Promotion; 2020. https://www.healthypeople.gov/2020/topics-objectives/topic/oral-health/objectives. Accessed May 20, 2019.
24. Hendryx M, Ducatman AM, Zulling KJ, et al. Adult tooth loss for residents of US coal mining and Appalachian counties. *Community Dent Oral Epidemiol.* 2012;40(6):488–497.
25. Hobdell M, Petersen PE, Clarkson J, Johnson N. Global goals for oral health 2020. *Int Dent J.* 2003;53:285–288.
26. Huang HC, Colditz G, Joshipura KJ. The association between tooth loss and the self-reported intake of selected CVD-related nutrients and foods among US women. *Community Dent Oral Epidemiol.* 2005;33(3):167–173.
27. Hung HC, Willett W, Ascherio A, et al. Tooth loss and dietary intake. *J Am Dent Assoc.* 2003;134(9):1185–1192.
28. Ismail AI, Szpunar SM. The prevalence of total tooth loss, dental caries, and periodontal diseases among Mexican Americans, Cuban Americans, and Puerto Ricans: findings from HHANES 1982–1984. *Am J Public Health.* 1990;80(suppl):66–70.
29. Jimenez M, Dietrich T, Shih MC, et al. Racial/ethnic variations in associations between socioeconomic factors and tooth loss. *Community Dent Oral Epidemiol.* 2009;37(3):267–275.
30. Joshipura KJ, Willett WC, Douglass CW. The impact of edentulousness on food and nutrient intake. *J Am Dent Assoc.* 1996;127(4):459–467.
31. Kassebaum NJ, Smith AGC, Bernabé E, et al. GBD 2015 Oral Health Collaborators. Global, regional, and national prevalence, incidence, and disability-adjusted life years for oral conditions for 195 countries, 1990-2015: a systematic analysis for the global burden of diseases, injuries, and risk factors. *J Dent Res.* 2017;96(4):380–387.
32. Kim JK, Baker LA, Seirawan H, et al. Prevalence of oral health problems in US adults, NHANES 1999–2004: exploring differences by age, education, and race/ethnicity. *Spec Care Dentist.* 2012;32(6):234–241.
33. Krall EA, Dawson-Hughes B, Garvey AJ, et al. Smoking, smoking cessation, and tooth loss. *J Dent Res.* 1997;76(10):1653–1659.
34. Luo H, Pan W, Sloan F, et al. Forty-year trends in tooth loss among American adults with and without Diabetes Mellitus: An age-period-cohort analysis. *Prev Chronic Dis.* 2015;12:E211.
35. Maisonneuve P, Amar S, Lowenfels AB. Periodontal disease, edentulism, and pancreatic cancer: a meta-analysis. *Ann Oncol.* 2017;28(5):985–995.
36. Manski RJ, Hyde JS, Chen H, et al. Differences among older adults in the types of dental services used in the United States. *Inquiry.* 2016 Jun 9;53.
37. Marcenes W, Kassebaum NJ, Bernabé E, et al. Global burden of oral conditions in 1990–2010: a systematic analysis. *J Dent Res.* 2013;92(7):592–597.
38. McGrath C, Bendi R. Influences of social support on the oral health of older people in Britain. *J Oral Rehabil.* 2002;29(10):918–922.
39. Meyer MS, JOshipura K, Giovannucci E, et al. A review of the relationship between tooth loss, periodontal disease, and cancer. *Cancer Causes Control.* 2008;19(9):895–907.
40. Moynihan P, Bradbury J. Compromised dental function and nutrition. *Nutrition.* 2001;17:177–178.
41. National Center for Health Statistics. Table 78. In: *Health, United States, 2016: With Chartbook on Long-Term Trends in Health.* Hyattsville, MD: National Center for Health Statistics; 2017.
42. Northridge ME, Ue FV, Borrell LN, et al. Tooth loss and dental caries in community-dwelling older adults in northern Manhattan. *Gerodontology.* 2012;29(2):e464–e473.
43. Naorungroj S, Slade GD, Divaris K, et al. Racial differences in periodontal disease and 10-year self-reported tooth loss among late middle-aged and older adults: the dental ARIC study. *J Public Health Dent.* 2017;77(4):372–382.
44. Nowjack-Raymer RE, Sheiham A. Association of edentulism and diet and nutrition in US adults. J Dent Res. 2003;82(2):123–126.
45. Okoro CA, Balluz LS, Eke PI, et al. Tooth loss and heart disease: findings from the Behavioral Risk Factor Surveillance System. *Am J Prev Med.* 2005;29(5):50–56.
46. Okoro CA, Strine TW, Eke PI, et al. The association between depression and anxiety and use of oral health services and tooth loss. *Community Dent Oral Epidemiol.* 2012;40(2):134–144.
47. Patel MH, Kumar JV, Moss ME. Diabetes and tooth loss: an analysis of data from the National Health and Nutrition Examination Survey, 2003–2004. *J Am Dent Assoc.* 2013;144(5):478–485.
48. Petersen PE. Global policy for improvement of oral health in the 21st century—implications to oral health research of World Health Assembly 2007, World Health Organization. *Community Dent Oral Epidemiol.* 2009;37:1–8.
49. Petersen PE. *The World Health Survey—The Global Burden of Oral Disease.* Geneva, Switzerland: World Health Organization; 2009.
50. Petersen PE, Kandelman D, Arpin S, et al. Global oral health of older people—call for public health action. Community Dent Health. 2010;27(supplement 2):257–268.
51. Rodrigues SM, Oliveira AC, Vargas AMD, et al. Implications of edentulism on quality of life among elderly. *Int J Environ Res Public Health.* 2012;9:100–109.
52. Rozier GR, White A, Slade GD. Trends in oral diseases in the U.S. *J Dent Educ.* 2017;eS97–eS109.
53. Saman DM, Lemieux A, Arevalo O, et al. A population-based study of edentulism in the US: does depression and rural residency matter after controlling for potential confounders? *BMC Public Health.* 2014;14(65).
54. Scannapieco FA, Cantos A. Oral inflammation and infection, and chronic medical diseases: implications for the elderly. *Periodontol 2000.* 2016;72(1):153–175.
55. Sheiham A, Steele JG, Marcenes W, et al. The relationship among dental status, nutrient intake, and nutritional status in older people. *J Dent Res.* 2001;80(2):408–413.
56. Singh A, Gupta A, Peres MA, et al. Association between tooth loss and hypertension among a primary rural middle aged and older Indian adult population. *J Public Health Dent.* 2016;76(3):198–205.
57. Slade GA, Akinkugbe AA, Sanders AE. Projections of U.S. edentulous prevalence following 5 decades of decline. *J Dent Res.* 2014;93(10):959–965.
58. Stewart DC, Ortega AN, Dausey D. Oral health and use of dental services among Hispanics. *J Public Health Dent.* 2002;62(2):84–91.
59. Stock C, Jurges H, Shen J, et al. A comparison of tooth retention and replacement across 15 countries in the over-50s. *Community Dent Oral Epidemiol.* 2016;44:223–231.
60. Wiener RC, Wiener MA, McNeil DW. Comorbid depression/anxiety and teeth removed: Behavioral Risk Factor Surveillance System 2010. *Community Dent Oral Epidemiol.* 2015;43(5):433–443.
61. WHO Expert Committee. *Recent Advances in Oral Health.* Geneva, Switzerland: World Health Organization; 1992.
62. Willet WC. Diet and health: what should we eat? *Science.* 1994;264(5158):532–537.
63. Wu B, Hybels C, Liang J, et al. Social stratification and tooth loss among middle-aged and older Americans from 1988 to 2004. *Community Dent Oral Epidemiol.* 2014;42(6):495–502.
64. Ziller S, Micheelis W, Oesterreich D. Goals for oral health in Germany 2020. *Int Dent J.* 2006;56:29–32.
65. Weintraub JA, Burt BA. Oral health status in the United States: tooth loss and edentulism. *J Dent Educ.* 1985;49:368–378.

# 18

# Measurement and Distribution of Malocclusion, Trauma, and Congenital Anomalies

JAGAN KUMAR BASKARADOSS, BDS, MPH, MJDF RCS (ENG)

PRADEEP BHAGAVATULA, BDS, MPH, MS

## Description and Etiology of Malocclusion

Malocclusion is a developmental condition where there is a deflection from the normal relation or alignment of the teeth to other teeth in the same arch and/or to the teeth in the opposing arch. Malocclusion has always been a source of concern for individuals since antiquity. Specimens dating back to the 8th century BCE indicate that Etruscans used orthodontic bands to improve the alignment of teeth.[22]

Unlike dental caries and periodontitis, malocclusion is not a disease; rather, it is more of a natural variation of the normal occlusion. The concept of "normal occlusion" as we know it today was described as early as in the 18th century by John Hunter. Carabelli, in the mid-19th century, described abnormal relationships of the upper and lower dental arches. Following this description, several theories were proposed to describe the pattern of malocclusion, although few provided a comprehensive picture of the condition.[1]

The most common causes for malocclusion are hereditary/genetic factors, environmental factors, and specific causes.[55] Malocclusion is primarily the result of disproportion between the size of the dental arches and the size of the permanent teeth, both of which are largely determined genetically.[38] An evolutionary reduction in jaw/tooth size and inheritance of discordant dental and facial characteristics are commonly cited genetic factors for an increase in the prevalence of malocclusion. Environmental influences affect the developing jaws and teeth mechanically via pressures or forces that move teeth or alter jaw growth. The pressures exerted by the tongue and lip, variations in jaw postures as a consequence of mouth breathing, etc., could affect the development of dental arch and cause malocclusion.

The specific causes of malocclusion can be grouped into four categories: (1) genetic syndromes (e.g., achondroplasia), (2) defects of embryologic development (e.g., cleft lip and palate), (3) trauma (e.g., perinatal or postnatal injuries), and (4) anomalies of postnatal development. (e.g., condylar hyperplasia). However, less than 5% of the population may have a pattern of malocclusion that can be attributed to a specific cause.[55]

## Measurement of Malocclusion

Since malocclusion is a deflection from normal, and "normal" occlusion is hard to define, there is no universally accepted index of malocclusion that can be used as an epidemiologic tool for measuring occlusal status.[69] In addition, there are no clear clinical guidelines to delineate the treatment need and timing for specific orthodontic interventions.[61] However, measuring the severity and prevalence of malocclusion is important for estimating the treatment need in the community and then prioritizing treatment with limited resources.

## Angle's Classification

Several malocclusion indices have been proposed, and these can be broadly placed in two categories: qualitative and quantitative. Qualitative indices provide nominal values for the types of malocclusion, for example, Angle's classification[7] and incisor classification.[13] Angle's classification is the most widely used index for evaluation of malocclusions. According to Angle, the upper first molars are the key to normal occlusion, and the mesiobuccal cusp of the upper first molars should occlude with the buccal groove of the lower first molars to attain normal occlusion. The other factor that Angle took into consideration for classifying malocclusion was the "line of occlusion." This line is a smooth curve passing through the central fossa of each upper molar and across the cingulum of the upper canine and incisor teeth. The same line runs along the buccal cusps and incisal edges of the lower teeth, thus specifying the occlusal as well as interarch relationships once the molar position is established.[57]

Angle described three classes of malocclusion:

Class I: There is a normal relationship of the molars, but the line of occlusion is incorrect because of malposed teeth, rotations, or other causes.

Class II: The lower molar is distally positioned relative to the upper molar, and the line of occlusion is not specified.

Class III: The lower molar is mesially positioned relative to the upper molar, and the line of occlusion is not specified.

However, the major drawback of these qualitative indices is that they do not provide an estimate of the severity of the condition or the treatment need. This limitation led to the development of several quantitative indices that not only categorize malocclusions but are also capable of providing estimates of the need for treatment.

Malocclusion indices can further be considered under the following five headings: (1) diagnostic—these indices are descriptive and aid in classifying malocclusion, (2) epidemiologic—these indices are useful in determining occlusal anomalies at the population level, (3) treatment need—these indices were developed in an attempt to categorize the treatment of malocclusion in groups according to urgency and need for treatment, (4) treatment success—these indices help in critically and objectively assessing treatment standards, and (5) treatment complexity—these indices help in grading the treatment complexity that could be useful to objectively set fee structure (Table 18.1).[52]

Several interesting indices were introduced In the 1960s and 1970s. Of these, the Handicapping Labio-Lingual Deviation (HLD) Index[26] received considerable public health attention when

## • TABLE 18.1  Malocclusion Indices

| Type of Measure | Type of Index | Name of Index | Author and Year of Development |
|---|---|---|---|
| Qualitative | Diagnostic | Angle's Classification | Angle 1899[7] |
| Quantitative | Treatment need | Handicapping Labio-Lingual Deviations (HLD) | Draker 1960[26] |
| Quantitative | Treatment need | Treatment Priority Index (TPI) | Grainger 1967[35] |
| Quantitative | Treatment need | Occlusal Index (OI) | Summers 1971[68] |
| Qualitative | Diagnostic | Incisor Classification | British Standard Institute 1983[13] |
| Quantitative | Treatment need | Dental Aesthetic Index (DAI) | Cons et al. 1986[18] |
| Quantitative | Treatment need | Index of Orthodontic Treatment Need (IOTN) | Brook and Shaw 1989[15] |
| Quantitative | Treatment success | Peer Assessment Rating (PAR) index | Richmond et al. 1992[58] |
| Quantitative | Treatment complexity | Index of Complexity, Outcome, and Need (ICON) | Daniels and Richmond 2000[24] |

it was applied to assess treatment needs for a public orthodontic program in New York state. The Treatment Priority Index developed by Grainger[35] and the Occlusal Index developed by Summers[68] were widely used in several epidemiologic studies.

Orthodontic indices developed in the late 1980s, however, take a different philosophical approach in that they aim to assess the aesthetics along with the other clinical aspects of function. One is the Dental Aesthetic Index, published in 1986 after years of testing.[18] In Europe, the Index of Orthodontic Treatment Need has received some use since it was first introduced in 1989.[15] The Peer Assessment Rating (PAR) index is designed to capture all the occlusal anomalies that might be found in malocclusion in a single score.[58] The Index of Complexity, Outcome, and Need (ICON),[24] which arrived with the new millennium, was shown to correlate well with patients' perceptions of aesthetics, speech, function, and need for treatment.[45] Most of these indices were never used after their introduction, but some are still being used for clinical and epidemiologic purposes.

## Treatment Priority Index

The Treatment Priority Index (TPI), proposed by Grainger,[35] is an epidemiologic tool used to rank malocclusions and assess the need for orthodontic treatment. The TPI has the advantage of being simple, efficient, and reproducible.[65] TPI was used for assessing treatment needs and provided the first national estimates of orthodontic needs in US children. Six occlusal features are assessed: (1) first molar relationship, (2) overjet, (3) overbite, (4) tooth displacement (crowding, rotations), (5) congenitally missing teeth, and (6) posterior crossbite.

## Occlusal Index

The Occlusal Index (OI) includes nine measurements: dental age, molar relation, overbite, overjet, posterior crossbite, posterior open bite, tooth displacement (actual and potential), midline relations, and congenitally missing permanent maxillary incisors. The index incorporates separate weighting mechanisms for deciduous, mixed, and permanent dentitions. The weighted score of individual components are added together to obtain the total OI score. Several studies on malocclusion in the 1970s used this index, and the index was reported to provide the best correlation with clinical standards and the greatest validity over time.[36,37]

## Index of Orthodontic Treatment Need

The Index of Orthodontic Treatment Need (IOTN) was developed to identify malocclusions that are most likely to benefit from orthodontic treatment.[15] It comprises two components, a dental health/functional component and an aesthetic component. The dental health component records the need for treatment on dental health and functional grounds, and the aesthetic component records the aesthetic impairment and, by implication, the justification for treatment on social-psychologic grounds.

The dental health component categorizes malocclusion in five grades based on the severity of the occlusal condition and its treatment need. Occlusal features assessed are missing teeth, overjet, crossbite, displacement of contact points (that is, crowding), and overbite. With practice, it is possible to ascribe reliably and easily the treatment need category to a given malocclusion. The aesthetic component of the IOTN uses a set of 10 intraoral photographs of anterior teeth in occlusion that range from no need for treatment on aesthetic grounds to definite need. The assessment is made by selecting the photograph thought to most closely match the aesthetics or alignment of the patient's anterior teeth, but the judgment is very subjective. Because of the lack of objectivity in assessing the aesthetic component, the treatment need is based primarily on the dental health component of the IOTN, which is more objective.

Epidemiologic studies that used the IOTN reported good reliability and ease of scoring. The simplicity in recording and the ease of training and calibrating examiners make IOTN an ideal instrument for large surveys. In the United States, the National Health and Nutrition Examination Survey (NHANES) III used IOTN to report on the treatment needs of the population.[56]

## Dental Aesthetic Index

Similar to the IOTN, the Dental Aesthetic Index (DAI) was developed to rank malocclusion according to the level of treatment need. The DAI starts from the premise that the impact of malocclusion on other oral pathologies is doubtful and that the main benefit of orthodontic treatment is its effect on the individual's social and psychologic well-being. The DAI has been adopted by several public health programs to screen and identify individuals who require orthodontic treatment.

The DAI measures 10 prominent traits of malocclusion, weighted on the basis of their relative importance, to produce a single score. It also aims to predict the clinical judgment of orthodontists by separating handicapping and non-handicapping malocclusions. Based on the total DAI score, the individual is categorized as follows: (1) no or slight treatment need (≤25);

(2) elective treatment need (26–30); (3) treatment highly desirable (31–35); and (4) treatment mandatory (≥36). For public health programs, a cut-off score of 31 or 36 is most commonly used to distinguish between handicapping and nonhandicapping occlusal conditions.[40]

DAI has been validated through a number of studies from different countries.[10,30,50] This validation has led to the acceptance of the DAI as a cross-cultural index. The World Health Organization (WHO) has also recommended the use of the DAI in its Pathfinder survey protocol.[74]

## Distribution of Malocclusion

Perfect interdigitation between teeth is seldom observed, and this leads to considerable disagreement on how much deviation from the ideal can be considered to be within acceptable limits. As a result, the prevalence of malocclusion in the United States between 1930 and 1965 was estimated to be 35% to 95%.[57] Currently, it is estimated that approximately two-thirds of the US population has some degree of malocclusion. More than half the population has Angle's Class I malocclusion, and approximately 15% have Angle's Class II malocclusion.[57]

The NHANES III,[56] conducted between 1988 and 1994 in the United States, measured several occlusal traits. According to the report, more than half the children (ages 8–11) had well-aligned incisors, and just over 40% of the youth (ages 12–17) had well-aligned incisors. In adults (ages 18–50), only approximately one-third of the lower incisors were well aligned. Approximately 15% of adolescents and adults had extremely irregular incisors. Additionally, more than one-quarter of the children had a midline diastema (>2 mm). There was a significant racial difference in relation to the midline diastema, with African Americans twice as likely to have a midline diastema compared with non-Hispanic Whites or Mexican Americans.

In terms of the occlusal contact discrepancy, approximately 30% of the children and 40% of the youth and adults had an ideal overjet (1–2 mm). An overjet of 5 mm or more, suggesting Angle's Class II malocclusion, occurred in approximately 23% of children, 15% of youth, and 13% of adults. Reverse overjet, indicative of Angle's Class III malocclusion, occurred in just over 3% of the population. Vertical deviations from the ideal overbite of 0 to 2 mm were observed in more than 50% of the population. Severe overbite (≥5 mm) was recorded for nearly 20% of the children, 15% of the youth, and 13% of the adults. As seen with the midline diastema, there was a significant racial difference for the vertical dental relationships as well. Severe deep bite was nearly twice as prevalent in non-Hispanic Whites as in African Americans or Mexican Americans.

The orthodontic treatment need of US population was reported in NHANES I[43,44] and NHANES III[56] (Figure 18.1). There has been an increase in children and youth not needing treatment and a decrease in those definitely needing treatment across racial groups. About 35% of adolescents were perceived by parents and peers as needing orthodontic treatment. One-third to half of the children and youth in the higher socioeconomic areas in the United States were receiving orthodontic care.[56] A higher proportion of non-Hispanic White youths had orthodontic treatment compared to African American and Mexican American youths. Perceived orthodontic treatment need is often influenced by aesthetic perceptions and socioecologic factors, which vary widely across different racial groups.

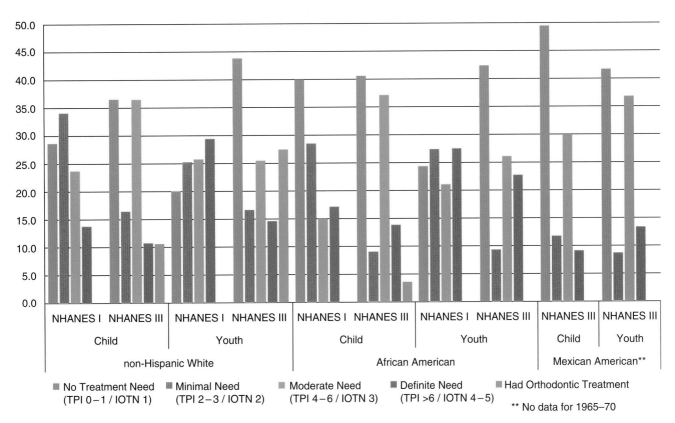

• **Figure 18.1** Percent of U.S. population estimated to need orthodontic treatment in NHANES I[29,30] versus NHANES III.[23,29,30]

## Malocclusion and Public Health

From a public health perspective, it is important to make a distinction between malocclusion as a handicapping anomaly versus an aesthetic discrepancy. Handicapping malocclusion has a profound impact on people's daily lives and well-being, with the greatest burden on the disadvantaged and marginalized population groups. The management of handicapping malocclusion is often time consuming and expensive, which poses a significant financial burden on the healthcare system. Complete prevention of malocclusion may be difficult to envision, as most malocclusion is an aesthetic discrepancy; however, timely interventions can help in minimizing the treatment needs at a later stage.

## Description and Etiology of Dental Trauma

In this chapter, dental trauma refers to injuries to the teeth and/or the periodontium (gums, periodontal ligament, and alveolar bone) and nearby soft tissues, such as the lips and tongue. The most frequent type of traumatic dental injuries (TDIs) are asymptomatic fractures restricted to the enamel,[5] yet TDIs are an important public health problem worldwide due to their high prevalence and

significant impact on those affected. The consequences of trauma to the teeth and orofacial structures can be wide ranging, from minor aesthetic concerns regarding an asymptomatic fracture to luxation leading to pulpal necrosis of the involved tooth or loss of function due to loss of the whole tooth. Consequently, TDIs can also negatively affect an individual's oral health–related quality of life (OHRQoL).[11]

Injuries to the head and neck region of the body can potentially be life threatening, as they may affect the brain. The Centers for Disease Control and Prevention estimated that in 2010, approximately, 2.5 million emergency department (ED) visits, hospitalizations, and deaths in the United States were due to traumatic brain injuries.[16] Reports based on a US Nationwide Emergency Department Sample found that more than 5 million ED visits were related to injuries of the head and neck region,[60] and more than 400,000 ED visits involved a facial fracture[3]. These data demonstrate the high frequency of injuries to the orofacial region. This section, however, focuses mainly on injuries to the teeth and not the other tissues of the orofacial region.

TDIs occur due to unintentional causes, such as falls or collisions, and also due to intentional infliction in acts of violence and abuse. Etiologic factors are very much related to the age of the individual. In preschool children, falls are the most common cause of oral injuries, whereas in school age children, injuries are most often caused by sports or hits by another person. In adolescents and young adults, assaults and traffic accidents are the most common etiologic factors.[4]

## Oral Factors

Inadequate lip coverage and increased overjet have often been associated with an increased risk of TDIs, with studies showing a doubling of risk among those with overjet larger than 3 mm.[51] Overjet remains significantly associated with TDIs even after adjusting for demographic factors such as age, sex, and race/ethnicity.[63] The threshold for overjet may differ across studies, however, with some using 3 mm but others using 5 mm to define a case of increased overjet.

## Sporting Activities

Participation in contact sports, especially without adequate protective gear such as mouth guards or other protective headgear, is also an important risk factor for TDIs. The Fédération Dentaire Internationale (FDI) World Dental Federation classified sports in two categories based on the risk of TDIs: high-risk sports (such as American football, hockey, ice hockey, lacrosse, martial arts, rugby, inline skating, skateboarding, and mountain biking) and medium-risk sports (such as basketball, soccer, team handball, diving, squash, gymnastics, parachuting, and water polo).[29]

## Health Conditions

Individuals who are obese are more likely to experience TDIs because they are more likely to experience falls,[20] although some studies have found fewer TDIs among obese individuals, likely due to a sedentary lifestyle. Attention deficit hyperactivity disorders, epilepsy, and cerebral palsy are some of the other conditions that have been found to increase the risk of TDIs.[8]

## Other Unintentional Causes of Traumatic Dental Injury (TDI)

Traffic accidents are another major cause of TDIs, especially among children who are not restrained in protective car seats and adults not wearing seatbelts.[75] Oral piercings, iatrogenic causes, and inappropriate use of teeth (as in biting into hard substances, using the teeth as tools to open bottles, etc.) have all been reported to a lesser extent in the literature as causes of TDI.

## Intentional Causes of Injury

Physical abuse and violence are also important causes of facial and dental injuries among adults and children.[32] Facial injuries are overrepresented in cases of physical assaults, with some studies reporting more than 50% of facial injuries are a result of an assault.[75]

## Measurement of Dental Trauma

Numerous classifications of dental trauma have been developed over the years, and many are intended for use in clinical settings and not epidemiologic studies. As many as 54 classification systems were used by various studies in the period from 1936 to 2003.[31] The classifications developed by WHO,[72] Ellis and Davey,[28] and Andreasen et al.[5] have been used widely and are described here along with the National Institute of Dental Research (NIDR) Trauma Index, a classification used in the NHANES III.[42] All of the listed classifications record trauma to all the teeth in the dentition, and for both primary and permanent teeth, except the NIDR Trauma Index, which is primarily applied for permanent incisor teeth.

## WHO Classification

The WHO proposed a TDI classification based on anatomical and therapeutic considerations in its *Application of the International Classification of Diseases to Dentistry and Stomatology* (ICD-DA) monograph.[72] The ICD classification is the international standard for reporting diseases and health conditions.[73] The ICD-10 code for injuries of the teeth and the paraoral structures is ICD-10-CM S02.5XXB and is based on the diagnosis, etiology, tissues involved, and severity of the injury.[73] The criteria for fracture of a tooth range from S02.50 to S02.59.[72] The WHO classification has some limitations. For example, luxation injuries are not separated as intrusive, extrusive, or lateral luxation injuries, and fractures of the alveolar process are listed separately as fractures of the jawbones and are not included in the classification of tooth fractures.

## Traumatic Dental Injury

Ellis and Davey proposed a classification for TDIs in 1970. The classification is based on a numerical system that describes the anatomical extent of the injury. In this classification, the injuries to the crowns and roots of the teeth are grouped into eight categories from Class 1 (simple fracture of the crown without dentin involvement) to Class 8 (fracture of the crown en masse).[28] It is a simple classification and, as noted by many researchers, allows subjective interpretations with the use of words such as "simple," "extensive," and "considerable."

## Andreasen's Clinical and Epidemiologic Classifications

Andreasen et al.[5] proposed two classifications. The first index is for use in clinical settings and is appropriate to use with diagnostic aids such as radiographs and pulp vitality testing. This classification overcomes certain limitations of the WHO classification, as it includes injuries to some of the tissues that are not included in the WHO classification.

It has four major categories: (1) injuries to the hard tissues, dental tissues, and the pulp; (2) injuries to periodontal tissues; (3) injuries to the supporting bone; and (4) injuries to the gingiva or oral mucosa. However, since most epidemiologic studies are conducted as field screenings and the use of certain diagnostic methods is not practical, Andreasen et al.[5] also proposed a second classification that is described in Table 18.2. This classification is similar to the Ellis and Davey classification[28] and is among the most widely used methods for classifying injuries to the teeth and supporting structures in epidemiologic studies.[31] There are seven categories, from Code 0 (indicating no injury) to Code 5 (indicating a tooth missing due to trauma) and Code 9 (for teeth that cannot be assessed due to the presence of appliances).

• **TABLE 18.2** **Commonly Used Classifications of Traumatic Dental Injuries**

| WHO Classification[72] | Ellis and Davey[28] | Andreasen Epidemiologic Classification[5] | NIDR Trauma Index[42] |
|---|---|---|---|
| Fracture of Tooth<br>S02.50 Fracture of enamel of tooth only, enamel chipping | Class 1 Simple fracture of the crown—involving little or no dentin | Code 0 No Injury | 0 No evidence of traumatic injury |
| S02.51 Fracture of crown of tooth without pulpal involvement | Class 2 Extensive fracture of the crown—involving considerable dentin but not the pulp | Code 1 Treated injury (presence of composite restorations or crowns or evidence of endodontic treatment) | 1 Unrestored enamel fracture that does not involve the dentin |
| S02.52 Fracture of crown of tooth with pulpal involvement | Class 3 Extensive fracture of the crown—involving considerable dentin and exposing the dental pulp | Code 2 Enamel fracture (loss of small portion of crown including only enamel) | 2 Unrestored fracture that involves the dentin |
| S02.53 Fracture of root of tooth | Class 4 The traumatized tooth which becomes nonvital—with or without loss of crown structure | Code 3 Enamel and dentin fracture not involving the pulp | 3 Untreated damage as evidenced by one of the following:<br>(a) dark discoloration as compared with the other teeth or<br>(b) presence of a swelling and/or fistula in the labial or lingual vestibule adjacent to an otherwise healthy tooth |
| S02.54 Fracture of crown with root of tooth | Class 5 Teeth lost due to trauma | Code 4 Injury involving pulp (presence of signs and symptoms of pulp exposure such as swelling, sinus tract, discoloration of tooth, and absence of dental caries) | |
| S02.57 Multiple fractures of teeth | Class 6 Fracture of the root—with or without loss of crown structure | Code 5 Missing tooth due to trauma (must ascertain that the tooth was lost due to trauma) | 4 Fracture restored, with either a full crown or a less extensive restoration |
| S02.59 Fracture of tooth, unspecified | Class 7 Displacement of the tooth—without fracture of crown or root | Code 9 Excluded tooth (signs of traumatic injury cannot be assed due to presence of appliances) | 5 Presence of a lingual restoration as a sign of endodontic therapy |
| Fracture of Alveolar Process<br>S02.40 Fracture of maxillary alveolar process<br>S02.60 Fracture mandibular of alveolar process | Class 8 Fracture of the crown en masse and its replacement | | 6 Tooth missing due to trauma<br><br>7 Any tooth or space that does not fall within the preceding categories |
| Dislocation of Tooth<br>S03.20 Luxation of tooth<br>S03.21 Intrusion or extrusion of tooth<br>S03.22 Avulsion of tooth (ex-articulation) | | | |

## NIDR Trauma Index

This index was developed in 1989 specifically for use in epidemiologic studies.[42] The classification scheme of the index is applied to each of the eight permanent incisor teeth or tooth spaces, with scores ranging from 0 to 6 used for the trauma classification and an exclusion score of Y. The index is based on clinical, nonradiographic evidence of tooth injury.[42] The examinee has to provide a positive history of injury and/or treatment received for assigning a score based on the criteria listed in Table 18.2.

## Distribution of Dental Trauma

TDIs are a relatively common occurrence worldwide, yet estimates of the prevalence and incidence of TDI are not as robust as one would expect. Most studies are based on small convenience samples, with very few studies of nationally representative samples like the NHANES. Differences in the methods of study, study designs, types of indices used, and type and number of teeth examined (e.g., NHANES only measures trauma to permanent incisors) are among some of the factors that make a comparison of statistics across studies and countries challenging.

The results from the few studies[9,17,34,64,66] that have reported incidence rates of traumatic dental injuries are provided in Table 18.3 and range from 1% to 3% per year in the general population. As expected, certain subgroups, such as athletes, may experience more injuries than the rest of the population.[17] In the primary dentition, the greatest incidence of trauma to the teeth occurs at ages 2 to 3 years, which is most likely because motor coordination is not fully developed at this age.[33] For the permanent dentition, age 9 to 12 years is considered the peak age for incidence. It is estimated that most (71%–92%) TDIs sustained occur among

**• TABLE 18.3 Incidence of Traumatic Dental Injuries**

| Author | Country/Region | Year | Age/Age Group (Years) | Sample Size | Incidence Rate | Place of Registration |
|---|---|---|---|---|---|---|
| **Australia** | | | | | | |
| Stockwell[66] | Australia | 1988 | 6–12 | 66,500 | 1.7 | At clinic |
| **Scandinavia** | | | | | | |
| Skaare and Jacobsen[64] | Norway | 2003 | 7–18 | ≈71,000 | 1.8 | At clinic |
| Glendor et al.[34] | Sweden | 1996 | 0–6 | 21,456 | 1.49 | At clinic |
| | | | 7–19 | 41,458 | 1.25 | At clinic |
| | | | 0–19 | 62,914 | 1.32 | At clinic |
| **Asia** | | | | | | |
| Basha et al.[9] | India | 2015 | 13 years | 782 | 3.0 | Public and private schools |
| **United States of America** | | | | | | |
| Cohenca et al.[17] | United States | 2007 | College athletes | 2040 males | 10.6 | At clinic |
| | | | | 1200 females | 5.0 | |

individuals under the age 19 years.[34] Incidence rates are higher among males than among females, with some studies reporting twice as many injuries among males.[34] Andreasen and Ravn[6] reported two peaks of incidences in boys: 2 to 4 years and 9 to 10 years; and among girls, the peak incidence was in the 2 to 3 years age group.

An often-cited statistic about the high frequency of dental trauma vis-à-vis trauma to other parts of the body is that the mouth and paraoral structures are 1% of the body area but sustain more than 5% of total injuries. Studies of both primary and permanent teeth have generally reported prevalence estimates in the range of 9% to 30%, with higher levels in some population subgroups. Data from NHANES III showed that one in every five children ages 6 to 20 experienced trauma to their incisors and that by the age of 50, the prevalence of TDIs is 28%.[42] Age, gender, race, and socioeconomic status are among some of the sociodemographic characteristics associated with TDIs.

The prevalence of dental trauma increases with age in both primary and permanent dentitions as the injuries are cumulative. Preschool-aged children 4 to 5 years old are more likely to have TDIs in the past when compared to children in the 1- to 3-year age group.[2] In the United States, the prevalence of TDIs is 2.9% among 6- to 8-year-old children and 11.1% among children who are 9 to 11 years old.[27] TDIs are also more prevalent among men than women.[27,42]

The relationship between socioeconomic status (SES) and traumatic dental injuries is uncertain, with some studies reporting that low SES children were at greater risk[12] and others reporting high SES children were at increased risk[23] and others showing no relationship.[19] Access to safe playing areas, likelihood of facing violence, or participation in sports such as skateboarding and horse riding have been posited as some of the reasons for differences. The impact of race/ethnicity on TDIs is also not clear, with conflicting results from studies likely because race is often correlated with SES.

Little is known about the exact global trends of TDI. In the United States, the prevalence of incisal trauma among both children and adolescents did not change significantly between the years 1988 to 1994 and 1999 to 2004, as reported by Dye et al.[27]

Analysis of the Children's Dental Health Surveys from 1973 to 2013 in the United Kingdom reported a nonsignificant decrease in prevalence among 8-year-old children (8% to 5%) and an overall decrease among 12-year-old (17% to 12.5%) and 15-year-old (17% to 9%) children.[12]

## Dental Trauma and Public Health

Traumatic dental injuries are predictable and preventable. Education of parents, teachers, school nurses, and other caregivers on methods of injury prevention—such as creating safe play areas where tripping, colliding, and falling are minimized—can help in preventing injuries. Education about care and first aid after an injury can also be very helpful in minimizing the long-term impacts of TDIs. Educational and regulatory interventions about use of protective gear during contact sports, efforts to increase compliance with seat belt laws, and use of appropriate child seats have significantly lowered the rates of all injuries, including TDIs. Additionally, interventions that decrease the instances of bullying and violence can decrease the risk of TDI.

Dental professionals can play an important role in preventing TDIs if they make injury prevention counseling a part of their anticipatory guidance plan. Facial and dental injuries are common among victims of abuse. Dentists are mandatory reporters of child abuse and neglect in most states in the United States, although laws on reporting abuse of adults are not clear. Thus dental providers should be watchful in identifying and reporting cases of child abuse to the appropriate authorities.

## Description and Etiology of Congenital Anomalies

Disturbances in normal head development during embryogenesis manifest clinically as malformations that affect orofacial and dental structures. The most common anomalies of public health importance are the orofacial clefts and tooth agenesis (oligodontia/hypodontia/anodontia).

## Orofacial Clefts

Orofacial clefts are the most common genetically determined craniofacial anomalies of the orofacial region. Clefts occur due to defects in the development or maturation of the embryonic processes and can affect the lips, palate, tongue, and other facial tissues. Clefts of the lips followed by the palate are by far the most common types of facial clefts. Orofacial clefts are classified as those that involve the lip with or without the palate (CL/P) or those that involve the palate only (CPO). Clefts are also divided into syndromic (associated with other abnormalities) and nonsyndromic (isolated). In the United States, orofacial clefts are recorded on the birth certificates of affected children, as they are congenital anomalies and reported in the birth defects registry.

Clefts mainly occur due to maternal exposure to teratogenic agents. Risk factors, such as maternal smoking during pregnancy, and use of certain medications, such as topiramate or valproic acid in the first trimester of pregnancy, cause orofacial clefts.[71] Additionally, interactions between certain genes and environmental factors, such as smoking, have also been shown to be important risk factors for the development of clefts.[62] Mothers with diabetes before the onset of pregnancy (not gestational onset), maternal overweight/obesity, and parental age at the time of birth have all been shown to increase the risk of having a child with CL/P.[21,67] Influenza in the first trimester is also a risk factor for cleft lip but not for cleft palate.[46]

Some of the features associated with the occurrence of orofacial clefts are as follows:
- Cleft lip only (CL) tends to be unilateral (approximately 90%), and approximately two-thirds occur on the left side regardless of gender, ethnic group, and severity of defect.
- There is a clear male predilection for CL/P and a tendency toward CP in females.
- The risk of clefts in stillbirths and abortions is approximately three times as frequent as in live births.
- Infant mortality rates are higher among children born with clefts, and the odds of mortality are two to nine times higher based on the presence of additional malformations.

## Tooth Agenesis

Different terms are used to describe the condition of congenitally missing teeth: hypodontia, oligodontia, anodontia, congenitally missing teeth, and dental agenesis. Anodontia refers to patients with the complete absence of teeth; oligodontia refers to patients with the absence of six or more teeth apart from the third molars.[54] Genetics, developmental anomalies, endocrine disturbances, and local factors such as pathology, facial trauma, and medical treatment have also been mentioned as etiologic factors.[14] Developmental anomalies associated with tooth agenesis include delayed tooth formation, prolonged primary tooth exfoliation, retained primary teeth, interdental spacing, reduced alveolar bone development, and increased freeway space.[70] Tooth agenesis has also been related to reduced jaw size.

## Distribution of Congenital Anomalies

As with other rare diseases and conditions, the incidence of orofacial clefts is reported as a proportion of total live births. The occurrence of cleft lip, cleft palate, or both in the United States has remained stable over the past few decades and is approximately 1 in 700 live births.[53] Each year, in the United States, approximately 2650 babies are born with a cleft palate, and 4440 babies are born with a cleft lip with or without a cleft palate.[53] Isolated orofacial clefts are one of the most common types of birth defects in the United States and represent almost 50% to 80% of all clefts.[53]

Regional variations in prevalence have been noted within the United States, with lower proportions of isolated cases in Alabama and Georgia and higher proportions of cases in Rhode Island, Tennessee, and West Virginia.[39] Racial/ethnic variations have also been reported in the incidence of clefts, with individuals of Japanese and Navajo Indian ancestries having the highest rates, followed by non-Hispanic Whites and African Americans.[39,49] Studies that examined rates of CL/P among various ethnic groups in the United States and United Kingdom found that the rates of CL/P among these groups were more similar to those in the countries of their origin than to those in the countries of their current residence, further suggesting a genetic role.[49] Globally, epidemiologic estimates of the true incidence and prevalence of orofacial clefts are tenuous, as most of the estimates come from countries with better access to medical care and nationwide registries of birth defects. Data from most developing countries come from studies on small convenience samples. Studies on the global prevalence of facial clefts have reported prevalence levels in the range of 1.38 to 1.7 per 1000 live births in low- and middle-income countries.[41] However, another report from WHO, which included data from 57 registries, found significant variations in prevalence between population groups, with a range of 3.4 to 22.9 cases per 10,000 births.[48]

Large differences in the prevalence of tooth agenesis have been reported, varying from 0.3%[59] to 36.5%.[47] The prevalence of third molar agenesis might be as high as approximately 50%, but agenesis of other teeth is less common, at 1% to 9.6% in the general non-Hispanic White population and 7.7% in the African American population. This is similar to the prevalence reported in Europe (5.5%) and Australia (6.3%).[54] There is no particular difference in the distribution of tooth agenesis across genders. The mandibular second premolar is clearly the most frequently absent tooth, followed by the maxillary lateral incisor (1%–4%) and the maxillary second premolar. Agenesis of the maxillary central incisors, maxillary and mandibular first molars, and mandibular cuspids is very rare. When deciduous tooth agenesis occurs, it is most often in the incisor region, followed by the first deciduous molars of the maxillary arch.[25]

## Congenital Anomalies and Public Health

The prevalence of congenital anomalies in the community is important from a public health perspective, as it is directly related to the dental service utilization. The management of congenital anomalies routinely requires a multidisciplinary team comprising surgeons, speech therapists, audiologists, dentists, orthodontists, psychologists, geneticists, and specialist nurses. The costs incurred for affected individuals in terms of treatment expenditures and exclusion from education, employment, and society in general are significant and affect not only the individual but also their families. A great deal of work needs to be done toward developing public health interventions that could alleviate the burden of disease and be delivered in a cost-effective manner.

# References

1. Ackerman JL, Proffit WR. The characteristics of malocclusion: a modern approach to classification and diagnosis. *Am J Orthod.* 1969;56:443–454.

2. Aldrigui JM, Jabbar NS, Bonecker M, Braga MM, Wanderley MT. Trends and associated factors in prevalence of dental trauma in Latin America and Caribbean: a systematic review and meta-analysis. *Community Dent Oral Epidemiol.* 2014;42:30–42.

3. Allareddy V, Nalliah RP. Epidemiology of facial fracture injuries. *J Oral Maxillofac Surg.* 2011;69:2613–2618.

4. Andersson L. Epidemiology of traumatic dental injuries. *J Endod.* 2013;39:S2–S5.

5. Andreasen JO, Andreasen FM, Andersson L. Textbook and color atlas of traumatic injuries to the teeth, 4th ed. Oxford, UK: Wiley-Blackwell; 2007.

6. Andreasen JO, Ravn JJ. Epidemiology of traumatic dental injuries to primary and permanent teeth in a Danish population sample. *Int J Oral Surg.* 1972;1:235–239.

7. Angle EH. Classification of malocclusion. *Dent Cosmos.* 1899;41:248–264.

8. Baca CB, Vickrey BG, Vassar SD, Cook A, Berg AT. Injuries in adolescents with childhood-onset epilepsy compared with sibling controls. *J Pediatr.* 2013;163. 1684–91.e4.

9. Basha S, Mohammad RN, Swamy HS, Sexena V. Association between Traumatic Dental Injury, Obesity, and Socioeconomic Status in 6- and 13-Year-Old Schoolchildren. *Soc Work Public Health.* 2015;30:336–344.

10. Baskaradoss JK, Geevarghese A, Roger C, et al. Prevalence of malocclusion and its relationship with caries among school children aged 11 - 15 years in southern India. *Korean J Orthod.* 2013;43:35–41.

11. Bendo CB, Paiva SM, Varni JW, et al. Oral health-related quality of life and traumatic dental injuries in Brazilian adolescents. *Community Dent Oral Epidemiol.* 2014;42:216–223.

12. Blokland A, Watt RG, Tsakos G, et al. Traumatic dental injuries and socioeconomic position—findings from the Children's Dental Health Survey 2013. *Community Dent Oral Epidemiol.* 2016;44:586–591.

13. British Standard Institute. In: British Standard Incisor Classification, Glossary of Dental Terms BS. London, UK: British Standard Institute; 1983:*4492*.

14. Brook AH. A unifying aetiological explanation for anomalies of human tooth number and size. *Arch Oral Biol.* 1984;29:373–378.

15. Brook PH, Shaw WC. The development of an index of orthodontic treatment priority. *Eur J Orthod.* 1989;11:309–320.

16. Centers for Disease Control and Prevention. Report to Congress on traumatic brain injury in the United States: epidemiology and rehabilitation. Washington, DC: Centers for Disease Control and Prevention; 2015.

17. Cohenca N, Roges RA, Roges R. The incidence and severity of dental trauma in intercollegiate athletes. *J Am Dent Assoc.* 2007;138:1121–1126.

18. Cons NC, Jenny J, Kohaut FJ. DAI: The Dental Aesthetic Index. Iowa City: University of Iowa; 1986.

19. Correa-Faria P, Martins CC, Bonecker M, et al. Absence of an association between socioeconomic indicators and traumatic dental injury: a systematic review and meta-analysis. *Dent Traumatol.* 2015;31:255–266.

20. Correa-Faria P, Martins CC, Bonecker M, et al. Clinical factors and socio-demographic characteristics associated with dental trauma in children: a systematic review and meta-analysis. *Dent Traumatol.* 2016;32:367–378.

21. Correa A, Gilboa SM, Besser LM, et al. Diabetes mellitus and birth defects. *Am J Obstet Gynecol.* 2008;199 237.e1–9.

22. Corruccini RS, Pacciani E. "Orthodontistry" and dental occlusion in Etruscans. *Angle Orthod.* 1989;59:61–64.

23. Da Rosa P, Rousseau MC, Edasseri A, et al. Investigating socioeconomic position in dental caries and traumatic dental injury among children in Quebec. *Community Dent Health.* 2017;34:226–233.

24. Daniels C, Richmond S. The development of the index of complexity, outcome and need (ICON). *J Orthod.* 2000;27:149–162.

25. Davis PJ, Darvell BW. Congenitally missing permanent mandibular incisors and their association with missing primary teeth in the southern Chinese (Hong Kong). *Community Dent Oral Epidemiol.* 1993;21:162–164.

26. Draker HL. Handicapping labio-lingual deviations: a proposed index for public health purposes. *Am J Orthod.* 1960;46:295–305.

27. Dye BA, Tan S, Smith V, et al. Trends in oral health status: United States, 1988-1994 and 1999-2004. *Vital Health Stat 11.* 2007;1–92.

28. Ellis GE, Davey KW. The Classification and Treatment of Injuries to the Teeth of Children: A Reference Manual for the Dental Student and the General Practitioner. Chicago, IL: Year Book Medical Publishers; 1970.

29. Fédération Dentaire Internationale. Commission on dental products. *Working Party No.* 1990;7:276.

30. Feldens CA, Dos Santos Dullius AI, Kramer PF, et al. Impact of malocclusion and dentofacial anomalies on the prevalence and severity of dental caries among adolescents. *Angle Orthod.* 2015;85:1027–1034.

31. Feliciano KM, de França Caldas A. A systematic review of the diagnostic classifications of traumatic dental injuries. *Dent Traumatol.* 2006;22:71–76.

32. Fisher-Owens SA, Lukefahr JL, Tate AR. Oral and dental aspects of child abuse and neglect. *Pediatr Dent.* 2017;39:278–283.

33. Flores MT. Traumatic injuries in the primary dentition. *Dent Traumatol.* 2002;18:287–298.

34. Glendor U, Halling A, Andersson L, Eilert-Petersson E. Incidence of traumatic tooth injuries in children and adolescents in the county of Västmanland. *Sweden Swed Dent J.* 1996;20:15–28.

35. Grainger RM. Orthodontic treatment priority index. *Vital Health Stat.* 1967;2:1–49.

36. Gray AS, Demirjian A. Indexing occlusions for dental public health programs. *Am J Orthod.* 1977;72:191–197.

37. Grewe JM, Hagan DV. Malocclusion indices: a comparative evaluation. *Am J Orthod.* 1972;61:286–294.

38. Harris EF, Johnson MG. Heritability of craniometric and occlusal variables: a longitudinal sib analysis. *Am J Orthod Dentofacial Orthop.* 1991;99:258–268.

39. IPDTOC Working Group. Prevalence at birth of cleft lip with or without cleft palate: data from the International Perinatal Database of Typical Oral Clefts (IPDTOC). *Cleft Palate Craniofac J.* 2011;48:66–81.

40. Jenny J, Cons NC. Establishing malocclusion severity levels on the Dental Aesthetic Index (DAI) scale. *Aust Dent J.* 1996;41:43–46.

41. Kadir A, Mossey PA, Blencowe H, Moorthie S, Lawn JE, Mastroiacovo P, et al. Systematic review and meta-analysis of the birth prevalence of orofacial clefts in low- and middle-income countries. *Cleft Palate Craniofac J.* 2017;54:571–581.

42. Kaste LM, Gift HC, Bhat M, Swango PA. Prevalence of incisor trauma in persons 6-50 years of age: United States, 1988-1991. *J Dent Res.* 1996;75. Spec No:696–705.

43. Kelly JE, Harvey CR. An assessment of the occlusion of the teeth of youths 12-17 years. *Vital Health Stat.* 1977;11:1–65.

44. Kelly JE, Sanchez M, Van Kirk LE. An assessment of the occlusion of the teeth of children 6-11 years. United States. *Vital Health Stat 11.* 1973;1–60.

45. Koochek AR, Yeh MS, Rolfe B, et al. The relationship between Index of Complexity, Outcome and Need, and patients' perceptions of malocclusion: a study in general dental practice. *Br Dent J.* 2001;191:325–329.

46. Luteijn JM, Brown MJ, Dolk H. Influenza and congenital anomalies: a systematic review and meta-analysis. *Hum Reprod.* 2014;29: 809–823.
47. Mahaney MC, Fujiwara TM, Morgan K. Dental agenesis in the Dariusleut Hutterite Brethren: comparisons to selected Caucasoid population surveys. *Am J Phys Anthropol.* 1990;82:165–177.
48. Mossey PA, Little J, Munger RG, Dixon MJ, Shaw WC. Cleft lip and palate. *Lancet.* 2009;374:1773–1785.
49. Mossey PA, Modell B. Epidemiology of oral clefts 2012: an international perspective. *Front Oral Biol.* 2012;16:1–18.
50. Nelson S, Armogan V, Abel Y, Broadbent BH, Hans M. Disparity in orthodontic utilization and treatment need among high school students. *J Public Health Dent.* 2004;64:26–30.
51. Nguyen QV, Bezemer PD, Habets L. A systematic review of the relationship between overjet size and traumatic dental injuries. *Eur J Orthod.* 1999;21:503–515.
52. Otuyemi OD, Jones SP. Methods of assessing and grading malocclusion: a review. *Aust Orthod J.* 1995;14:21–27.
53. Parker SE, Mai CT, Canfield MA, et al. Updated national birth prevalence estimates for selected birth defects in the United States, 2004-2006. *Birth Defects Res A Clin Mol Teratol.* 2010;88:1008–1016.
54. Polder BJ, Van't Hof MA, Van der Linden FP, et al. A meta-analysis of the prevalence of dental agenesis of permanent teeth. *Community Dent Oral Epidemiol.* 2004;32:217–226.
55. Proffit WR. On the aetiology of malocclusion. The Northcroft lecture, 1985, presented to the British Society for the Study of Orthodontics, Oxford, April 18. *Br J Orthod 1986.* 1985;13:1–11.
56. Proffit WR, Fields Jr HW, Moray LJ. Prevalence of malocclusion and orthodontic treatment need in the United States: estimates from the NHANES III survey. *Int J Adult Orthodon Orthognath Surg.* 1998;13:97–106.
57. Proffit WR, Fields HW, Sarver DM. *Contemporary Orthodontics.* 5th ed. St. Louis, MO: Mosby; 2013.
58. Richmond S, Shaw WC, O'Brien KD, et al. The development of the PAR Index (Peer Assessment Rating): reliability and validity. *Eur J Orthod.* 1992;14:125–139.
59. Rosenzweig KA, Garbarski D. Numerical aberrations in the permanent teeth of grade school children in Jerusalem. *Am J Phys Anthropol.* 1965;23:277–283.
60. Sethi RK, Kozin ED, Fagenholz PJ. Epidemiological survey of head and neck injuries and trauma in the United States. *Otolaryngol Head Neck Surg.* 2014;151:776–784.
61. Shaw WC, Richmond S, O'Brien KD. The use of occlusal indices: a European perspective. *Am J Orthod Dentofacial Orthop.* 1995;107:1–10.
62. Shi M, Wehby GL, Murray JC. Review on genetic variants and maternal smoking in the etiology of oral clefts and other birth defects. *Birth Defects Res C Embryo Today.* 2008;84:16–29.
63. Shulman JD, Peterson J. The association between incisor trauma and occlusal characteristics in individuals 8-50 years of age. *Dent Traumatol.* 2004;20:67–74.
64. Skaare AB, Jacobsen I. Dental injuries in Norwegians aged 7–18 years. *Dent Traumatol.* 2003;19:67–71.
65. Slakter MJ, Albino JE, Green LJ, et al. Validity of an orthodontic treatment priority index to measure need for treatment. *Am J Orthod.* 1980;78:421–425.
66. Stockwell AJ. Incidence of dental trauma in the Western Australian School Dental Service. *Community Dent Oral Epidemiol.* 1988;16:294–298.
67. Stothard KJ, Tennant PW, Bell R, Rankin J. Maternal overweight and obesity and the risk of congenital anomalies: a systematic review and meta-analysis. *JAMA.* 2009;301:636–650.
68. Summers CJ. The occlusal index: a system for identifying and scoring occlusal disorders. *Am J Orthod.* 1971;59:552–567.
69. Tang EL, Wei SH. Recording and measuring malocclusion: a review of the literature. *Am J Orthod Dentofacial Orthop.* 1993;103: 344–351.
70. Tavajohi-Kermani H, Kapur R, Sciote JJ. Tooth agenesis and craniofacial morphology in an orthodontic population. *Am J Orthod Dentofacial Orthop.* 2002;122:39–47.
71. Werler MM, Ahrens KA, Bosco JL, Mitchell AA, Anderka MT, Gilboa SM, et al. Use of antiepileptic medications in pregnancy in relation to risks of birth defects. *Ann Epidemiol.* 2011;21: 842–850.
72. World Health Organization. Application of the International Classification of Diseases to Dentistry and Stomatology. 3rd ed. Geneva, Switzerland: WHO; 1995.
73. World Health Organization. ICD-10: International Statistical Classification of Diseases and Related Health Problems. *10th rev.* Geneva, Switzerland: World Health Organization; 2004.
74. World Health Organization. Oral Health Survey: basic methods. Geneva, Switzerland: World Health Organization; 2013.
75. Zhou HH, Ongodia D, Liu Q, et al. Changing pattern in the characteristics of maxillofacial fractures. *J Craniofac Surg.* 2013;24: 929–933.

# 19

# Measurement and Distribution of Dental Fluorosis

JOHN J. WARREN, DDS, MS

STEVEN M. LEVY, DDS, MPH

## CHAPTER OUTLINE

## Description and Etiology of Dental Fluorosis

Dental fluorosis is a hypo-mineralization of enamel associated with elevated fluoride intake during the process of enamel formation. In its mildest form, dental fluorosis appears as barely discernable fine flecks or lines of opaque white enamel. Slightly more involved mild fluorosis often presents as lacy markings that follow the perikymata of the enamel.[16] More involved dental fluorosis is characterized by thicker lines or bands of opaque enamel that can coalesce to form larger areas of affected enamel. In severe cases, these coalesced areas sometimes break down to form discrete pits, which can be accompanied by areas that are stained orange to dark brown. As depicted in Figure 19.1, the appearance of dental fluorosis can range from such slight disturbances of enamel that it can be seen only on close examination with drying of the teeth to severe staining and pitting that can be a significant cosmetic concern.

At the structural level, dental fluorosis is characterized by subsurface porosity of the enamel surface, which is actually similar to what is seen in early dental caries lesions. Excess fluoride during enamel formation is believed to disrupt mineralization and promote the retention of enamel protein, yielding weaker enamel structures and thus subsurface porosity.[15] All developmental stages of enamel are thought to be susceptible to excess fluoride, but it appears the early maturation stage is when the enamel is most

sensitive to fluoride.[72] However, as described in this chapter, the precise ages when high fluoride intakes are most likely to result in dental fluorosis have not been firmly established.

Dental fluorosis is dose dependent—the greater the fluoride intake during tooth development, the more severe the fluorosis.[16] However, the exact amount necessary to cause fluorosis is unknown and can very among individuals. Data from the longitudinal Iowa Fluoride Study suggest that fluorosis prevalence on the maxillary incisors also varies with fluoride intake level early in life. That study found that fluorosis prevalence (mostly very mild) was 13% among those with average intakes of 0.04 mg of fluoride per kg of body weight from ages 0 to 36 months, and it increased to 23% when intakes were between 0.04 and 0.06 mg/kg and to 38% when fluoride intakes averaged 0.06 mg/kg or higher.[25]

As with the precise amounts needing to be ingested to produce dental fluorosis, the age periods when the maxillary incisors are most susceptible to fluoride ingestion resulting in fluorosis also are unclear. Various studies with different designs have estimated the most susceptible periods to be 0 to 12 months,[31] 12 to 36 months,[5] 15 to 30 months,[19,20] and 35 to 42 months.[29] Data from the Iowa Fluoride Study suggest that fluoride intakes during each of the first 4 years of life are important in fluorosis development but that the first year (0–12 months) is the most critical period followed by the second, third, and fourth years.[25]

Dental fluorosis can occur in the primary dentition, but it is less common and less commonly studied than in the permanent dentition. In areas of very high water fluoride concentrations, all primary teeth can be affected, but in most instances, only the later-erupting primary teeth are affected—mainly the primary second molars.[70]

## Measurement of Dental Fluorosis

"Mottled enamel," which was later understood to be caused by fluoride ingestion (i.e., dental fluorosis), was first described around 1900 by dentists in Germany and Italy who noted certain patients had black stained teeth, and it was speculated that the staining was related to the patients' drinking water.[18] However, the most systematic and noteworthy early description of mottled enamel was that made by Dr. Frederick McKay, who graduated from the University of Pennsylvania dental school in 1900 and shortly thereafter relocated to Colorado Springs, Colorado.[49] There he noted that

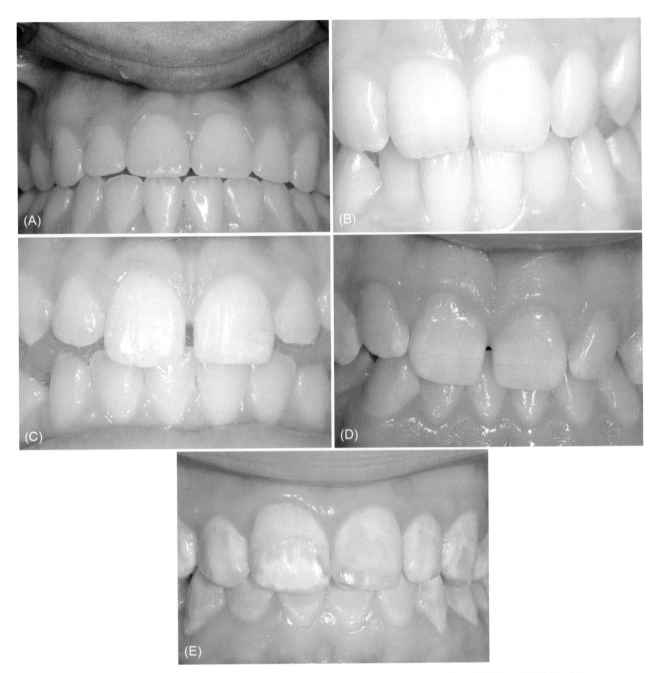

• **Figure 19.1** Examples of dental fluorosis. (A) Normal: Note the translucent enamel and lack of striations. (B) Mild Dental Fluorosis: Note thin striations along the buccal surfaces of the central incisors, with a small amount of surface area affected. (C) Mild Dental Fluorosis: This is a slightly more involved case of mild fluorosis, with more of the surface area affected. (D) Moderate Dental Fluorosis: Note coalesced areas on the buccal surfaces of the central incisors and most of the surface area affected. (E) Severe Dental Fluorosis: Note the enamel pitting, staining, and loss of some enamel.

many of his patients who had grown up in the area had white flecks or yellow or brown spots on their teeth and that some affected teeth were paper white and the enamel sometimes had shallow, stained pits.[41] Importantly, McKay also noted that many of these same patients had little, if any, dental caries experience.[42] In his work, McKay systematically examined nearly 3000 school children in the Colorado Springs area and found that nearly 90% of them were affected. Unfortunately, few details of how he and his colleagues assessed or measured the mottled enamel have survived.[42]

It should be noted that McKay suspected something in the water supplies around Colorado Springs was responsible for the mottled enamel, but while analyses of water samples were completed, the technology at the time did not allow for detection of trace elements. It was not until the early 1930s that Harry Churchill, a chemist with the Aluminum Company of America (ALCOA) and working with McKay, first identified fluoride as the likely culprit.[49] The identification of fluoride as the likely cause of lower dental caries rates and more dental fluorosis eventually led to a series of studies that evaluated fluorosis in school children in a number of communities with differing water fluoride concentrations. These studies were headed by Dr. H. Trendley Dean, the first dentist employed by the U.S. Public Health Service, who, in the mid-1930s, developed the first scheme to measure the prevalence and severity of dental fluorosis—Dean's Index.[12]

## Dean's Index

Dean had identified areas of mottled enamel from a survey of dentists across all 48 states,[11] and then followed up in selected areas by conducting clinical examinations of children. To assess dental fluorosis clinically, Dean initially devised a seven-point ordinal scale to score fluorosis with categories of normal, questionable, very mild, mild, moderate, moderately severe, and severe.[12] By the late 1930s, Dean modified his original index into a six-point scale by combining the moderately severe and severe categories of the original index (Box 19.1).[13] Dean's Index is based on the two most affected teeth in the mouth, although many studies and surveys have used a full-mouth assessment using the index as part of their protocols. Another aspect of Dean's measurement of fluorosis was his assignment of numerical scores to each fluorosis category to create the Community Fluorosis Index (CFI). Specifically, normal was scored as 0 for the CFI, questionable as 0.5, very mild as 1, mild as 2, and so on. While the assignment of numerical scores was arbitrary, his scheme resulted in a strong linear correlation of Dean's Index fluorosis scores with water fluoride concentrations in the communities he had studied (Figure 19.2).

Dean's Index continues to be used widely, including as part of examinations conducted by the U.S. National Health and Nutrition Examination Survey (NHANES), although the most recent NHANES examinations eliminated the "questionable" category by

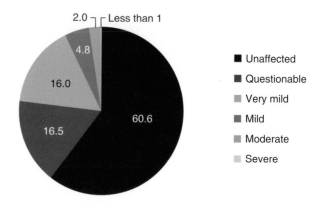

• **Figure 19.2** Distribution of dental fluorosis severity—U.S. National Health and Nutrition Examination Survey, 1999–2004. Note: Dental fluorosis is based on Dean's Fluorosis Index. Percentages do not sum to 100 due to rounding.[2]

considering such cases as normal.[48] Despite its wide use, Dean's Index has been criticized for having somewhat vague categories—including the "questionable" category—for not having any basis in histology or tooth development and for not being sensitive enough with either the very mild or very severe forms of the condition.[27] Because of these limitations, several other fluorosis indices have been developed. These are described briefly in the following sections.

## Tooth Surface Index of Fluorosis

The Tooth Surface Index of Fluorosis (TSIF) was developed in the 1980s by Herschel Horowitz and other researchers at the National Institute of Dental Research.[27] The TSIF is similar to the original Dean's Index in that it employs a seven-point scale, but as depicted in Box 19.2, it more completely differentiates categories of mild dental fluorosis and categorizes more severe forms based on staining with or without pitting. It should be noted that the TSIF does not use any drying of the teeth prior to scoring for fluorosis; thus this index is considered to be a measure of the public health impact of fluorosis rather than a precise scoring mechanism, and without drying, some very mild cases can be missed entirely or underscored. The TSIF has also been used as a means of scoring fluorosis in the primary dentition.[70]

## Thylstrup-Fejerskov Index

The Thylstrup-Fejerskov (TF) Index represents an attempt to develop a more sensitive and biologically based means of measuring dental fluorosis.[67] Unlike Dean's Index and TSIF, the scores are based on the histologic features of affected enamel and, as seen in Box 19.3, there are different descriptions for fluorosis appearance on smooth and occlusal tooth surfaces. The TF scores range from 0 to 9, and scoring requires examiners to estimate the extent of fluorosis (in mm) on a surface to make the score. Unlike other fluorosis measures, the TF Index requires thorough drying of the teeth, so even the mildest forms of fluorosis can be detected. Although the TF Index offers advantages in scoring fluorosis more precisely, it has not enjoyed widespread use in North America, and its use of thoroughly drying teeth makes it difficult to compare results to those obtained using other indices, particularly because the TF Index overestimates the prevalence as not all TF cases are aesthetically important.

---

• **BOX 19.1** **Criteria for Dean's Fluorosis Index**

**Normal**

The enamel represents the usual translucent semivitriform type of structure. The surface is smooth, glossy, and usually of a pale creamy white color.

**Questionable**

The enamel discloses slight aberrations from the translucency of normal enamel, ranging from a few white flecks to occasional white spots. This classification is used in those instances in which a definite diagnosis of the mildest form of fluorosis is not warranted and a classification of "normal" is not justified.

**Very Mild**

Small, opaque, paper-white areas scattered irregularly over the tooth but not involving as much as approximately 25% of the tooth surface. Frequently included in this classification are teeth showing no more than about 1 to 2 mm of white opacity at the tip of the summit of the cusps of the bicuspids or second molars.

**Mild**

The white opaque areas in the enamel of the teeth are more extensive but do not involve as much as 50% of the tooth.

**Moderate**

All enamel surfaces of the teeth are affected, and surfaces subject to attrition show marked wear. Brown stain is frequently a disfiguring feature.

**Severe**

Includes teeth formerly classified as "moderately severe" and "severe." All enamel surfaces are affected, and hypoplasia is so marked that the general form of the tooth may be altered. The major diagnostic sign of this classification is the discrete or confluent pitting. Brown stains are widespread and teeth often present a corroded appearance.

Dean HT, Dixon RM, Cohen C. Mottled enamel in Texas. *Public Health Rep.* 1935;50:424–442.

## • BOX 19.2  Clinical Criteria and Categorizations for the Tooth Surface Index of Fluorosis (TSIF)[27]

### Category 0
Enamel shows no evidence of fluorosis.

### Category 1
Enamel shows definite evidence of fluorosis, enamel has areas with parchment-white color that total less than one-third of the visible enamel surface. This category includes fluorosis confined only to incisal edges of anterior teeth and cusp tips of posterior teeth ("snowcapping").

### Category 2
Parchment-white fluorosis totals at least one-third of the visible surface but less than two-thirds.

### Category 3
Parchment-white fluorosis totals at least two-thirds of the visible surface.

### Category 4
Enamel shows staining in conjunction with any of the preceding levels of fluorosis. Staining is defined as an area of definite discoloration that may range from light to very dark brown.

### Category 5
Discrete pitting of the enamel exists, unaccompanied by evidence of staining of intact enamel. A pit is defined as a definite physical defect in the enamel surface with a rough floor that is surrounded by a wall of intact enamel. The pitted area is usually stained or differs in color from the surrounding enamel.

### Category 6
Both discrete pitting and staining of the intact enamel exist.

### Category 7
Confluent pitting of the enamel surface exists. Large areas of enamel may be missing and the anatomy of the tooth may be altered. Dark brown stain is usually present.

## • BOX 19.3  Clinical Criteria and Scoring for the Thylstrup-Fejerskov Fluorosis Index (TF)[66]

### Score 0
Normal translucency of enamel remains after prolonged air drying.

### Score 1
Narrow white lines located corresponding to the perikymata.

### Score 2
Smooth surfaces:
   More pronounced lines of opacity that follow the perikymata. Occasionally confluence of adjacent lines.
Occlusal surfaces:
   Scattered areas of opacity <2 mm in diameter and pronounced opacity of cuspal ridges.

### Score 3
Smooth surfaces:
   Merging and irregular cloudy areas of opacity. Accentuated drawing of perikymata often visible between opacities.
Occlusal surfaces:
   Confluent areas of marked opacity. Worn areas appear almost normal but usually circumscribed by a rim of opaque enamel.

### Score 4
Smooth surfaces:
   The entire surface exhibits marked opacity or appears chalky white. Parts of surface exposed to attrition appear less affected.
Occlusal surfaces:
   Entire surface exhibits marked opacity. Attrition is often pronounced shortly after eruption.

### Score 5
Smooth and occlusal surfaces:
   Entire surface displays marked opacity with focal loss of outermost enamel (pits) <2 mm in diameter.

### Score 6
Smooth surfaces:
   Pits are regularly arranged in horizontal bands <2 mm in vertical extension.
Occlusal surfaces:
   Confluent areas <3 mm in diameter exhibit loss of enamel. Marked attrition.

### Score 7
Smooth surfaces:
   Loss of outermost enamel in irregular areas involving less than half of entire surface.
Occlusal surfaces:
   Changes in the morphology caused by merging pits and marked attrition.

### Score 8
Smooth and occlusal surfaces:
   Loss of outermost enamel involving more than half of surface.

### Score 9
Smooth and occlusal surfaces:
   Loss of main part of enamel with change in anatomic appearance of the surface. Cervical rim of almost unaffected enamel is often noted.

## Fluorosis Risk Index

The Fluorosis Risk Index (FRI) was developed in the 1980s for a series of case-control studies of dental fluorosis risk factors conducted in New England.[53] As such, the FRI was developed to assess the presence of dental fluorosis on different teeth based on fluoride exposure during different phases of tooth development. This index is less concerned with scoring the severity of the condition, as it only has four categories—normal, questionable, definitive, and severe—but separately scores four zones per tooth to differentiate fluorosis scores related to periods of enamel formation. These four surface zones (incisal edge/occlusal, incisal, middle, and cervical thirds) are further categorized as FRI I zones and FRI II zones, corresponding to areas of early and late enamel mineralization, respectively.[53] The FRI has not been widely used because few studies have detailed, time-specific fluoride intake data for which it was designed.

## Developmental Defects of Enamel Index

Although not specific to dental fluorosis, the Developmental Defects of Enamel (DDE) index records both "diffuse" and "demarcated" opacities, along with hypoplasia.[8] The diffuse opacities are mostly attributable to dental fluorosis, but the index purposefully does not preclude etiologies other than excessive fluoride intake. The modified DDE includes a scoring scheme ranging from

1 (diffuse lines in the enamel) to 6 (pits of >2 mm in enamel along with confluent or patchy diffuse opacities). The modified DDE index also includes categorization of (nonfluoride) demarcated opacities (white/creamy or yellow/brown), and enamel hypoplasia. The "demarcated" enamel opacities described for the DDE Index can sometimes be mistaken for dental fluorosis, but because they have a different etiology (e.g., physical and/or biological trauma) not related to fluoride intake, they should not be recorded as fluorosis. Thus the DDE index offers a more comprehensive scoring of all types of enamel defects, although most studies have used it to measure dental fluorosis (diffuse opacities).

## Other Fluorosis Measurement Issues

To differentiate fluorosis from nonfluoride opacities, Russell[61] developed a series of criteria to distinguish fluoride opacities from nonfluoride opacities—sometimes referred to as Russell's criteria. Table 19.1 presents a summary of Russell's criteria. In brief, unlike dental fluorosis, nonfluoride opacities are well defined, do not follow the perikymata, and are more randomly distributed among the teeth.

Fluorosis can be difficult to assess, even in surveys such as NHANES that are highly standardized.[47] The various indices used for measuring dental fluorosis as described above are somewhat subjective and open to interpretation, and they vary in the degree of drying that is done when scoring. A quick review of the indices reveals that some indices require thorough drying of the teeth,[67] others do not dry the teeth at all,[8,12,27] and another minimally dries the teeth.[53] It is clear that drying of the teeth makes dental fluorosis stand out and become more detectable than is the case with wet teeth. This not only makes it problematic to compare studies using different indices but can also make it difficult for examiners to calibrate themselves to one another due to teeth becoming drier as the calibration sessions continue with subjects keeping their mouths open for longer periods. For these reasons, some have advocated using standardized photographs, with standardized drying regimens, for scoring of dental fluorosis.[71] A few studies that have assessed this approach have found photographic scoring to achieve reasonably high levels of reliability and generally good agreement with direct clinical scoring.[9,10,65] However, due to the drying necessary for high quality photographs, these approaches overestimate the prevalence of dental fluorosis compared to approaches that do not extensively dry the teeth.

## Risk Factors and Risk Indicators for Dental Fluorosis

As stated by Beltrán Aguilar et al.,[3] "the only known etiologic factor for enamel fluorosis is ingested fluoride." While there are other proposed etiologies for dental fluorosis as discussed below, the overwhelming majority of fluorosis occurs due to excessive total fluoride ingestion during tooth development. However, it remains unclear what amount is "excessive" and during which periods (ages) of tooth development higher fluoride intake is most likely to result in dental fluorosis. Because of these unknowns and the difficulty in assessing fluoride intake in children, most studies have assessed specific fluoride sources as risk factors for fluorosis rather than total fluoride intake.

Clearly, as first described by McKay,[41,42] high fluoride concentration of drinking water is a risk factor for dental fluorosis. His pioneering studies along with those of Dean et al.[11-14] demonstrated the positive relationship between water fluoride concentration and dental fluorosis prevalence, with fluorosis more prevalent in areas with higher water fluoride content. At the extreme, locales with water supplies having fluoride concentrations in excess of 6 parts per million (ppm), such as in areas of sub-Saharan Africa where water is often obtained from very deep wells, frequently have endemic severe dental fluorosis.[40,46,50,51,69]

| • TABLE 19.1 | Differential Diagnosis Between Milder Forms of Dental Fluorosis (Questionable, Very Mild, and Mild) and Nonfluoride Opacities of Enamel[60] | |
|---|---|---|

| Characteristic of Enamel Opacities | Milder Forms of Fluorosis | Nonfluoride Opacities |
|---|---|---|
| Area affected | Usually seen on or near tips of cusps or incisal edges | Usually centered in smooth surface; may affect entire crown |
| Shape of lesion | Resembles line shading in a pencil sketch; lines follow incremental lines in enamel; form irregular caps on cusps | Often round or oval |
| Demarcation | Shades off imperceptibly into surrounding normal enamel | Clearly differentiated from adjacent normal enamel |
| Color | Slightly more opaque than normal enamel; paper white incisal edges, tips of cusps may have frosted appearance; does not show stain at time of eruption (in these milder degrees, rarely at any time) | Usually pigmented at time of eruption; often creamy yellow to dark reddish orange |
| Teeth affected | Most frequent on teeth that calcify slowly (cuspids, bicuspids, second and third molars); rare on lower incisors; usually seen on six or eight homologous teeth; extremely rare in deciduous teeth | Any tooth may be affected; frequent on labial surfaces of lower incisors; may occur singly; usually one to three teeth affected; common in deciduous teeth |
| Gross hypoplasia | None; pitting of enamel does not occur in the milder forms; enamel surface has glazed appearance, is smooth to the point of explorer | Absent to severe; enamel surface may seem etched, be rough to explorer |
| Detection | Often invisible under strong light; most easily detected by line of sight tangential to tooth crown | Seen most easily under strong light on line of sight perpendicular to tooth surface |

During the time of the studies of McKay and Dean, fluoride from water was really the only source of ingested fluoride; there were no fluoride toothpastes or other fluoride products. Today, with numerous other sources of fluoride, risk factors for dental fluorosis are more numerous and varied, but water fluoride remains an important risk factor for dental fluorosis.[37] For example, a study by Burt et al.[5] demonstrated that the relationship between water fluoride concentration and fluorosis still remains valid. They studied the effects of an 11-month break in water fluoridation that occurred in the 1990s on subsequent fluorosis prevalence among children in a North Carolina community who were born before, during, and after the break in fluoridation. In this study, the overall prevalence of fluorosis was 44%, with a range from 32% to 62% depending on the age of the child when the break occurred; those born 4 to 5 years before the break had higher prevalence, whereas those who were up to 3 years of age at the time had lower prevalence.[5]

While there continues to be a strong association between fluoride concentration in tap water and dental fluorosis prevalence, in recent times, widespread consumption of bottled water, which typically has low fluoride concentrations,[33] has somewhat diluted this relationship in the United States and other industrialized countries. However, tap water, when mixed with infant formula concentrates, has been indicated as a risk factor for dental fluorosis,[28] and this finding is one of the reasons for the change in recommended community water fluoride concentration from a range of 0.7 to 1.2 ppm to a standard concentration of 0.7 ppm[68] and for recommendations to consider use of bottled water when mixing infant formula.[4]

Beyond water fluoride concentration, studies have reported that the use of dietary fluoride supplements increased the risk of dental fluorosis.[30,54,55,75] Other studies have found strong associations between fluorosis and early use and/or substantial ingestion of fluoride dentifrice.[7,35,45,52,56-58,60,64] In one such study, fluoridated dentifrice use before age 2 was found to be a risk factor for developing fluorosis, regardless of whether children resided in fluoridated or nonfluoridated communities.[58]

A series of well-designed case-control studies conducted by Pendrys et al.[53-56] used the Fluorosis Risk Index (FRI)[53] to identify risk factors for fluorosis. In these studies in both nonfluoridated and optimally fluoridated areas, risk factors for fluorosis included dietary fluoride supplement use from age 3 to 6 years, high household income levels, more frequent tooth brushing from 1 to 8 years, being non-Caucasian, use of powdered formula concentrates, and use of greater than a "pea-sized" amount of toothpaste more than once a day.

The Iowa Fluoride Study, a large longitudinal study of fluoride intake, dental fluorosis, and dental caries, has provided a great deal of information on fluoride intake in young children and the occurrence of dental fluorosis.[10,21,24-26,38,70] This study recruited more than 1300 newborns at hospital postpartum units and asked parents to periodically provide detailed information on their children's diets, fluoride product use, water sources, and other potential exposures beginning at 6 weeks of age and continuing through adolescence. Dental examinations for dental fluorosis and caries were conducted every 3 to 4 years beginning at age 5. This study found that early or improper dentifrice use,[21,38] along with higher water fluoride concentration and early use of infant formula,[38] were risk factors for fluorosis of the maxillary incisors. The study[24,26] also found a weak but significant association between amoxicillin use and dental fluorosis after anecdotal reports had suggested a link between dental fluorosis and

amoxicillin use. Subsequent study has supported this finding,[36] but a definitive link between amoxicillin use and fluorosis has not been established.

Some research has suggested that dental fluorosis occurs more frequently at higher altitudes. A few studies have found that, at roughly the same fluoride intake levels, children living at high altitudes had more prevalent and more severe dental fluorosis than their peers living near sea level.[39,62]

## Distribution of Dental Fluorosis

There is limited information on the overall prevalence and levels of severity of dental fluorosis on a worldwide scale, but a metaanalysis of more than 50 studies suggested that prevalence ranged from 16% to 32% depending on water fluoride concentration, and the authors concluded that fluorosis prevalence had increased substantially since the 1940s.[32]

Evidence also suggests that dental fluorosis prevalence and severity have increased in North America since the 1970s,[7] and specifically in the United States since the 1930s.[2,3] Studies conducted in various states during the 1980s and 1990s continued to show a relationship between water fluoride concentration and dental fluorosis prevalence, but the prevalence values were considerably higher than those reported by Dean[11-13] in communities with optimal water fluoride concentrations, presumably due to greater potential fluoride exposures than in Dean's era. These studies found prevalence of dental fluorosis in optimally fluoridated communities to be as high as 51% in Michigan,[66] 72% in Iowa,[64] 78% in North Carolina,[35] and 81% in Georgia.[73] These studies all used the TSIF index and considered any TSIF score greater than zero as "fluorosis," which probably explains, in part, the high prevalence; nevertheless, these findings clearly demonstrated evidence for increased prevalence.

On a nationwide scale in the United States, data from the 1986 to 1987 NIDR survey of schoolchildren, which used Dean's Index and a probability sample representing the entire US population, reported an overall prevalence of 23.5%, with fluorosis prevalence of nearly 30% among children in optimally fluoridated (0.7–1.2 ppm) areas and over 40% among children in areas with greater than 1.2 ppm fluoride concentrations.[23] In this study, only 1.4% of children had moderate or severe fluorosis overall, and 7.3% of those in areas of greater than 1.2 ppm fluoride had moderate or severe fluorosis. More recently, Beltrán-Aguilar et al.[2] reported that while less than 8% of people aged 6 to 49 had mild, moderate, or severe fluorosis as measured by Dean's Index (Figure 19.3), an additional 16% had very mild fluorosis, and a similar proportion (17%) had "questionable" fluorosis, leaving 61% unaffected. This study, which was based on NHANES 1999 to 2004 data, found that the highest prevalence was in adolescents, with 41% of 12- to 15-year-olds having mild, moderate, or severe fluorosis (Figure 19.4). Taken together, these findings again suggest that dental fluorosis prevalence continued to increase in the United States through the mid-2000s.

## Dental Fluorosis and Public Health

There has been considerable debate as to whether dental fluorosis constitutes a true public health problem in the United States. Stated differently: Does dental fluorosis pose a significant risk to

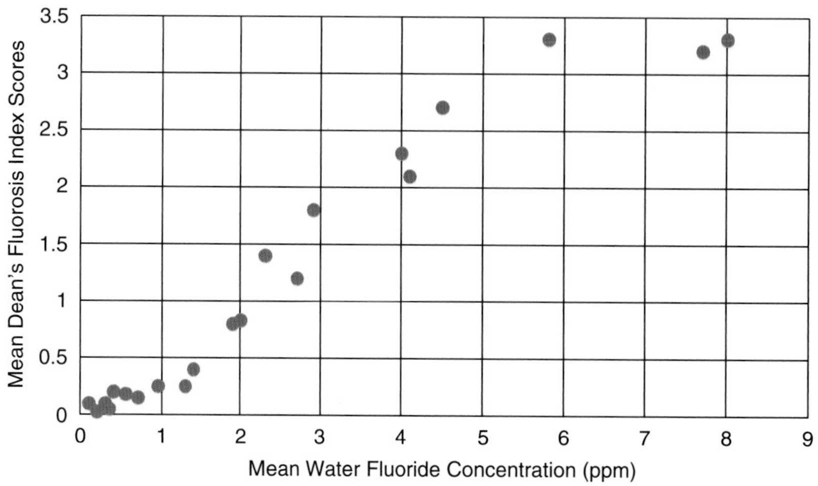

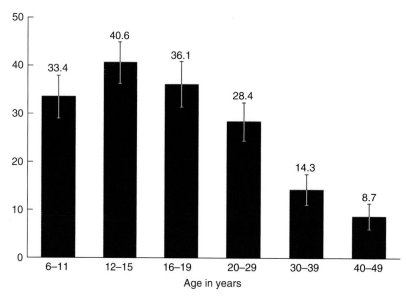

• **Figure 19.3** Data from Dean's studies to show the relation between mean Fluorosis Index scores and the fluoride concentration of the drinking water.[13]

• **Figure 19.4** Dental fluorosis prevalence by age – U.S. National Health and Nutrition Examination Survey, 1999–2004. Note: Dental fluorosis based on Dean's Fluorosis Index. Error bars represent 95% confidence intervals.[2]

the public's health? Given that the condition does not progress, is limited to only the oral cavity, and rarely has an effect on function, the answer to this question is "no"—it is not a true public health problem. However, for people with more severe forms of the condition, dental fluorosis can have an impact on aesthetics, in some cases to the point of requiring dental treatment to mask or cover affected anterior teeth. In severe dental fluorosis cases, loss of enamel due to pitting can leave the teeth more susceptible to caries. While aesthetic problems due to dental fluorosis have been estimated to affect about 2% of US schoolchildren,[22] in some places, such as East Africa where severe fluorosis is endemic,[50,51,69] the situation is different and dental fluorosis significantly affects a large number of people, making it a public health problem.

While dental fluorosis is not a true public health problem in the United States, in cases of moderate or severe fluorosis, it can affect aesthetic perceptions and quality of life.[6] In cases of very mild or mild fluorosis—by far the most common types of fluorosis in the United States (see Figure 19.3)—the impacts on aesthetic perceptions and quality of life have been found to be very modest[34,44] or nonexistent,[63] with at least one study finding that mild fluorosis can have a slight positive effect on aesthetics.[17] These and other studies have suggested that mild dental fluorosis is much less objectionable aesthetically than are malpositioned teeth, caries, or having spaces between anterior teeth.[43,44,74]

Given the trend in the United States toward higher dental fluorosis prevalence and aesthetic and quality of life concerns with severe fluorosis, several recommendations have been made to reduce systemic fluoride exposure and the risk of dental fluorosis. These recommendations have included a revised schedule for dietary fluoride supplements and use only for those at elevated caries risk,[59] recommendations to consider using bottled or other low-fluoride water for reconstituting infant formulas,[4] recommendations to limit the amount of toothpaste used with young children,[1] and the change in the recommended water fluoride concentration from a range of 0.7 to 1.2 ppm to a universal nationwide standard of 0.7 ppm.[68] The recommendation to reduce water fluoride concentration to 0.7 ppm was made specifically to reduce the risk of dental fluorosis while maintaining caries prevention and recognizing the many other sources of fluoride exposure.[68]

# References

1. American Dental Association Council on Scientific Affairs. Fluoride toothpaste use for young children. *J Am Dent Assoc.* 2014;145:190–191.
2. Beltrán-Aguilar ED, Barker L, Dye BA. *Prevalence and severity of dental fluorosis in the United States, 1999–2004; NCHS Data Brief No. 53.* Hyattsville, MD: National Center for Health Statistics; 2010.
3. Beltran-Aguilar ED, Griffin SO, Lockwood SA. Prevalence and trends in enamel fluorosis in the United States from the 1930s to the 1980s. *J Am Dent Assoc.* 2002;133:157–165.
4. Berg J, Gerweck C, Hujoel PP, et al. Evidence-based clinical recommendations regarding fluoride intake from reconstituted infant formula and enamel fluorosis: a report of the American Dental Association Council on Scientific Affairs. *J Am Dent Assoc.* 2011;142:79–87.
5. Burt BA, Keels MA, Heller KE. The effects of a break in water fluoridation on the development of dental caries and fluorosis. *J Dent Res.* 2000;79:761–769.
6. Chankanka O, Levy SM, Warren JJ, Chalmers JM. A literature review of esthetic perceptions of dental fluorosis and relationships with psychosocial aspects/oral health-related quality of life. *Community Dent Oral Epidemiol.* 2010;38:97–109.
7. Clark DC, Hann HJ, Williamson MF, et al. Influence of exposure to various fluoride technologies on the prevalence of dental fluorosis. *Community Dent Oral Epidemiol.* 1994;22:461–464.
8. Clarkson J, O'Mullane D. A modified DDE index for use in epidemiological studies of enamel defects. *J Dent Res.* 1989;68:445–450.
9. Cochran JA, Ketley CE, Sanches L, et al. A standardized photographic method for evaluating enamel opacities including fluorosis. *Community Dent Oral Epidemiol.* 2004;32(suppl 1):19–27.
10. Cruz-Orcutt N, Warren JJ, Broffitt B. Examiner reliability of fluorosis scoring: A comparison of photographic and clinical examination findings. *J Public Health Dent.* 2012;72:172–175.
11. Dean HT. Distribution of mottled enamel in the United States. *Public Health Rep.* 1933;703–734.
12. Dean HT, Dixon RM, Cohen C. Mottled enamel in Texas. *Public Health Rep.* 1935;50:424–442.
13. Dean HT, Elvove E, Poston RF. Mottled enamel in South Dakota. *Public Health Rep.* 1939;54:212–228.
14. Dean HT, Jay P, Arnold FA, et al. Domestic water and dental caries II—a study of 2,832 white children aged 12–14 years, of eight suburban Chicago communities, including L. Acidophilus studies of 1,761 children. *Public Health Rep.* 1941;56:761–792.
15. DenBesten PK, Thariani H. Biologicial mechanisms of fluorosis and level and timing of systemic exposure to fluoride with respect to fluorosis. *J Dent Res.* 1992;71:1238–1243.
16. DenBesten PK. Biological mechanisms of dental fluorosis relevant to the use of fluoride supplements. *Community Dent Oral Epidemiol.* 1999;27:41–47.
17. Do LG, Spencer A. Oral health-related quality of life of children by dental caries and fluorosis experience. *J Public Health Dent.* 2007;67:132–139.
18. Eager JM. Denti di Chiaie (Chiaie teeth). *Public Health Rep.* 1901;16:2576–2577.
19. Evans RW, Stamm JW. An epidemiologic estimate of the critical period during with human maxillary central incisors are most susceptible to fluorosis. *J Public Health Dent.* 1991;51:251–259.
20. Evans RW, Darvell BW. Refining the estimate of the critical period for susceptibility to enamel fluorosis in human maxillary central incisors. *J Public Health Dent.* 1995;55:238–249.
21. Franzman MR, Levy SM, Warren JJ, et al. Fluoride dentifrice ingestion and fluorosis of the permanent incisors. *J Am Dent Assoc.* 2006;137:645–652.
22. Griffin SO, Beltrán ED, Lockwood SA, Barker LK. Esthetically objectionable fluorosis attributable to water fluoridation. *Community Dent Oral Epidemiol.* 2002;30:199–209.
23. Heller KE, Eklund SA, Burt BA. Dental caries and dental fluorosis at varying water fluoride concentrations. *J Public Health Dent.* 1997;57:136–143.
24. Hong L, Levy SM, Warren JJ, et al. Association of amoxicillin use during early childhood with developmental tooth enamel defects. *Arch Pediatr Adolesc Med.* 2005;159:943–948.
25. Hong L, Levy SM, Warren JJ, et al. Fluoride intake levels in relation to fluorosis development in the permanent maxillary central incisors and first molars. *Caries Res.* 2006;40:494–500.
26. Hong L, Levy SM, Warren JJ, Broffitt B. Amoxicillin used during early childhood and fluorosis of later developing tooth zones. *J Public Health Dent.* 2011;73:229–235.
27. Horowitz HS, Heifets SB, Driscoll WS, et al. A new method for assessing the prevalence of dental fluorosis – the Tooth Surface Index of Fluorosis. *J Am Dent Assoc.* 1984;109:37–41.
28. Hujoel PP, Zina LG, Moimaz SAS, et al. Infant formula and enamel fluorosis—a systematic review. *J Am Dent Assoc.* 2009;140:841–854.
29. Ishii T, Suckling G. The appearance of tooth enamel in children ingesting water with a high fluoride content for a limited period during early tooth development. *J Dent Res.* 1986;65:974–977.
30. Ismail AI, Brodeur J-M, Kavanaugh M, et al. Prevalence of dental caries and dental fluorosis in students, 11–17 years of age, in fluoridated and non-fluoridated cities in Quebec. *Caries Res.* 1990;24:290–297.
31. Ismail AI, Messer JG. The risk of fluorosis in students exposed to a higher than optimal concentration of fluoride in well water. *J Public Health Dent.* 1996;56:22–27.
32. Khan A, Moola MH, Cleaton-Jones P. Global trends in dental fluorosis from 1980–2000: a systematic review. *J South African Dent Assoc.* 2005;60:418–421.
33. Lalumandier JA, Ayers LW. Fluoride and bacterial content of bottled water vs tap water. *Arch Fam Med.* 2000;9:246.
34. Lalumandier JA, Rozier RG. Parents' satisfaction with children's tooth color: fluorosis as a contributing factor. *J Am Dent Assoc.* 1998;129:1000–1006.
35. Lalumandier JA, Rozier RG. The prevalence and risk factors of fluorosis among patients in a pediatric dental practice. *Pediatr Dent.* 1995;17:19–25.
36. Laisi S, Ess A, Sahlberg C, et al. Amoxicillin may cause molar incisor hypomineralization. *J Dent Res.* 2009;88:132–136.
37. Leverett DH. Prevalence of dental fluorosis in fluoridated and nonfluoridated communities—a preliminary investigation. *J Public Health Dent.* 1986;46:184–187. Fall.
38. Levy SM, Broffitt B, Marshall TA, et al. Association between fluorosis of permanent incisors and fluoride intake from infant formula, other dietary sources and dentifrice during early childhood. *J Am Dent Assoc.* 2010;141:1190–1201.
39. Manji F, Baelum V, Fejerskov O. Fluoride, altitude and dental fluorosis. *Caries Res.* 1986;20:473–480.
40. Mann J, Mahmoud W, Ernest M, et al. Fluorosis and dental caries in 6–8 year-old children in a 5 ppm fluoride area. *Community Dent Oral Epidemiol.* 1990;18:77–79.
41. McKay FS, Black GV. An investigation of mottled teeth. *Dental Cosmos.* 1916;58:627–644, 781–792, 894–404.

42. McKay FS. The relation of mottled enamel to caries. *J Am Dent Assoc.* 1928;15:1429–1437.

43. McKnight CB, Levy SM, Cooper SE, et al. A pilot study of dental students' esthetic perceptions of computer-generated mild dental fluorosis compared to other conditions. *J Pub Health Dent.* 1999;59:18–23.

44. Meneghim MC, Kozlowski FC, Pereira AC, Assaf AV, Tagliaferro EPS. Perception of dental flouorosis and other oral health disorders by 12-year-old Brazilian children. *Int J Paediatr Dent.* 2007;17:205–210.

45. Milsom K, Mitropoulos CM. Enamel defects in 8-year-old children in fluoridated and non-fluoridated parts of Cheshire. *Caries Res.* 1990;24:286–289.

46. Ng'ang'a PM, Valderhaug J. Prevalence and severity of dental fluorosis in primary schoolchildren in Nairobi, Kenya. *Community Dent Oral Epidemiol.* 1993;21:15–18.

47. National Center for Health Statistics. Data quality evaluation of the dental fluorosis clinical assessment data from the National Health and Nutrition Examination Survey, 1999–2004 and 2011–2016. *Vital Health Stat.* 2019;2(183).

48. National Health and Nutrition Examination Survey (NHANES). *Oral Health Recorders Procedures Manual, Centers for Disease Control.* January 2015. https://wwwn.cdc.gov/nchs/data/nhanes/2015-2016/manuals/2015_Oral_Health_Recorders_Procedures_Manual.pdf.

49. National Institute of Dental and Craniofacial Research. The Story of Fluoridation. https://www.nidcr.nih.gov/OralHealth/Topics/Fluoride/TheStoryofFluoridation.htm. Accessed February 5, 2018.

50. Olsson B. Dental findings in high-fluoride areas in Ethiopia. *Community Dent Oral Epidemiol.* 1979;7:51–56.

51. Opinya GN, Valderhaug J, Birkeland JM. Fluorosis of deciduous teeth and first permanent molars in a rural Kenyan community. *Acta Odontol Scand.* 1991;49:197–202.

52. Osuji OO, Leake JL, Chipman ML, et al. Risk factors for dental fluorosis in a fluoridated community. *J Dent Res.* 1988;67:1488–1492.

53. Pendrys DG. The Fluorosis Risk Index: a method for investigating risk factors. *J Public Health Dent.* 1990;50:291–298.

54. Pendrys DG, Stamm JW. Relationship of total fluoride intake to beneficial effects and enamel fluorosis. *J Dent Res.* 1990;69(Special Issue):529–538.

55. Pendrys DG, Katz RV. Risk of enamel fluorosis associated with fluoride supplementation, infant formula, and fluoride dentifrice use. *Am J Epidemiol.* 1989;130:1199–1208.

56. Pendrys DG, Katz RV, Morse DE. Risk factors for enamel fluorosis in a fluoridated community. *Am J Epidemiol.* 1994;140:461–471.

57. Riordan PJ. Dental fluorosis, dental caries, and fluoride exposure among 7-year-olds. *Caries Res.* 1993;21:71–77.

58. Rock WP, Sabieha AM. The relationship between reported toothpaste usage in infancy and fluorosis of the permanent incisors. *Br Dent J.* 1997;183:165–170.

59. Rozier RG, Adair S, Graham F, et al. A report of the American Dental Association Council on Scientific Affairs: evidence based clinical recommendations on the prescription of dietary fluoride supplements for caries prevention. *J Am Dent Assoc.* 2010;141:1480–1489.

60. Rozier RG. Appropriate uses of fluoride: Considerations for the '90's. Reactor Paper. Presentation at 53rd Annual Meeting of American Association of Public Health Dentistry, Boston, MA, October 11, 1990.

61. Russell AL. The differential diagnosis of fluoride and nonfluoride enamel opacities. *J Public Health Dent.* 1961;21:143–146.

62. Rwenyonyi C, Bjorvatn K, Birkeland J. Altitude as a risk indicator of dental fluorosis in children residing in areas with 0.5 and 2.5 mg fluoride per litre in drinking water. *Caries Res.* 1999;33:267–274.

63. Sigurjóns H, Cochran JA, Ketley CE. Parental perception of fluorosis among 8-year-old children living in three communities in Iceland, Ireland and England. *Community Dent Oral Epidemiol.* 2004;32 (Suppl 1):34–38.

64. Skotowski MC, Hunt RJ, Levy SM. Risk factors for dental fluorosis in pediatric dental patients. *J Pub Health Dent.* 1995;55:154–159.

65. Soto-Rojas AE, Martínez-Mier EA, Ureña-Cirett JL, et al. Development of a standarisation device for photographic assessment of dental fluorosis in field studies. *Oral Health Prev Dent.* 2008;6:29–36.

66. Szpunar SM, Burt BA. Dental caries, fluorosis, and fluoride exposure in Michigan schoolchildren. *J Dent Res.* 1988;67:802–806.

67. Thylstrup A, Fejerskov O. Clinical appearance of dental fluorosis in permanent teeth in relation to histologic changes. *Community Dent Oral Epidemiol.* 1978;6:315–328.

68. United States Department of Health and Human Services Federal Panel on Community Water Fluoridation. US Public Health Service recommendation for fluoride concentration in drinking water for the prevention of dental caries. *Public Health Rep.* 2015;130:318–331.

69. Walvekar SV, Qureshi BA. Endemic fluorosis and partial defluoridation of water supplies—a public health concern in Kenya. *Community Dent Oral Epidemiol.* 1982;10:156–160.

70. Warren JJ, Levy SM, Kanellis. Prevalence of dental fluorosis in the primary dentition. *J Public Health Dent.* 2001;61:87–91.

71. Whelton HP, Ketley CE, McSweeney F. A review of fluorosis in the European Union: prevalence, risk factors and aesthetic issues. *Community Dent Oral Epidemiol.* 2004;32(suppl 1):9–18.

72. Whitford G. *Determinants and Mechanisms of Enamel Fluorosis. Ciba Foundation Symposium No. 205*, New York, NY: Wiley; 1997:226–245.

73. Williams JE, Zwemer JD. Community water fluoride levels, preschool dietary patterns, and the occurrence of fluoride enamel opacities. *J Pub Health Dent.* 1990;50:276–281.

74. Woodward GL, Main PA, Leake JL. Clinical determinants of a parent's satisfaction with the appearance of a child's teeth. *Community Dent Oral Epidemiol.* 1996;24:416–418.

75. Woolfolk MW, Faja BW, Bagramian RA. Relation of sources of systemic fluoride to prevalence of dental fluorosis. *J Public Health Dent.* 1989;49:78–82.

# 20

# Oral Health–Related Quality of Life

GEORGIA G. ROGERS, DMD, MPH

COLMAN MCGRATH, BA, BDentSc, DDPHRCS, MSc, FDSRCS,
FFDRCSI, MEd, PhD, FPH, FICD

## Introduction

The concept of oral health has evolved from a narrow reductive perspective, with a focus limited to disease/deformity, to broader considerations of the physical, social, and psychological aspects of oral health.[17] These developments followed from changes in the concept of health as "a state of complete physical, mental and social well-being and not merely the absence of disease or infirmity"; albeit almost half a century later.[42] The paradigm shift in the concept of health led to a focus on *quality of life* (QoL): as an "individual's perception of their position in life in the context of the culture and value systems in which they live and in relation to their goals."[40] In the context of health, QoL is the physical, social, and psychological aspects of one's health's state as deemed important by the individual.

The term *health-related quality of life* (HRQoL) was coined to distinguish it from the broader concept of QoL.[28] Recognizing the importance of oral health to general health, yet also acknowledging differences between them, the term *oral health–related quality of life* (OHRQoL) was subsequently coined. One useful definition of OHRQoL is "an individual's assessment of how the following aspects affect his or well-being-being: functional factors, psychological factors, social factors and experiences of pain/discomfort in relation to orofacial concerns."[14] OHRQoL highlights the intrinsic relationship between oral health and general health and their relationship with QoL.

In tandem, in the later decades of the 20th century there were considerable advances in the measurement (or rather assessment) of OHRQoL.[31] This facilitated our understanding of the impact of oral health on QoL, and evidence of the impact of oral healthcare on QoL increasingly became available. Despite the considerable advances, there remains considerable need for further advancements of the concept, measurement, and translation research within the field of OHRQoL.

## Concepts and Models of Health and Quality of Life

OHRQoL is a relatively new concept compared to HRQoL, and this in part has been attributed to the delay in its development or lack of consensus on a definition of oral health. The Surgeon General's report on oral health in 2000, for example, did not provide a concise definition of oral health, but it broadened the scope of oral health by stating that "Oral health means more than healthy teeth and the absence of disease. It involves the ability of individuals to carry out essential functions such as eating and speaking as well as to contribute fully to society."[7] The World Health Organization subsequently defined oral health as "a state of being free from chronic mouth and facial pain, oral and throat cancer, oral infection and sores, periodontal (gum) disease, tooth decay, tooth loss, and other diseases and disorders that limit an individual's capacity in biting, chewing, smiling, speaking, and psychosocial wellbeing."[43] More recently the FDI World Dental Federation proposed a universal definition of oral health unifying the physical, social, and psychological aspects of oral health that had evolved in recent decades (Figure 20.1).[11]

The call to develop socio-dental indicators to capture the physical, social, and psychological aspects of oral health has long been debated,[15] despite the delay from national and international organizations to reach a consensus on the definitions and concept of oral health. To this end the WHO's *International Classification of Impairment, Disability and Handicap* (ICIDH) of 1980 provided a useful framework for the concept of oral health and indeed the theoretical underpinning of several OHRQoL measures.[18] Twenty years later (2001), WHO proposed a revised model of health—*International Classification of Functioning, Disability and Health* (ICF or ICIDH-2), a unifying classification of how health states a effect body function and structure,

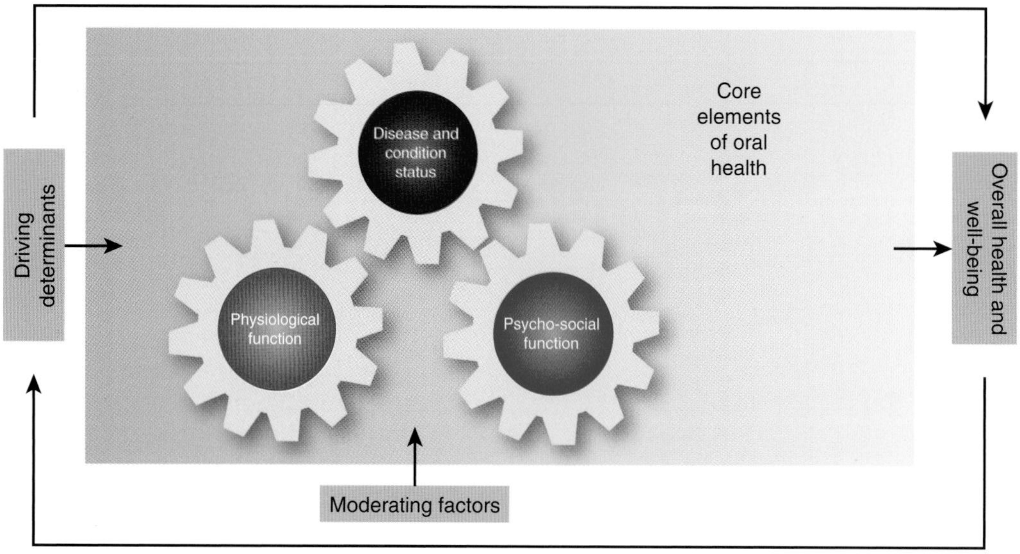

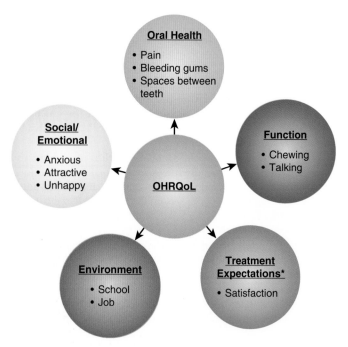

• **Figure 20.1** FDI (World Dental Federation) Definition and Framework of Oral Health, 2016.

activity and participation in the context of personal and environmental factors, and the negative and the positive effects. Unfortunately this has been less used or operationalized in the oral health context.[25]

There have been various theoretical models of HRQOL, and perhaps the most useful (or a least widely adapted and tested for OHRQoL) has been the Wilson and Cleary model.[39] This has highlighted the value and uses of OHRQoL—the what, why, how, and future implications for research and clinical practice (Figure 20.2).[30]

## Measuring the Impact of Oral Health on Quality of Life

It has long been acknowledged that oral health has an impact on QoL; calls for measurement of the social impact of oral health have been advocated in the literature from at least the 1970s.[15] The measurement—or the assessment, given its abstract nature—of the QoL impact of oral health followed suit. There are two broad approaches to the assessments of QoL: a hermeneutic and a functionalist approach.[24] These approaches differ in their schools of thought, methods of data collection and analyses, as well as methods of synthesis and presentation of findings.

The functionalist approach has been the dominant approach in response to calls to 'quantify' the overall impact, to simplify and standardize assessments, and to facilitate analysis and comparisons. Within the functionalist approach to assessing the impact of oral heath on QoL, a broad range of "instruments"—scales and batteries—exist that can be broadly classified into generic health-related quality of life instruments, (generic) oral health-related quality of life instruments, and condition-specific oral health-related quality of life instruments. Employing generic health-related quality of life instruments in the assessment of oral health's impact on QoL has obvious appeal, in that the impact of oral health states can be compared with the impact of other health states, generating clearer implications for policy and prioritization of need across health services.[2]

Although generic HRQoL has been useful in drawing attention to the impact of oral health on quality of life, there are many limitations to its ability to capture the subtle differences in oral health states. This in part (and perhaps in a major way) relates to the nature of the items (questions) within generic HRQoL—aspects of life not affected by one's oral health state. An array of (generic) OHRQoL instruments were developed to address these limitations (Table 20.1).[1] These differ in terms of underlying theoretical frameworks (or lack thereof), dimensions, domains, type and number of items, scoring methods (including "weighting"), and age group to be used with.

Despite such difference in OHRQoL instruments, there is no single measure that has proven to outperform others in all contexts. This in part relates to the fact that the key issue is not the instrument per se but what the instruments are being used

• **Figure 20.2** The five dimensions of influence of OHRQoL.[30]

## TABLE 20.1 The Development of Key Oral Health–Related Quality of Life Measures Over Time

| Year | Authors | OHRQoL Measures |
|------|---------|-----------------|
| 1986 | Cushing et al. | Social Impacts of Dental Disease |
| 1990 | Atchison and Dolan | Geriatric Oral Health Assessment Index |
| 1993 | Strauss and Hunt | Dental Impact Profile |
| 1994 | Slade and Spencer | Oral Health Impact Profile |
| 1994 | Locker and Miller | Subjective Oral Health Status Indicators |
| 1996 | Leao and Sheiham | Dental Impact on Daily Performances |
| 1997 | Adulyanon and Sheiham | Oral Impacts on Daily Performance |
| 2000 | McGrath and Bedi | The UK Oral Health–Related Quality of Life Measure |
| 2002 | Jokovic et al. | Child Perception Questionnaire |
| 2002 | Locker et al. | Family Impact Scale |
| 2003 | Jokovic et al. | Parental Perception Questionnaire |
| 2004 | Gherunpong et al. | Child-Oral Impacts on Daily Performance |
| 2007 | Broder et al. | Child Oral Health Impact Profile |
| 2007 | Pahel et al. | Early Childhood Oral Health Impact Scale |
| 2012 | Tsakos et al. | Scale of Oral Health Outcome (SOHO-5) |

Adapted from Allen PF. Assessment of oral health related quality of life. 2003 Sep 8;1:40. Gilchrist et al.: Assessment of the quality of measures of child oral health-related quality of life. BMC Oral Health 2014 14:40; Gilchrist et al., 2014.

for—intended use and type of studies. In selecting the most appropriate measure for use, it is important to consider the instruments' psychometric properties—essentially their validity and reliability.[19] There are various forms of validity (content, construct, criterion, concurrent, convergent, and divergent) and reliability (internal and external), to name a few. Moreover, in assessment of changes in OHRQoL as a result of treatment/care (or lack thereof) over time, there is a need to consider the longitudinal validity and stability; for this, psychometric properties of sensitivity and responsiveness are important to consider.[38] On the whole (generic) OHRQoL instruments have proved useful, but there are concerns that they may not capture the subtle experiences of different oral health states (e.g., orofacial deformities, xerostomia, dentine hypersensitivity), and condition-specific OHRQoL measures have been developed to this end.[6]

Assessment of the impact of oral health on the quality of life of infants, children, and adolescents has lagged behind assessments among adults. This has been attributed to the more complex nature of OHRQoL in younger age groups related to the conceptual difference in understanding, language, psychosocial awareness, and changing oral features among them—even among those of similar age.[26] Despite such complexities, there have been developments in assessing child OHRQoL. Again, an array of assessment approaches and methods have been employed using generic child-HRQoL, generic child-OHRQoL, and condition-specific child-OHRQoL instruments.

A number of instruments are widely used (Table 20.2), but again there is a need to consider their psychometric properties

in selecting the most appropriate measures for use depending on the task in hand.[36] A key issue is the use of a proxy (or proxies) in the assessments of the impact of child's oral health state on quality of life—the use of parent/primary caregiver views. Naturally there are concerns that a proxy's assessment may reflect their own views rather than that of the child.[22] Nonetheless, it is accepted that this may be the only feasible or practical approach for younger children and among those with special healthcare needs.

Another important issue is cross-cultural consideration. Although clinical indices have adapted readily for use internationally, the adaptation of OHRQoL instruments poses a number of challenges to employ internationally.[21] First, there is the issue of language and cultural differences and the need to develop culturally equivalent measures. Second, it is imperative that the psychometric properties of the instrument be assessed when employed in different settings, as they should exhibit consistent findings by different researchers in different settings. There are many conceptual and psychometric issues to consider, but it is not uncommon that these issues are overlooked in the rush to collect data. A key issue is whether the measures are to be used to facilitate cross-national research or cross-cultural research. Conventional translation strategies are limited because they enshrine deficiencies of the original questionnaire and do not permit modifications that reflect differences in culture and values. Using a conceptual definition of what one wanted to measure would allow flexibility in the methods to achieve this goal.[12]

## Impact of Oral Health and Oral Healthcare on Quality of Life

There has been an explosion of interest in assessing the impact of oral health on quality of life with more than a 100-fold increase in publications (in PubMed) within the new millennium compared to pre-2000. Fortunately, a growing understanding of the need to use standardized validated measures has made it feasible to synthesize the evidence of the impact of oral health on QoL by way of systematic reviews. A systematic review of the associations between oral conditions (tooth loss, periodontal disease, and dental caries) found that despite different definitions and measures of tooth loss and dental caries, the majority of the available evidence reported a negative impact of these conditions on HRQoL.[13] Mixed and inconclusive findings were observed in relation to the association between periodontal disease and HRQoL.

Longitudinal prospective studies were recommended to improve the strength of the findings. In terms of tooth loss/tooth retention, most studies showed a significant association between number of teeth and OHRQoL. After adjusting for other factors in the analyses, however, those studies found different cutoff points regarding the number of teeth that affect OHRQoL.[34] The number of occluding pairs and the location of remaining teeth have great impacts on OHRQoL. Having fewer anterior occluding pairs had a greater negative impact on aesthetics and thus affected OHRQoL considerably.

There is evidence that implant-supported prosthesis does improve OHRQoL among edentulous patients, but less evidence exists in support of implant-retained prosthesis among the partially dentate.[27] The benefits of rehabilitation/reconstruction for replacing missing teeth has long been of interest and in particular its impact on HRQoL/OHRQoL.[35] In edentulous patients, evidence suggests that implant over dentures are superior than complete dentures in terms of treatment-induced OHRQoL improvement, but only if OHRQoL at baseline is highly impaired and patients request implant treatment. For partially dentate patients, there is

• **TABLE 20.2** Child Oral Health–Related Quality of Life Measures

| Name/Author(s) | Number/Type of Questions | Dimensions Covered |
|---|---|---|
| Child Oral Health Quality of Life Questionnaire/Locker, Jokovic | 25 or 37/5 point scale<br><br>The final CPQ and PPQ contain 36 and 31 items | Child Perceptions Questionnaire (CPQ)—three versions: for children 6–7 years of age (CPQ6–7), for children 8–10 years of age (CPQ8–10), and for children 11–14 years of age (CPQ11–14). Items target functional limitations, oral symptoms, and emotional and social well-being. Parental-Caregiver's Perceptions Questionnaire (PPQ). Items target functional limitations, oral symptoms, and emotional and social well-being. Family Impact Section (FIS) measures the impact on the family. |
| Child Oral Impacts on Daily Performances (OIDP)/ Gherunpong | 8/3 point Likert scale | Frequency and severity of impact on eight daily performances: eating, speaking, cleaning teeth, smiling, emotional stability, relaxing, doing schoolwork, and social contact |
| Child Oral Health Impact Profile (COHIP)/Broder | 34/5 point Likert scale | Parental proxy report and child report (age 8+)—negative and positive impacts of five domains: oral health, functional well-being, social/emotional well-being, school environment, and self-image |
| Early Child Oral Health Impact Scale (ECOHIS)/Pahel | 13/5 point Likert scale | Proxy–parents/caregivers complete questions on behalf of children aged 3 and 5 years Child Impact Section (CIS) and the Family Impact Section (FIS)—six domains including symptoms, function, psychology, social interaction/self-image, parental distress, and family function |
| Scale of Oral Health Outcomes (SOHO)/Tsakos | 7/3 point scale | Age 5, frequency of difficulties with eating, drinking, speaking, smiling, playing, and sleeping due to oral problems |
| Pediatric Oral Health–Related Quality of Life (POQL)/Huntington | 10 × 2/5 point Likert scale | Each of 10 items asks for two responses: "how often" does it affect you and "how bothered" by it are you<br>Preschool: parent report on child (PRC) only<br>School age/preteen (8+): PRC and child self-report (CSR) |

not enough evidence that implant-supported fixed partial dentures (FPD) are superior in terms of OHRQoL to conventional FPD, but moderate evidence suggests that implant-supported FDP perform better than conventional removable partial dentures (RPD). "Patients can be informed that implant treatment is usually related to a significant improvement in OHRQoL. However, improvement is not necessarily higher than for conventional prosthodontic treatments but depends on patient's clinical and psychosocial characteristics."[35] A more recent systematic review found inconsistent evidence of the benefits of implant-supported fixed complete dentures or overdentures from patients' perspectives (including HRQoL and OHRQoL assessments) in the rehabilitation of edentulous patients.[44] This in part was attributed to the lack of standardized approach in assessing the impact of dental implant-supported removable and fixed appliances among edentulous patients.

As aforementioned, a systematic review of oral conditionals and HRQoL observed that "all studies" that informed the review identified that dental caries has a negative association with HRQoL.[26] Evidence of dental caries association with OHRQoL is more conflicting. There is ample evidence that dental caries places a considerable burden on the lives of children.[37] A systematic review of changes in OHRQoL following the management of dental caries among children under general anesthesia found that most studies identified significant improvement in OHRQoL.[16] Whereas all studies reported improved OHRQoL overall, some subscales showed changes that were not significant or worsened OHRQoL. The scientific quality of the studies varied considerably; only half of the studies used instruments validated in the study population.

In terms of malocclusion there is ample evidence that severe malocclusion, particularly for those with "an orthodontic treatment need," is associated with poorer OHRQoL.[33] However, this association depends on how malocclusion is assessed, how orthodontic treatment is assessed, and how OHRQoL is assessed. Surprisingly, despite much promotion and marketing of orthodontics to improve QoL, there is a paucity of evidence in the literature to support such claims. This can be attributed in part to the lack of patient-centered outcomes in orthodontics research, lack of standardized approach, and concerns about the appropriateness of using measures (in terms of psychometric appropriateness) across the relatively long treatment time, particularly when multiple treatment modalities are employed.[10] There is ample evidence of the benefits of orthognathic correction of severe dentofacial discrepancies.[32]

Conflicting evidence exists as to the negative impact of periodontal disease on HRQoL.[13] In terms of OHRQoL, a systematic review found that most studies identified that periodontal disease was associated with a negative impact on quality of life.[9] More severe periodontitis exerts the most significant impact on OHRQoL by compromising aspects related to function and aesthetics. Unlike periodontitis, gingivitis was associated with pain and difficulties performing oral hygiene and wearing dentures. Gingivitis was also negatively correlated with comfort. The results indicate that periodontal disease may exert an impact on the QoL of individuals, with greater severity of the disease related to greater impact. Longitudinal studies with representative samples are needed to ensure validity of the findings.

An earlier review found some evidence that nonsurgical periodontal treatment brought about an improvement in OHRQoL among patients with periodontal disease.[29] The effect size for this improvement in OHRQoL varied considerably. No significant differences were reported among different forms of nonsurgical periodontal treatment. Surgical periodontal therapy had a relatively lower impact on OHRQoL (although the number of studies reviewed was limited in terms of numbers of studies and number of participants). There is uncertainty about whether periodontal therapy improves OHRQoL because of serious limitations in systematic reviews addressing this question.[5]

## Further Developments and Future Directions

There have been considerable developments and advances in the definition and concept of oral health, QoL, and OHRQoL. Nonetheless there is a new definition of oral health developed by the FDI World Dental Federation with an aim of providing a universal definition of oral health.[3] It is important to consider the structural determinants of such definitions and models—particularly the "upstream" factors that determine oral health and OHRQoL.[8] Of note, there have been considerable limitations in understanding the impact of oral health (as opposed to disease) on QoL. WHO's revised model of health provides a useful framework for understanding and studying health and health-related states, not just disease/deformity. The revised model provides a useful approach to operationalizing and identifying common factors of function, participation, and environment associated with oral health.[8]

The use of psychometrics has enabled considerable advancements in validating and testing models of oral health and OHQoL,[4] improved the consistency and stability of OHRQoL measures over time,[41] and expedited the development of "short form" measures that easier to use in clinical settings.[20] Further advances in methodologies to examine the psychometric properties of OHRQoL measures in terms of configural structure, factor loadings, error variances, factor variances and covariance, and intercept invariance will refine and standardize these instruments. The issue of cross-national versus cross-cultural use of OHRQoL measures needs to be reexamined. The value of alternative approaches over the one-size-fits-all approaches associated with functionalists ought to be considered in these investigations.

As OHRQoL is increasingly regarded as a true outcome measure rather than a surrogate outcome measure, the importance of determining the benefits of oral healthcare cannot be overemphasized—in particular the need to determine the "minimal important difference" or "minimal important clinical difference" associated with oral healthcare interventions. Evidence-based practice requires information on the magnitude of change in OHRQoL and effect sizes associated with an array of oral healthcare treatment modalities and different practice settings.[23]

## Summary

In summary, there have been considerable advances, success, and interest in assessing the impact of oral health on QoL and of oral healthcare's impact on QoL. For the most part, assessment has focused on the burden (negative impacts) associated with oral disease and deformity. There is evidence that oral disease has a negative impact on the QoL of many around the world, irrespective of how or where it is studied. Evidence of the impact of oral healthcare in reducing the negative experiences of OHRQoL associated with oral diseases and deformities is less readily available, but promising findings are emerging. With advances in technologies and methodologies, contemporary and advanced psychometric testing of OHRQoL instruments is informing and redefining assessments. Rather than focusing on the negative effects of oral diseases and conditions, researchers are seeking to quantify the positive effects of oral health on QOL, and the roles of prevention, interceptive care, and minimally Invasive treatment in safeguarding OHRQoL.

## References

1. Allen PF. Assessment of oral health related quality of life. *Health Qual Life Outcomes*. 2003;1:40.
2. Allen PF, McMillan AS, Walshaw D, et al. A comparison of the validity of generic- and disease-specific measures in the assessment of oral health-related quality of life. *Community Dent Oral Epidemiol*. 1999;27:344–352.
3. Baker SR, Foster Page L, Thomson WM, et al. Structural determinants and children's oral health: a cross-national study. *J Dent Res*. 2018;97:1129–1136.
4. Baker SR. Testing a conceptual model of oral health: a structural equation modeling approach. *J Dent Res*. 2007;86:708–712.
5. Brignardello-Petersen R. Uncertainty about whether periodontal therapy improves oral health-related quality of life owing to serious limitations in systematic review addressing this question. *J Am Dent Assoc*. 2018;149:e35.
6. Cunningham SJ, Hunt NP. Quality of life and its importance in orthodontics. *J Orthod*. 2001;28:152–158.
7. DHHS, US Department of Health and Human Services. *Oral Health in America: a Report of the Surgeon General*. Rockville, MD: US Department of Health and Human Services, National Institute of Dental and Craniofacial Research, National Institutes of Health; 2000.
8. Dougall A, Molina GF, Eschevins C, et al. A global oral health survey of professional opinion using the International Classification of Functioning, Disability and Health. *J Dent*. 2015;43:683–694.
9. Ferreira MC, Dias-Pereira AC, Branco-de-Almeida LS, et al. Impact of periodontal disease on quality of life: a systematic review. *J Periodontal Res*. 2017;52:651–665.
10. Fleming PS, Koletsi D, O'Brien K, et al. Are dental researchers asking patient-important questions? A scoping review. *J Dent*. 2016;49:9–13.
11. Glick M, Williams D, Kleinman D, et al. A new definition for oral health developed by the FDI World Dental Federation opens the door to a universal definition of oral health. *JADA*. 2016;147:915–917.
12. Guyatt GH. The philosophy of health-related quality of life translation. *Qual Life Res*. 1993;2:461–465.
13. Haag DG, Peres KG, Balasubramanian M, et al. Oral conditions and health-related quality of life: a systematic review. *J Dent Res*. 2017;96:864–874.
14. Inglehart MR, Bagramian RA. Oral health-related quality of life: an introduction. In: Inglehart MR, Bagramian RA, eds. *Oral Health-Related Quality of Life*. Chicago, IL: Quintessence Publishing; 2002:1–6.
15. Jago JD. Toward formulation of socio-dental indicators. *Int J Health Services*. 1976;6:681–698.
16. Knapp R, Gilchrist F, Rodd HD, et al. Change in children's oral health-related quality of life following dental treatment under general anesthesia for the management of dental caries: a systematic review. *Int J Paediatr Dent*. 2017;27:302–312.
17. Locker D. Measuring oral health: a conceptual framework. *Community Dental Health*. 1988;5:3–18.
18. Locker D. Concepts of oral health, disease and the quality of life. In: Slade GD, ed. *Measuring Oral Health and Quality of Life*. Chapel Hill: University of North Carolina, Dental Ecology 1997.
19. Locker D. Oral health and quality of life. *Oral Health Prev Dent*. 2004;2(suppl 1):247–253.
20. Locker D, Allen PF. Developing short-form measures of oral health-related quality of life. *J Public Health Dent*. 2002;62:13–20.

21. MacEntee MI, Brondani M. Cross-cultural equivalence in translations of the oral health impact profile. *Community Dent Oral Epidemiol.* 2016;44:109–118.

22. Marshman Z, Gibson BJ, Owens J, et al. Seen but not heard: a systematic review of the place of the child in 21st-century dental research. *Int J Paediatr Dent.* 2007;17:320–327.

23. Masood M, Masood Y, Saub R, et al. Need of minimal important difference of oral health-related quality of life measures. *J Public Health Dent.* 2014;74:13–20.

24. McGrath C, Bedi R. Measuring the impact of oral health on life quality in two national surveys—functionalist versus hermeneutic approaches. *Community Dent Oral Epidemiol.* 2002;30:254–259.

25. McGrath C, Bedi R. The association between dental anxiety and oral health-related quality of life in Britain. *Community Dent Oral Epidemiol.* 2004;32:67–72.

26. McGrath C, Broder H, Wilson-Genderson M. Assessing the impact of oral health on the life quality of children: implications for research and practice. *Community Dent Oral Epidemiol.* 2004;32:81–85.

27. Reissmann DR, Dard M, Lamprecht R, et al. Oral health-related quality of life in subjects with implant-supported prostheses: a systematic review. *J Dent.* 2017;65:22–40.

28. Ronen GM. Reflections on the usefulness of the term "health-related quality of life". *Dev Med Child Neurol.* 2017;59:1105–1106.

29. Shanbhag S, Dahiya M, Croucher R. The impact of periodontal therapy on oral health-related quality of life in adults: a systematic review. *J Clin Periodontol.* 2012;39:725–735.

30. Sischo L, Broder H. Oral health-related quality of life: what, why, how, and future implications. *J Dent Res.* 2011;90:1264–1270.

31. Slade GD, ed. *Measuring Oral Health and Quality of Life.* Chapel Hill, NC: University of North Carolina; 1997.

32. Soh CL, Narayanan V. Quality of life assessment in patients with dentofacial deformity undergoing orthognathic surgery–a systematic review. *Int J Oral Maxillofac Surg.* 2013;42:974–980.

33. Sun L, Wong HM, McGrath CPJ. The factors that influence oral health-related quality of life in 15-year-old children. *Health Qual Life Outcomes.* 2018;16:19.

34. Tan H, Peres KG, Peres MA. Retention of teeth and oral health-related quality of life. *J Dent Res.* 2016;95:1350–1357.

35. Thomason JM, Kelly SA, Bendkowski A, et al. Two implant retained overdentures—a review of the literature supporting the McGill and York consensus statements. *J Dent.* 2012;40(1):22–34.

36. Thomson WM, Broder HL. Oral-health-related quality of life in children and adolescents. *Pediatr Clin North Am.* 2018;65:1073–1084.

37. Tinanoff N, Baez RJ, Diaz Guillory C, et al. Early childhood caries epidemiology, etiology, risk assessment, societal burden, management, education, and policy: global perspective. *Int J Pediatr Dent.* 2019;29:238–248.

38. Tsakos G, Allen PF, Steele JG, et al. Interpreting oral health-related quality of life data. *Community Dent Oral Epidemiol.* 2012;40:193–200.

39. Wilson I, Cleary P. Linking clinical variables with health-related quality of life. A conceptual model of patient outcomes. *J Am Med Assoc.* 1995;273:59–65.

40. WHOQOL. The World Health Organization quality of life assessment: position paper from the World Health Organization. *Soc Sci Med.* 1995;41:1403–1409.

41. Wong MC, Lau AW, Lam KF, et al. Assessing consistency in oral health-related quality of life (OHRQoL) across gender and stability of OHRQoL over time for adolescents using Structural Equation Modeling. *Community Dent Oral Epidemiol.* 2011;39:325–335.

42. World Health Organization. *Constitution of the World Health Organization* as adopted by the International Health Conference, New York, 19–22 June 1946; signed on 22 July 1946 by the representatives of 61 States (Official Records of the World Health Organization, no. 2, p. 100) and entered into force on 7 April 1948. Geneva: WHO.

43. Petersen PE. WHO Oral Health Programme. In: *The World Oral Health Report 2003: Continuous Improvement of Oral Health in the 21st Century—The Approach of the WHO Global Oral Health Programme.* World Health Organization; 2003. Available from: https://www.who.int/oral_health/publications/world-oral-health-report-2003/en/.

44. Yao CJ, Cao C, Bornstein MM, et al. Patient-reported outcome measures of edentulous patients restored with implant-supported removable and fixed prostheses: a systematic review. *Clin Oral Implants Res.* 2018;29(suppl 16):241–254.

# Health Promotion and Prevention of Oral Diseases

# 21

# Oral Health Behavior Change and Oral Health Promotion

MARITA ROHR INGLEHART, Dipl Psych, Dr phil, Dr phil habil

## Introduction

Since the early 1960s, the National Center for Health Statistics (NCHS)—which is part of the Centers for Disease Control and Prevention (CDC)—has conducted National Health and Nutrition Examination Surveys (NHANES). This magnificent effort allowed to collect comprehensive health-related information and to then publish health statistics for the United States.[83] Over the years, oral health–related survey data and examination results have provided an excellent and highly reliable resource for dental public health and oral health researchers who studied the oral health of children and adults in the United States.[30] For example, in 2017, Dye and colleagues used NHANES data from 1999 through 2004 and from 2011 through 2014 and found that untreated dental caries in primary teeth among 2- to 8-year-old children had decreased from the earlier period to the later period from 24% to 14%, but there was little change in the prevalence of caries in older children and adolescents.[31] Concerning the oral health of dentate adults 30 years of age or older, Eke and colleagues analyzed data from 2009 through 2014 and estimated that 42% had periodontitis, with 7.8% having severe periodontitis.[34] Most recently, in January 2019, Dye and colleagues also reported that while edentulism among adults 50 years or older was lower in 2009 through 2014 than in 1999 through 2004, 11% still experienced this condition.[32]

These statistics come to life when considering their consequences. Research concerning the consequences of poor oral health for children's lives showed that it does not only affect children's future oral health,[47] but also their general health,[8,119] quality of life,[38,51] school attendance[45] and the use of emergency services.[107] Negative effects of adults' poor oral health on these patients' general health (e.g., cardiovascular health[44] and preterm deliveries[85]) and quality of life[56] are also well documented. The key question therefore is how oral disease in children and adults can be prevented and how these patients' oral health can be improved.

## Oral Health and Oral Health Promotion: The Role of Health Behavior

Oral disease prevention and the improvement of oral health are functions of oral health promotion efforts. The World Health Organization (WHO) states that "health promotion enables people to increase control over their own health. It covers a wide range of social and environmental interventions that are designed to benefit and protect individual people's health and quality of life by addressing and preventing the root causes of ill health, not just focusing on treatment and cure."[125] This definition points to some central aspects of health promotion.

First, it stresses people's autonomy and the ultimate objective to allow them to have control over their own health. When considering patients' oral health, it is clear that patients have control over their oral health not only by engaging in good oral hygiene but also by having a healthy diet (see Chapter 23) and abstaining from tobacco use (see Chapter 28).

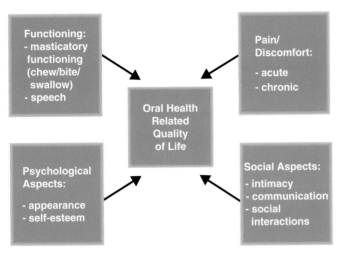

• **Figure 21.1** Oral health–related quality of life.

Second, this definition also draws attention to the fact that social and environmental interventions are part of health promotion. For example, water fluoridation (see Chapters 24 and 25) is one environmental factor that contributed significantly to preventing oral disease in the United States.

Third, the fact that not only health but also quality of life is addressed in this definition is crucial. In the context of oral health, Inglehart and Bagramian defined oral health–related quality of life (OHR-QoL) as assessments of how oral health affects quality of life related to (1) oral functioning (such as being able to chew, bite, swallow, or speak), (2) psychological well-being (such as a person's satisfaction with the appearance of their teeth and smile and self-esteem), (3) social well-being (such as the level of comfort when eating or speaking in front of others), and (4) pain/discomfort (Figure 21.1).[55]

In 2000, Inglehart & Bagramian organized an international workshop at the University of Michigan, funded by the National Institutes of Health (NIH), that brought together nearly 100 researchers from around the world to discuss the role that oral health–related quality of life can play in oral health–related research, practice, and education. In 2002, they then edited a volume titled *Oral Health–Related Quality of Life*[56] that highlighted the wide range of applications of oral health–related quality of life in clinical practice, research, and education.[61] Since then, hundreds of publications have explored the role of quality of life when treating patients with periodontal diseases, caries, and oral cancer.[53,54] Ensuring that patients are not only free of pain and discomfort but can also function and experience a good psychological and social quality of life has been embraced increasingly over time in dentistry.

Fourth, the WHO definition of health promotion[125] also drew attention to the fact that prevention is of central importance in addition to the treatment and cure of disease.

When applying this WHO definition to oral health, this chapter clearly embraces the fact that patients' autonomy and ability to have control over the prevention of disease is important. It will describe a motivational communication approach that has as the central assumption that patients' oral health depends on their oral health-related knowledge, their sense of self-efficacy and their own behavior. It considers good health and good oral health–related quality of life as the ultimate outcome of oral healthcare and stresses the importance of preventing oral diseases. However, this chapter focuses primarily on health behavior change, the patient-centered and social aspect of oral health promotion, while later

chapters focus on environmental factors (see Chapters 24 and 25) and treatment-related factors (see Chapters 26 and 27).

Focusing centrally on behavior change begins with the reflection of the fact that both dental caries and periodontal disease are related to behavioral factors such as a lack of patients' self-care efforts, the use of tobacco products, and diet-related behavior—in short: to patients' lack of constructive oral health–related behavior. Unfortunately, research by Rosania and colleagues found that 56% of adults reported that stress led them to neglect regular brushing and flossing.[104] These percentages can be contrasted with results of systematic reviews that analyzed the relationships between tooth brushing frequency and gingival recession,[97] head and neck cancer,[126] periodontitis,[127] and incident and increment of dental caries,[68] which provided at least some evidence for the benefits of tooth brushing. Research also showed that smoking is a leading risk factor for periodontal disease[66] and increases the risk of periodontitis by 85%.[70] The relationship between diet and nutrition and oral health has also been explored extensively,[86] and the many ways in which oral health is affected by diet and nutrition are well documented.

Given this empirical evidence for the role of behavioral factors for the etiology of oral diseases, the question arises why such large percentages of the US population still suffer from oral diseases that could be potentially prevented with oral health promotion efforts.

## Oral Health Behavior Change: Three Problems and Potential Solutions

Observations in clinical settings might provide some insight into potential answers to the question of why there is a disconnect between dentists' and dental hygienists' efforts to educate their patients about oral health promotion and patients' oral health–related behavior—and ultimately their oral health.

Scenario 1 takes place in a dental school clinic. A dental student provided a dental cleaning for a male patient in his late 70s. Towards the end of the appointment, the dental student tells the patient: "Now I am going to teach you how to brush your teeth" and then proceeds to explain good brushing techniques such as the benefits of circular brush strokes and spending at least 30 seconds brushing each quadrant of the mouth. The dental patient looks unenthusiastic, listens, and then leaves. This scenario is exemplary for a **general** approach to oral health education. The student knows what tooth brushing should look like and explains it to every patient in more or less the same general way. In contrast, a patient-centered **tailored** approach would carefully explain first why a certain type of health education is offered to this particular patient and then tailor it to the patient's situation.

Scenario 2 is used to describe a "**one shot**" versus a "**story line**" approach of education about oral health promotion. A dental student provides a prophylaxis for a female patient in her 50s. The student finds considerable interproximal plaque during the dental cleaning and decides to educate the patient about flossing. The patient does not floss and does not think that flossing would be helpful. The student explains the benefits of flossing and shows the patient how to do it. The patient leaves with a new tooth brush and floss. Two weeks later, the patient returns for an operative appointment and the student is surprised that the patient had not used the floss. This scenario illustrates the importance of using a story line approach instead of a one shot approach. Providing education about flossing or any other oral health–related behavior only once and independent of the patient's considerations of a potential behavior change not very likely to succeed. Instead, assessing the patient's readiness for change and then starting to build on this readiness to change in a systematic way over time is more likely to result in the desired change. More concretely, if a patient does not think about flossing at all, it is unlikely that a short intervention will result in a major behavior change. Creating motivation in a patient and then building on that motivation over time might be a more promising approach.

Scenario 3 focuses on the question of how to best approach behavior change. Research shows that "pushing" a patient to changing a behavior might be perceived by the patient as having his or her freedom limited and thus might result in reactance.[16,18,114] Understanding how to create a **process of change in a cooperative manner** therefore seems to be more promising.

## Motivational Communication: One-on-One Oral Health Promotion in Dental Offices

Identifying (1) that a tailored approach might be more successful than a general approach, (2) that a story line approach might be more realistic than a one shot approach, and (3) that gaining a clearer understanding of how to best cooperate with a patient to create behavior change is the starting point for the following analysis of how an approach called *motivational communication* can be used for oral health promotion efforts in one-on-one situations such as in dental offices. It postulates that motivational communication consists on one hand of a clear analysis of the **content** that is addressed and on the other hand of having a clear understanding of the psychologic **processes** that allow behavior change. To understand this approach, it is helpful to reflect on **what** should be changed, **when** it should be changed, and **how** it can be changed.

### What? Content Considerations: From a General to a Tailored Approach

When dentists develop a treatment plan for a patient, they carefully consider information they collected when taking a medical/dental history, doing an oral exam, taking x-rays, etc. Deciding on the content of an educational intervention aimed at increasing patients' oral health promotion efforts is quite similar. It has to start with collecting information and then identifying which behavior change is a top priority for this particular patient. Figure 21.2 shows that a patient's oral health might be affected by oral health–related behaviors such as tooth brushing or flossing, by lifestyle-related behaviors such as using tobacco products or having a high sugar diet, and by general health-related factors such as taking medication that results in xerostomia. Identifying which specific behavior change might be most important is crucial because trying to change more than one behavior at a time is not likely to succeed.[50,78]

Once a behavior has been identified as being important to be changed to improve oral health or prevent oral disease, the next step is to explore the patient's considerations related to this particular behavior change. These considerations can be categorized as being related to the patient's affective (**A**), behavioral (**B**), and cognitive (**C**) responses related to the targeted behavior.[59] Figure 21.3 provides an overview of these three components.

**Affective** factors are related to how patients feel about the behavior they should change, how motivated they are to change this behavior, and how motivated they are to engage in constructive oral health promotion. For example, patients' responses to the simple question "How do you feel about your teeth?" differ widely and can be quite informative. Answers can range from "I don't want to keep my teeth. Pull them out and give me dentures." to "My teeth

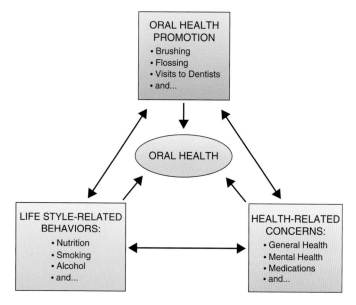

• **Figure 21.2** Behaviors related to oral health.

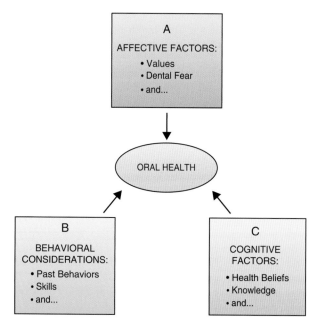

• **Figure 21.3** A – B – C considerations and oral health.

are extremely important to me and losing a tooth would be awful." Their responses also differ in content, addressing such diverse aspects as aesthetics ("My teeth give me the nicest smile!"), functionality ("My teeth are great. I can eat and bite everything I want."), or other quality of life–related concerns ("My teeth do not hurt me and that is great."). Understanding the content of these affective factors is crucial when planning how to motivate a person to change a specific oral health–related behavior. Considering patients' apprehension and dental fear in addition to their motivation to change is also quite beneficial when trying to understand a patient's affective responses to a dental visit and health behavior change.[24]

**Behavioral** factors constitute a second group of patient-related factors that need to be understood if behavior change is to be successful. Important considerations are to explore whether a patient ever engaged in a certain behavior in the past or if a patient has the skills to engage in a behavior. For example, patients with severe arthritis in their hands will need a distinctly different behavior-change approach to ensuring good oral hygiene compared to patients with excellent manual skills.

**Cognitions** or patients' thoughts are also of crucial importance. A review of research related to behavior change shows that researchers considered cognitions such as health beliefs,[12-14] attitudes and intentions,[40] and expectations[37] when they explained behavior change. One additional cognitive factor is a patient's knowledge about oral health–related matters. Research showed that it cannot be assumed that dental patients have the necessary knowledge concerning how to promote good oral health for themselves[9] or for their children.[1] Understanding which oral health–related knowledge needs to be provided can therefore be important when determining how to communicate with this patient and which information to introduce.

Once a provider has decided on a behavior that needs to be changed to improve a patient's oral health or prevent oral disease and has an understanding of what the patient's affective, behavioral, and cognitive considerations are, the next step is to explore at which stage of change the patient is.

## When? Content and Process: From a One Shot to a Story Line Approach

The question at which stage of change a patient is was most explicitly addressed by Prochaska and DiClemente.[27,92-96] When these researchers introduced their trans theoretical theory in 1982, they used it to explain how therapy with addicts unfolds. They identified five stages in the therapy process, namely the stages of precontemplation, contemplation, preparation, action, and maintenance. While they intermittently only focused on the first four of these stages,[91,94] they returned to the five-stage model later on.[28,92,93] Table 21.1 shows that while the patient has no motivation for change in the first stage, motivation has to increase to move a patient through the five stages and achieve the maintenance of the targeted behavior.

In the first stage of precontemplation, a dental patient might not think about stopping to smoke or beginning to floss. A patient in this stage does not contemplate/consider that a behavior (e.g., smoking) or a lack of behavior (e.g., not flossing) could affect their oral health negatively. The provider's objective has to be to engage the patient in contemplation of this fact to create a motivation to change. Stage 2 is the stage of contemplation. In this stage, patients are aware that a problem exists and are contemplating how they could solve this problem. However, they are not really committed to making a behavior change and can get stuck in this stage for a considerable amount of time. The fact that contemplators usually struggle with the pros and cons of behavior change should inform dental providers to help patients increase the numbers of pros and reduce the number of cons.

Once patients begin to get ready for change, they move into Stage 3, the stage of preparation. Patients in this stage have an intention to change their behavior and begin to make small changes. Prochaska, DiClemente, and Norcross[92] refer to this stage also as the phase of decision-making. In some way, the patients make the decision to change but are not following through yet. Dental care providers need to acknowledge that patients in this phase are on the right track. Stage 4 is the stage of action. Now patients actually show the targeted behavior. They might have stopped smoking, begun to floss, or discontinued drinking sugary drinks. Dental providers might assume that their work is done at this point.

However, they need to consider Marlatt and Gordon's relapse prevention theory,[74] which describes very vividly that permanent behavior change is unlikely to occur right away. Relapsing into old behavior patterns is quite likely. Dental care providers therefore need to continue to reinforce the new behavior. They might even prepare their patients for the fact that they might relapse—but emphasize that the only important behavior at this point is to get back to the targeted behavior as quickly as possible. Once patients have actually well established the new behavior, they are in the final stage, the maintenance stage. In this stage, the patients have shown the targeted behavior consistently over a longer period. Dental care providers who see their patients reach this stage need to consider that even in this stage, positive reinforcement is helpful.

What do these considerations contribute to the process of behavior change? First, they allow dentists and dental hygienists to communicate with a patient at the stage of change the patient is in. Realizing that change is slow and moves gradually from stage to stage can help providers not to have unrealistic expectations for change. Change is an ongoing story and not a one shot event. The Chinese saying that "One drop of water can make a hole in a stone if it continues over time" is a reminder that behavior change is

| • TABLE 21.1 | Exemplifying the Trans Theoretical Model of Change on Tobacco Use Cessation Efforts | | | | |
| --- | --- | --- | --- | --- | --- |
| | | EXAMPLE: TOBACCO USE CESSATION INTERVENTION | | | |
| Your patient might say: | Trans theoretical model: Stages of change | A Affective factors: Motivation | B Change-related behavior | C Cognitive factors: Thinking |
| "I am not interested in talking about stopping to smoke." | Pre-contemplation | None | None | None |
| "Every now and then I think I should stop smoking." | Contemplation | Low | None | Yes |
| "I also talked with my husband and told him I would stop on January 1." | Preparation | Moderate | Low to moderate | Yes |
| "I stopped smoking 3 weeks and 2 days ago – but I had a few cigarettes at a party on Saturday." | Action | High | High | Selective information seeking? |
| "I stopped smoking about 2 years ago and have not smoked since then." | Maintenance | Excellent | Excellent | Consistent with behavior |

likely to occur over time and not as a result of a one-time educational intervention.

After identifying the behavior that is most important to be changed; getting to know the patient's affective, behavioral, and cognitive considerations; and identifying the stage of change a patient is in, the next step is to consider how change unfolds. The theory of motivational interviewing is a successful approach to behavior change that can be applied to oral health–related behavior change.

## How? Process Considerations: Motivational Interviewing

Motivational interviewing (MI) was originally developed to address the change of addictive behavior.[80] This fact is reflected in the title of the original monograph *Motivational Interviewing: Preparing People to Change Addictive Behavior* that Miller and Rollnick published in 1991.[80] When research showed that this technique can be applied to changing behavior in amazingly different contexts, the authors changed the title of the second edition to *Motivational Interviewing: Preparing People for Change*.[81] They published their latest edition in 2013, with the title *Motivational Interviewing: Helping People Change*.[82]

Since 2003, research has focused on how MI can be used to change the behavior of patients in dental healthcare settings. Some of these studies explore how providers could use MI to change their patients' smoking behavior[23,67,98-100] or engage in a brief intervention with patients who abuse/are dependent on alcohol to change their behavior concerning the use of alcohol.[112] Other oral health–related studies focused on the possibility of using MI to change patients' behavior to increase oral health promotion and prevent oral diseases.[48,111,122-124]

The general assumption that unites these different MI-based oral health–related projects is the belief that the two most prevalent oral diseases, caries and periodontal disease, are largely preventable by engaging patients in positive oral health–promotion efforts, thus proposing that dental care providers can make a difference by communicating with their patients about changing behaviors. In this chapter, however, we argue that focusing on the process of communication and change has to start with content considerations: What is the most important behavioral aspect that needs to be changed? What are patients' affective, behavioral, and cognitive considerations related to this behavior? And where is a specific patient in the process of change? Combining these content considerations with MI process considerations is offered as the new and comprehensive approach to behavior change referred to as the Motivational Communication approach.

Once the content questions are answered, the actual process of behavior change can begin. Figure 21.4 provides an interpretation of the way in which Miller and Rollnick's four principles[81] guide behavior change–related communication. However, before discussing the four principles of MI, it is crucial to create an understanding of its spirit. The definition of MI provided by Miller and Rollnick[70] (p. 25) describes motivational interviewing as "a client-centered, directive method for enhancing intrinsic motivations to change by exploring and resolving ambivalence." The first part of this short sentence points to the clear connection between MI and Carl Rogers's client-centered approach to therapy. Rogers introduced the term "client-centered" over half a century ago[101-103] as a response against Freud's psychoanalysis,[41] the dominant approach to therapy at that time. Rogers looked at psychoanalysis, the first approach to engaging patients in talking therapy, and developed a revolutionary alternative. The philosophy underlying Rogers's approach can best be captured by considering the

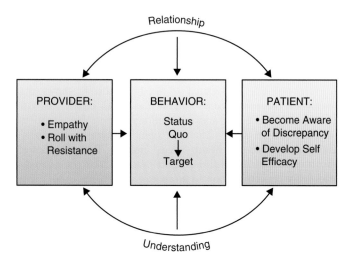

• **Figure 21.4** The process of motivational interviewing.

paradigm shift that he introduced when he refused to use the term "patient" and replaced it with the term "client." In Freud's perspective of his relationship with his patients, he was in charge and the patient benefitted from his expertise and was healed by Freud. The provider was in the driver's seat and had the knowledge and expertise to heal, while the patient was the passenger, the object that was healed by the powerful and all-knowing provider.

When Rogers introduced the term "client," he clearly moved away from accepting this old power differential.[101-103] In Rogers's therapeutic alliance, the client is in charge and hires the provider. The client is the only person who has the in-depth understanding of what is happening and causing the distress and pain the client experiences. The power differential between a client and a provider is thus redefined from a relationship that focuses on the patient's compliance with the provider's instructions and directions to a relationship of cooperation. Rogers believed that the role of the provider was to be empathetic and genuinely interested in understanding the client's situation. By being empathetic, accepting, and understanding of the client's inner struggles, the provider allows the client to approach and face the threatening, embarrassing, and painful issues that cause the mental despair. The client is thus in control of initiating behavior change and makes the decisions about change.

Motivational interviewing clearly accepts this client-centered perspective when Miller and Rollnick[81] stress the value of Rogers's approach to provide an empathetic setting. Applying this client-centered approach to the interaction between a dental healthcare provider and a dental patient thus points to a shift in treatment philosophy away from a provider-centered approach that requires patient compliance to a partnership and cooperative approach between a provider and a client/patient. It stresses the absolute significance of the power of the therapeutic alliance and the rapport between a provider and a patient as the basis for behavior change. In dentistry, research concerning patients' acceptance of treatment recommendations such as having periodontal surgery instead of nonsurgical treatment[88] and their cooperation with treatment recommendations such as wearing a bite splint[62] demonstrate the ultimate importance of this fact.

With a basic humanistic approach to behavior change comes the first of the four principles that Miller and Rollnick introduced, the principle that the provider needs to show empathy for the client as a starting point of MI.[81] Empathy can be communicated both nonverbally and verbally. Nonverbal cues can be for example nodding in agreement; verbally communicating empathy can range from sharing one's own personal experiences to sharing information about another person's similar experiences or statistical supportive information.

The second principle outlined by Miller and Rollnick is referred to as creating a discrepancy in the client's mind.[81] The power of cognitive dissonance as a means to change behavior was previously introduced by consistency theorists such as Festinger in 1957.[37] In his theory of cognitive dissonance, Festinger offered a parsimonious approach to explaining behavior change. It allowed hundreds of researchers to use his theory to explain behavior in many different contexts (see Inglehart, 1991, for an overview).[58] Festinger postulated that dissonance, a tension motivating the person to make changes in a situation, arises when an event occurs that contradicts a person's expectations. For example, a person expects to get wet when standing in the rain. If the person stands in the rain and does not get wet, the person experiences dissonance, an inner tension driving the person to find an explanation for this situation. Realizing that somebody else holds an umbrella over the person or that a tree is protecting the person from getting wet would provide such an explanation and would allow the person to reduce the dissonance and return to a state of consonance.

When a provider creates a discrepancy in a client's mind between the present status (example: "I smoke" or "I do not floss") and the targeted goal ("I should stop smoking; it is unhealthy" or "I should floss daily to prevent periodontal disease"), this discrepancy creates the motivation that fuels the change. Miller and Rollnick[81] (p. 22) therefore state explicitly "no discrepancy, no motivation"—and thus no change.[81]

As a third principle, Miller and Rollnick discuss that a provider should "roll with resistance." In addition to considering the value of a client centered approach and the power of empathy for bringing about change, clinical psychologists introduced resistance to change as an additional central element that affects the complexity of behavior change. Miller and Rollnick adopted this concept as a fundamental principle from clinical psychology.[81] This principle is concerned with the fact that patients are likely to resist change and that the provider's rolling with the patient's resistance will ultimately result in change. The original term "resistance" was introduced by Freud to describe his patients' unwillingness to accept his interpretations of their psychologic situation (p. 289).[41] However, in 1966, Brehm[18] pointed out that resistance is not only an issue in therapeutic situations but that it applies to all types of situations where attempts are made to change a person's behavior. Brehm postulated that any attempt to limit a person's freedom of choice by forcing them to change a behavior will result in reactance, a powerful motivation to resist change. The applicability of this principle to a situation in which messages about changing the consumption of alcohol were given showed that this general principle can easily be applied to health-related behavior changes.[16]

Miller and Rollnick[81] therefore realized very acutely that in a situation that focuses on behavior change, resistance might prevent this exact change. A provider's rolling with resistance will therefore be crucial to diffuse this negative energy and thus allow the patient to reflect on the possible potential that a behavior change might have for their lives. In addition, the term "rolling with resistance" takes on an additional meaning when considering the fact that behavior change is often not a one-time and final step but might be part of a process in which behavior change is followed by relapse into the old behavior.

Two clinical psychologists, Marlatt and Gordon,[74] originally introduced the concept of relapse and relapse prevention when they analyzed the recovering behavior of alcoholics and drug addicts. They stressed the importance of understanding that behavior change might not be established at once but might take on a cycle of change and relapse until the new behavior is ultimately established. Tedesco and colleagues suggested considering this concept in the context of oral healthcare.[116] In regard to MI, rolling with resistance might include the realization that behavior change is a process that consists of positive behavior change and relapse into old behavior patterns. One basic assumption here is that a client will not progress through behavior change efforts without resisting the change. However, when a client shows signs of resistance, the provider needs to roll with this resistance instead of arguing against it.

Miller and Rollnick's fourth and final principle is related to creating a sense of self-efficacy in the client. This term was previously extensively discussed by Bandura,[10] an educational psychologist who showed that behavior change can be the result of observing others and imitating their behavior.[10] In 2004, Do applied these principles to the behavior of children during dental visits.[29] Later on, Bandura developed his approach further by describing the internal processes that will facilitate behavior change.[11] He introduced the importance of understanding the role of self-efficacy for a person's willingness to engage in a new behavior.[11,39] Self-efficacy is an internal awareness that assures the person that he or she is able to successfully engage in a certain behavior and thus sets the stage to actually perform the behavior. For example, if a patient tells the provider "I cannot floss," this statement signals that the person has a minimal sense of self-efficacy. Unless the provider supports the client and turns this lack of self-efficacy into a positive sense of self-efficacy, this patient is not likely to engage in flossing behavior.[76] Miller and Rollnick adopted this concept of self-efficacy as one of the four essential components that explain how change is brought about.[81]

While showing empathy, creating discrepancy, rolling with resistance, and increasing self-efficacy are the four principles of MI, Miller and Rollnick[81] also mention four tools or techniques that help to use the four principles and create behavior change. The acronym the authors use for these core interviewing skills is OARS, which stands for asking open-ended questions, being affirmative, being reflective, and summarizing.[81] They described asking open-ended questions as opening a door for the client, giving the client time to think and consider the answer. In some way, open-ended questions provide an opportunity to learn something new. Being affirmative instead of critical or judgmental is one way to create a humanistic environment. Reflectively responding to a client's statement can offer an opportunity to find out if the client's perspective is accurately perceived and to portray that understanding to the client. Summarizing what was communicated at the end of a communication ensures that client and provider have the same understanding and expectations of the situation.

## Application: "What," "When," and "How" During a Dental Visit

After discussing the "what," "when," and "how" of behavior change aimed at increasing oral health–promotion efforts and/or reducing oral disease, it might be helpful to reflect on how this approach can be applied concretely to one-on-one dentist/dental hygienist–patient encounters.

A patient's first dental visit offers an opportunity to collect relevant information about the **content** of needed health behavior changes throughout the visit. Taking a medical/dental history allows getting to know the person, establishing rapport, and collecting the information needed to treat the patient safely.

Additional information collected during the oral exam and based on radiographs will complement the understanding of which behavior change education might be the top priority for this patient. Using open-ended questions, affirmative statements, and reflective responding can further support establishing rapport and increasing understanding of the patient's situation.

Once a needed behavior change is identified and information has been collected about the patient's affective, behavioral, and cognitive considerations concerning this targeted behavior and its change,[59] an assessment of the patient's stage of change should follow.[27,28,91-96] Collecting this content-related information is ongoing throughout the appointment; informing the patient about oral health–related findings during the oral examination and while gathering information can create a basis for the upcoming educational intervention.

Once a baseline of content considerations is established, the actual **process** of behavior change can unfold. Using the four principles of MI and the four tools begins with showing empathy throughout the process.[81] Beginning the behavior change communication with an explanation of why a specific health behavior change is discussed is helpful for creating an understanding in the patient and using a patient-centered approach. This explanation can also begin the process of creating a discrepancy in the patient's mind between the patient's perception of the status quo and the targeted changed behavior and its benefits for the patient's oral health. Engaging the patient actively, for example by letting the patient demonstrate tooth brushing or flossing (if these are behaviors targeted in the behavior change process), can provide concrete opportunities to make discrepancies between current destructive or unhelpful behavior and more constructive

behavior salient and thus can create a clear sense of why behavior change should occur. Using open-ended questions, affirmative statements, and reflective responding throughout this process is helpful.[81]

Optimally, a cooperative effort will be made to create a plan for concrete next steps by the end of the oral health behavior change intervention. Summarizing at the end, providing an opportunity for the patient to share any additional information and to ask any questions will be useful to ensure that provider and patients have shared expectations for next steps. Adding information to the clinical chart about the health behavior change efforts will allow following up over time and taking a story line approach.

## From the Cradle to the Grave: Oral Health Promotion Over the Course of Life

When Inglehart and Tedesco suggested that a patient's affective, behavioral, and cognitive considerations are information that healthcare providers can use to better understand the patient's oral health–related behavior and to engage in more informed and patient-centered behavior change interventions,[59] they also pointed out that oral health promotion efforts have to consider the time in a patient's life at which the oral behavior change occurs (Figure 21.5). A discussion of the role of the impact of the patient's stage in life on oral health behavior change can complement the general motivational communication considerations.

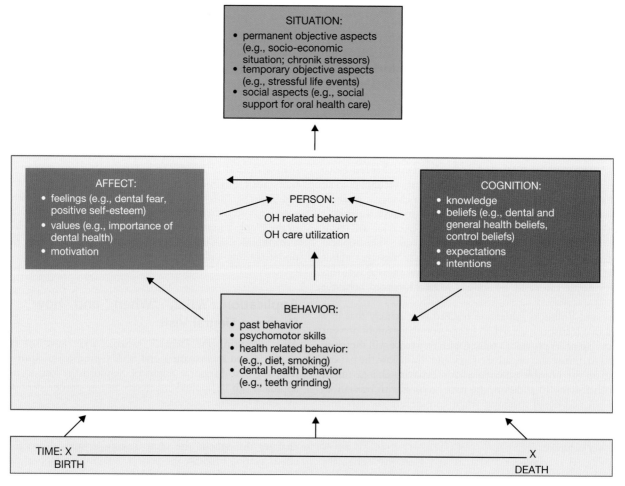

• **Figure 21.5** The new century model of oral health promotion.

## Infant Oral Health Exams: Anticipatory Guidance and the Power of Establishing a Dental Home

The first ever U.S. Surgeon General's Report on Oral Health, in 2000,[118] drew attention to the fact that dental caries was the most common chronic childhood disease and was five times more common than asthma, seven times more common than hay fever, and 14 times more common than chronic bronchitis. Ensuring that parents engage in preventive oral health promotion is therefore crucial. Already in 1986, the American Academy of Pediatric Dentistry (AAPD) adopted a policy on infant oral healthcare as a way to promote oral health and prevent oral disease in these very young children.[5] More recently in 2006[4] and 2014,[3] the AAPD revisited this guideline on infant oral healthcare and again stressed the importance of establishing a dental home for infants by their first birthday.[3]

Once an infant has a dental home, the AAPD recommended that a first visit should include not only taking the infant's medical/dental history and the parents' dental history, conducting an oral examination, demonstrating age-appropriate tooth brushing, assessing the infant's risk of developing caries, and determining a prevention plan, but the visit should also focus on providing anticipatory guidance for the parent.[3,84] The AAPD recommended that the content of this educational intervention should include information for the parent about their infant's dental and oral development, the role of fluoride for the prevention of oral disease, nonnutritive sucking habits, teething, injury prevention, oral hygiene instruction, and the effects of diet on their infant's dentition.[3]

These recommendations should alert dental care providers to the important role that families play in oral health promotion for their children.[60] More specifically, they can complement providers' content considerations when they approach an oral health behavior change intervention for parents and their infants. Therefore it is important that dentists seize the opportunity to get infants off to an early start for good oral health by offering dental homes and infant oral health examinations for infants while engaging parents in anticipatory guidance.[6,19,73]

## Early Childhood: Using Visual Information to Improve Communication with Parents of Young Children

According to the 2003 National Assessment of Adult Literacy (NAAL), 36% of US adults are unable to perform "basic" child preventive health tasks such as using an immunization schedule, following recommendations from a preventive health brochure, and interpreting a growth chart.[69] In addition, research also showed that there was a relationship between caregivers' oral health literacy and their children's oral health status[20] and that adults with lower oral health literacy were less likely to seek dental care for their children.[79] Additionally, even if parents sought oral healthcare for their child, the information they received during this visit did not necessarily affect their oral health–related attitudes and behaviors.[64] Benitez and colleagues showed, for example, that informing parents in conversations about the hazard of a specific behavior (namely that putting their child to sleep with a bottle containing juice can cause early childhood caries) did not successfully affect this behavior.[15] Tinanoff and colleagues also found that educating parents by verbally informing them about the hazards of frequent and prolonged feeding with the bottle also proved ineffective.[117] Despite this evidence, dental providers often rely solely on verbal communication to educate parents about oral health promotion for their child.

One alternative to using only verbal motivational communication could be to use visual information during health behavior change interventions. Using illustrations when conveying information is supported by research that showed that humans have a preference for picture-based, rather than text-based, information.[106] Health-related research found that illustrations can be very effective when they are used to take advantage of the patients' "teachable moment," the time when they are ready to accept new information because of their increased interest during the discussion of their health status.[75]

In addition to using general illustrations in patient education, research also showed that individualizing patient instruction was more effective.[49] Wang and colleagues therefore explored the effects of educating parents of young children in the dental office about their child's upcoming operative appointment by using standardized and/or individualized illustrations or a traditional verbal approach.[121] The standardized visual information consisted of a flip chart that showed pictures of healthy primary teeth versus teeth with different oral health problems. Individualized visual information was provided on an odontogram of primary teeth as depicted in Figure 21.6. Dental hygienists used a green marker to indicate on this chart which dental care the child had received at a visit and used a red marker to circle which dental care was still needed at a next operative visit. The results showed that 46.9% of verbally informed parents missed the next operative appointment compared to 19.1% of parents who had received information with the help of standardized illustrations, 15.6% who had received individualized illustrations, and 10.4% who had received both individualized and standardized visual information.[121]

A follow-up study by Picard and colleagues in 2014[90] explored whether educating parents with visual aids versus verbally after their child's treatment under general anesthesia would improve their attendance at follow-up appointments. The results showed that 78% of the parents who had been educated with the help of visual information returned, while only 52% of the parents who had received traditional verbal instructions returned for follow-up appointments. The results of these two studies point to the significance of informing parents about the very basic disease process of dental caries with the aid of individualized illustrations to increase parents' compliance with the recommended dental treatment for their children. Using illustrations for oral health education about oral health promotion plus individualizing this information for the specific child such as by using an odontogram with specific information as well as upcoming treatment can therefore be highly recommended.[90] Complementing motivational communication efforts with the use of individualized and standardized visual information can clearly increase the effectiveness of these educational interventions.

## Oral Health Education for Children in Kindergarten Through Grade 5: Experiential Learning at Its Best

Given the high percentages of US children with oral disease and the significant consequences of caries, it seems obvious that major efforts are needed to find better ways to educate children about oral health promotion. Developmental psychology points to the fact that children in kindergarten and elementary school grades are likely to benefit from hands-on, experiential learning.[89] Research on the benefits of experiential oral health education in classroom settings showed that this type of instruction resulted in increased learning compared to traditional lecturing for children.[7] Inglehart and colleagues therefore explored the effectiveness of an

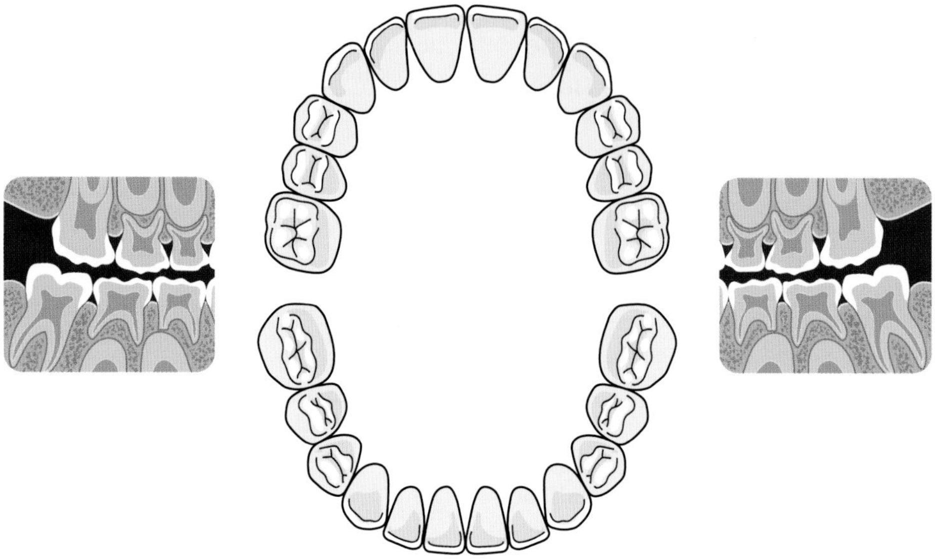

• **Figure 21.6** Odontogram of primary dentition.

experiential approach to educating kindergarten and elementary school–age children in a dental office.[57] The objectives of their study were to determine if practice-based experiential oral health education for 5- to 10-year-old children affected their oral health–related behavioral intentions, parents/guardians' perceptions of children's oral health–related behavior two weeks later, and parents' satisfaction with their child's dental visit and their preferences for communication modalities. The results showed that children who had received experiential educational intervention were more likely to brush their teeth on their own, to provide oral health–related reasons for brushing, to floss their teeth, and to floss more frequently and by themselves than children before the experiential intervention and children who had received traditional verbal oral health education. At a 2-week follow-up phone call, parents of children in the experiential group brushed and flossed more frequently, reported that their children brushed and flossed more independently and flossed more frequently, and had improved dental visit evaluations and increased preferences for using pictures and hands-on activities compared to parents of children who had received traditional verbal oral health education. While these results concerning the effects of practice-based experiential oral hygiene–related instruction for young children can be considered just a first step in exploring the value of experiential learning, future research should investigate its benefits and ways to complement the general motivational communication approach with experiential learning efforts. The fact that the experiential intervention for the children had also shown positive results for parents was encouraging given the fact that not all parents are sufficiently knowledgeable about oral health promotion efforts for their child and are the gate keepers who might prevent their child from receiving oral health care by not utilizing oral health care services.[1]

## Adolescence: Keeping Oral Health Promotion Alive and Well

Dental researchers and clinicians recognize that adolescent patients have distinctive characteristics and needs.[2,35] For example, adolescents have high caries rates,[2,33,36] an increased risk for traumatic injuries,[2] a tendency for poor nutritional habits[2] such as drinking excessive amounts of soft drinks,[72] an increased interest in appearance-related aesthetics,[22] high rates of dental phobia,[109-111] and special social and psychological needs.[2] Given the characteristics of this population, it seems important to explore how oral health promotion education can be best structured for patients in this age group to ensure adolescents maintain good oral hygiene efforts and engage in solid oral health promotion. Brukiene and Aleksejuniene's[21] 2009 review of the literature about the effectiveness of different strategies to promote oral health among 12- to 18-year-old adolescents found that in most studies only a slight or no improvement was reported in the adolescents' attitudes and that a deterioration of oral hygiene efforts was observed over time. Based on this literature review, the authors concluded that research on alternative methods for educating adolescents about oral health–related issues should be explored. Using visual information might be one way to educate pediatric patients in this age group more successfully.[35] However, any motivational communication efforts should consider the unique characteristics and needs of this age group.

## Oral Health Behavior Change and Adults: Addressing Destructive Habits While Considering Health Literacy Concerns

Prior to considering the specific content areas of behavior change that need to be addressed with adults, the topic of health literacy needs to be revisited. The Institute of Medicine defined health literacy as the degree to which patients are able to obtain, process, and understand basic health information and services needed to make appropriate health decisions.[63] Research showed that almost half (43%) of the adults in the United States were unable to comprehend and navigate printed materials related to everyday issues such as health, safety, and finance.[69,105] Adults with lower health literacy were 1.5 to 3 times more likely to encounter poorer health, to underuse health resources, to have higher rates of chronic diseases, and to engage in unhealthy behavior.[26] Health literacy is also relevant in connection with patients' knowledge about oral health–related issues,[120,71] oral health–related behavior,[120] their use of oral healthcare services,[87] and their dental fear.[108] In addition, adults with lower oral health literacy were also less likely to seek dental care for their children.[79] Given this significant impact of oral health literacy in the context of preventing oral diseases and ensuring oral healthcare use, dental care providers and any other professionals engaging in behavior change communication need to carefully consider how to ensure that the communication unfolds on a level of health literacy that is appropriate for the patient addressed. Chapter 22 will provide more in-depth considerations of this topic.

When considering oral health behavior change in adults, two central areas are of concern. The first area is the change of destructive lifestyle-related behaviors such as smoking or chewing tobacco and diet-related behaviors such as the consumption of foods and beverages with high sugar contents. Chapter 28 will address the detrimental effects of tobacco use and Chapter 23 the role of diet for oral health.

The second area of concern focuses on the relationship between oral health and systemic health, such as diabetes, and mental health, such as eating disorders[42] and depression.[77] While the relationships between for example periodontal disease and diabetes are widely discussed, consideration of the role of dental care providers in engaging patients with mental health issues in constructive oral health–promotion efforts receives much less attention. This situation is unfortunate because mental health issues such as addictions, anxiety disorders, and affective disorders can have a significant effect on patients' oral health and oral healthcare use. More research is needed to ensure that educational efforts will be developed for dental care providers to realize the crucial role they can play in promoting good oral health among patients with mental health concerns.

## Oral Health Behavior Change and Dental Patients 65 Years of Age and Older

When dental care providers engage in oral health promotion efforts with adults over 65 years of age, special considerations concerning sensory and cognitive changes related to aging should be considered when engaging in motivational communication.[46,113] These communication efforts become especially challenging when communicating with patients with mild, moderate, or severe neurocognitive deficits (previously referred to as dementia)[17] or patients who have been recently bereaved or face death.[43,65]

## Outlook: Benefits and Challenges

The humanistic model of professional behavior (Figure 21.7) suggests that professional behavior is a function of dental care providers' awareness, skills, and knowledge related to the behavior at hand.[61] In the case of oral health behavior change related communication, research shows that while constructive oral health behavior can clearly prevent oral disease and improve oral health, increased professional education efforts are needed to gain a better understanding of how to best create optimal change. This chapter proposes the motivational communication model that analyzes the two central components of behavior change—**content and process**—and tries to answer the questions how we know *what* to change, *when* change is likely to occur, and *how* we best achieve the process of change. The argument can be made that the newly introduced comprehensive approach to oral health behavior change

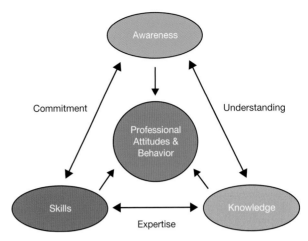

• **Figure 21.7** The humanistic model of professional education.

called Motivational Communication might provide a basis for more organized and deliberate efforts in this arena.

However, three challenges should be described as well. The first is the fact that cultural influences such as unconscious biases[25] might affect our oral health behavior change communication with patients from different socioeconomic and/or ethnic/racial backgrounds, with different gender identities or sexual orientations,[52] or with different abilities or from different religious backgrounds—to name just a few of the many social identities that patients have. Education about cross-cultural communication and communication breakdowns is clearly needed to raise dental care providers' awareness concerning these issues when communicating and treating patients.

Second, time and financial constraints limit the efforts that dentists and dental hygienists can devote to oral health behavior change in one-on-one settings. Taking oral health education to the community such as to Head Start programs, kindergarten classes, and other schools; to community groups with adults; and to residential homes for older adults and nursing homes is clearly important. A comprehensive motivational communication approach for community-based education is therefore being developed.

Third, deliberate efforts to connect motivational communication efforts with preventive dentistry strategies such as fluoride applications (see Chapter 25) and the use of dental sealants and other preventive treatments (Chapter 26) are crucial because they would clearly increase the effectiveness of these efforts. Future research in this context is needed.

Finally, returning to the WHO definition of health promotion,[125] it is obvious that oral health behavior change efforts are just one part of the efforts needed to promote good oral health. However, these efforts undoubtedly can be highly effective and deserve scientific scrutiny to understand how to use and apply the best possible and effective approaches. Ultimately, they also need to be considered in an ethical framework, taking into account the role of professional responsibilities and ethical practice in the context of oral health promotion.[115]

## Acknowledgment

I want to thank Dr. Philip S. Richards, my colleague at the University of Michigan School of Dentistry, who is a master clinician who inspired me to think about these issues from the first time we talked about patient–dentist interactions in the 1990s.

# References

1. Akpabio A, Klausner CP, Inglehart MR. Mothers' knowledge about promoting their children's oral health—who knows what? *J Dent Hyg.* 2008;82(1):12.
2. American Academy of Pediatric Dentistry. Adolescent Oral Health Care. Oral health Policies and Recommendations. The Reference Manual of Pediatric Dentistry. 2019–2020. https://www.aapd.org/research/oral-health-policies–recommendations/adolescent-oral-health-care/
3. American Academy of Pediatric Dentistry. Guideline on perinatal and infant oral health care. Reference Manual. *Pediatr Dent.* 2016;38(6):150–154.
4. American Academy of Pediatric Dentistry. Guideline on infant oral health care. Reference Manual 2006–07. *Pediatr Dent.* 2006;28(suppl):73–76.
5. American Academy of Pediatric Dentistry. Policy on infant oral health care. Reference Manual. Adopted in 1986; https://www.aapd.org/assets/1/7/G_InfantOralHealthCare.pdf.
6. Ananaba N, Malcheff S, Briskie D, Inglehart MR. Infant oral health examinations—general and pediatric dentists' attitudes and professional behavior. *J Michigan Dent Assoc.* 2010;92(12):38–43.
7. Angelopoulou MV, Kavvadia K, Taoufik K, et al. Comparative clinical study testing the effectiveness of school based oral health education using experiential learning or traditional lecturing in 10 year-old children. *BMC Oral Health.* 2015;28(15):51.
8. Ayhan H, Suskan E, Yildirim S. The effect of nursing or rampant caries on height, body weight and head circumference. *J Clin Pediatr Dent.* 1996;20:209–212.
9. Bagramian RA, Narendran S, Khavari AM. Oral health status, knowledge, and practices in an Amish population. *J Public Health Dent.* 1988;48(3):147–151.
10. Bandura A. Influence of models' reinforcement contingencies on the acquisition of imitative responses. *J Pers Soc Psychol.* 1965;1(6):589–595.
11. Bandura A. Self-efficacy: toward a unifying theory of behavioral change. *Psychol Rev.* 1977;84:191–215.
12. Becker MH, ed. The health belief model and personal health behavior. *Health Ed Monogr.* 1974;2:324–473.
13. Becker MH. Understanding patient compliance: the contributions of attitudes and other psychosocial factors. In: Cohen SJ, ed. *New Directions in Patient Compliance.* Lexington, MA: Health; 1979.
14. Becker MH, Rosenstock IM. Compliance with medical advice. In: Steptoe A, Mathews A, eds. *Health Care and Human Behavior.* London: Academic Press; 1984.
15. Benitez C, O'Sullivan D, Tinanoff N. Effect of a preventive approach for the treatment of nursing bottle caries. *ASDC J Dent Child.* 1994;61(1):46–49.
16. Bensley SL, Wu R. 1991. The role of psychological reactance in drinking following alcohol prevention messages. *J Appl Soc Psych.* 1991;21(13):1111–1124.
17. Black WD, Andreasen NC. *Introductory Textbook of Psychiatry.* 6th ed. Washington, DC: American Psychiatric Publishing; 2014:439–458.
18. Brehm JWA. *Theory of Psychological Reactance.* Oxford, UK: Academic Press; 1966.
19. Brickhouse TH, Unkel JH, Kancitis I, et al. Infant oral health care: a survey of general dentists, pediatric dentists, and pediatricians in Virginia. *Pediatr Dent.* 2008;30(2):147–153.
20. Bridges SM, Parthasarathy DS, Wong HM, Yiu CK, Au TK, McGrath CP. The relationship between caregiver functional oral health literacy and child oral health status. *Patient Educ Couns.* 2014;94(3):411–416.
21. Brukiene V, Aleksejuniene J. An overview of oral health promotion in adolescents. *Int J Paediatr Dent.* 2009;19:163–171.
22. Christopherson EA, Briskie D, Inglehart MR. Objective, subjective, and self-assessment of preadolescent orthodontic treatment need - A function of age, gender, and ethnic/racial background? *J Public Health Dent.* 2009;69(1):9–17.
23. Davis JM, Stockdale MS, Cropper M. The need for tobacco education: studies of collegiate dental hygiene patients and faculty. *J Dent Educ.* 2005;69(12):1340–1352.
24. de Jongh A, Muris P, ter Horst G, Duyx MP. Acquisition and maintenance of dental anxiety: the role of conditioning experiences and cognitive factors. *Behav Res Therapy.* 1995;33(2):205–210.
25. Devine PG, Forscher PS, Austin AJ, Cox TL. Long-term reduction in implicit race bias: a prejudice habit breaking intervention. *J Exp Soc Psychol.* 2012;48(6):1267–1278.
26. DeWalt DA, Berkman ND, Sheridan S, Rohr KN, Pignone MP. Literacy and health outcomes: a systematic review of the literature. *J Gen Intern Med.* 2004;19:1228–1239.
27. DiClemente CC, Prochaska JO. Self-change and therapy change of smoking behavior: A comparison of processes of change in cessation and maintenance. *Addict Behav.* 1982;7(2):133–142.
28. DiClemente CC, Prochaska JO, Fairhurst SK, Velicer WF, Velasquez MM, Rossi JS. The process of smoking cessation: an analysis of precontemplation, contemplation, and preparation stages of change. *J Consult Clin Psychol.* 1991;59(2):295–304.
29. Do C. Applying social learning theory to children with dental anxiety. *J Contemp Dental Pract.* 2004;5(1):126–135.
30. Dye BA, Li X, Lewis BG, Iafolla T, Beltran-Aguilar ED, Eke PI. Overview and quality assurance for the oral health component of the National Health and Nutrition Examination Survey (NHANES), 2009–2010. *J Public Health Dent.* 2014;74(3):248–256.
31. Dye BA, Mitnik GL, Iafolla TJ, Vargas CM. Trends in dental caries in children and adolescents according to poverty status in the United States from 1999 through 2004 and from 2011 through 2014. *J Am Dent Assoc.* 2017 Aug;148(8):550–565.e7.
32. Dye BA, Weatherspoon DJ, Lopez Mitnik G. Tooth loss among older adults according to poverty status in the United States from 1999 through 2004 and 2009 through 2014. *J Am Dent Assoc.* 2019 Jan;150(1):9–23.e3.
33. Edelstein BL. Disparities in oral health and access to care: findings of national surveys. *Ambul Pediatr.* 2002;2(2 suppl):141–147.
34. Eke PI, Thornton-Evans GO, Wei L, et al. Periodontitis in US Adults: National Health and Nutrition Examination Survey 2009–2014. *J Am Dent Assoc.* 2018 Jul;149(7):576–588.e6.
35. Ertugrul HZ. *Informing Adolescent Dental Patients and Their Parents about Oral Health Care Needs – Analyzing the Effects of Using Visual Aides. [master's thesis].* Ann Arbor, MI: University of Michigan; 2010.
36. Featherstone JDB. The science and practice of caries prevention. *J Am Dent Assoc.* 2000;131(7):887–899.
37. Festinger L. *A Theory of Cognitive Dissonance.* Evanston, IL: Row, Peterson; 1957.
38. Filstrup SL, Briskie D, da Fonseca M, et al. Early childhood caries and quality of life—child and parent perspectives. *J Pediatr Dent.* 2003;25(5):431–440.
39. Finlayson TL, Siefert K, Ismail AI, et al. Reliability and validity of brief measures of oral health-related knowledge, fatalism, and self-efficacy in mothers of African American children. *Pediatr Dent.* 2005;27(5):422–428.
40. Fishbein M, Ajzen I. Attitudes towards toward objects as predictors of single and multiple behavioral criteria. *Psychol Rev.* 1974;81(1):59–74.
41. Freud S. *A General Introduction to Psychoanalysis.* Riviere J, trans. New York: Washington Square Press; 1952.
42. Frimenko KM, Murdoch-Kinch CA, Inglehart MR. Education about eating disorders: dental students' perceptions and practice of interprofessional care. *J Dent Educ.* 2017;81(11):1327–1337.
43. Gawande A. *Being Mortal: Medicine and What Matters in the End.* New York, NY: Metropolitan Books, Henry Holt and Company; 2014.
44. Genco R, Offenbacher S, disease Beck S Periodontal, disease cardiovascular. Epidemiology and possible mechanisms. *J Am Dent Assoc.* 2002;133(suppl):14S–22S.
45. Gift HC, Reisine ST, Larach DC. The social impact of dental problems and visits. *Am J Public Health.* 1992;82(12):1663–1668.

46. Goldblatt RS, Yellowitz JA. The senior friendly office. In: Friedman PK, ed. *Geriatric Dentistry: Caring for Our Aging Population*. New York, NY: Wiley; 2014:43–58.

47. Greenwall AL, Johnsen D, DiSantis TA, et al. Longitudinal evaluation of caries patterns from the primary to the mixed dentition. *Pediatr Dent*. 1990;12:278–282.

48. Harrison R, Benton T, Everson-Stewart S, Weinstein P. Effect of motivational interviewing on rates of early childhood caries: a randomized trial. *Pediatr Dent*. 2007;29(1):16–22.

49. Hayes KS. Randomized trial of geragogy-based medication instruction in the emergency department. *Nursing Res*. 1998;47(4):211–218.

50. Hovland CI, Janis IL, Kelley HH. *Communication and Persuasion: Psychological Studies of Opinion Change*. New Haven, CT: Yale University Press; 1953.

51. Inglehart MR. *Reactions to Critical Life Events. A Social Psychological Analysis*. New York: Praeger Publishing; 1991.

52. Inglehart MR. Quality of life and oral health. In: Mostofsky DI, Forgione AG, Giddon DB, eds. *Behavioral Dentistry. Blackwell-Munksgaard*; Copenhagen, Denmark. Publishers; 2006:19–28.

53. Inglehart MR. Patient – provider communication: Does gender matter? In: Kaste LM, Halpern L, eds. *Gender Disparities in Oral Health and Disease. Dent Clin North Am*. 2013;57(2):357–370.

54. Inglehart MR. Quality of life and oral health. In: Mostofsky DI, Farida F, eds. *Behavioral Dentistry*. 2nd ed. Hoboken, NJ: Wiley; 2014.

55. Inglehart MR. Bagramian RA. Oral health related quality of life—introduction and overview. In: Inglehart MR, Bagramian RA, eds. *Oral Health and Quality of Life*. Chicago, IL: Quintessence; 2002:1.

56. Inglehart MR, Bagramian RA, eds. *Oral Health and Quality of Life*. Chicago, IL: Quintessence; 2002.

57. Inglehart MR, Filstrup SL, Wandera A. Oral health related quality of life and children. In: Inglehart MR, Bagramian RA, eds. *Oral Health and Quality of Life*. Chicago, IL: Quintessence; 2002. chap 8.

58. Inglehart MR, Maples S, Boynton J, et al. *Practice-based experiential oral health education for 5-10 year old children*. Fort Lauderdale, FL: American Association of Dental Research Meeting; March 2018.

59. Inglehart MR, Tedesco LA. Behavioral research related to oral hygiene practices: a new century model of oral health promotion. *Periodontol. 2000*. 1995;8:15–23.

60. Inglehart MR, Tedesco LA. The role of the family in preventing oral diseases. In: Cohen LK, Gift HC, eds. *Disease Prevention and Oral Health Promotion—Socio-Dental Sciences in Action*. Copenhagen, Denmark: Munksgaard; 1995:271–307.

61. Inglehart MR, Tedesco LA, Valachovic RW. Quality of life—refocusing dental education. In: Inglehart MR, Bagramian RA, eds. *Oral Health and Quality of Life*. Chicago, IL: Quintessence; 2002: chap 16.

62. Inglehart MR, Widmalm SE, Syriac PJ. Occlusal splints and quality of life—does the quality of the patient-provider relationship matter? *Oral Health Prev Dent*. 2014;12(3):249–258.

63. Institute of Medicine. *Health Literacy: A Prescription to End Confusion*. Washington, DC: National Academies Press; 200413.

64. Kanellis MJ, Logan HL, Jakobsen J. Changes in maternal attitude toward baby bottle tooth decay. *Pediatr Dent*. 1997;19(1):56–60.

65. Kessler D. *The Needs of the Dying: A Guide for Bringing Hope, Comfort, and Love to Life's Final Chapter*. New York, NY: Harper Collins; 2000.

66. Kinane DF, Chestnutt LG. Smoking and periodontal disease. *Crit Rev Oral Biol Med*. 2000;11(3):356–365.

67. Koerber A, Crawford J, O'Connell K. The effects of teaching dental students brief motivational interviewing for smoking-cessation counseling: a pilot study. *J Dent Educ*. 2003;67(4):439–447.

68. Kumar S, Tadakamadla J, Johnson NW. Effect of tooth brushing frequency on incidence and increment of dental caries: a systematic review and meta-analysis. *J Dent Res*. 2016;95(11):1230–1236.

69. Kutner ME, Greenberg E, Jin Y, et al. The Health Literacy of America's Adults: Results from the 2003 National Assessment of Adult Literacy. Publication 2006-2483. Washington, DC: National Center for Education. *Statistics*. 2006;.

70. Leite FRM, Nascimento GG, Scheutz F, et al. Effect of smoking on periodontitis: a systematic review and meta-regression. *Am J Prev Med*. 2018;54(6):831–841.

71. Macek MD, Manski MC, Schneiderman MT, et al. Knowledge of oral health issues among low-income Baltimore adults: a pilot study. *J Dent Hyg*. 2011;85:49–56.

72. Majewski RF. Dental caries in adolescents associated with caffeinated carbonated beverages. *Pediatr Dent*. 2001;23(3):198–203.

73. Malcheff S, Pink TC, Sohn W, et al. Infant oral health examinations: pediatric dentists' professional behavior and attitudes. *Pediatr Dent*. 2009;31(3):202–209.

74. Marlatt GA, Gordon JR. Theoretical rationale and overview of the model. In: Marlatt GA, Gordon JR, eds. *Relapse Prevention: Maintenance Strategies in Addictive Behavior Change*. New York, NY: The Guilford Press; 1985:3–70.

75. McBride CM, Emmons KM, Lipkus IM. Understanding the potential of teachable moments: the case of smoking cessation. *Health Educ Res*. 2003;18(2):156–170.

76. McCaul KD, O'Neill HK, Glasgow RE. Predicting the performance of dental hygiene behaviors: an examination of the Fishbein and Ajzen model and self-efficacy. *J Appl Soc*. 1988;18(2):114–128.

77. McFarland M, Inglehart M. Depression, self efficacy, and oral health—an exploration. *Oral Health Dent Manage*. 2010;9(4):214–222.

78. McGuire WJ. The Yale communication and attitude change program in the 1950s. In: Dennis EE, Wartella EA, eds. *American Communication Research: The Remembered History*. Mahwah, NJ: Lawrence Erlbaum Associates; 1996:39–59.

79. Miller E, Lee JY, DeWalt DA. Impact of caregiver literacy on children's oral health outcomes. *Pediatrics*. 2010;126:107–114.

80. Miller WR, Rollnick S. *Motivational Interviewing: Preparing People to Change Addictive Behavior*. New York: Guilford Press; 1991.

81. Miller WR, Rollnick S. *Motivational Interviewing: Preparing People to Change*. 2nd ed. New York, NY: Guilford Press; 2002.

82. Miller WR, Rollnick S. *Motivational Interviewing: Helping People Change*. 3rd ed. New York, NY: Guilford Press; 2013.

83. National Center for Health Statistics. National Health and Nutrition Examination Survey—Overview. https://www.cdc.gov/nchs/data/nhanes/nhanes_13_14/NHANES_Overview_Brochure.pdf. Accessed January 15, 2019.

84. Nowak AJ, Casamassimo PS. Using anticipatory guidance to provide early dental intervention. *J Am Dent Assoc*. 1995;126(8):1156–1163.

85. Offenbacher S, Boggess KA, Murtha AP, Jared HL, Lieff S, McKaig RG, Mauriello SM, Moss KL, Beck JD. Progressive periodontal disease and risk of very preterm delivery. *Obstet Gynecol*. 2006;107(1):29–36.

86. Palmer CA, Diet Boyd LD. *Nutrition in Oral Health*. 3rd ed. New York, NY: Pearson; 2017.

87. Parker EJ, Jamieson LM. Associations between indigenous Australian oral health literacy and self-reported oral health outcomes. *BMC Oral Health*. 2010;10:3.

88. Patel AM, Richards RS, Wang H, et al. Surgical or non-surgical periodontal treatment? Factors affecting patient decision making. *J Periodontol*. 2006;77(4):678–683.

89. Piaget J, Inhelder B. *The Psychology of the Child*. 2nd ed. New York, NY: Basic Books; 1969.

90. Picard AJ, Estrella MR, Boynton J. Educating parents of children receiving comprehensive dental care under general anesthesia with visual aids. *Pediatr Dent*. 2014;36(4):329–335.

91. Prochaska JO, DiClemente CC. Common processes of change in smoking, weight control, and psychological distress. In: Shiffman S, Wills T, eds. *Coping and Substance Abuse*. San Diego, CA: Academic Press; 1985:345–363.

92. Prochaska JO, DiClemente CC, Norcross JC. In search of how people change: applications to addictive behaviors. *Am Psychol.* 1992; 47(9):1102–1114.

93. Prochaska JO, DiClemente CC. Stages of change in the modification of problem behaviors. In: Hersen M, Eisler RM, Miller PM, eds. *Progress in Behavior Modification.* Sycamore, IL: Sycamore Press; 1992:184–214.

94. Prochaska JO, DiClemente CC. Stages and processes of self-change in smoking: toward an integrative model of change. *J Consult Clin Psychol.* 1983;51(3):390–395.

95. Prochaska JO, DiClemente CC. *The Transtheoretical Approach: Crossing Traditional Boundaries of Change.* Homewood, IL: Dorsey Press; 1984.

96. Prochaska JO, DiClemente CC. Toward a comprehensive model of change. In: Miller WR, Heather N, eds. *Treating Addictive Behaviors: Processes of Change.* New York: Plenum Press; 1986:3–27.

97. Rajapakse PS, McCracken GI, Gwynnett E. Does tooth brushing influence the development and progression of non-inflammatory gingival recession? A systematic review. *J Clin Periodontol.* 2007;34(12): 1046–1061.

98. Ramseier CA, Bornstein MM, Saxer UP, et al. Tobacco use prevention and cessation in the dental practice. *Schweizer Monatsschrift für Zahnmedizin.* 2007;117(3):253–278.

99. Ramseier CA, Christen A, McGowan J, et al. Tobacco use prevention and cessation in dental and dental hygiene undergraduate education. *Oral Health Prev Dent.* 2006;4(1):49–60.

100. Ramseier CA, Mattheos N, Needleman I, Watt R, Wickholm S. Consensus report: first European Workshop on tobacco use prevention and cessation for oral health professionals. *Oral Health Prev Dent.* 2006;4(1):7–18.

101. Rogers C. A theory of therapy, personality and interpersonal relationships as developed in the client-centered framework. In: Koch S, ed. Psychology: *A Study of a Science. Vol. 3: Formulations of the Person and the Social Context.* New York, NY: McGraw Hill; 1959.

102. Rogers C. *Client-Centered Therapy: Its Current Practice, Implications and Theory.* London, UK: Constable; 1951.

103. Rogers C. *On Becoming a Person: A Therapist's View of Psychotherapy.* London, UK: Constable; 1961.

104. Rosania AE, Low KG, McCormick CM, et al. Stress, depression, cortisol, and periodontal disease. *J Periodontol.* 2009;80(2):260–266.

105. Rudd RE. Health literacy skills of U.S. adults. *Am J Health Behav.* 2007;31(suppl 1):S8–S18.

106. Sansgiry SS, Cady PS, Adamcik BA. Consumer comprehension of information on over-the-counter medication labels: effects of picture superiority and individual differences based on age. *J Pharm Mark Manage.* 1997;11:63–76.

107. Sheller B, Williams BJ, Lombardi SM. Diagnosis and treatment of dental caries-related emergencies in a children's hospital. *Pediatr Dent.* 1997;19(8):470–475.

108. Shin WK, Braun T, Inglehart MR. Parents' dental anxiety and oral health literacy: effects on parents' and children's oral health-related experiences. *J Public Health Dent.* 2014;74(3):195–201.

109. Skaret E, Raadal M, Berg E, et al. Dental anxiety among 18-year-olds in Norway: prevalence and related factors. *Eur J Oral Sci.* 1998;106(4):835–843.

110. Skaret E, Raadal M, Berg E, et al. Dental anxiety and dental avoidance among 12 to 18 year olds in Norway. *Eur J Oral Sci.* 1999;107(6):422–428.

111. Skaret E, Weinstein P, Kvale G, et al. An intervention program to reduce dental avoidance behaviour among adolescents: a pilot study. *Eur J Paediatric Dent.* 2003;4(4):191–196.

112. Smith AJ, Shepherd JP, Hodgson RJ. Brief interventions for patients with alcohol-related trauma. *Br J Oral Maxillofac Surg.* 1998;36(6): 408–415.

113. Stein PS, Aalboe JA, Savage MW, Scott AM. Strategies for communicating with older dental patients. *J Am Dent Assoc.* 2014;145(2): 159–164.

114. Steindl C, Jonas E, Sittenthaler S. Understanding psychological reactance: new developments and findings. *Zeitschrift für Psychologie.* 2015;223(4):205–214.

115. Tannahill A. Beyond evidence—to ethics: a decision-making framework for health promotion, public health and health improvement. *Health Promot Int.* 2008;23(4):380–390.

116. Tedesco LA, Keffer MA, Davis EL. Social cognitive theory and relapse prevention: reforming patient compliance. *J Dent Educ.* 1991;55(9):575–582.

117. Tinanoff N, Daley NS, O'Sullivan DM, Douglass JM. Failure of intense preventive efforts to arrest early childhood and rampant caries: three case reports. *Pediatr Dent.* 1999;21(3):160–163.

118. United States Department of Health and Human Services. Oral Health in America. A Report of the Surgeon General. Rockville, MD: US Department of Health and Human Services. In: *National Institutes of Health*; 2000.

119. Van Gemert-Schriks MCM, van Amerongen EW, Aartman IHA, et al. The influence of dental caries on body growth in prepubertal children. *Clin Oral Invest.* 2011;15:141–149.

120. Vann WF, Lee JY, Baker D, Divaris K. Oral health literacy among female caregivers: impact on oral health outcomes in early childhood. *J Dent Res.* 2010;89:1395–1400.

121. Wang SJ, Briskie D, Hu J, Majewski R, Inglehart MR. Illustrated information for parent education—parent and patient responses. *Pediatr Dent.* 2010;32:295–303.

122. Weinstein P, Harrison R, Benton T. Motivating parents to prevent caries in their young children: one-year findings. *J Am Dent Assoc.* 2004;135(6):731–738.

123. Weinstein P, Harrison R, Benton T. *J Am Dent Assoc.* 2004;135(9): 1224. Author reply in: 2004b;1224–1226;135(6):731–738.

124. Weinstein P, Harrison R, Benton T. Motivating mothers to prevent caries: confirming the beneficial effect of counseling. *J Am Dent Assoc.* 2006;137(6):789–793.

125. World Health Organization (WHO). *What is Health Promotion?* https://www.who.int/features/qa/health-promotion/en/. Accessed September 9, 2019.

126. Zeng XT, Leng WD, Zhang C. Meta-analysis on the association between tooth brushing and head and neck cancer. *Oral Oncol.* 2015;51(5):446–451.

127. Zimmermann H, Zimmermann N, Hagenfeld D, et al. Is frequency of tooth brushing a risk factor for periodontitis? A systematic review and meta-analysis. *Community Dent Oral Epidemiol.* 2015;43(2): 116–127.

# 22

# Health Education and Health Literacy in Dental Public Health

RICHIE KOHLI, BDS, MS

ELI SCHWARZ, DDS, MPH, PhD, FHKAM, FHKCDS, FACD, FRACDS

## CHAPTER OUTLINE

## Introduction

Health promotion is defined by the Ottawa Charter as the process of enabling people to increase control over and to improve their health.[15] Health promotion is a combination of health education activities and the adoption of healthy public policies.[15] Health education focuses on building individuals' capacities through educational, motivational, skill-building, and consciousness-raising techniques.[15] Healthy public policies provide the environmental supports that will encourage and enhance behavior change.[15] By influencing both individuals' capacities and providing environmental support, meaningful and sustained change in the health of individuals and communities can occur.[15] Health literacy is an outcome of effective health education, increasing individuals' capacities to access and use health information to make appropriate health decisions and maintain basic health.[15] Figure 22.1 highlights the interlinkages between health education, health promotion, and health literacy.[15] Health promotion is discussed in detail in Chapter 21. The focus of the present chapter is to discuss health literacy and oral health education.

## What Is Health Literacy?

### Definition

Health literacy is an important issue that is being addressed at the national level as demonstrated in recent Institute of Medicine (IOM) reports[20,21] and Healthy People 2020 objectives.[16] The term "health literacy" was first used in 1974 by S.K. Simonds in the monograph *Health Education as Social Policy* in the Proceedings of the Will Rogers Conference on Health Education.[45] Since then the health literacy concept—especially its definition and measurement—has gained interest. The most commonly used definition of health literacy is the one given by Ratzan and Parker in 2000,[40] according to which health literacy is an individual's capacity to obtain, process, and understand basic (written or oral) health information and services needed to make appropriate health decisions.

A working group sponsored by the National Institute of Dental and Craniofacial Research (NIDCR) adapted this definition to the context of oral health and defined oral health literacy as the degree to which individuals have the capacity to obtain, process, and understand basic health information and services needed to make appropriate oral health decisions.[32] Recently, a 2016[37] discussion paper by Pleasant et al. published by the National Academy of Medicine pointed out that current definitions of health literacy have limitations as confirmed by the literature. This is because current definitions focus on defining health literacy as an individual skill or ability, which is in fact not solely an individual characteristic.[37] Further, it doesn't explain and distinguish understanding versus acting.[37] The authors recommended that four components should be considered in a definition of health literacy.[37]

Component 1: Include system demands and complexities as well as individual skills and abilities
Component 2: Include measurable components, processes, and outcomes
Component 3: Recognize potential for an analysis of change
Component 4: Demonstrate linkage between informed decisions and action

This is in line with the oral health literacy model[21] (Figure 22.2) that illustrates the potential influence of health literacy as

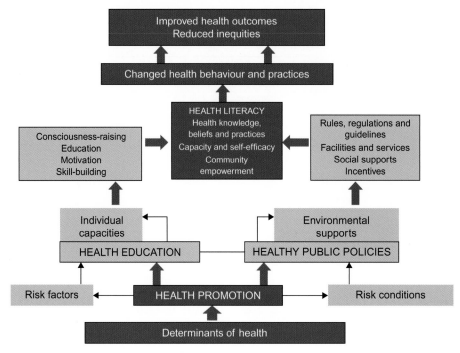

• **Figure 22.1** Relationship between major health concepts.[15]

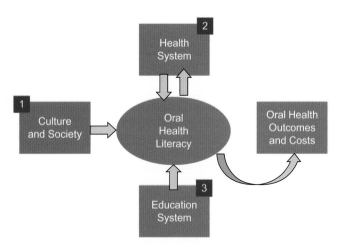

• **Figure 22.2** Oral health literacy framework from IOM, 2004. (Institute of Medicine [IOM]. *Oral Health Literacy: Workshop Summary.* Washington, DC: the National Academies Press; 2013.)

individuals interact with (1) cultural and social factors, (2) health system, and (3) educational systems and suggests that these factors may ultimately contribute to health outcomes and costs.

Thus, health literacy can be a very effective tool in preventing disease, eliminating health inequity, increasing treatment and medical care diagnosis and effectiveness, lowering barriers to access, and improving health outcomes at a lower cost overall.[37]

## Types of Health Literacy

Based on what health literacy enables us to do, there are three types of literacy[9,33]:

1. Basic/functional health literacy: sufficient basic skills in reading and writing to be able to function effectively in everyday situations

2. Interactive health literacy: more advanced cognitive and literacy skills that, together with social skills, can be used to actively participate in everyday activities, to extract information and derive meaning from different forms of communication, and to apply new information to changing circumstances

3. Critical health literacy: the ability to critically analyze information and use this information to influence, inspire, and take action to create change in the community

The 2003 National Assessment of Adult Literacy (NAAL) was a nationally representative assessment of English literacy among American adults age 16 and older that measured literacy directly through tasks completed by adults (in contrast to relying on indirect measures of literacy such as self-reports and other subjective evaluations).[47] NAAL provided the first-ever national assessment of adults' ability to use their literacy skills to understand health-related materials and forms.[47]

Three literacy scales were used in the NAAL assessment:

*The prose literacy scale* measured the knowledge and skills needed to search, comprehend, and use information from texts that were organized in sentences or paragraphs (12 items).

*The document literacy scale* measured the knowledge and skills needed to search, comprehend, and use information from noncontinuous texts in various formats (12 items).

*The quantitative literacy scale* measured the knowledge and skills needed to identify and perform computations using numbers embedded in printed materials (four items).

NAAL used 28 tasks to measure health literacy organized around three domains of health and healthcare information and services: *clinical* domain (three items), *prevention* domain (14 items), and *navigation of the health system* (11 items). NAAL results indicated that the majority of adults (53%) had intermediate health literacy. An additional 12% of adults had proficient health literacy. Among the remaining adults, 22% had basic health literacy, and

14% had below basic health literacy. As stated in the NAAL report,[47] starting with adults who had graduated from high school or obtained a GED or high school equivalency certificate, average health literacy increased with each higher level of education. Adults living below the poverty level had lower average health literacy than adults living above the poverty threshold. Women had higher average health literacy than men. White and Asian/Pacific Islander adults had higher average health literacy than black, Hispanic, American Indian/Alaska Native, and multiracial adults. Hispanic adults had lower average health literacy than adults in any of the other racial/ethnic groups. Adults who spoke only English before starting school had a higher average health literacy than adults who spoke only Spanish or another non-English language. Adults ages 65 and older had lower average health literacy than adults in younger age groups. More adults ages 65 and older also had below basic health literacy than adults in any of the younger age groups.[47]

## Oral Health Literacy Tools

The most common oral health literacy measurement tools used in the literature are based on either the Rapid Estimate of Adult Literacy in Medicine (REALM)[6] or the Test of Functional Health Literacy in Adults (TOFHLA).[35] The REALM assesses participants' ability to read from a list of medical terms, whereas TOFHLA assesses participants' literacy and numeracy skills. REALM was adapted as the Rapid Estimate of Adult Literacy in Dentistry (REALD),[10] and TOFHLA was adapted as Test of Functional Health Literacy in Dentistry (TOFHLiD).[13] Table 22.1 from Dickson-Swift et al.[7] provides a chronologic overview of oral health

literacy tools used in the literature. In a recent review of oral health literacy tools by Dickson-Swift et al.,[7] the authors pointed out that the majority of the health literacy tools are heavily biased toward word recognition, numeracy, and reading skills, rather than what it means in terms of health behavior and service utilization. More recent tools focusing on decision-making and service navigation require formal validation work.[7] There is also a need to develop tools adapted for specific populations for acceptability and cultural competence.[7]

## Implications of Low Oral Health Literacy

It is estimated that in the United States, 44% of adults with less than basic health literacy skills had a dental visit in the preceding year compared to 77% of those with proficient health literacy skills.[41] Low health literacy is associated with increased use of emergency care,[21] less use of preventive regimens and screenings,[21] poor oral health outcomes,[3] and missed dental appointments.[17] Low health literacy also results in increased costs to the population in general,[18] ranging between $106 billion and $238 billion annually.[50] The case examples in Box 22.1 depict the importance of patient understanding and acting on the instructions provided by the physician or dental provider.

## Improving Oral Health Literacy in Clinical Practice

Recognizing that limited health literacy is a barrier and that effective communication skills, including those of the dental team, could impede oral disease management and the public's health

## • TABLE 22.1 Chronologic Overview of Oral Health Literacy Tools[7]

| Abbreviation | Name of Tool | Year | Authors | Type of Tool |
|---|---|---|---|---|
| REALD-99 | Rapid Estimate of Adult Literacy in Dentistry | 2007 | Richman et al. | 99-item word recognition |
| REALD-30 | Rapid Estimate of Adult Literacy in Dentistry −30 | 2007 | Lee et al. | 30-item word recognition common dental words |
| ToFHLiD | Test of Functional Health Literacy in Dentistry | 2007 | Gong et al. | Reading comprehension and numeracy 68-item reading comprehension and 12-item numeracy |
| OHLI | Oral Health Literacy Instrument | 2009 | Sabbahi et al. | Reading comprehension and numeracy |
| REALM-D | Rapid Estimate of Adult Literacy in Medicine and Dentistry | 2010 | Atchinson et al. | 84-item word recognition |
| CMOHK | Comprehensive Measure of Oral Health Knowledge | 2010 | Macek et al. | 44 questions conceptual knowledge |
| BHLOHKP | Baltimore Health Literacy and Oral Health Knowledge Project survey | 2011 | Macek et al. | 44-item questionnaire conceptual knowledge across four domains |
| HKREALD-30 | Hong Kong Rapid Estimate of Adult Literacy in Dentistry | 2012 | Wong et al. | Adaptation of the REALD-99 translated |
| OHLA-S | Oral Health Literacy Assessment-Spanish | 2012 | Lee et al. | Developed using the REALD-30 word |
| OHLA-E | Oral Health Literacy Assessment-English | 2012 | Lee et al. | Developed using the REALD-30 word recognition and comprehension |
| REALMD-20 | Rapid Estimate of Adult Literacy in Dentistry- 20 | 2013 | Gironda et al. | 20-item word recognition |
| HKOHLAT-P | Hong Kong Oral Health Literacy Assessment Task | 2013 | Wong et al. | Mainly literacy and numeracy tasks |
| OHL-AQ | Oral Health Literacy Adults Questionnaire | 2013 | Sistani et al. | 17 items in four sections, reading, comprehension, numeracy, literacy, and decision-making |
| HeLD | Health Literacy in Dentistry | 2013 | Jones et al. | Modeled on the Health Literacy Management Scale (HeLMS) |

### • BOX 22.1   Case Examples of Health Literacy

- A 2-year-old is diagnosed with an inner ear infection and is prescribed an antibiotic. Her mother understands that her daughter should take the prescribed medication twice a day. After carefully studying the label on the bottle and deciding that it doesn't tell how to take the medicine, she fills a teaspoon and pours the antibiotic in her daughter's painful ear.[36]

- A 35-year-old man came in for a dental hygiene appointment. It has been 2 years since he was last seen in your office. When you begin to examine his teeth you notice pronounced "notches" worn into the proximal surfaces of virtually all of his teeth. When questioned, he says, "Well, you told me to use a see-sawing motion with the dental floss for 10 seconds on each tooth."[28]

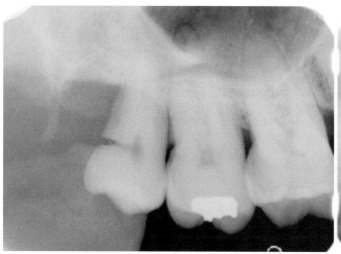
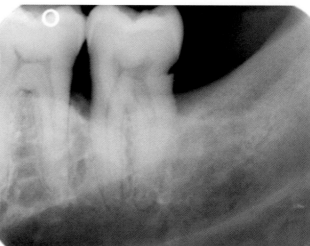

Radiographic view of notches before extraction

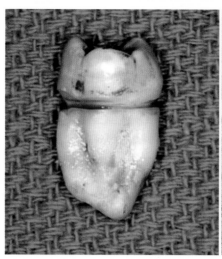
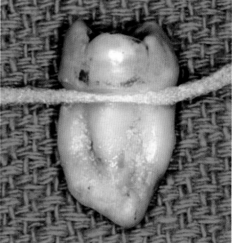

Notches as seen on extracted teeth due to incorrect flossing

literacy, the American Dental Association (ADA) conducted a survey[38] of their membership to (1) determine techniques used by dentists and dental team members to ensure effective patient communication and understanding and (2) identify the variation in routine use of these techniques. Out of 6300 mailed surveys to a sample of dentists, 2010 dentists responded (33.4% response rate). Responses from 1994 were used for analysis. Respondents indicated on a 5-point Likert scale how often—from never to always—during a typical work week they used certain communication techniques that affect patient understanding. The 18 questions were distributed among the following five domains:

1. Patient-friendly environment (three questions)
2. Teach-back method (two questions)
3. Help understanding (five questions)
4. Patient-friendly materials (three questions)
5. Understandable language (five questions)

The results from this survey showed that less than one-quarter of dentists routinely used the techniques listed in the patient-friendly practice or teach-back method domains (Table 22.2).

The most frequently used techniques by the dentists included assistance techniques, the use of materials and aids, and interpersonal communication techniques. As seen from the table, less than half of the dentists used health literacy techniques considered basic. Based on these results, the authors recommended[38]: the dental profession needs to

- develop and disseminate communication guidelines and programs, such as continuing education courses and toolkits;

● **TABLE 22.2** Dentists' Routine Use of Oral Health Literacy[38]

| Technique | Percent Routinely Used |
|---|---|
| **Patient-Friendly Environment** | |
| 1. Ask patients how they learn best | 4.9 |
| 2. Refer patients to internet | 11.1 |
| 3. Use interpreter | 15.3 |
| **Teach-Back Method** | |
| 4. Ask patient to repeat information or instructions[a] | 16.0 |
| 5. Ask patient to tell you what they will do at home to follow instructions[a] | 23.5 |
| **Help Understanding** | |
| 6. Underline key points in printed materials | 31.5 |
| 7. Follow up by phone to check understanding | 35.1 |
| 8. Read instructions out loud | 48.1 |
| 9. Ask staff to follow up on post-care instructions | 53.3 |
| 10. Write or print out instructions | 54.5 |
| **Patient-Friendly Materials** | |
| 11. Use video or DVD | 15.8 |
| 12. Hand out printed materials | 65.9 |
| 13. Use models or x-rays to explain | 73.1 |
| **Understandable Language** | |
| 14. Present only 2 or 3 concepts at a time[a] | 29.8 |
| 15. Ask family member or friend to participate[a] | 34.3 |
| 16. Draw or use pictures[a] | 42.5 |
| 17. Speak slowly[a] | 67.8 |
| 18. Use simple language[a] | 90.6 |

Note: Techniques indicated by an [a] are considered basic techniques.

- advance dentist–patient communication effectiveness;
- develop oral health literacy tools; and
- implement policies and programs to ensure that graduating dental care professionals and dentists already in practice are meeting the information needs of all their patients.

According to Chew et al.,[5] three validated questions can be used to identify individuals who need extra help in understanding their oral health needs and the required skills they need to practice for improved oral health:

1. "How often do you have someone (like a family member, friend, hospital/clinic worker or caregiver) help you read hospital materials?" (Help Read)
2. "How often do you have problems learning about your medical condition because of difficulty understanding written information?" (Problems Reading)
3. "How confident are you filling out forms by yourself?" (Confident with Forms).

Responses are scored on a Likert scale from 0 to 4, and participants are asked to choose between all of the time, most of the time, some of the time, a little of the time, or none of the time. Based on the patient responses (e.g., all of the time, most of the time, some of the time), the provider can determine if extra assistance is needed to ensure that the patient understands what is being conveyed.

For patients' feedback and to assess how dentists and dental staff are doing, one can use the communication tool based on the tool developed by Makoul et al.[18,31] (Box 22.2). This tool can also be used for practice changes as needed.

The Partnership for Clear Health Communication (PCHC) of the National Patient Safety Foundation launched the Ask Me 3 program[19] to help improve health literacy through clear communication between patients and healthcare providers. It encourages patients and families to ask three specific questions of their providers to better understand their condition and what they need to do to stay healthy: (1) What is my main problem?, (2) What do I need to do?, and (3) Why is it important for me to do this?

## What Is Oral Health Education?

Health education forms an important part of health promotion activities. As indicated in Figure 22.1, the linkage between health promotion, health education, and health literacy is strong. Health education's contribution to improved health outcomes is really predicated on ensuring as high a level of health literacy as possible. The traditional World Health Organization (WHO) definition of health education is "any combination of learning opportunities designed to facilitate voluntary changes of behavior which lead to improved health. The behaviors of individuals, families, communities, or institutions may need to be changed. Education is needed during the initiation and at all subsequent stages of any community health measure."[39]

We can deepen the understanding of the definition by further dissecting its important terms. *Combination* emphasizes the importance of matching the multiple determinants of behavior with multiple learning experiences or educational experiences. *Designed* distinguishes health education from incidental learning experiences as a systematically planned activity. *Facilitate* means predispose, enable, and reinforce. *Voluntary* means without coercion and with full understanding and acceptance of the purposes of the action. *Changes* mean behavioral steps taken by an individual, group, or community to achieve an intended health effect. Health education therefore provides the consciousness-raising, concern-arousing, action-stimulating impetus for public involvement and commitment to social reform. It emphasizes the imparting of accurate information to set the stage for the adoption of sound health practices or the abandonment of poor ones. It focuses on acquainting people with the causes of disease, on health practices to reduce and avoid risk, and on ways to detect a developing problem. Health education is usually embedded in health promotion or other programs, such as patient education in medical care programs, occupational health education in industrial safety programs, or school health education in school programs. Alternative labels used for health education programs and activities include social marketing, mass communications, behavior modification, in-service training, patient education, and some forms of health counseling, as will be discussed later.

Although education is distinct from promotion, both are necessary components of programs to prevent oral disease. Education helps to gain and maintain interest, provides new information, and

• BOX 22.2 **Communication Assessment Tool Based on Makoul et al.[18,31]**

Communication with patients is a very important part of quality oral health care. We would like to know how you feel about the way your dental care provider communicated with you. Your answers are completely confidential, so please be open and honest.

| 1 | 2 | 3 | 4 | 5 |
|---|---|---|---|---|
| poor | fair | good | very good | excellent |

Please use this scale to rate the way the dentist or dental hygienist communicated with you.
Circle your answer for each item below.
The dentist/dental hygienist

| | | poor | | | | excellent |
|---|---|---|---|---|---|---|
| 1. | Greeted me in a way that made me feel comfortable | 1 | 2 | 3 | 4 | 5 |
| 2. | Treated me with respect | 1 | 2 | 3 | 4 | 5 |
| 3. | Showed interest in my ideas about my oral health | 1 | 2 | 3 | 4 | 5 |
| 4. | Understood my main health concerns | 1 | 2 | 3 | 4 | 5 |
| 5. | Paid attention to me (looked at me, listened carefully) | 1 | 2 | 3 | 4 | 5 |
| 6. | Let me talk without interruptions | 1 | 2 | 3 | 4 | 5 |
| 7. | Gave me as much information as I wanted | 1 | 2 | 3 | 4 | 5 |
| 8. | Talked in terms I could understand | 1 | 2 | 3 | 4 | 5 |
| 9. | Showed me how to do oral hygiene procedures | 1 | 2 | 3 | 4 | 5 |
| 10. | Had me demonstrate how to do oral hygiene procedures | 1 | 2 | 3 | 4 | 5 |
| 11. | Checked to be sure I understood everything | 1 | 2 | 3 | 4 | 5 |
| 12. | Encouraged me to ask questions | 1 | 2 | 3 | 4 | 5 |
| 13. | Involved me in decisions as much as I wanted | 1 | 2 | 3 | 4 | 5 |
| 14. | Discussed next steps, including any follow-up plans | 1 | 2 | 3 | 4 | 5 |
| 15. | Showed care and concern | 1 | 2 | 3 | 4 | 5 |
| 16. | Spent the right amount of time with me | 1 | 2 | 3 | 4 | 5 |
| 17. | The dentist's staff treated me with respect | 1 | 2 | 3 | 4 | 5 |

reinforces preexisting knowledge. Health promotion provides the preventive procedure and at the same time offers the opportunity to educate individuals, communities, and other health professionals about the value of the measure introduced.[48]

In a way, these definitions highlight how our perceptions of health education and promotion have evolved during the last 30 to 40 years and how we as professional health educators have changed roles in relation to the individuals, communities, and organizations we are trying to affect. The roots of the paternalistic approach to health education can be found in the health propaganda campaigns of the 1920s and 1930s focused on eradicating serious infectious diseases.[48] With the declining rates of these threats, campaigns for healthy lifestyles to address the increasing burden of chronic disease took over in the 1960s and 1970s. Originally, the prevailing educational and preventive approach was the "doctor knows best" method. But increasingly, the shortcomings of this approach were demonstrated by the obvious lack of effect of campaigns and programs and the increasing realization of the complex sociobehavioral mechanisms that influenced these outcomes.[33,44] Watt[51] has questioned the traditional practice of focusing on those behaviors that were seen to be the cause of dental diseases. He has emphasized that human behavior is extremely complex and that knowledge gain alone rarely leads to sustained behavioral change. In addition, people's behaviors are enmeshed within the social, economic, and environmental conditions under which they are living, and we need to understand the entire context of these factors.

## Health Education Planning

Previously it was emphasized that health education was a planned activity. The typical steps of creating a health education activity are illustrated in Figure 22.3.

Health educators will use this generic planning model as a stepwise guide to create a health education intervention and to ensure that clear goals and strategies are defined prior to initiating the intervention. Part of the preparation for such a planning process is often to identify and select an appropriate theoretical framework for the activity, which may depend on what the education process aims to achieve. These theoretical frameworks are known as health behavior theories.

Since the 1960s, social scientists have taken an interest in the field of dentistry, leading to the development of particular health behavior theories (please refer to Chapter 21 on health behaviors).[25] Examples of these are the health belief model,[2,26] the transtheoretical model of change,[49] and the theory of reasoned action.[30] Several of these frameworks have underpinned applied health education activities with a focus on explaining why recipients of the educational efforts did or did not change their behavior as expected, for instance in relation to preventive dental behavior, diet changes, or tobacco cessation. Most recently, other theoretical frameworks, such as the PRECEDE-PROCEED model, have been applied to oral health education interventions.[4] The extent to which these approaches have led to successful outcomes is discussed in the next section.

## Evidence for Oral Health Education Effectiveness

As indicated in Figure 22.3, evaluation of the impact of the health education intervention is an important component of the entire planning cycle. Therefore it is also important to consider what evidence exists for the impact of health education activities in general. This can be applied to health education in the clinical setting or in population groups, such as health education campaigns or broader education programs. Several Cochrane and other systematic reviews have been conducted to identify successful health education programs or approaches used by dental professionals or lay people to improve the oral health situation.[22-24,42,43] These reviews cover a span of several decades and comprise both systematic reviews and more narrative literature reviews.

• BOX 22.3    Health Literacy Activity

The Newest Vital Sign[52] is a tool designed to quickly and simply assess a patient's health literacy skills. It can be administered in only 3 minutes and is available in English and Spanish. The patient is given a specially designed ice cream nutrition label to review and is asked a series of questions about it. Based on the number of correct answers, healthcare providers can assess the patient's health literacy level and adjust the way they communicate to ensure patient understanding. As an exercise on health literacy, please answer the following questions based on ice cream nutrition label below:

**Nutrition Facts**

| | | |
|---|---|---|
| Serving Size | | ½ cup |
| Servings per container | | 4 |
| Amount per serving | | |
| Calories   250 | Fat Cal | 120 |
| | | %Dy |
| **Total Fat** 13g | | 20% |
| Sat Fat 9g | | 40% |
| **Cholesterol** 28mg | | 12% |
| **Sodium** 55mg | | 2% |
| **Total Carbohydrate** 30g | | 12% |
| Dietary Fiber 2g | | |
| Sugars 23g | | |
| **Protein** 4g | | 8% |

*Percentage Daily Values (DV) are based on a 2,000 calorie diet. Your daily values may be higher or lower depending on your calorie needs.
**Ingredients:** Cream, Skim Milk, Liquid Sugar, Water, Egg Yolks, Brown Sugar, Milktat, Peanut Oil, Sugar, Butter, Salt, Carrageenan, Vanilla Extract.

**Score by giving 1 point for each correct answer (maximum 6 points).**

**Score of 0-1** suggests high likelihood (50% or more) of limited literacy.

**Score of 2-3** indicates the possibility of limited literacy.

**Score of 4-6** almost always indicates adequate literacy.

Answer Keys:

1) b  2) d  3) c  4) c  5) b  6) c

1. If you eat the entire container, how many calories will you eat?
   a. 250
   b. 1000
   c. 120
   d. 480

2. If you are allowed to eat 60 grams of carbohydrates as a snack, how much ice cream could you have?
   a. Half the container
   b. ½ cup
   c. One cup
   d. A and C are both correct

3. Your doctor advises you to reduce the amount of saturated fat in your diet. You usually have 42 grams of saturated fat each day, which includes one serving of ice cream. If you stop eating ice cream, how many grams of saturated fat would you be consuming each day?
   a. 31
   b. 0
   c. 33
   d. 29

4. If you usually eat 2500 calories in a day, what percentage of your daily value of calories will you be eating if you eat one serving?
   a. 5%
   b. 8%
   c. 10%
   d. 12.5%

5. Pretend you are allergic to the following substances: penicillin, peanuts, latex gloves, and bee stings.
   Is it safe to eat this ice cream?
   a. Yes
   b. No

6. If you answered that is it is not safe to eat this ice cream, explain why. Because the ice cream contains:
   a. Carrageenan
   b. high levels of carbohydrates
   c. Peanut oil
   d. high level of fat

From Weiss BD, Mays MZ, Martz W. Quick assessment of literacy in primary care: the newest vital sign. *Ann Fam Med.* 2005;3:514–522.

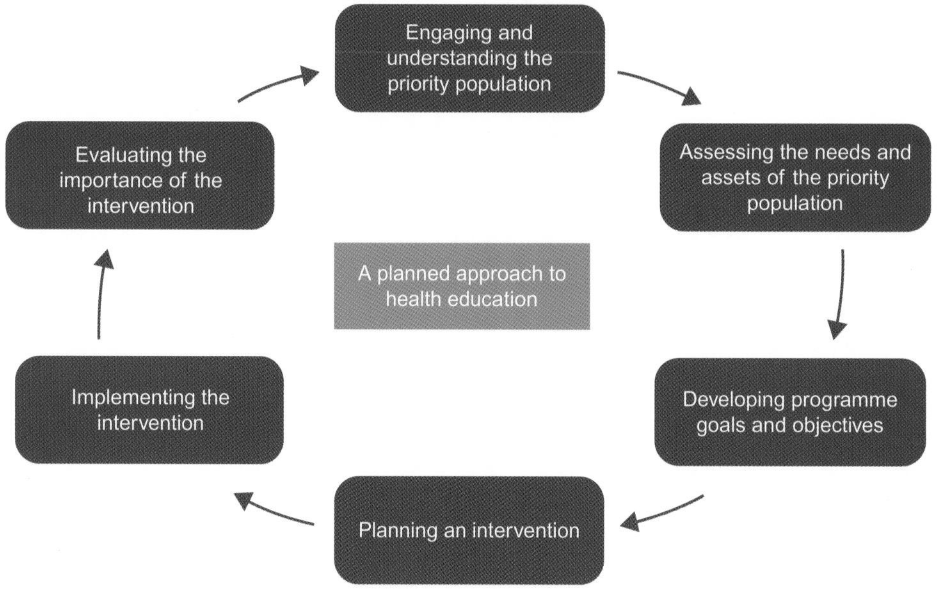

• **Figure 22.3** Common components of health education planning cycle.

Overall, they paint a picture of concern for the success of health education in changing people's behavior and improving the oral health outcomes of individuals and groups. Some of the challenges are methodologic, which means that a particular oral health education activity may not be as well planned as it could be. This could be in terms of an unclear goal or a lack of a theoretical context. For instance, a fluoride toothbrushing program is initiated without a clear picture of what the outcome measure will be—reduced dental caries, reduced plaque score, gingival bleeding, or oral health knowledge—and how the data are going to be collected and analyzed. The variability of methods used makes it difficult to generalize from one intervention study to other areas or populations. Other challenges relate to funding of the intervention, which may be sufficient for oral health education activities but not for an evaluation process, which means that outcome data may become an afterthought or not be done at all.

Related to these challenges are the duration of the intervention and the sustainability. An intervention that is initiated to run for a brief period may be less effective, because the behavioral changes we intend simply take a long time to take effect or measure. There is also the question of what happens when funding for the intervention ceases: Has the activity been built into the structure of a more comprehensive health education program or has it been a standalone program that simply stops when funding runs out? The British Health Education Authority produced a publication in the 1970s on the scientific basis of oral health education that is now in its seventh edition. Initially it summarized a few recommendations for what to do and how to do it, but it has since expanded to be a solid oral health education guide for the entire oral health team.[29]

In their extensive review on Promoting oral health in populations[22] Kay and Craven address the requirements for successful outcomes of population and individual oral health education activities. They conclude with the following:
• Fluoride remains the most potent preventive measure against caries.

• One-on-one tailored advice may be helpful for particular high-risk groups, such as new mothers of young children and members of minority ethnic groups.
• Combining population-based programs with more traditional health education may hold promise.
• School-based programs can improve oral hygiene in the short term, but the impact on caries is uncertain.
• More research is needed on improving oral health of older adults.
• More research is required on the comparative costs of programs.
• Appropriate evaluation of health education needs more emphasis and proper funding.

In particular with regard to individual patients, Kay and Craven emphasize that if end goals and outcomes are not made clear, behavioral change will not occur.[22] Statements such as "improve your diet" or "you need to brush better" do not make anything clear. The patient is left not knowing exactly what they are supposed to do or why they may want to do it.

When advising patients on behavioral change, the dental care provider needs to:
• Give the patient a personally relevant reason for taking action; for example: "That is three fillings you have needed in the last year. I can tell you how to stop the white-spot lesion becoming a hole."
• Make it clear what is to be achieved; for example: "Limit sugar intake to mealtimes and completely stop taking any sweetened drinks."
• Offer them a technique whereby the goal can be achieved; for example: "Why not try using sweetener instead of sugar and eat your sweets at mealtimes?"

Making precise statements about why the person might want to change, offering precise and achievable goals, and describing exactly what changes to make means behavioral change is more likely. All three steps are vital if patients are to benefit from the professional's knowledge about the causes of oral diseases and their prevention.[22]

To conclude, it should be recognized that considerable oral health and disease disparities exist. Satur et al. comment that while there is health education work in progress in many areas, challenges still exist in finding workable approaches for low-income groups, adolescents, native communities, older adults, and those affected by disability, mental illness, and drug and alcohol addictions.[42] Many of these groups are also the ones with the greatest disease and care-access challenges.

## Health Educators

Health educators are a defined group of individuals. To a certain extent most health professionals, such as dentists or dental hygienists, might be considered dental health educators when they engage in educational activities. At the chair side, they may be discussing tobacco cessation with a patient, or in a school or other institutional environment, they may be explaining how to maintain a healthy mouth and teeth through toothbrushing with fluoride toothpaste. In that instance, their role goes beyond their clinical activities. However, in spite of the perceived importance of this role, oftentimes it remains accessory to their main clinical role, and the formal training of dentists and dental hygienists in health education takes up a relatively small part of their professional curriculum.

The Australian bachelor of oral health, which is the modernized version of the original dental therapist, has recognized this evolution by defining the oral health therapist's triple role as a dental hygienist, a dental therapist, and an oral health educator with rather equal components of these areas included in their education. There is, however, a formal training for general health educators in the United States and similar roles, for instance, in Canada, the United Kingdom, and Australia. University-trained health educators, sometimes called health education specialists, will typically complete a bachelor's degree and may continue with a master's degree in health education. Some employers require health educators to be a Certified Health Education Specialist (CHES).[53] This certification is offered by the National Commission for Health Education Credentialing (NCHEC) on the basis of an exam, and continued certification is predicated on ongoing completion of continuing education similar to what dentists and dental hygienists do in their own fields.

Of particular importance in the ongoing healthcare transformation during the beginning of the 21st century has been the inclusion of community health workers or traditional health workers who are recruited from the local community and are employed to facilitate the access of especially low-income and other vulnerable population groups to an increasingly complex healthcare system. Community health workers typically have a high school diploma, although some jobs may require postsecondary education. Education programs may lead to a 1-year certificate or a 2-year associate's degree and cover topics such as wellness, ethics, and cultural awareness, among others. Community health workers typically have a shared language or life experience with and an understanding of the community that they serve.[14] An example of how one US state has regulated its approach to traditional health workers including community health workers and others is provided by the Oregon Health Authority regulations, which among other topics include oral health training requirements.[34] Most states do not require health education certification for community health workers.

## Health Education Advancement by Technology

One of the most disruptive changes to people's everyday lives over the last decade has been the introduction and influence of social media. The ubiquitous existence of mobile technology is fast becoming an important addition to the way healthcare is being delivered through telehealth/teledentistry methodologies and the application of eHealth and mHealth (mobile health). The overarching term *telehealth* is defined by the Centers for Medicare and Medicaid Services as "the use of telecommunications and information technology to provide access to health assessment, diagnosis, intervention, consultation, supervision and information across distance."[46]

The ADA has established that telehealth is not a specific service but refers to a broad variety of technologies and tactics to deliver virtual medical, health, and education services in dentistry. It can include patient care and education delivery through live video (synchronous), store-and-forward (asynchronous), and remote patient monitoring (RPM).[1] Within dental practice, teledentistry is used extensively in disciplines like preventive dentistry, orthodontics, endodontics, oral surgery, periodontal conditions, detection of early dental caries, patient education, oral medicine, and diagnosis. Some of the key modes and methods used in teledentistry are electronic health records, electronic referral systems, digitizing images, teleconsultations, and telediagnosis. All the applications used in teledentistry aim to bring about efficiency, provide access to underserved population, improve quality of care, and reduce oral disease burden.[27] Two codes have been defined for synchronous and asynchronous services in the Current Dental Terminology (CDT) code set. But in its guidance the ADA has stated that although current dental benefit plan coverage and reimbursement provisions should apply to services delivered in office and via teledentistry, there is no expectation that commercial and government dental benefit plans must create new coverage provisions pertaining to teledentistry. Further, coverage and reimbursement for D9995 and D9996 is likely to vary between commercial benefit plan offerings and by state for government programs (e.g., Medicaid).[1]

At the time of writing, these methodologies are innovative and have not been tested in major controlled clinical trials, but a series of demonstration trials have been carried out in California, Oregon, and Colorado. They have focused on providing access to underserved populations (rural, Medicaid) through dental care teams where a dental hygienist and assistant conduct outreach activities in a local community (origination site), such as oral health screenings and preventive activities, but at the same time collect clinical data (clinical assessment, x-ray, intra- and extraoral photos) that are uploaded to a secure cloud-based site from where a dentist at a distant site can download the information and make a diagnostic decision based on the electronic health record information. The dental hygienist can then be instructed in a plan of action that may involve the placement of an interim restorative treatment or possibly referral to a dental clinic. This model has been called the virtual dental home.[11,12] Other telehealth-supported models have been described with midlevel providers such as dental therapists in Alaska and Australia.[8]

The potential for providing health education messages to populations in low-income countries and other locations where there are serious access challenges to dental care and dental health personnel but a wide ranging use of mobile phones and other technology has been recognized by the WHO, which has initiated a series of mHealth initiatives, among them mOralHealth.[54,55] The potential for communicating health messages, recalls, reminders, etc. through the use of mobile technology is clearly limitless. The effectiveness of these methodologies in improving the oral health of individuals and populations and addressing some of the shortcomings that have been documented in the previous pages is yet to be evaluated.

# References

1. ADA guide to understanding and documenting teledentistry events. Available from: http://www.ada.org/en/~/media/ADA/Publications/Files/D9995andD9996_ADAGuidetoUnderstandingandDocumenting TeledentistryEvents_v1_2017Jul17; 2017. Accessed May 21, 2019.

2. Becker MH, ed. *The Health Belief Model and Personal Health Behavior*. Thorofare, NJ: Slack; 1974.

3. Berkman ND, Sheridan SL, Donahue KE, et al. Low health literacy and health outcomes: an updated systematic review. Ann Intern Med. 2011;155(2):97–116.

4. Binkley CJ, Johnson KW. Application of the PRECEDE-PROCEED Planning Model in Designing an Oral Health Strategy. *J Theory Pract Dent Public Health*. 2013;1(3). Available from: http://www.sharmilachatterjee.com/ojs-2.3.8/index.php/JTPDPH/article/view/89. Accessed May 21, 2019.

5. Chew LD, Griffin JM, Partin MR, et al. Validation of screening questions for limited health literacy in a large VA outpatient population. J Gen Internal Med. 2008;23(5):561–566.

6. Davis TC, Long SW, Jackson RH, et al. Rapid estimate of adult literacy in medicine: a shortened screening instrument. *Fam Med*. 1993;25:391–395.

7. Dickson-Swift V, Kenny A, Farmer J, et al. Measuring oral health literacy: a scoping review of existing tools. BMC Oral Health. 2014;14(1):148.

8. Estai M, Winters J, Kanagasingam Y, et al. Validity and reliability of remote dental screening by different oral health professionals using a store-and-forward telehealth model. *Br Dent J*. 2016 Oct 7;221(7):411–414.

9. Freebody P, Luke A. Literacies programs: Debates and demands in cultural context. Prospect: An Australian Journal of TESOL. 1990;5(3):7–16.

10. Gironda M, Der-Martirosian C, Messadi D, Holtzman J, Atchison K. A brief 20-item dental/medical health literacy screen (REALMD-20). *J Public Health Dent*. 2013;73:50–55.

11. Glassman P, Harrington M, Namakiah M, et al. The virtual dental home: Bringing oral health to vulnerable and underserved populations. *California Dent J*. 2012;40:569–577.

12. Glassman P, Helgeson M, Kattlove J. Using telehealth technologies to improve oral health for vulnerable and underserved populations. *California Dent J*. 2012;40:579–585.

13. Gong DA, Lee JY, Rozier RG, et al. Development and testing of the Test of Functional Health Literacy in Dentistry (TOFHLiD). *J Public Health Dent*. 2007;67:105–112.

14. Health Educator or Community Health Worker. Available from: https://www.truity.com/career-profile/health-educator-or-community-health-worker. Accessed February 15, 2018.

15. Health Education. *Theoretical Concepts, Effective Strategies and Core Competencies*. World Health Organization. Regional Office for the Eastern Mediterranean: Cairo, Egypt; 2012.

16. Healthy People 2020. Office of Disease Prevention and Health Promotion. Available from: http://www.cdc.gov/nchs/healthy_people/hp2020.htm.

17. Holtzman JS, Atchison KA, Gironda MW, et al. The association between oral health literacy and failed appointments in adults attending a university-based general dental clinic. *Community Dent Oral Epidemiol*. 2013 June;42(3):263–270.

18. Horowitz A, Kleinman D. Oral health literacy: the new imperative to better oral health. Dent Clin N Am. 2008;52:333–344.

19. Institute for Healthcare Improvement/National Patient Safety Foundation, Boston, Massachusetts, USA. Available from: http://www.ihi.

org/resources/Pages/Tools/Ask-Me-3-Good-Questions-for-Your-Good-Health.aspx. Accessed May 21, 2019.

20. Institute of Medicine. *Health Literacy: A Prescription to End Confusion*. Washington, DC: The National Academies Press; 2004.

21. Institute of Medicine. *Oral Health Literacy: Workshop Summary*. Washington, DC: The National Academies Press; 2013.

22. Kay E, Craven R. Promoting oral health in populations. In: Fejerskov O, Kidd E, eds. *Dental Caries—The Disease and Its Clinical Management*. 2nd ed. Oxford, UK: Blackwell Munksgaard; 2008:476–486.

23. Kay E, Locker D. A systematic review of the effectiveness of health promotion aimed at improving oral health. *Community Dent Health*. 1998;15:132–144.

24. Kay EJ, Locker D. Is dental health education effective? A systematic review of current evidence. *Community Dent Oral Epidemiol*. 1996;24:231–235.

25. Kegeles SS, Cohen LK. Role of social sciences in dentistry. In: Richards ND, Cohen LK, eds. *Social Sciences in Dentistry, A Critical Bibliography*. The Hague, Netherlands: Federation Dentaire Internationale; 1971.

26. Kegeles SS. Why people seek dental care: A review of present knowledge. *Am J Public Health*. 1961;51:1306–1311.

27. Khan SA, Omar H. Teledentistry in practice: literature review. *Telemed J E Health*. 2013;19:565–567.

28. Lenton PA, Ridpath J. Health Literacy for the Dental Team. What Does This Mean For Us As Dental Professionals and Clinicians? Available from: https://www.dentalcare.com/en-us/professional-education/ce-courses/ce335/what-does-this-mean-for-us-as-dental-professionals-and-clinicians. Accessed May 21, 2019.

29. Levine RS, Stillman-Lowe C. *The Scientific Basis of Oral Health Education*. 7th ed. London, UK: BDJ Books; 2014.

30. Madden TJ, Ellen PS, Ajzen I. A comparison of the theory of planned behavior and the theory of reasoned action. *Personality and Soc Psych Bull*. 1992;18:3–9.

31. Makoul G, Krupat E, Chang CH. Measuring patient views of physician communication skills: development and testing of the communication assessment tool. *Patient Educ Couns*. 2007;67:333–342.

32. National Institute of Dental and Craniofacial Research, National Institutes of Health. The invisible barrier: literacy and its relationship with oral health. A report of a workgroup sponsored by the National Institute of Dental and Craniofacial Research, National Institutes of Health, US Public Health Service, US Dept of Health and Human Services. J Public Health Dent. 2005;65(3):174–182.

33. Nutbeam D. Health literacy as a public health goal: A challenge for contemporary health education and communication strategies into the 21st century. *Health Promot Int*. 2000;15:259–267.

34. Oregon Health Authority, Health Systems Division: Medical Assistance Programs, ORS division 180, Traditional Health Workers. Available from: https://secure.sos.state.or.us/oard/displayDivisionRules.action;JSESSIONID_OARD=wJOXSWRw3w4KD3CNQ_3kgc3s3F87Q pNh2qcEXCqmt8Kc5dcVjx-O!-268141702?selectedDivision=1741. Accessed May 21, 2019.

35. Parker R, Baker D, Williams M, et al. The test of functional health literacy in adults: a new instrument for measuring patients' literacy skills. *J Gen Intern Med*. 1995;10:537–541.

36. Parker RM, Ratzan SC, Lurie N. Health literacy: A policy challenge for advancing high-quality health care. Health Affairs. 2003;22(4):147.

37. Pleasant A, Rudd RE, O'Leary C, et al. *Considerations for a new definition of health literacy*. Washington, DC: National Academy of Medicine; 2016. Available from: http://nam.edu/wp-content/uploads/2016/04/Considerations-for-a-New-Definition-of-Health-Literacy.pdf. Accessed May 21, 2019.

38. Podschun GP. Dentist-patient communication techniques used in the United States: The results of a national survey. In: *IOM (Institute of Medicine). 2013. Oral Health Literacy: Workshop Summary*. Washington, DC: The National Academies Press; 2013:41–49.

39. Prevention of oral diseases. *WHO Offset Publication No. 103*. Geneva, Switzerland: World Health Organization; 1987.

40. Ratzan SC, Parker RM, Selden CR, et al. *Introduction, National Library of Medicine Current Bibliographies in Medicine: Health Literacy,*

*2000. NLM Pub. No. CBM 2000-1.* National Institutes of Health, US Department of Health and Human Services: Bethesda, MD; 2000.

41. Rozier RG. Oral health in North Carolina: Innovations, opportunities, and challenges. Oral Health. 2012;73(2):100–107.

42. Satur JG, Gussy MG, Morgan MV, et al. Review of the evidence for oral health promotion effectiveness. *Health Educ J.* 2010;69: 257–266.

43. Schou L, Locker D. *Oral Health: A Review of the Effectiveness of Health Education and Health Promotion.* Dutch Center for Health Promotion and Health Education: Amsterdam, Netherlands; 1994.

44. Silversin JB, Kornacki MJ. Controlling dental disease through prevention: Individuals, institutional and community dimensions. In: Cohen LK, Bryant PS, eds. *Social Sciences and Dentistry—A Critical Bibliography.* Quintessence: London, UK; 1984.

45. Simonds SK. Health education as social policy. Health Ed Monogr. 1974;21:1–10.

46. Telemedicine. Available from: https://www.medicaid.gov/medicaid/benefits/telemed/index.html. Accessed September 21, 2018.

47. The Health Literacy of America's Adults: Results from the 2003 National Assessment of Adult Literacy (NAAL), website. Available from: https://nces.ed.gov/pubsearch/pubsinfo.asp?pubid=2006483.

48. Towner E. The history of dental health education: A case study of Britain. In: Schou L, Blinkhorn A, eds. *Oral Health Promotion.* Oxford, UK: Oxford University Press; 1993.

49. Transtheoretical Model from Board Review in Preventive Medicine and Public Health. Available from: https://www.sciencedirect.com/topics/nursing-and-health-professions/transtheoretical-model; 2017. Accessed May 21, 2019.

50. University of Connecticut School of Business. New report estimates cost of low health literacy between $106–$236 billion dollars annually. https://www.medicalnewstoday.com/releases/85542.php. Accessed May 21, 2018.

51. Watt RG. Strategies and approaches in oral disease prevention and health promotion. *Bull WHO.* 2005;83:711–718.

52. Weiss BD, Mays MZ, Martz W. Quick Assessment of Literacy in Primary Care: The Newest Vital Sign. *Ann Fam Med.* 2005;3: 514–522.

53. What is Health Education? Coalition of National Health Education Organizations. Available from: http://www.cnheo.org/files/health_ed.pdf. Accessed May 21, 2019.

54. World Health Organization. Be He@lthy, Be mobile. A handbook on how to implement mBreetheFreely. mHealth for asthma and COPD. Geneva, Switzerland: World Health Organization and International Telecommunication Union; 2017. Available from: http://www.who.int/ncds/prevention/be-healthy-be-mobile/handbooks/en/. Accessed May 21, 2019.

55. World Health Organization. Report of the Global mOralHealth Workshop, October 2018. World Health Organization, Geneva: 2019. Available from: https://apps.who.int/iris/bitstream/handle/10665/326149/WHO-NMH-PND-2019.6-eng.pdf. Accessed December 2019.

# 23

# Diet and Oral Health

**ELIZABETH KRALL KAYE, PhD, MPH**

**TERESA A. MARSHALL, PhD, RD/LD**

## CHAPTER OUTLINE

## Introduction

Proper nutrition plays an important role in achieving and maintaining both oral health and overall health.[67] There is growing awareness that guidelines for good oral health are entirely consistent with those for systemic health. Dental professionals can play a role in delivering dietary advice to patients, not only to limit sugar and between-meal snacking but also to reinforce health-related messages given by medical providers.[4]

Human diets are composed of a complex mixture of nutrients and other food substances. Contrasting approaches have been used to study the role of diet in health, and the approach frames how the results are interpreted and used to formulate recommendations for patients and the public. A common approach uses classic experimental or epidemiologic methods to isolate intake levels of one nutrient or food at a time and observe the effects on health status or surrogate biomarkers. This approach is useful for identifying biological mechanisms and the consensus results contribute to the formulation of dietary guidelines and recommendations, but it does not account for the fact that people consume mixed diets in which nutrients may interact with one another. A complementary alternate approach describes food and beverage patterns as they actually occur in the population and relates the patterns, rather than individual nutrients, to health outcomes.[34] The different approaches may result in conflicting results and confusion regarding the best dietary advice to give patients. The goal of this chapter is to summarize the literature on diet and common oral conditions and provide suggestions for effectively conveying that information to patients.

## Dental Caries

Dental caries is a multifactorial disease that affects more than 20% of children and adolescents[17] and over 90% of adults in the United States.[18] The development and progression of caries require a susceptible tooth surface, presence of oral bacteria, and a substrate the bacteria can use to form acids that demineralize enamel and cementum. That substrate is dietary carbohydrate.

*Carbohydrates.* The forms in which the major nutritionally important carbohydrates exist in foods are the monosaccharides, disaccharides, and polysaccharides. Carbohydrates typically contribute at least half of an individual's total daily intake of calories. Monosaccharides are the basic building blocks of carbohydrates, of which four—glucose, galactose, fructose, and mannose—are the most common in the human diet. Disaccharides consist of monosaccharide pairs joined by a glycosidic bond. Important naturally occurring disaccharides are sucrose, lactose, and maltose. All monosaccharides, and sometimes disaccharides, are considered simple sugars. The complex polysaccharides include starches and fiber, both of which are chains of glucose molecules.

Starches are joined by alpha glycosidic bonds, whereas fiber's glucose molecules are linked in the beta orientation. Alpha and beta refer to the spatial orientation of the individual glucose molecules around a bond, and different enzymes are required to break the linkages. Humans possess salivary and intestinal enzymes to digest alpha but lack the enzymes for beta linkages. Therefore, starch is digestible in the oral cavity and intestinal tract, but fiber is not. The food industry produces "modified starches" with properties of enhanced emulsification, stabilizing, thickening, and prolonged shelf life for use in bakery, confectionary, and other convenience food products. The modified starches contain a mixture of simple sugars and oligosaccharides (i.e., short chain glucose units) that are digestible in the oral cavity.

Carbohydrates play a key role in caries development because many are metabolized, or "fermented," by plaque bacteria. Monosaccharides obtained directly from foods or formed by digestion of disaccharides, oligosaccharides, and polysaccharides in the mouth by salivary $\alpha$-amylase are used by bacteria to produce acids that erode mineralized dental tissues. Tooth enamel will begin to demineralize when plaque pH decreases to approximately 5.5 or below. Cementum covering the root surfaces demineralizes in a less acidic environment, around 6.0 to 6.2. Upon ingestion of a carbohydrate, the pH of plaque follows an established pattern; pH decreases sharply within a few minutes then gradually returns to neutral over the span of 20 to 40 minutes as saliva buffers the acid and clears it from the oral cavity.[68] The type and amount of carbohydrate consumed, frequency of consumption, and combination of carbohydrate with other nutrients and food components determine the degree to which plaque pH falls and the length of time it remains below the critical pH levels. In addition to producing acid, oral bacteria use sucrose to form insoluble polysaccharides that underlie the structure of dental biofilm and promote bacterial adherence to the tooth surface.[54]

*Simple sugars.* Mono- and disaccharides are digested more rapidly than starch and thus have higher cariogenic potential. Studies of sugar and caries risk carried out in the mid-20th century established sugar intake as a risk factor for dental caries,[28,38] and numerous intervention or longitudinal studies since then have confirmed that the amount and/or frequency of intake of sugars is associated with increased risk of developing caries.[5,49,55] It is difficult to determine if the amount of sugar or frequency of consumption has a greater impact on caries development. However, the distinction is probably moot because in a typical daily eating pattern, the two measures are highly interrelated.

The strength of the association between sugar intake and caries risk appears to be diminished when fluoridated water or fluoride toothpaste are used.[7,9] As sugar intake has increased in recent decades in both industrialized and developing countries, different patterns between per capita sugar intake and caries prevalence have emerged. In developed countries, where fluoride exposure is more widespread, there tends to be an inverse or flat association between sugar intake and caries, whereas in developing countries high sugar intake is still associated with greater caries prevalence.[47]

Mono- and disaccharides are found naturally in the food supply, primarily in fruits, vegetables, grains, honey, and syrups such as maple and agave. They are also frequently added during food and beverage processing to provide sweetness, enhance texture, and act as preservatives. Simple sugars that are added at the table or during processing are referred to as added sugars and accounted for 14% to 17% of total calorie intake by children and adults in the United States in 2011 and 2012.[57]

Sugar-sweetened beverages (SSBs) deserve prominent mention because they are often consumed by themselves between meals and sipped over a long period, prolonging the length of time oral bacteria have to digest carbohydrates and produce acids. SSBs include a wide range of products, such as carbonated sodas and noncarbonated fruit juices, fruit drinks, energy drinks, sweetened tea and coffee, and flavored sweetened water. More than one-third of children ages 19 to 23 months consume an SSB on any given day,[26] and almost two-thirds of children ages 2 to 19 years consume at least one SSB each day.[60] Although consumption of sodas by children and adults in the United States has been decreasing since 1999, use of energy and sports drinks has risen during the same time period.[27] Confirming results of cross-sectional studies, frequent consumption of SSBs other than 100% fruit juice is consistently associated with increased incidence of caries among children and adults.[7,13,36,74] The association of 100% fruit juice, which the World Health Organization (WHO) considers a "free" sugar whose consumption should be limited,[49] is unclear, with some studies showing a decreased risk of caries[1,13,22] and others showing an increased risk.[37]

*Complex carbohydrates.* Because they need time to be digested in the mouth, starches are considered mildly cariogenic or noncariogenic. Some research has suggested that the combination of sugar and starch may enhance a food's cariogenic potential, causing a reduction in biofilm pH and resulting in more mineral loss relative to sugar alone,[59] but others find no difference between sugar alone and sugar–starch combinations.[3] Starches are the most abundant carbohydrate in the typical diet and are derived primarily from grains, vegetables, and fruits. Breads and starchy grain-based desserts (e.g., cakes, cookies, pies) are the top contributors of total calories in the diets of US adults,[53] whereas SSBs and processed desserts are the major contributors of calories from added sugars.[46]

It is commonly believed that fiber cleanses the tooth surface of plaque and removes food debris between teeth. However, there is little evidence supporting this mechanism. One study reported inverse associations between calculus score and dietary fiber or servings of fibrous foods.[65] High-fiber foods do require longer or more vigorous mastication, which stimulates salivary flow. Natural food sources of dietary fiber are limited to plants.

*Effect of Other Foods and Nutrients on Caries.* When sugar is consumed with or immediately before a nonfermentable food, the drop in plaque pH and length of time below the critical level are attenuated[61] due to the presence of other nutrients with cariostatic or neutral properties. Calcium and phosphorus are the two main minerals incorporated into the crystalline structure of enamel and cementum. Presence of these ions in the diet and saliva promotes remineralization of incipient caries. Intake of dairy foods rich in calcium is inversely associated with caries incidence in children and adolescents[41] and with the number of incident root caries over a 6-year period in the elderly.[76] Although the disaccharide lactose has cariogenic potential, that potential may be offset by casein and other proteins, fats, and vitamins found in milk and particularly in cheese products.[35] Some dairy foods, such as yogurt, also contain probiotic bacteria that compete with and inhibit mutans streptococci growth.[11]

*Dietary Quality Indices and Dietary Patterns.* Mixed diets are the norm. There are many reasons why examining the total diet rather than focusing on individual nutrients is a more intuitive approach to studying associations of diet with caries and other oral conditions. Other nutrients consumed in combination with simple sugars may intensify or attenuate the effect of sugars. Intakes of individual nutrients are highly intercorrelated. Nutrients with similar functions tend to cluster within foods groups, for example, fruits and vegetables are excellent sources of many antioxidant vitamins. Finally, the findings may be better understood by the public for whom it is more practical to track their intake of a few major food groups rather than dozens of nutrients. However, few studies of diet and caries have used this holistic approach.

Several dietary quality indices have been developed that are based on guidelines for general health. The Healthy Eating Index (HEI)[72] was originally developed in 1995 by the US Department of Agriculture to monitor the quality of the diet of the US population in relation to the Dietary Guidelines for Americans (DGA).[73] It has also been useful for examining relationships between total diet and health-related outcomes. Among children, HEI scores were significantly lower in those with early childhood caries (ECC) or severe ECC than caries-free children.[1,52,77] In addition to having lower total HEI scores, children with ECC frequently fail to meet recommendations for many HEI components, including grain, meat, cholesterol, fruit, dairy, and sodium.[52,77] Reducing the amount of SSBs in the diet led to increased consumption of vegetables, less saturated fat, and improvements in overall dietary quality.[29] The Dietary Approaches to Stop Hypertension (DASH) diet score is another index that assesses compliance to a diet that emphasizes whole grains, fruits, vegetables, and low-fat dairy foods and has been shown to lower blood pressure. Low compliance scores with the DASH diet were associated with higher root caries increments in a cohort of older men.[36]

Dietary pattern analysis describes how foods are consumed in a population without reference to a predetermined set of guidelines. A low sugar/high starch dietary pattern, characterized by bread, pastries, crackers, muffins, and chips, was significantly associated with higher caries incidence among Australian adolescents.[12] Surprisingly, the high sugar/low starch (e.g., syrups, confectionery, jam, dried fruit) and medium sugar/low starch (which included sodas) patterns were not related to caries increment. Although these findings represent only one cohort of limited age range, they do challenge the notion that only sugars are important dietary risk factors for caries and suggest that when counseling patients to reduce caries risk, the total diet needs to be considered.

*Meal Patterns.* A traditional meal pattern includes three meals and two to three snacks per day. A structured meal pattern enables delivery of adequate nutrition for growth and development while limiting exposure to fermentable carbohydrates. More recently, the traditional meal pattern has been replaced by frequent snacking, including prolonged SSB consumption, with less emphasis on meals. Frequent snacking is associated with lower overall diet quality and increased risk of dental caries.[56]

## Sugar Substitutes

A number of chemical compounds that taste sweet but have little or no caloric value are common flavor additives, either alone or in combination, to foods, beverages, and oral hygiene products such as mouthwash and toothpaste. The sugar alcohols such as xylitol, sorbitol, erythritol, and mannitol are reduced-calorie sweeteners with caloric values ranging from 0.2 to 2.7 kcal/g. Their sweetness in relation to sucrose ranges from 35% to 100%. Sugar alcohols cannot be metabolized by oral bacteria or are metabolized very slowly (i.e., sorbitol) and therefore have reduced demineralization and cariogenic potential when compared to sucrose and fructose.[10] Xylitol has caries-preventive properties and its use as a therapeutic agent has been extensively investigated. Treatment protocols generally include four to five gum or lozenge exposures per day; effectiveness is complicated by compliance and gastrointestinal side effects associated with the sugar alcohol.

Nonnutritive sweeteners have zero or minuscule calories and are used widely in manufactured foods and beverages and as tabletop sweeteners. Although they are largely marketed as aids for weight loss, these products are also noncariogenic, either because oral bacteria cannot digest them or they are used in such small quantities as to have minimal effect on acid production.[23] Nonnutritive sweeteners approved for use in the United States are saccharin, acesulfame potassium (ace-K), aspartame, neotame, advantame, sucralose, and rebaudioside A.

Aspartame is a peptide consisting of two amino acids, aspartic acid, and phenylalanine and has a caloric value of 4 kcal/g. However, because it is 180 times as sweet as sucrose, the quantity needed to sweeten foods and beverages is so small that the calorie content becomes negligible. When broken down by peptidases, it yields the two component amino acids and methanol. Aspartame ingestion must be monitored and limited by persons with the genetic disease phenylketonuria (PKU), which is characterized by difficulty metabolizing phenylalanine, and a warning label is placed on foods containing this sweetener. Advantame is structurally related to aspartame and is the sweetest of all sugar substitutes, about 20,000 times sweeter than sucrose. Because advantame is used in such small quantity, the availability of

phenylalanine from its use is considered insignificant and warning labels for persons with PKU are not required.

Rebaudioside A (Reb A) is a purified glycoside extract of *stevia rebaudiana*, a plant native to South America that has been used there as a sweetener for several hundred years. Reb A is about 200 times sweeter than sucrose. Stevia leaf is also available commercially, but it is not approved by the US Food and Drug Administration as a food additive.

## Dental Acid Erosion

Acid erosion of the teeth refers to the irreversible loss of tooth enamel that occurs following exposure to acids other than those produced by bacteria. Although some acids are of endogenous origin, such as gastric acids associated with gastroesophageal reflux or vomiting, most acid exposures are of exogenous origin. The main dietary sources of acid associated with dental erosion are found in soda, fruit juice, and whole fruit. The dietary behavior of holding or swishing acidic beverages in the mouth and xerostomia increase the risk of erosion. Phosphoric, citric, and carbonic acids are the most common acids added to foods and beverages and provide tartness, enhance flavors, and/or act as preservatives. Carbon dioxide is added to provide fizz, or carbonation, and when it dissolves in water, carbonic acid is formed. Carbonated beverages generally have a pH in the range of 2.0 to 3.5 (pH 7.0 is neutral), so diet sodas might affect teeth by erosion. Many other types of beverages, such as sports drinks, flavored water, vitamin water, energy drinks, and fruit juices and cocktails, are also acidic.[58] Citric acid is found naturally in fruits and used as an additive. Fruits contain necessary vitamins and minerals in addition to acid, so acidity should not be the foremost reason for avoiding fruit; proper dental hygiene after eating will mitigate any harmful effects. Although it is not clear if erosion leads to caries, the two conditions often coexist, especially in persons who consume a lot of soft drinks and fruit juices.

## Periodontal Diseases

Periodontal disease affects nearly half of the adult US population.[20] It is an inflammatory, multifactorial disease that involves destruction of the periodontal ligament and alveolar bone tissues that support the teeth, and it is one of the major reasons for tooth loss among adults. Based on the known biological roles of various nutrients in the body, one would predict that many nutrients play a role in maintaining the integrity of these tissues. Vitamin C is necessary for the formation of collagen, vitamin A for maintenance and differentiation of epithelial cells, and calcium and phosphorus for bone mineralization. Other vitamins and fatty acids have roles in regulating inflammation, cell repair, and limiting damage to cells from reactive oxygen species. Observational studies have shown inverse associations of periodontal disease prevalence and incidence with higher intakes of omega-3 fatty acid,[50] vitamin C,[40] and dietary fiber.[51,65]

Increased refined carbohydrate intake may affect the level of plaque, which harbors periodontal pathogens. The highest tertile of added sugar intake level was related to greater periodontal disease prevalence among young adults.[44] In a pilot study, lowering the amount of starchy and refined carbohydrate to a very low level (<103 g/day) resulted in reductions in gingival bleeding and total periodontal inflamed surface area.[75] Although mostly from observational studies, the evidence suggests patients with periodontal diseases can benefit from advice to increase their dietary intakes of fiber, fish oils, fruits, and vegetables and to reduce intakes of refined sugars.[70]

## Oral and Pharyngeal Cancers

Approximately 50,000 cases of cancers of the oral cavity and pharynx occur each year and account for roughly 3% of total annual incident cancer cases in the United States. The risk factors that explain the majority of cases of oral and pharyngeal cancers (OPC) are tobacco use, infection with the human papilloma virus, and two major dietary factors—alcohol use and inadequate fruit and vegetable consumption.[24]

Ethanol, the active ingredient in alcoholic beverages, is a small 2-carbon structure that can easily diffuse from the stomach or intestine into the bloodstream without having to be broken down. Ethanol is produced by fermentation by anaerobic microorganisms of carbohydrates found in fruits, honey, grains, vegetables, and other plants. Common forms of alcohol consumed include the fermented beverages beer and wine, in which yeasts digest carbohydrates and convert them into ethanol, and distilled beverages such as liquors and brandies, which are concentrated and often aged after fermentation. Although the ethanol content by weight of the different beverages can vary, one drink or unit of alcohol has been defined as 14 g of ethanol (0.6 oz), which is approximately the amount contained in 12 oz of beer, 5 oz of wine, or 1.5 oz of liquor.

Risk of oral cancers increases in a dose-response manner as alcohol consumption increases.[6] Several mechanisms are potentially involved. Acetaldehyde, which is an intermediate of ethanol metabolism, is a probable human carcinogen. A number of contaminants identified in alcoholic beverages that result from the production and aging processes are also carcinogens. For example, roasting grains over an open fire, which is done for beer and some whiskies, results in a reaction between nitrogen oxide gases in smoke and proteins in the grain to form nitrosamines. In some countries, asbestos-containing filters are used to remove impurities from wine. Liquors stored in charred wood barrels absorb hydrocarbons from the wood. In addition, alcohol impairs the body's ability to absorb or metabolize some nutrients, and liver damage caused by chronic overconsumption of alcohol interferes with endogenous production of immunologic products and transport proteins. Excess alcohol consumption tends to displace nutritious foods and decreases the likelihood of meeting dietary guidelines for intake of antioxidant vitamins and minerals.

Reactive oxygen species (ROS), or free radicals, are unstable molecules that are formed during normal metabolism and by cellular responses to inflammation. Accumulation of ROS causes damage to cell DNA, RNA, lipids, and proteins. Many nutrients function as antioxidants to scavenge free radicals before they can accumulate. Vitamins C, E, and A; carotenoids; and polyphenol compounds—all of which are found predominantly in fruits and vegetables—and the minerals selenium and zinc can all act as antioxidants. Large-scale case-control and prospective studies have reported reduced risk of OPC among persons with the highest dietary intakes of vitamin C,[16] vitamin E,[19] carotenoids,[42] allium compounds,[21] and total fruits and vegetables.[45] High intakes of antioxidants such as folate may attenuate the risk of OPC associated with high alcohol intake.[66] Taking multivitamin and mineral supplements has not been shown to be beneficial in lowering OPC risk.[43]

## Dentition Status and Dietary Intake

Loss of teeth interferes with mastication and may adversely affect one's ability to consume a balanced diet. In particular, the ability to chew dry, fibrous, or hard foods such as whole grains and fresh fruits and vegetables is compromised, and the likelihood of meeting intake recommendations for fiber and many vitamins and minerals is reduced. The degree of dietary deficiency may depend on the extent of tooth loss and location of the missing teeth. In cross-sectional studies, having 20 or fewer total teeth, fewer than nine total occluding tooth pairs or fewer than five posterior occluding pairs was associated with reduced consumption of fruits and vegetables,[8,63,64] fiber,[32] and multiple vitamins and minerals.[15,79] Lower intakes of these foods and nutrients are especially evident among edentate persons even when the teeth are replaced with conventional dentures.[30,33]

Prospective studies have suggested that as people lose teeth, they tend toward a less healthy dietary pattern. Overall, women participating in the Nurses' Health Study made beneficial dietary changes, such as reducing their intakes of saturated fat, trans fats, cholesterol, and vitamin B12, over a 4-year interval while increasing beta-carotene, vitamin C, and fiber. However, these changes were less dramatic among the women who lost any teeth compared to those who lost none.[30] A similar trend was observed with loss of five or more teeth in a cohort of men followed for 8 years.[31]

Rehabilitation with conventional dentures, whether full or partial, does not guarantee an improvement in dietary intake or nutritional status. Persons with ill-fitting dentures consume a less varied and nutritionally poorer diet than persons with good-fitting dentures.[62] There may be more improvement in dietary quality with the use of implant-supported dentures, but results are mixed, and most intervention studies have had follow-up periods of 1 year or less. One longer term study followed patients rehabilitated with an implant-supported mandibular denture for 5 years and saw significant improvements in vegetable intake.[69] Tailored dietary counseling may be needed to sustain beneficial dietary changes beyond the short term.[78]

The association between diet and tooth loss is likely bidirectional. On the one hand, tooth loss can result in poor dietary quality. On the other, insufficiency of essential nutrients in the diet may indirectly increase the risk of tooth loss by caries and periodontal diseases. Calcium from dairy sources was inversely related to the risk of losing teeth in men and women.[2] Higher consumption of high-fiber foods was associated with less bleeding on probing and lower risk of tooth loss among older men.[65]

## Dietary Guidelines and Recommendations

*Overall diet.* The US Departments of Agriculture and Health and Human Services publish dietary guidelines every 5 years that incorporate the latest research on diet and health. The focus is primarily on healthy dietary patterns with recommendations for only a few individual nutrients, such as sugar, saturated fat, sodium, and alcohol (Box 23.1).

*Sugar Intake.* Based on studies showing associations between sugar intake and multiple diseases, the DGA, WHO, and several medical organizations recommend that for optimal health, adults and children reduce their sugar intake. However, there are a number of barriers that deter patients and the public from fully complying with and implementing the recommendations.

• BOX 23.1 Key 2015–2020 Dietary Guidelines and Recommendations for Americans[73]

**Guidelines**
- Follow a healthy eating pattern across the life span.
- Focus on variety, nutrient density, and amount.
- Limit calories from added sugars and saturated fats and reduce sodium intake.
- Shift to healthier food and beverage choices.
- Support healthy eating patterns for all.

**Recommendations**
The 2 major Recommendations are:
1. Consume a healthy eating pattern that accounts for all food and beverages within an appropriate calorie level.
   - A healthy eating pattern includes:
     - A variety of vegetables from all of the subgroups—dark green, red and orange, legumes (beans and peas), starchy, and other
     - Fruits, especially whole fruits

- Grains, at least half of which are whole grains
- Fat-free or low-fat dairy, including milk, yogurt, cheese, and/or fortified soy beverages
- A variety of protein foods, including seafood, lean meats and poultry, eggs, legumes (beans and peas), and nuts, seeds, and soy products
- Oils
- A healthy eating pattern limits saturated and trans fats, added sugars, sodium and alcohol.
  - Consume less than 10% of calories per day from added sugars
  - Consume less than 10% of calories per day from saturated fats
  - Consume less than 2300 mg/day of sodium
  - If alcohol is consumed, it should be consumed in moderation—up to one drink per day for women and up to two drinks per day for men—and only by adults of legal drinking age.
2. Meet the Physical Activity Guidelines for Americans.

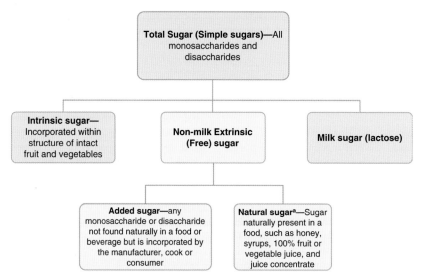

a Honey, syrup and, in some circumstances juice/concentrate, that are incorporated into foods by the manufacturer, cook or consumer may be considered added sugar.

• **Figure 23.1** Types of sugar.

One source of confusion is the different terminology used to describe sugar[48] (Figure 23.1). The US DGA recommend that less than 10% of caloric intake is derived from "added" sugar, whereas the WHO guideline states that less than 10% of calories should come from "free" sugar. Sugars are added to a large number and variety of food products and must be identified in the ingredient list on food labels, but manufacturers can list sugars under multiple different names.[71] Food labels list grams of total sugar in a serving, but many do not break down total sugar into added versus naturally occurring. Additional information about added sugars has begun to appear on more food labels in recent years, but the extra detail does not necessarily make the label more understandable.[39] Furthermore, by framing the recommendation in terms of percent of calorie, consumers need to know how many calories they consume daily and the caloric value of sugar (4 kcal/g) to calculate their own percentage. Knowing that these many barriers exist, an alternative approach is to shift the narrow focus away from sugar and provide advice to patients that encompasses the total diet. An individual's calorie

intake is not unlimited, so when the diet meets recommended levels of whole grains, fruits, and vegetables, other less nutrient-dense foods are displaced.

*Public Health Efforts to Reduce Sugar Intake.* Improvements and clarity in food labeling will ideally help to educate the public about their diet and give them the necessary information to change eating habits. However, public health officials recognize that focusing only on individual behaviors has limited success when socioeconomic forces compete with and override health concerns. The wide availability of sugar in processed foods and beverages and the lower cost of processed foods relative to "healthy" or natural products make it difficult for patients to change their diet even when they are motivated to do so. Modeling the public policy efforts that have been successful in reducing tobacco consumption, Mexico and several US cities have tried to reduce sugar intake by implementing additional taxes on high-sugar foods and beverages or restricting the purchase of large soda portions. Outcomes have been inconsistent. After Mexico began taxing SSBs, consumption during the following 2 years declined more than 5%,[14] and despite fears of lost

**• TABLE 23.1** Dietary Screening for the Dental Office

| Screening Area | Ideal Behavior | Recommended Behavior Change | Rationale for Behavioral Change |
|---|---|---|---|
| Meal patterns | 3 meals and 2–3 snacks | Work toward consumption of all foods and beverages (except water) at 3 meals and 2–3 snacks | Reduced exposures will decrease caries risk |
| | | Aim for similar meal and snack times every day | Structured meals are associated with improved diet quality |
| Food groups | ChooseMyPlate[a] age and gender guidelines met | Gradually modify food choices till compliant with ChooseMyPlate[a] | Compliance with ChooseMyPlate[a] will ensure adequate nutrient intake for periodontal tissue health, systemic health, and reduced oral cancer risk |
| | | Consider referral to registered dietitian | |
| Sugar-sweetened beverages (SSBs) | <12 oz/day consumed in <20 min | Replace SSB with sugar free beverages | Reduced SSB exposure will decrease caries risk and improve overall diet quality |
| | | Consume SSB in <20 min | |
| | | If routine SSB consumption is >20 oz/day, provide anticipatory guidance for energy replacement (ChooseMyPlate[a]) | Individuals consuming significant energy from SSB will be hungry; prepare individuals for the hunger by suggesting healthy food choices |
| | | If preferred SSB is caffeinated, suggest caffeine replacement or gradually wean from SSB | Headaches associated with caffeine withdrawal reduce likelihood of successful behavior change |

[a]Reference 73.

jobs voiced by the opposition, there was minimal impact on beverage manufacturing and commercial sales jobs.[25] Several US cities and states attempted to institute higher taxes on sugary beverages, but only a few have been successful so far; in others, the laws were not approved by voters or overturned shortly after going into effect. An effort in New York City to restrict the sale of super-sized sodas was overturned by the state Court of Appeals. If sugar consumption is to be reduced, it will take a combination of better nutrition education at all ages, health promotion, and public policy.

*Dietary Screening in the Dental Office*: Caries risk assessment generally includes evaluation of dietary exposures to fermentable carbohydrate. However, the oral healthcare practitioner is in a unique position to expand a patient's dietary evaluation to consider periodontal health, oral cancer prevention, and systemic health. Three key areas to evaluate include meal structure, food group intakes, and SSB exposures. Table 23.1 identifies desired diet-related behaviors, recommended changes for improved dietary habits, and the rationale for behavior change. Nutrient supplements are often recommended for patients who are missing food groups, but such supplementation does not correct dietary habits or reduce caries risk. Patients with significant dietary issues and/or nutrition-related systemic disease should be referred to registered dietitians for additional dietary guidance.

## Summary

An optimal diet is one of many factors that play roles in reducing the risks of caries, oral cancer, periodontal disease, and tooth loss. Dental professionals should provide dietary guidance that goes beyond sugar restriction and provide patients with resources to improve their overall diet. This will have benefits to the oral cavity and the total body. Research supports the idea that dietary recommendations for lowering risk of many chronic systemic diseases are entirely consistent with promoting good oral health.

## References

1. AbdelAziz WE, Dowidar KML, El Tantawi MMA. Association of healthy eating, juice consumption, and bacterial counts with early childhood caries. *Pediatr Dent.* 2015;37:462–467.
2. Adegboye AR, Twetman S, Christensen LB, et al. Intake of dairy calcium and tooth loss among adult Danish men and women. *Nutrition.* 2012;28:779–784.
3. Aires CP, Del Bel Cury AA, Tenuta LM, et al. Effect of starch and sucrose on dental biofilm formation and on root dentine demineralization. *Caries Res.* 2008;42:380–386.
4. American Dental Association. Policies and recommendations on diet and nutrition. Available from: http://www.ada.org/en/about-the-ada/ada-positions-policies-and-statements/policies-and-recommendations-on-diet-and-nutrition; 2016. Accessed 22 May, 2019.
5. Anderson CA, Curzon ME, Van Loveren C, et al. Sucrose and dental caries: a review of the evidence. *Obes Rev.* 2009;10(suppl 1):41–54.
6. Bagnardi V, Rota M, Botteri E, et al. Alcohol consumption and site-specific cancer risk: a comprehensive dose-response meta-analysis. *Br J Cancer.* 2015;112:580–593.
7. Bernabe E, Vehkalahti MM, Sheiham A, et al. The shape of the dose-response relationship between sugars and caries in adults. *J Dent Res.* 2016;95:167–172.
8. Brennan DS, Singh KA, Liu P, et al. Fruit and vegetable consumption among older adults by tooth loss and socio-economic status. *Aust Dent J.* 2010;55:143–149.
9. Burt BA, Pai S. Sugar consumption and caries risk: a systematic review. *J Dent Educ.* 2001;65:1017–1023.

10. Burt BA. The use of sorbitol- and xylitol-sweetened chewing gum in caries control. *J Am Dent Assoc.* 2006;137:190–196.

11. Cagetti MG, Mastroberardino S, Milia E, et al. The use of probiotic strains in caries prevention: a systematic review. *Nutrients.* 2013;5: 2530–2550.

12. Campain AC, Morgan MV, Evans RW, et al. Sugar-starch combinations in food and the relationship to dental caries in low-risk adolescents. *Eur J Oral Sci.* 2003;111:316–325.

13. Chankanka O, Marshall TA, Levy SM, et al. Mixed dentition cavitated caries incidence and dietary intake frequencies. *Pediatr Dent.* 2011;33:233–240.

14. Colchero MA, Rivera-Dommarco J, Popkin BM, et al. In: Mexico, evidence of sustained consumer response two years after implementing a sugar-sweetened beverage tax. *Health Aff (Millwood).* 2017;36: 564–571.

15. de Andrade FB, de Franca Caldas A Jr, Kitoko PM. Relationship between oral health, nutrient intake and nutritional status in a sample of Brazilian elderly people. *Gerodontology.* 2009;26:40–45.

16. De Munter L, Maasland DH, van den Brandt PA, et al. Vitamin and carotenoid intake and risk of head-neck cancer subtypes in the Netherlands Cohort Study. *Am J Clin Nutr.* 2015;102:420–432.

17. Dye BA, Thornton-Evans G, Li X, et al. *Dental Caries and Sealant Prevalence in Children and Adolescents in the United States, 2011–2012.* NCHS Data Brief No. 191. 2015/05/02 ed. Hyattsville, MD: National Center for Health Statistics; 2015;1–8.

18. Dye BA, Thornton-Evans G, Li X, et al. *Dental Caries and Tooth Loss in Adults in the United States, 2011–2012.* NCHS Data Brief No. 197. Hyattsville, MD: National Center for Health Statistics; 2015.

19. Edefonti V, Hashibe M, Parpinel M, et al. Vitamin E intake from natural sources and head and neck cancer risk: a pooled analysis in the International Head and Neck Cancer Epidemiology consortium. *Br J Cancer.* 2015;113:182–192.

20. Eke PI, Zhang X, Lu H, et al. Predicting periodontitis at state and local levels in the United States. *J Dent Res.* 2016;95:515–522.

21. Galeone C, Turati F, Zhang ZF, et al. Relation of allium vegetables intake with head and neck cancers: evidence from the INHANCE consortium. *Mol Nutr Food Res.* 2015;59:1641–1650.

22. Ghazal T, Levy SM, Childers NK, et al. Factors associated with early childhood caries incidence among high caries-risk children. *Community Dent Oral Epidemiol.* 2015;43:366–374.

23. Giacaman RA, Campos P, Munoz-Sandoval C, et al. Cariogenic potential of commercial sweeteners in an experimental biofilm caries model on enamel. *Arch Oral Biol.* 2013;58:1116–1122.

24. Grundy A, Poirier AE, Khandwala F, et al. Cancer incidence attributable to lifestyle and environmental factors in Alberta in 2012: summary of results. *CMAJ Open.* 2017;5:E540–E545.

25. Guerrero-Lopez CM, Molina M, Colchero MA. Employment changes associated with the introduction of taxes on sugar-sweetened beverages and nonessential energy-dense food in Mexico. *Prev Med.* 2017;105S:S43–S49.

26. Hamner HC, Perrine CG, Gupta PM, et al. Food consumption patterns among U.S. children from birth to 23 months of age, 2009-2014. *Nutrients.* 2017;(9).

27. Han E, Powell LM. Consumption patterns of sugar-sweetened beverages in the United States. *J Acad Nutr Diet.* 2013;113:43–53.

28. Harris R. Biology of the children of Hopewood House, Bowral, Australia. 4. Observations on dental-caries experience extending over five years (1957-61). *J Dent Res.* 1963;42:1387–1399.

29. Hedrick VE, Davy BM, Myers EA, et al. Changes in the healthy beverage index in response to an intervention targeting a reduction in sugar-sweetened beverage consumption as compared to an intervention targeting improvements in physical activity: results from the Talking Health Trial. *Nutrients.* 2015;7:10168–10178.

30. Hung HC, Colditz G, Joshipura KJ. The association between tooth loss and the self-reported intake of selected CVD-related nutrients and foods among US women. *Community Dent Oral Epidemiol.* 2005;33:167–173.

31. Hung HC, Willett W, Ascherio A, et al. Tooth loss and dietary intake. *J Am Dent Assoc.* 2003;134:1185–1192.

32. Iwasaki M, Taylor GW, Manz MC, et al. Oral health status: relationship to nutrient and food intake among 80-year-old Japanese adults. *Community Dent Oral Epidemiol.* 2014;42:441–450.

33. Joshipura KJ, Willett WC, Douglass CW. The impact of edentulousness on food and nutrient intake. *J Am Dent Assoc.* 1996;127: 459–467.

34. Kant AK. Dietary patterns and health outcomes. *J Am Diet Assoc.* 2004;104:615–635.

35. Kashket S, DePaola DP. Cheese consumption and the development and progression of dental caries. *Nutr Rev.* 2002;60:97–103.

36. Kaye EK, Heaton B, Sohn W, et al. The Dietary Approaches to Stop Hypertension Diet and new and recurrent root caries events in men. *J Am Geriatr Soc.* 2015;63:1812–1819.

37. Kolker JL, Yuan Y, Burt BA, et al. Dental caries and dietary patterns in low-income African American children. *Pediatr Dent.* 2007;29:457–464.

38. Krasse B. The Vipeholm Dental Caries Study: recollections and reflections 50 years later. *J Dent Res.* 2001;80:1785–1788.

39. Laquatra I, Sollid K, Smith Edge M, et al. Including "added sugars" on the nutrition facts panel: How consumers perceive the proposed change. *J Acad Nutr Diet.* 2015;115:1758–1763.

40. Lee JH, Shin MS, Kim EJ, et al. The association of dietary vitamin C intake with periodontitis among Korean adults: Results from KNHANES. *PLoS One.* 2017;12. e0177074.

41. Lempert SM, Christensen LB, Froberg K, et al. Association between dairy intake and caries among children and adolescents. results from the Danish EYHS follow-up study. *Caries Res.* 2015;49:251–258.

42. Leoncini E, Edefonti V, Hashibe M, et al. Carotenoid intake and head and neck cancer: a pooled analysis in the International Head and Neck Cancer Epidemiology Consortium. *Eur J Epidemiol.* 2016;31:369–383.

43. Li Q, Chuang SC, Eluf-Neto J, et al. Vitamin or mineral supplement intake and the risk of head and neck cancer: pooled analysis in the INHANCE consortium. *Int J Cancer.* 2012;131:1686–1699.

44. Lula EC, Ribeiro CC, Hugo FN, et al. Added sugars and periodontal disease in young adults: an analysis of NHANES III data. *Am J Clin Nutr.* 2014;100:1182–1187.

45. Maasland DH, van den Brandt PA, Kremer B, et al. Consumption of vegetables and fruits and risk of subtypes of head-neck cancer in the Netherlands Cohort Study. *Int J Cancer.* 2015;136:E396–E409.

46. Martinez Steele E, Baraldi LG, Louzada ML, et al. Ultra-processed foods and added sugars in the US diet: evidence from a nationally representative cross-sectional study. *BMJ Open.* 2016;6. e009892.

47. Masood M, Masood Y, Newton T. Impact of national income and inequality on sugar and caries relationship. *Caries Res.* 2012;46:581–588.

48. Mela DJ, Woolner EM. Perspective: Total, added or free? What kind of sugars should we be talking about? *Adv Nutr.* 2018;9:63–69.

49. Moynihan P. Sugars and dental caries: Evidence for setting a recommended threshold for intake. *Adv Nutr.* 2016;7:149–156.

50. Naqvi AZ, Buettner C, Phillips RS, et al. n-3 Fatty acids and periodontitis in US adults. *J Am Diet Assoc.* 2010;110:1669–1675.

51. Nielsen SJ, Trak-Fellermeier MA, Joshipura K, et al. Dietary fiber intake is inversely associated with periodontal disease among US adults. *J Nutr.* 2016;146:2530–2536.

52. Nunn ME, Braunstein NS, Kaye EAK, et al. Healthy Eating Index is a predictor of early childhood caries. *J Dent Res.* 2009;88: 361–366.

53. O'Neil CE, Keast DR, Fulgoni VL, et al. Food sources of energy and nutrients among adults in the US: NHANES 2003-2006. *Nutrients.* 2012;4:2097–2120.

54. Paes Leme AF, Koo H, Bellato CM, et al. The role of sucrose in cariogenic dental biofilm formation–new insight. *J Dent Res.* 2006;85:878–887.

55. Palacios C, Rivas-Tumanyan S, Morou-Bermudez E, et al. Association between type, amount, and pattern of carbohydrate consumption with dental caries in 12-year-olds in Puerto Rico. *Caries Res.* 2016;50:560–570.

56. Palmer CA, Kent R, Loo CY Jr, et al. Diet and caries-associated bacteria in severe early childhood caries. *J Dent Res.* 2010; 89:1224–1229.
57. Powell ES, Smith-Taillie LP, Popkin BM. Added sugars intake across the distribution of US children and adult consumers: 1977-2012. *J Acad Nutr Diet.* 2016;116:1543–1550. e1541.
58. Reddy A, Norris DF, Momeni SS, et al. The pH of beverages in the United States. *J Am Dent Assoc.* 2016;147:255–263.
59. Ribeiro CC, Tabchoury CP, Del Bel Cury AA, et al. Effect of starch on the cariogenic potential of sucrose. *Br J Nutr.* 2005;94:44–50.
60. Rosinger A, Herrick K, Gahche J, et al. *Sugar-Sweetened Beverage Consumption Among U.S. Youth, 2011–2014.* NCHS Data Brief, No. 271. Hyattsville, MD. National Center for Health Statistics; 2017.
61. Rugg-Gunn AJ, Edgar WM, Jenkins GN. The effect of altering the position of a sugary food in a meal upon plaque pH in human subjects. *J Dent Res.* 1981;60:867–872.
62. Sahyoun NR, Krall E. Low dietary quality among older adults with self-perceived ill-fitting dentures. *J Am Diet Assoc.* 2003;103: 1494–1499.
63. Sahyoun NR, Lin CL, Krall E. Nutritional status of the older adult is associated with dentition status. *J Am Diet Assoc.* 2003;103:61–66.
64. Savoca MR, Arcury TA, Leng X, et al. Severe tooth loss in older adults as a key indicator of compromised dietary quality. *Public Health Nutr.* 2010;13:466–474.
65. Schwartz N, Kaye EK, Nunn ME, et al. High-fiber foods reduce periodontal disease progression in men aged 65 and older: The Veterans Affairs Normative Aging Study/Dental Longitudinal Study. *J Am Geriatr Soc.* 2012;60:676–683.
66. Shanmugham JR, Zavras AI, Rosner BA, et al. Alcohol-folate interactions in the risk of oral cancer in women: a prospective cohort study. *Cancer Epidemiol Biomarkers Prev.* 2010;19:2516–2524.
67. Sheiham A, Watt RG. The common risk factor approach: a rational basis for promoting oral health. *Community Dent Oral Epidemiol.* 2000;28:399–406.
68. Sreebny LM, Chatterjee R, Kleinberg I. Clearance of glucose and sucrose from the saliva of human subjects. *Arch Oral Biol.* 1985;30:269–274.
69. Tajbakhsh S, Rubenstein JE, Faine MP, et al. Selection patterns of dietary foods in edentulous participants rehabilitated with maxillary complete dentures opposed by mandibular implant-supported prostheses: a multicenter longitudinal assessment. *J Prosthet Dent.* 2013;110:252–258.
70. Tonetti MS, Chapple IL. Biological approaches to the development of novel periodontal therapies—consensus of the Seventh European Workshop on Periodontology. *J Clin Periodontol.* 2011;38(suppl 11): 114–118.
71. US Department of Agriculture. ChooseMyPlate.gov Website. Washington DC. Added Sugars. Available from: https://www.choosemyplate.gov/eathealthy/added-sugars. Accessed December 9, 2019.
72. Food and Nutrition Service. fns.usda.gov Website. Washington DC. Healthy Eating Index (HEI). Available from: https://www.fns.usda.gov/resource/healthy-eating-index-hei. 2019. Accessed December 9, 2019.
73. U.S. Department of Health and Human Services and U.S. Department of Agriculture. 2015–2020 Dietary Guidelines for Americans. 8th Edition. December 2015. Available from: https://health.gov/dietaryguidelines/2015/guidelines/executive-summary/. Accessed December 9, 2019.
74. Warren JJ, Weber-Gasparoni K, Marshall TA, et al. A longitudinal study of dental caries risk among very young low SES children. *Community Dent Oral Epidemiol.* 2009;37:116–122.
75. Woelber JP, Bremer K, Vach K, et al. An oral health optimized diet can reduce gingival and periodontal inflammation in humans - a randomized controlled pilot study. *BMC Oral Health.* 2016;17:28.
76. Yoshihara A, Watanabe R, Hanada N, et al. A longitudinal study of the relationship between diet intake and dental caries and periodontal disease in elderly Japanese subjects. *Gerodontology.* 2009;26:130–136.
77. Zaki NAA, Dowidar KML, Abdelaziz WEE. Assessment of the Healthy Eating Index-2005 as a predictor of early childhood caries. *Int J Paediatr Dent.* 2015;25:436–443.
78. Zare Javid A, Seal CJ, Heasman P, et al. Impact of a customised dietary intervention on antioxidant status, dietary intakes and periodontal indices in patients with adult periodontitis. *J Hum Nutr Diet.* 2014;27:523–532.
79. Zhu Y, Hollis JH. Tooth loss and its association with dietary intake and diet quality in American adults. *J Dent.* 2014;42:1428–1435.

# 24

# Fluoride and Human Health

MARK E. MOSS, DDS, PhD

JAYANTH KUMAR, DDS, MPH

## Introduction

The story of fluoride in dentistry (see Box 24.1, A Classic Epidemiologic Study), begins with the observation that teeth were cosmetically affected by drinking water that contained relatively higher concentrations of the agent. While this pattern was being investigated, it became clear that the caries levels were lower in communities that had more fluoride in the drinking water. Research was then conducted to identify a therapeutic window for optimizing benefits and minimizing the negative cosmetic impact on the community. Once this therapeutic window was identified, studies were conducted to test whether a community benefit could be demonstrated.

The fact that high concentrations of fluoride occur naturally in drinking water in some communities and low concentrations of fluoride are added to drinking water in some communities demonstrates that it has both beneficial and detrimental effects. These effects require that governmental agencies, professional organizations, and practitioners use the best available evidence to ensure its safety and effective use. The assurance of safety is a pillar of public health practice. This chapter directs our attention toward this dimension with a particular focus on our current understanding of the safety of fluoride in human health.

This chapter summarizes the literature on fluoride in drinking water and its effects. As there are many governmental and professional organizational reports and a few systematic reviews, we relied largely on these comprehensive reports. Where comprehensive reviews were not available, we used individual studies to assess the effect of fluoride.

## Fluoride Intake

Fluorine is one of the most reactive elements and therefore is never found naturally in its elemental form. The fluoride ion, however, is abundant in nature and occurs almost universally in soils and waters in varying, but generally low, concentrations. Seawater contains 1.2 to 1.4 ppm fluoride.[73] Fresh surface water generally has very low concentrations, 0.2 ppm fluoride or less, whereas concentrations of up to 29.5 ppm fluoride have been recorded in deep well water in Arizona[47] and concentrations of over 40 ppm in boreholes in Kenya.[46] Fluoride's ubiquity in soil and water means that all plants and animals contain fluoride to some extent.

Humans absorb fluoride from air, food, and water. Fluoride intake from air is usually negligible, around 0.04 mg fluoride/day.[72,73] Exceptions can occur around some industrial plants that work with fluoride-rich material, such as aluminum smelters with inadequate safeguards to prevent the escape of fluoride-containing compounds. Such environmental hazards should be controlled to the extent possible, an issue that has nothing whatever to do with the use of fluoride to control caries.

Fluoride's abundance in soils and plants means that everyone consumes it to some extent. Despite both the variability of the human diet and methodologic difficulties inherent in analyzing such minute amounts of fluoride consumed by everyone, studies to estimate the average daily intake of fluoride from all sources have provided fairly consistent results. Estimates for an adult North American male in an area with fluoridated water fall within the range of 1 to 3 mg fluoride/day from food and beverages, decreasing to 1 mg fluoride/day or less in an area without fluoridation.[20,41,55,60,62,63,67]

In the 1970s, the United States Congress enacted the Safe Drinking Water Act, the main federal law that ensures the quality of Americans' drinking water. It authorizes the Environmental

**• BOX 24.1   A Classic Epidemiologic Study**

As a new dental graduate in the early 1900s, Dr. Frederick McKay headed west and opened a practice in Colorado Springs, Colorado. He soon noticed that many of his patients had a curious blotching of the enamel that he had not encountered before. People in the area called it Colorado brown stain, and to them it was just a local oddity. McKay was clearly a born scientist; he had an inquiring mind and fine powers of observation, and Colorado brown stain piqued his curiosity. In 1908 he began to investigate the extent of Colorado brown stain in the surrounding area.

In his travels over the next few years, McKay found that the condition was highly prevalent in the Colorado Springs area. It was found only in long-term residents, individuals who had been born there, or who had come to the area as babies. Because the stain was difficult to polish off, McKay reasoned that it must be caused by an environmental agent that was active during the period of enamel formation. To ensure that his findings attracted some attention, McKay was shrewd enough to enlist the collaboration of G.V. Black, a major figure in dental history, in writing the first description of what then came to be called *mottled enamel*.[11]

McKay found that mottled enamel was endemic in many other communities along the Continental Divide and the plains to the east. It was most prevalent where deep artesian wells were the source of drinking water, and within any community the persons affected had almost invariably been users of the same water supply. By the 1920s McKay had reached the conclusion that the etiologic agent had to be a constituent of some community water supplies, despite the fact that chemical analyses all failed to identify likely constituents. In communities such as Andover and Britton, South Dakota, where he found severe mottling, he advised mothers to obtain their children's drinking water from sources other than the community supply. In Oakley, Idaho, McKay found that children living on the outskirts of the city, using water from a private spring, were free of mottling. He advised the citizens of Oakley to abandon their old supply and tap this spring for a new source, which the community did in 1925. McKay was right, as children born in Oakley subsequent to the change were free of mottled enamel.[50]

By 1930, new methods of spectrographic analysis of water had been developed. In 1931 McKay sent several samples of suspected water to an Alcoa Company chemist named Churchill, who was using these new methods. Churchill identified fluoride in each of the samples, in amounts ranging up to 14 parts per million (ppm).[18] At around the same time, similar findings were reported by investigators at the University of Arizona[15] and by a veterinary group in Morocco (then still a French colony) that was studying *le darmous*, the local name given to an extreme degree of mottled enamel found in Moroccan sheep.[70]

The immediate reaction of the scientific community to the identification of fluoride in drinking water was one of concern, because fluoride in high concentrations was known to be a protoplasmic poison. The discovery led to the appointment in 1931 of the first dentist to the newly established National Institute of Health. This was H. Trendley Dean, who was transferred from elsewhere in the U.S. Public Health Service to become the one-person Dental Hygiene Unit, an odd name for a unit formed to investigate mottled enamel (it subsequently became the National Institute of Dental Research in 1948).

Amidst this flurry of concern, however, McKay had also noted some benefits that seemed to accompany mottled enamel. In 1928, 3 years before fluoride was identified in drinking water, he was confident enough to publish his view that caries experience was reduced by the same waters that produced mottled enamel.[49] A similar observation was made shortly afterward in England by Ainsworth,[2] who like McKay was an observant dentist with an inquiring mind. Although McKay was not the first to make this observation, none of the earlier observers took the idea any further. McKay and Dean are good examples of the right people being in the right place at the right time.

The task of defining the relationship of fluoride to mottled enamel now passed to Dean. His first job was to map out the prevalence of mottled enamel in the United States. Dean began using the term *fluorosis* to replace *mottled enamel* in the mid-1930s.[24] By the mid-1930s, Dean had concluded that this "minimal threshold" level was 1 ppm fluoride[21] and that fluorosis seen in communities with water below 1 ppm fluoride was "of no public health significance."[25] In the mid-1930s Dean shifted his focus to examine a beneficial role of fluoride, using fluorosis data for children in parts of South Dakota, Colorado, and Wisconsin and caries data from an earlier 26-state survey in what today would be called an ecologic study (see Chapter 12). Although he could hardly have failed to notice the low caries experience in communities with fluoride-bearing water during his early surveys, this was his first report in which he commented on the inverse relationship between fluorosis and caries.[23] The work was republished in 2006 highlighting its importance in public health.

Encouraged by these preliminary data, Dean chose four cities in central Illinois as study sites in which to test the hypothesis that consumption of fluoride-containing water was associated with a reduced prevalence of caries. Galesburg and Monmouth, where Dean had already studied fluorosis,[25] used water from deep wells that averaged 1.8 and 1.7 ppm fluoride. Macomb and Quincy used surface water averaging 0.2 ppm fluoride. Clinical examinations of children ages 12 to 14 years, all with lifetime residence in their respective cities, showed that more than twice as many children in Galesburg and Monmouth were free of detectable caries than in the two cities with low-fluoride water, and the mean number of permanent teeth affected by caries in Galesburg and Monmouth was half of that in the two cities with low-fluoride water.[26] The evidence to support the fluoride–caries hypothesis was now stronger.

The next logical step was therefore to define the lowest fluoride level at which caries was clearly inhibited. This was done through a series of investigations that have become known collectively as the 21 cities study and that are rightly considered a landmark in dental research. The first part consisted of the results of clinical examinations of children ages 12 to 14 with lifetime residence in eight suburban Chicago communities with various but stable mean fluoride levels in their domestic water.[27] The project was later expanded by adding data from 13 additional cities in Illinois, Colorado, Ohio, and Indiana.[22] The collective findings of the 21 cities study are depicted graphically in Figures 24.1 and 24.2. Figure 24.1 shows that dental caries experience in different communities dropped sharply as fluoride concentration rose toward 1 ppm then leveled off. Figure 24.2 shows the dental fluorosis experience that Dean found among the 12- to 14-year-olds in the 21 cities. Dean's practice was to show questionable fluorosis separately in his reports, as we have done in Figure 24.2. The data in Figure 24.2 suggest that, had "questionable" fluorosis been included in the prevalence figures, then the level for "acceptable" fluorosis might have been set at concentrations lower than 1 ppm fluoride.

Because the 21 cities study had a cross-sectional design, the results confirmed the association but could not by themselves establish the cause-and-effect relationship between fluoridated water and reduced caries prevalence. But the data in Figures 24.1 and 24.2 did lead to the adoption of 1.0 to 1.2 ppm as the appropriate concentration of fluoride in drinking water in temperate climates, a standard that remained in place in the United States until 2015. These results also set the stage for a prospective test of the fluoride–caries hypothesis, first suggested in 1943.[3] The years of study of people using water with fluoride levels much higher than the proposed 1 ppm were sufficient to convince public authorities that the prospective tests could be carried out in safety. These first prospective studies are described in Chapter 25.

Protection Agency (EPA) to set national standards for drinking water to protect against health effects from exposure to naturally occurring and manmade contaminants. It requires periodic reassessment of regulations for drinking water contaminants. To fulfill this requirement, EPA's Office of Water (OW) published a report[31] in 2010 on the various sources that contribute to fluoride exposure in the United States for the purpose of estimating total exposures for children during the period of sensitivity to severe dental fluorosis (6 months to 14 years) and for the adult population because of the potential for bone fractures and skeletal fluorosis.

According to this report, the main sources of fluoride are water, beverages, solid food, and toothpaste. As noted by the National Research Council in 2006,[53] fluoride intake from drinking water depends on individual water consumption and fluoride concentration in the water. The intake will be lower if water purification or

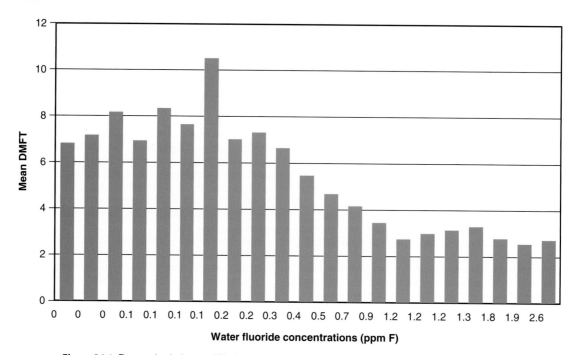

• **Figure 24.1** Decayed, missing, and filled permanent teeth (DMFT) in children ages 12 to 14 in 21 cities in the late 1930s, related to the fluoride concentration.[22,27]

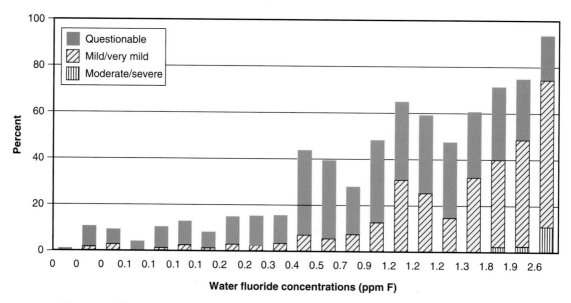

• **Figure 24.2** Fluorosis experience of children ages 12 to 14 in 21 cities in the late 1930s, related to the fluoride concentration of drinking water.[22,27]

**• TABLE 24.1** Representative Values for Fluoride Intakes Used in Calculation of the Relative Source Contribution (RSC) for Drinking Water

| Age Group (Years) | Drinking Water Intake[a] (mg/day) | Food Intake (mg/day) | Beverage Intake (mg/day) | Toothpaste Intake (mg/day) | Soil Intake (mg/day) | Total (mg/day) | RSC (%) |
|---|---|---|---|---|---|---|---|
| 0.5–<1 | 0.84 | 0.25[b] | — | 0.07 | 0.02 | 1.19 | 71 |
| 1–<4 | 0.63 | 0.16 | 0.36 | 0.34 | 0.04 | 1.53 | 41 |
| 4–<7 | 0.82 | 0.35 | 0.54 | 0.22 | 0.04 | 1.97 | 42 |
| 7–<11 | 0.86 | 0.41 | 0.60 | 0.18 | 0.04 | 2.09 | 41 |
| 11–14 | 1.23 | 0.47 | 0.38 | 0.20 | 0.04 | 2.32 | 53 |
| >14 | 1.74 | 0.38 | 0.59 | 0.10[c] | 0.02 | 2.83 | 61 |

[a]Consumers only: 90th percentile intake except for >14 years. The >14 value is based on the Environmental Protection Agency Office of Water policy of 2 L/day.
[b]Includes foods, fluoride in powdered formula, and fruit juices; no allocation for other beverages.
[c]Assumed to be 50% of the value for the 11- to 14-year-old age group.[31]
Reproduction of Table 7-1 From EPA Office of Water 2010 Report.

filtration systems are used to remove fluoride. Some individuals could be exposed to substantially higher amounts of fluoride from drinking water because of specific types of activities that increase water intake (e.g., athletes or outdoor laborers in warm climates), life stage (e.g., pregnant or lactating women), or as a result of medical conditions such as diabetes mellitus, diabetes insipidus, or renal problems. Table 24.1 is a reproduction of Table 7.1 from the EPA report[31] and shows the representative values derived for typical individuals under age 14 exposed to 0.87 mg/L of fluoride in municipal water systems whose water intake is in the 90th percentile (high water consumers). For the adult population, the estimation is based on consumption of 2 L of water per day. This table was used by EPA to frame discussions around safety related to risk of skeletal fluorosis in adults and severe dental fluorosis in children. It shows that at the 90th percentile of exposure, adults (and children under age 14) would be exposed to less than 3 mg fluoride daily and children age 7 to 14 would be exposed to less than 2.5 mg fluoride daily. Fluoride intake among children under age 7 would be about 2 mg or less daily.

Because fluoridation of public drinking water systems has been demonstrated as effective in reducing dental caries, the U.S. Public Health Service (PHS) provides recommendations regarding optimal fluoride concentrations in drinking water for community water systems.[69] Based on the EPA OW estimate, the U.S. Department of Health and Human Services (HHS) published an updated PHS recommendation in 2015 because of new data that address changes in the prevalence of dental fluorosis, the relationship between water intake and outdoor temperature in children,[8] and the contribution of fluoride in drinking water to total fluoride exposure in the United States. The current recommendation for the optimal fluoride concentration in drinking water for prevention of dental caries in the United States has been set at 0.7 mg/L (reduced from the previous range of 0.7–1.2 mg/L set in 1962).[69]

This policy change will have an impact on estimates of exposure used in EPA's analysis. With fluoride concentration in water reduced to a uniform level of 0.7 mg/L—from the average concentration of 0.87 mg/L (a 19.5% reduction)—the total fluoride intake will be lower. For those consumers who are drinking the upper limit of the recommended amount of water (instead of 90th percentile for water systems under the old upper limit), the

**• TABLE 24.2** Revised Estimates of Fluoride Exposure Attributable to Drinking Water Under the 2015 Recommendation of 0.7 mg/L

| Age Group (Years) | Drinking Water Fluoride Intake at 0.7 mg/L (mg/day) | Total Fluoride Intake (mg/day) | Relative Source Contribution From Drinking Water (%) |
|---|---|---|---|
| 0.5 to <1 | 0.68 | 1.02 | 67 |
| 1 to <4 | 0.51 | 1.41 | 36 |
| 4 to <7 | 0.66 | 1.81 | 37 |
| 7 to <11 | 0.69 | 1.92 | 36 |
| 11 to 14 | 0.99 | 2.08 | 48 |
| >14 | 1.40 | 2.49 | 56 |

estimated total mg/day of fluoride is likely to be as shown in Table 24.2. The table shows that the reduced level of fluoride in drinking water will result in a substantial change in the amount of fluoride intake for all age groups. However, the proportion of fluoride intake that comes from drinking water is only modestly reduced because of the prominent role that drinking water holds compared to other sources of fluoride.

## Infancy

Fluoride ingestion in infancy is a matter of some concern because of the risk of dental fluorosis. A source of high fluoride intake for infants has been identified as powdered infant formula reconstituted with fluoridated drinking water.[9,14] Methodical estimates of fluoride intake by infants have come from the Iowa Fluoride Studies, initiated in the 1990s, which showed that fluoride exposure among infants is extensive and variable. The Iowa studies documented the fluoride exposures of newborn infants at periodic intervals through extensive interviews about fluoride exposure from drinking water, toothpaste, and dietary supplements. During the first 3 years of life, fluoride ingestion from these sources averaged 0.37 to 0.45 mg daily from birth to 3 months, 0.5 mg at 6 to 9 months, 0.36 mg at 12 and 16 months, and 0.5 to 0.63 mg from 16 to 36 months.[43] Although mean intakes in Iowa were similar to those estimated in the earlier market basket surveys, there was a considerable range of intakes, with 90th percentile values well above the means and medians. When values were expressed as fluoride intake per kg of body weight, nearly half of the children up to 6 months of age were found to be exceeding the desirable limits, although this proportion dropped considerably at later ages. The desirable upper limit of intake for 12-month-old children, beyond which fluorosis risk is greatly increased, has been estimated at 0.43 mg fluoride/day.[13] The 12-month-old children in the Iowa studies averaged 0.36 mg fluoride/day,[43] but more than 25% of them were ingesting fluoride above that upper limit.

## Early Childhood

As children age, fluoride intake is reduced when the tendency to swallow toothpaste diminishes. A recent paper from the Iowa group examined fluorosis in permanent canines, premolars, and second molars with fluoride intake patterns while the children were followed from ages 2 to 8.[10] The investigators found that while children tended to reduce their fluoride intake after age 5, a relatively high proportion of these so-called late-erupting permanent teeth had fluorosis (mostly mild or very mild). Only four children had moderate/severe fluorosis. The authors stated that the main source of fluoride ingestion was from drinking water. The recent reduction in optimum fluoride level from 1.0 to 0.7 mg/L will result in a 30% decrease in fluoride intake attributable to drinking water for most children. The impact of this will be to effectively shift the risk of fluorosis downward.

For example, in the Iowa cohort, the proportion of children that had fluorosis in a canine tooth was 6.7% in the lowest tertile of exposure, 20.9% in the middle tertile of exposure, and 25.5% in the highest tertile of exposure. By reducing fluoride intake, the risk distribution will shift downward so that the vast majority of children would be shifted into an exposure level that is equivalent to the lowest exposure tertile defined in this study, assuming that children continue to drink about the same amount of water.

The wide variation in consumption patterns is also highlighted among children ages 2 to 8 years followed longitudinally in the Iowa Fluoride Study. Only 62% of children who were classified by tertile of fluoride intake (i.e., high, moderate, or low) between ages 2 to 5 years remained in that same relative tertile class when they were ages 5 to 8 years. In other words, 38% of children are not consistently consuming more or less fluoride than their peers up to age 8.

## Intake After Tooth Development Is Complete: Adolescence and Adulthood

For most people, water and other beverages provide some 75% of fluoride intake, regardless of whether the drinking water is fluoridated.[63] This may occur because many soft drinks and fruit juices are processed in cities with fluoridated water, or it may reflect variable fluoride content of the ingredients. One brand of grape juice in North Carolina, for example, was found to contain more than 1.6 ppm fluoride, even when reconstituted with deionized water.[57] Even in soft drinks of the same brand, fluoride levels can vary considerably due to production at different sites.[34]

For a typical adult living in a fluoridated community, fluoride exposure in North America arises from consumption of: water (61% of daily fluoride intake), other beverages (22% of daily fluoride intake), solid food (13% of daily fluoride intake), and toothpaste (4% of daily fluoride intake). They were derived by the EPA from studies of the general population ages 14 years or older using generally accepted methods of estimating dietary intake. Notable in this is the EPA's emphasis on assessing safety and the EPA's use of data for the 90th percentile of water consumption for children. The estimates assume that individuals consume 2 L/day of water that has 0.87 ppm fluoride. Total intake of fluoride for this hypothetical individual would be less than 3 mg of fluoride per day. As stated earlier, now that the level of fluoride in drinking water has been reduced, the estimate of total daily fluoride intake will now be lower, by nearly 20% $[(0.87-0.7)/0.87 = 0.195]$. Box 24.2 addresses the risk of fluorosis from toothpaste.

## Absorption, Retention, and Excretion

Ingested fluoride is absorbed mainly from the upper gastrointestinal tract, and some 95% of ingested fluoride is absorbed. Absorbed fluoride is transported in the plasma and is either excreted or deposited in the calcified tissues. Most absorbed fluoride is excreted in the urine; a single ingestion of 5 mg fluoride by an adult is absorbed and cleared from the blood in 8 to 9 hours.[72] Fluoride ingested on an empty stomach produces a peak plasma level within 30 minutes. The time of the plasma peak is extended, and the level of the peak reduced, if the fluoride is taken with food. This is probably because of the binding of some fluoride with calcium and other divalent and trivalent cations. When fluoride absorption is inhibited in this way, fecal excretion of fluoride increases.[29]

Studies of what is called the *body burden* of fluoride—meaning the amount that can be safely absorbed and the point at which fluoride absorption becomes a health concern—have relied mostly on urinary volumes and plasma concentrations as the primary

---

### • BOX 24.2  Risk of Fluorosis From Toothpaste

Fluorosis results from too much fluoride during tooth development. Longitudinal studies done in Iowa have shown that the period from 12 to 24 months after birth appears to be critical for risk of fluorosis in permanent maxillary central incisors.[35] It is known that this age group tends to ingest a relatively greater amount of toothpaste when brushing. Estimates from the EPA report on fluoride intake as shown below suggest that the proportion of fluoride intake from toothpaste varies by the child's age. This underscores the importance of proper toothbrushing supervision and management of the amount of toothpaste applied to the toothbrush for preventing fluorosis in young children.

| | |
|---|---|
| Age 6–11 months | 6% |
| Age 1–4 years | 22% |
| Age 4–7 years | 11% |
| Above age 7 | 9% |

Note: Estimates are based on water consumption at 90th percentile for age and water of 0.87 ppm fluoride. As water consumption decreases and fluoride level in water is reduced to 0.7 ppm fluoride, the proportion of total ingested fluoride from toothpaste will increase.
See Chapter 14 for discussion of fluorosis.

measures. Samples of both are relatively simple to obtain, although both measures reflect only recent fluoride intake (i.e., during the previous 3–4 weeks) rather than lifetime intakes. Urinary concentrations can vary considerably with fluid intake during the period of fluoride exposure,[28] and a 24-hour sample is required for accuracy. Accurate monitoring of plasma levels in individuals also requires frequent measurement because of normal hour-to-hour fluctuations. Plasma fluoride concentrations are more closely correlated with urinary flow rates than with urinary fluoride concentrations.[30] Measurement of fluoride in body fluids has relied on use of a fluoride-specific electrode and this is known to be unreliable at concentrations below about 0.019 mg/L, a level that is typical for individuals consuming water with optimal fluoride. As a result, studies that rely on this method tend to overestimate levels of fluoride in plasma or urine.[53]

Although there is no absolute measure of lifetime fluoride intake, even theoretically, the closest measure of long-term fluoride intake would be based on bone fluoride content. At any point in time, it is estimated that 99% of fluoride in the body is in bone.[53] However, for research purposes, this is a theoretical concept only; people typically do not volunteer to give bone samples! Pharmacokinetic modeling is a tool for integration of estimates from research studies to make predictions. This methodology is well established for bone fluoride modeling, such that bone resorption and formation can be estimated in rats if the fluoride values are known.[45] Using pharmacokinetic models, bone levels of fluoride have been predicted based on chronic exposure to fluoride in water. These models also perform well for patients who underwent osteoporosis treatment involving intakes of 25 mg fluoride per day for up to 6 years.[53] Recently, some initial work using physiologically based pharmacokinetic (PBPK) models has been developed for children in fluoridated and nonfluoridated communities in Canada.[38] As refinements to the input values become validated, these models will allow public health policy makers to examine the impact of approaches to manage fluoride exposure from multiple sources to balance risks of fluorosis and the beneficial reduction of dental caries in the population.

Metabolism of fluoride is essentially the pharmacokinetics of fluoride as it travels through our bodies from ingestion to deposition in tissue, removal from tissue, and excretion. For fluoride, mobilization into and out of tissue is largely influenced by pH. *Fluoride balance* is the net result from the accumulated effects of fluoride ingestion, degree of fluoride deposition in bones and teeth, mobilization rate of fluoride from bone, and efficiency of the kidneys in clearing absorbed fluoride.

Plasma fluoride is found in inorganic and organic forms. The biologic significance of the organic form has not yet been determined, and its concentration is independent of fluoride intake from inorganic, bioavailable sources. Discussions of fluoride physiology in the literature primarily focus on inorganic fluoride. Absorbed fluoride is transported by plasma as ionic fluoride, or "acid-labile fluoride," not bound to proteins in plasma or at least readily available when pH changes.[61] It is the level of this ionic fluoride that rises temporarily after fluoride ingestion and then drops rapidly; ionic fluoride levels are not homeostatically regulated but reflect exposure. In a healthy adult male living in an area with fluoridated water, plasma fluoride levels are around 0.019 ppm (1 μmol/L), although this level fluctuates throughout the day.[29] Plasma levels are generally higher in persons living in fluoridated communities than in those living in nonfluoridated communities. Plasma fluoride levels in persons with chronic kidney failure can rise to 0.05 to 0.09 ppm fluoride (2.6–4.7 μmol/L)

without affecting health.[39] Nephrotoxic plasma fluoride values in healthy individuals have been estimated at 0.95 ppm fluoride (50 μmol/L).

Fluoride has an affinity for calcified tissues, that is, bone and developing teeth. Fluoride that is not excreted is deposited in these hard tissues, although storage is dynamic rather than inert. Bone fluoride levels (from postmortem assays) range from 800 to 10,000 ppm, depending on many factors, including age and fluoride intake. Fluoride levels in the outer few microns of dental enamel range from 400 to 3000 ppm and decrease rapidly with greater enamel depth. Fluoride concentrations in soft tissue rise or fall in parallel with plasma fluoride levels, but because healthy excretion and deposition mechanisms operate so rapidly, there is negligible retention of fluoride in the fluids of soft tissues other than the kidney.[72] Some fluoride has been found in the aorta and the pineal gland, associated with calcification of these tissues.[53] The blood–brain barrier limits fluoride transfer, and the pineal gland lies outside of it. Deposition in the placenta is also associated with islets of calcified tissue.[32] A greater proportion of ingested fluoride is excreted in older persons than in the young because the growing skeleton in young people absorbs more fluoride[71,74] and probably because children have lower renal clearance rates than adults.[65]

Because of the importance of the kidneys in maintaining fluoride balance, the only disease condition that requires medical consideration with regard to fluoride ingestion is chronic kidney failure. Patients who receive renal dialysis for long periods with fluoride-free water have maintained plasma levels of 0.06 ppm fluoride, whereas in some inadvertently receiving dialysis with fluoridated water (definitely not a recommended procedure) levels as high as 0.24 ppm fluoride have been recorded. Although a plasma level of around 0.09 ppm fluoride had been suggested as the upper limit before a kidney patient undergoing dialysis should reduce fluoride intake, evidence for this recommendation has come from only a few case studies.[39] With today's standards for dialysate fluid, current medical opinion is that even persons with severe renal impairment can consume fluoridated water without ill effects as long as they are receiving regular dialysis treatment. Aluminum, iron, and other minerals create greater technical problems for the renal dialysis process than does fluoride. The standard for dialysate water set by the Association for the Advancement of Medical Instrumentation is that the fluoride content should not exceed 0.2 ppm.[19] Water used in renal dialysis should first be treated by reverse osmosis, which is superior to the older process of deionization in that it removes fluoride and other minerals almost entirely.[40]

## Optimal Fluoride Intake

Discussions concerning optimizing fluoride intake have largely been framed in terms of balancing risks and benefits for the population.[66] Table 24.3 is a reproduction of recommended total dietary fluoride published in 2001.[16] In the table, age-specific recommendations for total dietary intake of fluoride are summarized in terms of adequate intake to prevent caries and also avoid the occurrence of moderate enamel fluorosis in developing teeth or skeletal fluorosis in adults.

Discussions about "optimal" intake are vague about what this intake is optimal for. The implication is that this degree of ingestion is optimal for caries resistance (see Spencer et al.[66] for discussion and research gaps). It is also worth noting that McClure's

| • TABLE 24.3 | Recommendations for Using Fluoride to Prevent and Control Dental Caries in the United States. Fluoride Recommendations Work Group MMWR August 17, 2001/50 (RR14);1–42 |
|---|---|

| Age | REFERENCE WEIGHT[a] | | ADEQUATE INTAKE[b] | TOLERABLE UPPER INTAKE[c] |
|---|---|---|---|---|
| | kg | lb | mg/day | mg/day |
| 0–6 months | 7 | 16 | 0.01 | 0.7 |
| 6–12 months | 9 | 20 | 0.5 | 0.9 |
| 1–3 years | 13 | 29 | 0.7 | 1.3 |
| 4–8 years | 22 | 48 | 1.1 | 2.2 |
| ≥9 years | 40–76 | 88–166 | 2.0–3.8 | 10.0 |

[a]Values based on data collected during 1988–1994 as part of the third National Health and Nutrition Examination Survey.

[b]Intake that maximally reduces occurrence of dental caries without causing unwanted side effects, including moderate enamel fluorosis.

[c]Highest level of nutrient intake that is likely to pose no risks for adverse health effects in almost all persons.

1943 comment was observational, although it somehow was turned into a recommendation over time. Empirical evidence suggests that fluoride intake of 0.05 to 0.07 mg/fluoride/kg/day in childhood is a broad upper limit if unesthetic fluorosis is to be avoided.[13] There is no evidence to link this range of fluoride ingestion with caries inhibition, so we suggest that the term *optimal intake* be dropped from common usage. It may be more instructive to think in terms of optimizing fluoride to address risk at the level of the individual. Balancing the benefits of fluoride for caries prevention with risks for fluorosis is in alignment with the practice of precision healthcare—matching age-specific windows of risk to tailored care. In this manner, tailoring fluoride delivery to stages of development reflects management of dental caries as a chronic disease.

## Fluoride and Human Health

The Federal Safe Drinking Water Act requires periodic assessment of our knowledge base "to identify research needed to fill data gaps on total exposures to fluoride and its toxicity." Thus, in 2006, the National Research Council published a comprehensive assessment of the scientific basis for recommendations about the safety and toxicology of fluoride in a 500-page document.[28] The charge to the committee was to review the scientific adequacy of the recommendations for community drinking water standards and identify data gaps and make recommendations for further research. The brief overview below summarizes aspects of public health research and fluoride exposure around the relevant biologic systems.

### Musculoskeletal Effects

The musculoskeletal system is important with respect to fluoride due largely to fluoride's affinity for bone.

### Bone Density, Fracture Experience, and Osteoporosis

Bone fragility conditions (e.g., preventing spontaneous vertebral fracture in the elderly as a result of osteoporosis) have been treated for years with high doses of fluoride combined with calcium, estrogen, and vitamin D. This is because fluoride stimulates osteoblastic activity, whereas other drugs used in the treatment of osteoporosis inhibit bone resorption. Controlled clinical trials have shown that high doses of fluoride (30–60 mg/day), administered under medical supervision, can increase vertebral bone mass and reduce the vertebral fracture rate.[53,56] Haguenauer et al.[33] conducted a meta-analysis of randomized controlled trials and concluded that fluoride has the ability to increase bone mineral density at the lumber spine, but it does not result in a reduction in vertebral fractures.

These studies answer one prominent question about the health effects of fluoride: they show that even frail elderly people can tolerate large fluoride intakes (e.g., 30–60 mg fluoride/day) vastly higher than anyone would experience with fluoridated drinking water. Day-to-day use of fluoridated water obviously results in much lower daily intakes (1–3 mg fluoride/day for adults, see earlier) than those seen at the therapeutic doses just described. In some communities in the United States and in other countries, fluoride occurs naturally at a much higher level in drinking water and therefore the intake can be higher. This varying concentration of naturally occurring fluoride in drinking water has provided an opportunity to compare bone fracture rates between populations exposed to different concentrations of fluoride in drinking water. To assess if water fluoridation increased the risk of fracture, McDonagh et al.[48] included 29 studies in their systematic analysis on the association with bone fracture or problems with bone development and water fluoride. The authors did not find an effect of fluoride on bone fracture at concentrations generally found in fluoridated communities. There were four analyses that indicated a significant increase in risk of fracture and five that indicated a significant decrease in risk at the 5% significance level, with studies that were 10 years or longer in duration associated with a protective effect of water fluoridation on bone fractures.

The U.S. National Research Council's (NRC) review of the effect of fluoride on bone fractures focused its review on studies involving exposure to fluoride in drinking water near or within the range of 2 to 4 mg/L. The review suggested that several strong studies indicated an increased risk of bone fracture.[53] The one study using serum fluoride concentrations found no appreciable relationship to fractures.[64] Li et al.[44] studied bone fractures rates in six Chinese populations with water fluoride concentrations ranging from 0.25 to 7.97 ppm. The authors reported a U-shaped exposure-response curve for all fractures combined (but not hip fractures) for this population of individuals. The prevalence of overall bone fracture was lowest in the population of 1.00 to 1.06 ppm fluoride in drinking water, which was significantly lower ($P < .05$) than that of the groups exposed to water fluoride levels above 4.32 and below 0.34 ppm. Water fluoride levels at 1.00 to 1.06 ppm decreased the risk of overall fractures but not for hip fractures relative to negligible fluoride in water. It should be noted that the total daily fluoride intake in relation to fluoride concentration in drinking water in these Chinese populations is relatively higher compared to that of the US populations. Research continues, but it can be stated that the evidence supports only marginal benefits to bone from fluoridated water, and there is no evidence that bone fracture experience is altered by exposure to drinking water containing 1.0 ppm fluoride.[37,59,68,75]

## Skeletal Fluorosis

Skeletal fluorosis is a condition associated with prolonged ingestion or inhalation of high amounts of fluoride. It is characterized by sporadic pain, stiffness of the joints, and osteosclerosis of the pelvis and spine. The condition is progressive and in advanced stages, it is characterized by calcification of ligaments, limitation of joint movement and crippling deformities of the spine and major joints. It has been reported in individuals residing in India, China, and Africa, where the fluoride intake is exceptionally high from a variety of sources including high concentration of fluoride in drinking water and indoor burning of fluoride-rich coal resulting in a high indoor fluoride concentration. The early stages of the condition are reversible by reducing fluoride intake.

Very few reports of skeletal fluorosis have been documented in the United States. Based on limited studies of these individuals, it is suggested that a daily fluoride dose in excess of 10 mg over a period of 10 years may be required to produce signs of skeletal fluorosis. Izuora and colleagues[36] reported a case of a 48-year-old white woman from Georgia who reported throbbing, severe bone and joint discomfort over the previous decade. Painful areas included her elbows, wrists, hips, knees, and ankles. According to the authors, her dietary history disclosed that she imbibed 1 to 2 gallons of brewed orange-pekoe and pekoe-cut black tea daily since age 12 years. The authors estimated a daily intake of 14.6 or 29.3 mg of fluoride depending on the amount of water consumed. The patient reported complete resolution of pain 6 months after cessation of tea drinking and while continuing ergocalciferol (vitamin D2).

## Reproductive and Developmental Effects

The NRC report concluded that high-quality studies in laboratory animals over a range of fluoride concentrations (0–250 mg/L in drinking water) indicate that adverse reproductive and developmental outcomes occur only at very high concentrations.[53] The studies of human populations have design limitations that make them of little value for risk evaluation at levels below 4 mg/L of fluoride in drinking water.

The focus of the early human studies has been on the role of fluoride in the birth of children with Down syndrome. Down syndrome is a genetic disorder caused by an extra copy of all or part of chromosome 21. Advanced maternal age is a known risk factor of having a child with Down syndrome. The 2000 McDonagh review[48] included six studies that considered the relationship between fluoride exposure and Down syndrome. All six studies were assessed as being of poor quality and most did not control for confounders. The authors concluded that the evidence for an association between water fluoride level and the incidence of Down syndrome is weak. Public Health England (PHE), an expert national public health agency, analyzed data collected in England and found that after adjusting for maternal age, there was no evidence of an association between fluoridation and Down syndrome.[59] Because of routine genetic testing and early diagnosis in the United States and other countries, it will be difficult to study the incidence of Down syndrome and conduct analysis to assess the effect of exposure to fluoride.

## Neurotoxicity and Neurobehavioral Effects

In the National Research Council report it was recommended that further research be conducted to assess the role of fluoride exposure in neurodevelopment, specifically on measures of intelligence such as IQ deficits resulting from fluoride exposure.[53] In 2012, a systematic review of relatively obscure cross-sectional studies—mostly conducted in areas of China where fluoride levels were 2.5 to 4 times higher than United States—raised concerns.[17] However, the fundamental concern is whether results from these cross-sectional studies conducted in high-fluoride areas are relevant to humans at the level of fluoride exposure in the United States.

Broadbent et al.[12] conducted an analysis of longitudinal data collected in New Zealand for IQ measures over 30 years. The study provided no evidence of risk in IQ deficits attributable to community water fluoride at ages 7 to 13 years and age 38 years. The exposures in the study were similar to those in developed countries such as the United States. In 2017, a study in Mexico was published that raised concerns about fluoride exposure during pregnancy.[6] The study found that urinary fluoride during pregnancy was associated with a decline in cognitive ability at age 4 among 287 children and at ages 6 to 12 among 211 children.

Another study[5] published in 2017 provided assurance that fluoride exposure at levels relevant for the general population was not linked to learning disabilities in children. Researchers in Canada used population-based data to assess a subsample of children who had tap water and urinary samples collected and analyzed for fluoride content. The investigators did not find an association between fluoride exposure and self-reported measures of learning disabilities in families of children ages 3 to 12. Research conducted in Sweden on a large registry of more than 40,000 individuals provides some compelling evidence for the safety of fluoride in drinking water.[1] They concluded that there was essentially no evidence of an effect of fluoride on these neurodevelopmental outcomes.

Animal data also provide assurance of safety with respect to fluoride exposure and neurodevelopmental outcomes. In 2018 the National Toxicology Program (NTP) of the U.S. Department of Health and Human Services published results from animal studies that were designed to address limitations identified in the NRC report.[51] These results did not find exposure-related differences in motor, sensory, or learning and memory performances in rats.

Although the evidence for significant detrimental effects arising from fluoride exposure in the perinatal period is weak, further research continues because child development is an important topic known to vary based on a wide range of exposures.[76,77] Data on fluoride will be among the array of variables that researchers will examine since it is relatively straightforward to analyze fluoride with the other environmental measures that are collected.

## Effects on the Endocrine Systems

Endocrine systems play roles in a variety of hormonal interactions that have an impact on a range of biologic processes such as sexual maturity and regulation of metabolism. Some studies of fluoride exposure in drinking water at levels below 4 mg/L have demonstrated associations between fluoride level and thyroid function. However, the changes observed in thyroid function are not linked to an adverse health condition. For example, calcitonin and parathyroid hormone levels may be observed to be higher in individuals exposed to fluoride, but normal physiologic functions are not impaired. Most studies of the impact of fluoride exposure on the endocrine system are primarily focused on thyroid function. Two recent studies are described here.

One is an ecologic study from the United Kingdom,[58] and the other is a cross-sectional study from Canada.[4] Both had limitations, but the ecologic design is inferior in that the exposure—fluoride in this case—is not measured at the level of the individual.

The Canadian study[4] had good measures of exposure at the level of individual, but being a cross-sectional study, the exposure only reflected the current level fluoride and did not provide longitudinal exposure history, although the study participants did provide residence histories going back 3 years so that exposure histories could be constructed. The cross-sectional design is a limitation. However, the study did make use of a population-based sample that is representative of the Canadian population. It showed no association between fluoride level and thyroid stimulating hormone or self-reported thyroid disorders. In addition to residence histories for the past 3 years, tap water samples and urine samples from study participants were used to assess fluoride exposure. The study provides good evidence that at the level of the individual, fluoride exposure at levels common to the general population does not impair thyroid function.

In 2015 researchers from England conducted an ecologic study that looked at the association between locations with fluoridated water and prevalence of hypothyroidism from a registry kept by the national health system.[58] The data showed an association between diagnosis of hypothyroidism and living in an area where public water is fluoridated. The authors note that only 10% of the population has exposure to public water systems that are fluoridated. This raises concerns that people living in communities that fluoridate the water may also differ in other ways from the 90% of the people living in other nonfluoride communities.

The thyroid gland is of importance to fluoride safety largely because we know that fluoride (fluorine) and iodine have similar chemical properties, and iodine is clearly linked to healthy thyroid function. The two studies that were published since the NRC report each had limitations, and taken together they did not demonstrate any adverse health outcomes attributable to fluoride.

## Effects on the Gastrointestinal, Renal, Hepatic, and Immune Systems

The National Research Council reviewed effects of fluoride in drinking water on a variety of other organ systems, including the gastrointestinal system, kidneys, liver, and the immune system. It is clear that fluoride concentrations above 4 mg/L can be irritating to the gastrointestinal tract.[53] However, the NRC concluded that effects on the gastrointestinal system, including renal and hepatic tissues, are unlikely for exposures below 4 mg/L. Individuals on renal dialysis are a special population and care must be taken to ensure that water is properly handled to avoid exposure to a variety of agents found in tap water, including fluoride.[40]

## Genotoxicity and Carcinogenicity

Concerns about cancer incidence and mortality due to exposure to fluoride have been raised for many years, but these studies have been of low quality and lacked scientific rigor. Of particular concern in these studies is the assessment of exposure to fluoride that occurred at the community level or group level and did not consider total fluoride intake at the individual level. Many difficulties are encountered in conducting studies of cancer. Cancers arise in different tissues and organ systems by different pathways. Because of the long latency period that can take 10 years or longer before a diagnosis of cancer is made, it is difficult to assess exposure to causal factors in human populations. Many cancers like osteosarcomas are rare, and statistical inference is difficult when associations are weak. Animal studies can yield information that helps to focus hypotheses about risk factors for specific cancers in humans. However,

there are limits to the generalizability of findings in animal studies for humans.

The NRC report identified osteosarcoma, a form of bone cancer, as the cancer endpoint that met criteria for biologic plausibility.[52,53] Biological plausibility is one component of a method of reasoning that provides an explanation for the underlying mechanism of the effect, as fluoride in high doses has the ability to stimulate osteoblasts. The stimulation of cell division or mitogenicity may lead to carcinogenesis by facilitation of mutational changes. Animal studies, however, have yielded both positive and negative results.[52]

In 1990, an animal study conducted as part of the NTP raised concern about the potential for fluoride to cause osteosarcoma.[54] The findings from the NTP study were determined to be "equivocal" and indicated a need for further evaluation. A follow-up NTP study found no treatment-related increases at a higher dose of fluoride exposure (250 ppm) in male F344/N rats. Since then a number of cross-sectional and case-control epidemiologic studies of osteosarcoma have been conducted in varying parts of the world with both positive and negative findings. In a 2000 systematic review, McDonagh et al.[48] found that of nine studies comprising 20 analyses of bone cancers, one found a significant negative effect in both men and boys (more cancers).

In 2006, a study reported by Bassin and colleagues attracted considerable media attention because the authors concluded that their exploratory analysis found an association between fluoride exposure in drinking water during childhood and the incidence of osteosarcoma among boys but not consistently among girls.[7] The exposure to fluoride was determined by interviewing subjects to determine whether they had resided in a fluoridated or a nonfluoridated community. A follow-up study conducted by Kim and colleagues used bone fluoride levels to determine fluoride exposure and showed no significant association between bone fluoride levels and osteosarcoma.[42]

In 2016, the National Health and Medical Research Council (NHMRC) of Australia conducted a comprehensive evaluation of health effects of fluoride in drinking water, NHMRC Evidence Evaluation.[37] This evaluation included six studies that assessed osteosarcoma and water fluoridation. Five of these studies were conducted in four different countries (the United Kingdom, United States, Republic of Ireland, and New Zealand) and found no association between water fluoridation and osteosarcoma. The sixth study suggested that osteosarcoma was related to fluoride levels in drinking water. However, unlike the five studies that were based on large and well-established cancer registries, the sixth study included only 10 people with osteosarcoma and 10 without and was considered low quality. This led to the conclusion that there is no association between water fluoridation at current Australian levels of fluoride in drinking water and incidence of osteosarcoma.

Overall, more recent high-quality studies have not shown consistent evidence that fluoride is a risk factor for cancer incidence in humans. This is further bolstered by the fact that osteosarcoma remains a rare cancer and is not increasing either in countries where community water fluoridation is practiced or in countries such as China, India, and African nations where endemic areas with occurrence of skeletal fluorosis is common.

## Fluoride: Public Health Considerations

Acute toxicity from fluoride exposure at levels found in drinking water does not occur, but water operators work with concentrations of fluoride that are highly toxic before they are diluted. Work processes to ensure safety are followed and verified by testing of water prior to leaving the water plant. Guidelines for water operators are well established.

Assurance of the safety of chronic exposure to low levels of fluoride has been a pillar of public health practice, and the knowledge base continues to grow. For more than 70 years, community water fluoridation has met rigorous scientific standards for safety. The role of fluoride in caries prevention has grown, and multiple sources of fluoride exposure have emerged. To date, the accumulated studies do not demonstrate cause for concern beyond the adverse cosmetic effect of enamel fluorosis. Efforts to prevent enamel fluorosis at the population level have led to a revision of the Centers for Disease Control and Prevention guideline for fluoride in public water systems to 0.7 ppm (mg/L). This revision represents active engagement and a collaborative approach toward policy development and assurance based on surveillance data. Collaboration between public health officials, the dental profession, and community stakeholders led to the change.

As a profession, dentistry is committed to public health. Dental professionals act as both advocates for patients and as citizen-scientists in their communities. These two roles play out quite clearly around the topic of fluoride. In large measure, these roles share a common commitment to the ethical principles of beneficence and nonmaleficence—optimizing benefits and minimizing risks (see Chapter 3) in public health practice - assuring the public of safety and improving population health.

# References

1. Aggeborn L, Ohman M. *The Effects of Fluoride in the Drinking Water.* Uppsala, Sweden: Institute for Evaluation of Labour Market and Education Policy; 2017.
2. Ainsworth NJ. Mottled teeth. *Br Dent J.* 1933;55:233–250.
3. Ast DB. The caries-fluorine hypothesis and a suggested study to test its application. *Public Health Rep (1896–1970).* 1943;58(23): 857–879.
4. Barberio AM, Hosein FS, Quiñonez C, et al. Fluoride exposure and indicators of thyroid functioning in the Canadian population: implications for community water fluoridation. *J Epidemiol Commun Health.* 2017;71(10):1019–1025.
5. Barberio AM, Quiñonez C, Hosein FS, McLaren L. Fluoride exposure and reported learning disability diagnosis among Canadian children: implications for community water fluoridation. *Can J Pub Health.* 2017;108(3):e229–e239.
6. Bashash M, Thomas D, Hu H, et al. Prenatal fluoride exposure and cognitive outcomes in children at 4 and 6–12 years of age in Mexico. *Environ Health Perspect.* 2017;125(9).
7. Bassin EB, Wypij D, Davis RB, Mittleman MA. Age-specific fluoride exposure in drinking water and osteosarcoma (United States). *Cancer Cause Control.* 2006;17(4):421–428.
8. Beltrán-Aguilar ED, Barker L, Sohn W, Wei L. Water intake by outdoor temperature among children aged 1–10 years: implications for community water fluoridation in the U.S. *Public Health Rep.* 2015;130(4):362–371.
9. Berg J, Gerweck C, Hujoel PP, et al. Evidence-based clinical recommendations regarding fluoride intake from reconstituted infant formula and enamel fluorosis: a report of the American Dental Association Council on Scientific Affairs. *J Am Dent Assoc.* 2011;142(1):79–87.
10. Bhagavatula P, Curtis A, Broffitt B, et al. The relationships between fluoride intake levels and fluorosis of late-erupting permanent teeth. *J Public Health Dent.* 2018;78(2):165–174.
11. Black GV, McKay FS. Mottled teeth—an endemic developmental imperfection of the teeth heretofore unknown in the literature of dentistry. *Dent Cosmos.* 1916;58:129–156.
12. Broadbent JM, Thomson WM, Ramrakha S, et al. Community water fluoridation and intelligence: prospective study in New Zealand. *Am J Public Health.* 2015;105(1):72–76.
13. Burt BA. The changing patterns of systemic fluoride intake. *J Dent Res.* 1992;71(5):1228–1237.
14. Buzalaf MAR, Granjeiro JM, Damante CA, et al. Fluoride content of infant formulas prepared with deionized, bottled mineral and fluoridated drinking water. *J Dent Children.* 2001;68(1):37–41.
15. Cammack Smith M, Lantz E, Smith HV. The cause of mottled enamel. *J Dent Res.* 1932;12(1):149–159.
16. CDC Fluoride Recommendations Work Group. Recommendations for using fluoride to prevent and control dental caries in the United States. *Morb Mortal Weekly Rep.* 2001;50:1–42.
17. Choi AL, Sun G, Zhang Y, Grandjean P. Developmental fluoride neurotoxicity: a systematic review and meta-analysis. *Environ Health Perspect.* 2012;120(10):1362–1368.
18. Churchill HV. Occurrence of fluorides in some waters of the United States. *J Ind Eng Chem.* 1931;23(9):996–998.
19. Coulliette AD, Arduino MJ. Hemodialysis and water quality. *Sem Dialysis.* 2013;26(4):427–438.
20. Dabeka RW, McKenzie AD, Lacroix GMA. Dietary intakes of lead, cadmium, arsenic and fluoride by Canadian adults: a 24-hour duplicate diet study. *Food Add Contam.* 1987;4(1):89–101.
21. Dean HT. Chronic endemic dentaln fluorosis: (mottled enamel). *JAMA.* 1936;107(16):1269–1273.
22. Dean HT, Arnold FA Jr, Elvove E. Domestic water and dental caries: V. Additional studies of the relation of fluoride domestic waters to dental caries experience in 4,425 white children, aged 12 to 14 years, of 13 cities in 4 states. *Public Health Rep (1896–1970).* 1942;57(32): 1155–1179.
23. Dean HT, Brandt EN. Endemic fluorosis and its relation to dental caries (1938) [with Commentary]. *Public Health Rep (1974–).* 2006;121:212–219.
24. Dean HT, Elvove E. Studies on the minimal threshold of the dental sign of chronic endemic fluorosis (mottled enamel). *Public Health Rep (1896–1970).* 1935;50(49):1719–1729.
25. Dean HT, Elvove E. Some epidemiological aspects of chronic endemic dental fluorosis. *Am J Public Health Nations Health.* 1936;26(6):567–575.
26. Dean HT, Jay P, Arnold F Jr, et al. Domestic water and dental caries, including certain epidemiological aspects of oral L. acidophilus. *Public Health Rep (1896–1970).* 1939;54(21):862–888.
27. Dean HT, Jay P, Arnold FA Jr, et al. Domestic water and dental caries: II. A study of 2,832 white children, aged 12–14 years, of 8 suburban Chicago communities, including Lactobacillus acidophilus studies of 1,761 children. *Public Health Rep (1896–1970).* 1941;56 (15):761–792.
28. Ehrnebo M, Ekstrand J. Occupational fluoride exposure and plasma fluoride levels in man. *Int Arch Occup Environ Health.* 1986;58(3): 179–190.
29. Ekstrand J. *Fluoride Metabolism.* Copenhagen, Denmark: Munksgaard; 1996.
30. Ekstrand J, Ehrnebo M. The relationship between plasma fluoride, urinary excretion rate and urine fluoride concentration in man. *J Occup Med.* 1983;25(10):745–748.
31. EPA, Health and Ecological Criteria Division Office of Water. *Fluoride: Exposure and Relative Source Contribution Analysis.* Washington, DC: US Environmental Protection Agency; 2010.
32. Ericsson Y, Malmnäs C. Placental transfer of fluorine investigated with F18 in man and rabbit. *Acta Obstet Gyn Scan.* 1962;41(2):144–158.
33. Haguenauer D, Welch V, Shea B, et al. Fluoride for the treatment of postmenopausal osteoporotic fractures: a meta-analysis. *Osteoporosis Int.* 2000;11(9):727–738.
34. Heilman JR, Kiritsy MC, Levy SM, et al. Assessing fluoride levels of carbonated soft drinks. *J Am Dent Assoc.* 1999;130(11):1593–1599.

35. Hong L, Levy SM, Broffitt B, et al. Timing of fluoride intake in relation to development of fluorosis on maxillary central incisors. *Community Dent Oral Epidemiol.* 2006;34(4):299–309.

36. Izuora K, Twombly JG, Whitford GM, et al. Skeletal fluorosis from brewed tea. *J Clin Endocrin Metab.* 2011;96(8):2318–2324.

37. Jack B, Ayson M, Lewis S, et al. *Health Effects of Water Fluoridation: Evidence Evaluation Report.* Sydney, Australia: University of Sydney, NHRMC Clinical Trials Centre; 2016.

38. Jean KJ, Wassef N, Gagnon F. A physiologically-based pharmacokinetic modeling approach using biomonitoring data in order to assess the contribution of drinking water for the achievement of an optimal fluoride dose for dental health in children. *Int J Environ Res Public Health.* 2018;15(7):1358.

39. Johnson WJ, Taves DR, Jowsey J. Fluoridation and bone disease in renal patients. In: *Oral Presentation at: AAAS Selected Symposium Number 11;* 1979. Boulder, CO.

40. Kasparek T, Rodriguez OE. What medical directors need to know about dialysis facility water management. *Clin J Am Soc Nephr.* 2015;10(6):1061–1071.

41. Kramer L, Osis D, Wiatrowski E, Spencer H. Dietary fluoride in different areas in the United States. *Am J Clin Nutr.* 1974;27(6):590–594.

42. Lee JY, Divaris K, Baker AD, Rozier RG, Lee S-YD, Vann WF Jr. Oral health literacy levels among a low-income WIC population. *J Public Health Dent.* 2011;71(2):152–160.

43. Levy SM, Warren JJ, Davis CS, Kirchner HL, Kanellis MJ, Wefel JS. Patterns of fluoride intake from birth to 36 months. *J Public Health Dent.* 2007;61(2):70–77.

44. Li Y, Liang C, Slemenda CW, et al. Effect of long-term exposure to fluoride in drinking water on risks of bone fractures. *J Bone Mineral Res.* 2001;16(5):932–939.

45. Lupo M, Brance ML, Fina BL, Brun LR, Rigalli A. Methodology developed for the simultaneous measurement of bone formation and bone resorption in rats based on the pharmacokinetics of fluoride. *J Bone Mineral Metab.* 2014;33(1):16–22.

46. Manji F, Kapila S. Fluorides and fluorosis in Kenya. Part I: The occurrence of fluorides. *Odonto-stoma tropicale.* 1986;9(1):15–20.

47. McClure FJ. *Water Fluoridation: The Search and the Victory.* Bethesda, MD: US Department of Health, Education, and Welfare; 1970.

48. McDonagh MS, Kleijnen J, Whiting PF, et al. Systematic review of water fluoridation. *Br Med J.* 2000;321(7265):855–859.

49. McKay FS. The relation of mottled enamel to caries. *J Am Dent Assoc.* 1928;15(8):1429–1437.

50. McKay FS. Mottled enamel: the prevention of its further production through a change of the water supply at Oakley, Ida. *J Am Dent Assoc.* 1933;20(7):1137–1149.

51. McPherson CA, Zhang G, Gilliam R, et al. An evaluation of neurotoxicity following fluoride exposure from gestational through adult ages in Long-Evans hooded rats. *Neurotoxicity Res.* 2018;1–18.

52. Morry DW, Steinmaus C. *Evidence on the Carcinogenicity of Fluoride and Its Salts.* Sacramento, CA: Office of Environmental Health Hazard Assessment's Reproductive and Cancer Hazard Assessment Branch; 2011.

53. National Research Council. *Fluoride in Drinking Water: A Scientific Review of EPA's Standards.* Washington, DC: The National Academies Press; 2006.

54. National Toxicology Program. *Toxicology and Carcinogenesis Studies of Sodium Fluoride in F344/N Rats and B6C3F1 Mice.* Research Triangle Park, NC: National Toxicology Program (NTP); 1990.

55. Osis D, Kramer L, Wiatrowski E, Spencer H. Dietary fluoride intake in man. *J Nutr.* 1974;104(10):1313–1318.

56. Pak CYC, Sakhaee K, Piziak V, et al. Slow-release sodium fluoride in the management of postmenopausal osteoporosis. A randomized controlled trial. *Ann Int Med.* 1994;120(8):625–632.

57. Pang DTY, Phillips CL, Bawden JW. Fluoride intake from beverage consumption in a sample of North Carolina children. *J Dent Res.* 1992;71(7):1382–1388.

58. Peckham S, Lowery D, Spencer S. Are fluoride levels in drinking water associated with hypothyroidism prevalence in england? A large observational study of GP practice data and fluoride levels in drinking water. *J Epidemiol Commun Health.* 2015;69(7):619–624.

59. Public Health England. *Water Fluoridation. Health monitoring report for England.* London, England: PHE Publications; 2018. 2018.

60. San Filippo FA, Battistone GC. The fluoride content of a representative diet of the young adult male. *Clin Chimica Acta.* 1971;31(2):453–457.

61. Singer L, Ophaug R, Myers HM. Ionic and nonionic fluoride in plasma (or serum). *CRC Critical Rev Clin Lab Sci.* 1982;18(2):111–140.

62. Singer L, Ophaug RH, Harland BF. Fluoride intakes of young male adults in the United States. *The. Am J Clin Nutr.* 1980;33(2):328–332.

63. Singer L, Ophaug RH, Harland BF. Dietary fluoride intake of 15–19-year-old male adults residing in the United States. *J Dent Res.* 1985;64(11):1302–1305.

64. Sowers M, Whitford GM, Clark MK, et al. Elevated serum fluoride concentrations in women are not related to fractures and bone mineral density. *J Nutr.* 2005;135(9):2247–2252.

65. Spak CJ, Berg U, Ekstrand J. Renal clearance of fluoride in children and adolescents. *Pediatrics.* 1985;75(3):575–579.

66. Spencer AJ, Do LG, Mueller U, et al. Understanding optimum fluoride intake from population-level evidence. *Adv Dent Res.* 2018;29(2):144–156.

67. Spencer H, Osis D, Lender M. Studies of fluoride metabolism in man: a review and report of original data. *Sci Total Environ.* 1981;17(1):1–12.

68. Sutton M, Kiersey R, Farragher L, et al. Health effects of water fluoridation. In: *An Evidence Review.* Dublin, Ireland: Health Research Board, 2015.

69. USDHHS Federal Panel on Community Water Fluoridation. US Public Health Service recommendation for fluoride concentration in drinking water for the prevention of dental caries. *Public Health Rep.* 2015;130(4):318–331.

70. Velu HBL. Darmous (dystrophie dentaire) du mouton et solubilité du principé actif des phosphates naturels qui le provique. *Bull Soc Pathol Exot.* 1931;24:848–851.

71. Villa A, Anabalón M, Cabezas L. The fractional urinary fluoride excretion in young children under stable fluoride intake conditions. *Community Dent Oral Epidemiol.* 2000;28(5):344–355.

72. Whitford GM. Fluoride metabolism. In: Newbrun E, ed. *Fluorides and Dental Caries: Contemporary Concepts for Practioners and Students.* 3rd ed. Springfield, IL: Thomas; 1986:174–198.

73. Whitford GM. The metabolism and toxicity of fluoride. *Monogr Oral Sci.* 1996;16:1–153. Rev 2.

74. Whitford GM. Fluoride metabolism and excretion in children. *J Public Health Dent.* 1999;59(4):224–228.

75. Yin XH, Huang GL, Lin DR, et al. Exposure to fluoride in drinking water and hip fracture risk: a meta-analysis of observational studies. *PLoS One.* 2015;10(5).

76. National Toxicology Program. *Draft NTP Monograph on the Systematic Review of Fluoride Exposure and Neurodevelopmental and Cognitive Health Effects.* Washington, DC: USDHHS, September 6, 2019. https://www.asdwa.org/wp-content/uploads/2019/10/draft_fluoride_monograph_20190906_5081.pdf.

77. Green R, Lanphear B, Hornung R, Flora D, Martinez-Mier A, Neufeld R, Ayotte P, Muckle G, Till C. Association Between Maternal Fluoride Exposure During Pregnancy and IQ Scores in Offspring in Canada. *JAMA Pediatr.* 2019;173(10):940–948. https://doi.org/10.1001/jamapediatrics.2019.1729.

# 25

# Fluoride and Caries Prevention

MARK E. MOSS, DDS, PhD

DOMENICK T. ZERO, DDS, MS

## Introduction

The benefits of fluoride not only in public water systems but also in a wide variety of formulations and delivery vehicles are generally accepted by the public health community, dental researchers, and practicing professionals worldwide.[56,102,105] This chapter presents an overview of the role of fluoride in preventing dental caries. It summarizes material from systematic reviews and clinical recommendations published by panels who developed evidence-based guidelines. The reader is encouraged to track these sources because updates occur frequently, and new evidence is routinely integrated into our knowledge base for fluoride.

The chapter begins with a mechanistic view of fluoride in caries prevention then describes the ways prevention can be tailored to address health across different settings beginning with the population level and then focusing on clinical dental practice uses of fluoride before finally expanding beyond the traditional dental practice setting to address high-risk groups outside of the dental clinical using innovative approaches to extend prevention.

The remarkable therapeutic anticaries effect of fluoride is now recognized to be primarily mediated by its posteruptive (topical) interaction with the tooth structure. Early observational studies identified a role for fluoride in enamel formation because of a condition known as dental fluorosis (see Chapter 24). This led to studies that focused on fluoride reactivity with tooth mineral and its incorporation into the developing tooth structure, which forms a more stable mineral phase, known as fluorapatite, thus decreasing acid solubility and preventing dental decay. However, the earlier emphasis on the importance of fluoride incorporation during tooth formation (its preeruptive effect) has been overshadowed by more recent studies, and it is now generally accepted that the posteruptive (topical) interaction of fluoride with the tooth structure accounts for the vast majority of fluoride's anticaries benefit.[66] At recommended levels in drinking water, fluoride provides a low-cost, steady-state background level of protection that shifts the distribution of dental caries in a favorable manner for an entire community.

Over-the-counter (OTC) oral care products, purchased by individuals, have fluoride levels at concentrations sufficient to penetrate the dental biofilm that forms on tooth surfaces, delivering therapeutic levels of fluoride to the enamel and more importantly concentrating fluoride in incipient lesions. To a large extent, community water fluoridation at the population level and OTC oral care products with fluoride at the individual level are sufficient for caries prevention for many individuals. However, for some high-risk groups and individuals, targeted approaches can be beneficial. This chapter highlights the ways that fluoride can be used in different formulations and in a range of settings to prevent dental caries. For each fluoride modality, there is a biomechanical context for effective delivery of the fluoride agent as well as a policy-societal context. The aim is to provide the reader with knowledge to support effective options for dental caries prevention using fluoride modalities.

## Fluoride and the Science of Prevention

Prevention can be described in a variety of ways. Some preventive interventions target entire populations and others are focused on individuals who are at the highest level of risk.[113] Recently, Auerbach[14] has conceptualized prevention across three broad settings with clinical care (an individual-based approach) at one extreme and traditional public health or population-based approaches at the other extreme. In the middle, Auerbach identifies innovative hybrid approaches that seek to extend clinical preventive interventions into nontraditional community settings. This conceptualization highlights a role for targeting high-risk groups such as children attending schools in communities with low socioeconomic status or children on Medicaid. Because fluoride has been adapted for simple applications that are effective, it has helped bridge the gap between public health and traditional clinical care to offer options for Auerbach's middle prevention "bucket" outside the clinical setting (Figure 25.1).

The figure shows how extending evidence-based interventions into nontraditional settings can increase the number of high-risk individuals who have access to the intervention. These efforts typically involve partnerships or collaborations to provide services in new settings or innovative ways, such as application of fluoride varnish in schools with a high proportion of children at high risk for caries because of low socioeconomic status. Table 25.1 shows how caries prevention can be structured in each of Auerbach's settings.

The delivery of a preventive intervention can target individuals, whole populations, or groups within a population. In a population-based approach, the preventive intervention is applied to shift the entire population risk profile to a more favorable distribution.[113] Community water fluoridation is an excellent example of the population-based approach to prevention. In the high-risk approach, a preventive intervention is applied to individuals who have been identified as having a greater risk for the condition of interest. A fluoride varnish application for a child with white-spot lesions is an

example of a high-risk approach. Since the high-risk approach requires a determination of risk status to identify individuals to be targeted, a clinical evaluation is often required, and this can limit the public health application of the high-risk approach. However, high-risk groups can be identified using other measures that occur at the level of the population. Socioeconomic status can be used to identify schools with high-risk children. School-based dental caries prevention programs that target high-risk schools–where more than 50% of the children are in a free or reduced lunch program–are examples of the high risk approach applied to groups in community settings. A range of approaches can complement one another and be used together, especially for a condition like dental caries in which nearly the entire population is at risk.

Prevention affects a disease process at different levels. In terms of dental caries, primary prevention aims to keep healthy people from developing carious lesions. In secondary prevention, we are screening to detect caries at an early stage to intervene to stop or reverse lesion progression. In tertiary prevention we are addressing advanced disease to minimize the impact on quality of life and function. Until recently, restorative dentistry was the only form of tertiary prevention for dental caries, in that it seeks to restore function and prevent pain and tooth loss. Evidence now exists to support a role for silver diamine fluoride (SDF) within the context of nonrestorative treatment for carious lesions that can be fairly advanced.[123] In addition to a role in secondary prevention, use of SDF extends options for tertiary prevention by halting disease progression in teeth that have severe carious breakdown as part of care management. The next section provides an overview of the caries process to provide an understanding of the mechanistic role of fluoride in prevention of dental caries.

## Overview of Dental Caries

To fully appreciate the role of fluoride in caries prevention, we must understand the caries process. Traditionally, this has followed a path built around the concepts of agent, host, and environment that permeate public health. In 1962, Keyes[75] outlined the triad for dental caries as (1) host and teeth, (2) diet and substrate, and (3) microflora. Keyes stressed the interconnections between these domains and laid the framework for research around them. For fluoride, a role in "host fortification" was described. This conceptual framework has served to underscore the importance of interactions among the components of the triad. For example, diet emphasizes the complexity of the host–substrate interaction, and

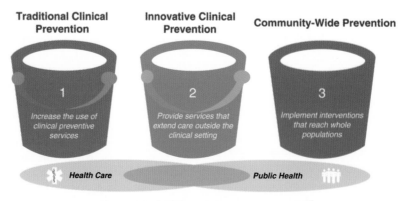

• **Figure 25.1** The Three Buckets of Prevention.[14]

## • TABLE 25.1  Framing Use of Fluoride Into Auerbach's "Three Buckets of Prevention"[14]

| Setting | Target Group | Dental Professional's Role | Intervention Goal |
|---|---|---|---|
| **Traditional Clinical Setting** | | | |
| Examples:<br>Silver diamine fluoride application<br>High fluoride toothpaste prescription | High-risk individuals | Clinical management | • Shift risk status of individual<br>• Empower individual to manage oral health |
| **Nontraditional Community Setting** | | | |
| Examples:<br>Fluoride varnish or fluoride mouth rinse program in schools | High-risk groups—defined by social determinants such as schools with high proportion of children from families with low socioeconomic status, or children on Medicaid | Delegated and collaborative—shared with community partner | • Improve access to prevention<br>• Shift risk distribution in group<br>• Triage and case management of those needing clinical care<br>• Improve oral health literacy |
| **Traditional Public Health Setting** | | | |
| Examples:<br>Water fluoridation<br>Salt fluoridation<br>Milk fluoridation | Whole population | Advisory and advocacy—promote policies that address health equity | Shift risk distribution in population |

the substrate–microflora interaction emphasizes the factors that lead to the production of acids that damage the surfaces that are in close proximity. This dietomicrobial challenge remains the driving force of dental caries activity. Today we have a greater appreciation for the complexity of these interactions and the difficulty in designing effective preventive interventions to address them. Building from Keyes' triad, the interaction of host and microflora is now better understood as the oral microbiome and the tooth–microflora interaction is better understood as the oral biofilm.

The concept of the oral microbiome represents the idea that bacteria are part of a complex host–microbe community where the oral cavity serves as an ecologic niche for a diverse array of microorganisms that will behave differently under different conditions.[81] Many of these complex interactions help maintain a steady state of health by providing a barrier of protection and through supporting our immune system. When this complex ecologic balance is disturbed, a shift can occur that favors conditions that can cause disease.[114]

The microflora in dental plaque is properly understood as the manifestation of a biofilm that covers the teeth. Biofilm is a general term for a surface-attached microbial colony.[130] The biofilm describes the characteristics of the layer of microorganisms and debris that covers our teeth and gums. This biofilm is intrinsically linked to the health of our mouths. The biofilm serves as a mediator between the external environment and oral hard and soft tissues that are covered by the biofilm.

Preventive strategies aim to address the ecology of the biofilm to favor conditions that ensure healthy interactions with tooth surfaces. Elimination of specific microflora has proven difficult, and mechanical dislodgment of biofilm through toothbrushing can disrupt some pathogenic biofilm accumulation but will not eliminate the biofilm completely, especially in areas that are difficult to access. Current interventions that use fluoride take advantage of its ability to play a therapeutic role under the pH conditions that are found in the biofilm.[77] A large part of the clinical effectiveness of fluoride is based on its capacity to concentrate in the biofilm and serve as a reservoir for fluoride, where it can be readily available to modify the dynamic caries process in favor of arresting and

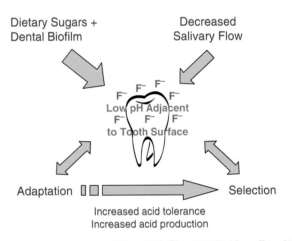

Dynamic Ecology of Dental Biofilm   Modified from Zero (1993)

• **Figure 25.2**  Conceptual model of the primary drivers of dental caries.

reversing caries progression. In this chapter, we describe how fluoride functions within this paradigm.

Dental caries is primarily the consequence of a physiologic process of adaptation by (endogenous) bacteria in the biofilm to a low pH environment (Figure 25.2).[145] Dental caries can be described best as a complex biofilm-mediated disease that can be mostly ascribed to behaviors involving frequent ingestion of fermentable carbohydrate (sugars such as glucose, fructose, sucrose, and maltose) and poor oral hygiene in combination with inadequate fluoride exposure.[107]

## Components of Biofilm Dynamics of Importance to Dental Caries

### Dietary Sugars

Dietary sugars play a prominent role in driving the caries process.[120,147] Certain oral microorganisms are equipped to ferment sugars and create a protective matrix of extracellular polymeric substances, and this sets the stage for a cascade of events that transform the microenvironment within the biofilm. Acids generated by sugar metabolism lower the pH, favoring species that can adapt and tolerate (aciduric) low pH conditions, thus shifting the ecology of the biofilm to favor a dominant role for greater acid production in areas of the biofilm that are anatomically well suited to avoid mechanical debridement from toothbrushing. The protective effects of saliva also depend on the sufficiency of the salivary glands to produce saliva and the ability for an adequate amount of saliva to reach the biofilm to buffer the acid challenge to the enamel surface of the tooth. Saliva also plays a key role in the process of mineralization that occurs in enamel.[29,34]

From a pragmatic perspective, interventions that do not rely heavily on individual behavior are more likely to be effective.[60] It is clearly difficult to change dietary patterns at the level of the individual to limit frequent ingestion of sugar due to its ubiquitous presence in the environment, heavy advertising, and the biologic preference for sweets. Similarly, efforts to alter the microflora have been unsuccessful. An array of fluoride interventions have been developed to effectively raise the threshold for injury to tooth structure from diet–microbial acid challenges. Each challenge represents a transaction of mineral content at the outer layer of enamel. As long as there is a sufficient supply of fluoride available, conditions favor tooth preservation and remineralize. If the diet–microbial challenge increases in frequency or magnitude and exceeds the ability of fluoride to remineralize, then caries lesions will form.

In this conceptual model, fluoride's role is central to preventing and reversing the loss of mineral in the caries process, effectively stopping or slowing down the progress of lesion development.[54] Slowing down the process allows the dental professional the opportunity to adopt a more conservative approach and delay surgical (operative) intervention until it's absolutely necessary to prevent further caries progression. In essence, prevention is about biofilm conditioning to support enamel health so that adequate fluoride is available when acid attacks occur.[146]

### Fluoride and Remineralization

Mechanistically, fluoride has been shown to decrease the rate of enamel demineralization and increase the rate of enamel remineralization.[57] More importantly, tooth structure that has been remineralized in the presence of fluoride is more resistant to subsequent acid challenges. Thus, not only does fluoride help reverse the caries process, but it also helps mitigate future disease progression. The evidence to support anticaries effectiveness of fluoride can be found in several sources, including the Cochrane Library, the American Dental Association (ADA), and the Guide to Community Preventive Services.

Evidence for fluoride toothpaste and mouthrinse comes from several systematic quantitative evaluations of the scientific literature. These reviews have concluded that there is reasonably strong scientific evidence supporting the frequent use of dentifrice products with fluoride concentrations of 1000 ppm and above and for the use of fluoride mouthrinses for individuals who are at a higher risk of developing dental caries.[148]

### Fluoride and Conditioning of Dental Biofilm

Fluoride's role within dental biofilm is very important for replacing lost mineral in dental enamel. The biofilm is a key reservoir for fluoride that is bioavailable for remineralization of enamel. Social factors that determine a person's dietary patterns over time have an important influence on both the growth of deleterious microbial populations in the mouth and the way these bacteria affect the

biofilm pathogenicity or virulence. Similarly, social and behavioral factors can influence exposure to fluoride that can, in turn, determine the availability of biofilm fluoride during the remineralization cycle.

Within the dental biofilm, intracellular fluoride can directly affect microbial metabolism and reduce acid production by certain bacteria. Although several studies have demonstrated a role for fluoride within the pathophysiology of acid production by *S. mutans*,[77,92] the practical application of these findings to prevent and/or reduce decay is not clear at this time. Fluoride levels in the plaque fluid—the space around the bacterial cell surfaces—is readily available for remineralization and thus is the most important reservoir for fluoride. Studies have shown that caries progression is tied to the level of fluoride in plaque fluid.[85,133] Mature biofilms may contain calcium fluoride ($CaF_2$) mineral complexes, which are considered to be important sources of bioavailable fluoride under low pH conditions.[140]

Using our conceptual model, we can understand dental caries as a chronic process that can be managed.[74,107,116] As such, management of dental caries falls within the same paradigm as management of other chronic conditions, such as diabetes mellitus or asthma. Typically, a chronic disease management strategy represents a collaborative approach to care that empowers the patient and their family in self-management within a system of clinical and community support. For caries management, fluoride levels need to be maintained, since levels drop after brushing due to salivary clearance and swallowing.[150] Salivary fluoride levels can be considered a marker of fluoride retention in the oral cavity after topical fluoride use; these levels reflect the fluoride retained by the teeth, biofilm, and the oral mucosa at a point in time after fluoride use.[148,150] In a chronic disease management framework, dental professionals seek to guide patients and inform them about ways to maintain a steady-state fluoride concentration in their oral cavity. Dental professionals can help patients become empowered in managing their caries risk by working with them to select a fluoride product and method of delivery. This approach should also take into consideration salivary flow rate and behavioral factors that influence fluoride retention and thus fluoride effectiveness.

### Fluoride and the Biofilm Effects on Different Tooth Surfaces

The landscape of the dental biofilm varies tremendously within the mouth. It has different properties that are largely determined by the location of the tooth surface that the biofilm covers and the anatomy of the tooth. For example, the buccal pits on a lower first molar offer both a unique ecologic niche for microorganisms and debris to escape contact with a toothbrush bristle and reduced exposure to saliva relative to other parts of the dentition. Areas that are not easily cleansed tend to harbor plaque biofilm that has had an opportunity to age. If adequate fluoride levels can be sufficiently maintained, these areas can play a role in remineralization.

## Optimizing Environmental Exposure Using a Population-Based Approach

Public health policies for reducing disease can be generally classed as population-based strategies or high-risk strategies.[60,113] The primary difference is whether it is intended to shift the entire population distribution of a disease or only those at the highest risk for disease. Innovative approaches seek to target high-risk groups to improve access to preventive interventions. The "3 bucket" conceptualization mentioned earlier shows how all three approaches—targeting individuals, targeting high-risk groups, and community-wide prevention—can work together to reduce the burden of disease in a community.

Community water fluoridation is the controlled addition of a fluoride compound to a public water supply to bring its fluoride concentration up to a level that will best prevent dental caries while avoiding unsightly fluorosis. It is a population-based prevention strategy that serves to shift the distribution of dental caries in the community so that more people are caries free and that those who experience caries have a reduction in the number of decayed teeth. Community water fluoridation has been described fittingly as an interplay of epidemiologic science, science dissemination, communication, and policy development.[4] The epidemiologic origin with its population health focus forms the basis for public health policy. The fluoride–caries relationship was first discovered in studies of communities with naturally fluoridated water and because of this water fluoridation is the purest public health use of fluoride. Community water fluoridation is not a high-risk approach to caries prevention, rather, it is population based; its use means fluoride reaches everyone in the community. This feature is both the measure's greatest strength and its greatest challenge in terms of social policy with inherent challenges of science dissemination and communication. The next section discusses the science specific to water fluoridation as a means of controlling a chronic disease, specifically, caries at the community level.

The unit usually used in the United States for expressing the fluoride concentration in drinking water is parts per million (ppm), although countries using metric measurements usually express it in milligrams per liter (mg/L). Fortunately, the numerical values are the same in both measuring units; that is, 1.2 ppm is the same as 1.2 mg/L. We use parts per million in this book.

## Optimal Fluoride Concentrations in Drinking Water

Public policy for controlled water fluoride levels in the United States takes the form of nonenforceable guidelines set by the U.S. Public Health Service (PHS) (Box 25.1). As of 2015, current policy is that the optimal level for the United States should be 0.7 ppm fluoride. This PHS recommendation replaces an earlier recommendation that varied by geographic area ranging from 0.7 to 1.2 ppm fluoride that had been in place since 1962.[139]

Reasons for revising the recommendation included:
- Drinking water is one of several available sources of fluoride.
- An increase in the prevalence of fluorosis since the time the guidelines were developed (see Chapter 19) indicates that young people are ingesting more fluoride than they used to. Increased use of commercial juice drinks in place of milk and water could be a factor.[93]
- Air conditioning is widespread and has been a major factor in promoting population growth in hotter parts of the country. Because we live in an increasingly climate-controlled environment, the original premise that people drink more water in hotter parts of the country becomes weaker.[20,69,125]

## BOX 25.1 Drinking Water Standards

The U.S. Environmental Protection Agency (EPA) is the regulatory agency with responsibility for setting national standards for acceptable drinking water under the Safe Drinking Water Act (Public Law 93-523). This act first passed in 1974 and has been renewed several times since. Most of these standards deal with defining acceptable levels of bacterial and chemical contaminants. In the 1975–76 National Interim Primary Drinking Water Regulations, promulgated soon after passage of the Act, the EPA referred to naturally occurring fluoride above 2 ppm as a "contaminant" requiring removal from drinking water. This requirement, intended to reduce dental fluorosis in affected areas, was criticized by many local authorities because of cost (defluoridation is more expensive than fluoridation). Many communities that used drinking water naturally fluoridated at more than 2 ppm were small and could not afford the cost of meeting the standard. In addition, few seemed interested in defluoridating: The resulting fluorosis did not concern them and they were not aware of any other ill effects.

The 1980 Interim Primary Drinking Water Regulations[51] left the recommended maximum contaminant level (RMCL) at 2 ppm fluoride but included an explanatory statement that this standard did not contradict the beneficial effects of fluoride in reducing dental decay. Whether this statement really helped clarify things, especially because that unfortunate word contaminant was retained, is doubtful. Public discussion on establishing the final standards became intense during the mid-1980s; the EPA was deluged with demands from both proponents and opponents of fluoridation. The state of South Carolina, for whom compliance with the RMCL of 2 ppm fluoride would have been very expensive, brought suit against the EPA in 1981 to attempt to force it to revoke the interim RMCL. The EPA, in response, promised to rule on the issue when its studies were complete.

Eventually the EPA settled this seemingly irresolvable issue by ducking underneath it. Concluding after its studies that dental fluorosis in the United States was a cosmetic defect rather than a health problem, the EPA proposed an RMCL for fluoride of 4.0 ppm on the grounds that this level was sufficiently low to protect against crippling skeletal fluorosis.[52] By late 1986, this RMCL became the maximum contaminant level for 4.0 ppm fluoride, meaning that the EPA now had a standard to enforce. The original level of 2.0 ppm fluoride became a secondary standard; that is, it was a nonenforceable recommended maximum, in effect a guideline. This secondary standard was justified on the grounds that "2 mg/L would prevent the majority of cases of water-related cosmetically objectionable dental fluorosis while still allowing for the beneficial effects of fluoride (prevention of dental caries)."[53]

Although some aspects of this debate resembled a Gilbert and Sullivan operetta, it raised the serious question of whether control of dental fluorosis should be a subject for national standards or whether the issue should be left to states or localities to handle. State dental directors have to carry much of the regulatory load, and many are unhappy with the requirement that local communities must be notified when their fluoride levels are between 2 and 4 ppm, especially because the EPA mandates that the word contaminant (again!) must appear in the letters of notification.[47]

Standards of this sort quite properly need reexamination from time to time. In 1992 and again in 2006, the EPA requested the National Research Council to review the issue of primary and secondary standards for fluoride in drinking water. Expert committees whose members had a variety of backgrounds (most were from outside dentistry) concluded that there was no current evidence to justify a change in the standards.[100] The committee recommendations support the issue of the relationship of fluoride exposure to health be revisited at regular intervals because new evidence was appearing continuously. Following these reports, the EPA decided not to change what was then called the maximum contaminant level goal of 4.0 ppm fluoride. This standard still holds, and the EPA deemed that the standard has low priority and is not appropriate for revision.[48]

## Early Studies of Fluoridated Water

All the early research on the safety of fluoride use and its impact on human health and function studied fluoride in drinking water. By the time the first controlled fluoridation trials were begun in 1945, research had established the following facts:

- The healthy human body possesses a prompt and efficient excretory mechanism for fluoride that minimizes the danger of long-term accumulation, at least at the low fluoride levels usually found naturally in drinking water in the United States.
- Although ingested fluoride is partly deposited in bone, and although skeletal fluoride concentrations increase with age, skeletal damage could not be demonstrated in users of fluoride-bearing domestic water in the United States.
- No impairment in general health could be found among people who had drunk water with up to 8 ppm fluoride for long periods.

Four independent studies of controlled fluoridation—in which the fluoride concentration in the water supplies of the communities ranged from negligible levels to 1.0 to 1.2 ppm—were begun in 1945 and 1946. They followed a long series of epidemiologic studies of caries experience related to fluoride concentration in drinking water.

The four communities originally studied were:

1. Grand Rapids, Michigan. This study was begun in January 1945 with nearby Muskegon as the control city and was directed by Dean and his colleagues.[36]
2. Newburgh, New York, with Kingston as the control city.[10]
3. Evanston, Illinois, with Oak Park as control.[24]
4. Brantford, Ontario, with Sarnia as control. Naturally fluoridated Stratford, Ontario, was also included in this study.[70]

At the end of study durations, ranging up to 15 years, caries experience was shown to be sharply reduced in each of the study populations despite some differences in study design and examination criteria.[8,11,22,71] These pioneer studies also found that dental fluorosis occurred to about the same extent[12,119] as Dean had described earlier[35]: namely, some 7% to 16% of the population was found to have mild to very mild fluorosis when the fluoride exposure came from drinking water containing 1.0 ppm fluoride.

The four original studies in which fluoride was added to drinking water are sometimes called "classic" studies, although "pioneering" might be a better term. By present-day standards of field trials, they were rather crude. Although they are often referred to as "longitudinal" studies, none of them was; all were of sequential cross-sectional design. Sampling methods and dental examiners tended to vary from year to year,[7] which risked bias and unnecessary random error. Methods of statistical analysis were primitive by today's standards. Data from the control communities were largely neglected after the initial reports, and conclusions were based on the much weaker before–after analysis in the test cities. (Among the early studies, the only true longitudinal study of fluoridation's effects was the Tiel-Culemborg study in the Netherlands.)[15]

Perhaps too much emphasis has been given to these four pioneering studies, as they really just confirmed prospectively what had already been demonstrated through Dean's research, which still stands as a model of how to apply the epidemiologic method. But despite the design flaws in the original four studies, it is difficult for an open-minded observer to reject their conclusions that fluoridation was effective in reducing the prevalence and severity of caries.

Public policy on any issue usually has to be established based on current evidence, and water fluoridation is no exception. When one considers that adults, on average, ingest 1 to 3 mg fluoride/day in their normal diets, that 9 to 10 million Americans (and many other peoples around the world) have been drinking naturally fluoridated water for a century or so, and that over 100 million Americans have been drinking fluoride-supplemented water for generations, there is a lot of empirical evidence that fluoridation at 1 ppm is not harmful. Certainly, there is no credible evidence that fluoride in these amounts leads to serious ill health. The scientific method cannot prove a negative; we take inability to reject the null hypothesis for specific conditions (see Chapter 13) as evidence of safety. There is strong basis to support the policy of the PHS that fluoride should be added to drinking water at the recommended concentration of 0.7 ppm.

## Fluoridation in the United States

The Division of Oral Health of the Centers for Disease Control and Prevention (CDC) in Atlanta maintains fluoridation surveillance for the United States. The Water Fluoridation Reporting System, a voluntary program, forwards data from the states to the CDC, which then publishes the information periodically on its website. Extent of fluoridation is one of the eight indicators used in the National Oral Health Surveillance System.

At the end of 2014, the CDC estimated that fluoridated water was reaching some 211 million people in the United States, 66% of the total population and 74% of those receiving municipal water.[138] Nearly 12 million of these people were receiving water naturally fluoridated at 0.7 ppm fluoride or more; the greatest concentrations of naturally fluoridated communities are found in Texas, Illinois, and New Mexico.[100] In 2014 there were more than 18,000 water systems with controlled or natural fluoride levels of 0.7 ppm fluoride or more; these represent less than one-third of all public water systems in the country. This may not sound like much, but a large majority of public water systems serve communities with fewer than 1000 people, where fluoridation is not cost-effective on a per capita basis. Drinking water is fluoridated in 44 of the 50 largest American cities.[2] Over 130 communities have had continuous water fluoridation for 50 years, and 700 communities in the United States have been fluoridating the water for 30 years or longer. Many of the naturally fluoridated communities have been using the same water source for more than three generations. The proportion of state populations reached by fluoridation ranges from close to 100% in Kentucky, Minnesota, Illinois, North Dakota, Maryland, Georgia, and Virginia (plus the District of Columbia) to 12% in Hawaii. In 2014, 20 states had reached the Healthy People 2020 objective of 79.6% of the population served by community water systems having optimal fluoride levels.

### Role of Federal, State, and Local Governments in Fluoridation

The decision to fluoridate is usually made by the local community, although a number of jurisdictions can be involved when water service district boundaries do not coincide with city and county boundaries. In 2009, state laws mandating fluoridation were present in 12 states; at the other end of the spectrum, there are four states that have laws requiring referenda.[16] The fluoridation laws generally have been successful, because a high proportion of the population is receiving fluoridated water in all states with them. Some of the states, however, have provisions in their laws that can frustrate progress. These provisions reflect the political compromises necessary to get the law passed. For example, the California law, passed after a vigorous political battle in 1996, cannot be enforced unless outside funds (i.e., state or federal funds) are made available to the local community for the purchase, installation, and operation of the fluoridation system.

The PHS, initially through its Division of Dental Health (now defunct) and later through the CDC, provides consultative expertise to promote fluoridation and has periodically provided funding through several mechanisms. In 2017, a partnership between the National Association of County and City Health Officials and the CDC provided funds in a pilot program to support equipment for community water fluoridation. Future funding remains uncertain.

## Caries Reductions From Fluoridation

For many years, the statement that "water fluoridation reduces dental caries experience by half" was hardly questioned within dentistry. At a time when drinking water was the only significant source of fluoride, that statement was probably true enough. Its basis was Dean's 21 cities epidemiologic study of naturally fluoridated areas,[37,38] supplemented by the results of the initial four controlled fluoridation projects begun in 1945 and 1946. A summary of the results of these four pioneering studies is presented in Table 25.2. The table shows that after 13 to 15 years of fluoridation, decayed, missing, and filled (DMF) scores in 12- to 14-year-old permanent-resident children favored fluoridation by 48% to 70%. In absolute terms, average DMF levels in the fluoridated communities dropped from seven to nine teeth at the start of the studies to three to four teeth per child after 13 to 15 years.

Since those studies, exposure to fluoride from toothpaste, other dental products, and food and drink has essentially become universal. As a result, water fluoridation has moved from being the sole fluoride exposure, as it was in those early days, to one of a number of fluoride exposures. Caries status overall has continued to improve, and overall fluoride exposure has to take much of the credit for that. Another reason for the inability to attribute 50% reductions in caries to water fluoridation today is that the effects of fluoride in drinking water diffuse into surrounding communities and raise the baseline. This diffusion or "halo" effect has important implications for accurate estimation of the benefit of an intervention to a community since the comparison group is likely also receiving a benefit indirectly. Nonetheless, 12-year-old children living in states where more than half of the communities have fluoridated water have 26% fewer decayed tooth surfaces per year than 12-year-old children living in states where less than one-quarter of the communities are fluoridated.[65] A rigorous systematic review in Britain, carried out by an expert group at the University of York, concluded that the median increase in the proportion of persons with decayed, missing, and filled permanent teeth (DMFT) score of 0 attributable to water fluoridation was 15%.[95] Because the review had strict criteria for inclusion and exclusion of studies, this conclusion was reached from a fairly small number of studies. (One of the conclusions of the systematic review was that the large body of literature on the effectiveness of water fluoridation was generally of poor quality, as was the literature claiming harm from fluoridation.)

It would thus be unreasonable to expect continuation of 50% reductions in caries levels from fluoridated water alone; the generally reduced caries levels we enjoy today are a result of total fluoride exposure from all sources. The continuing importance of water fluoridation as a cornerstone of public policy, however, is indicated by the fact that the CDC lists it as one of the top 10 public health achievements of the 20th century[136] and is listed as one of the 14 community-wide interventions that can have a positive health impact in 5 years (the HI-5 Interventions).[137]

## Reducing the Disparities in Caries Through Fluoridation

*Disparities* refers to the differences in health status between favored and unfavored groups in our society, arising from social factors and determinants that vary among racial-ethnic groups and those of different socioeconomic status (SES). Disparities are a complex and persistent problem, with economic costs and political and moral implications that are tied to notions of social justice. Fluoridation has the major social advantage of benefiting children in lower SES areas relatively more than those in higher SES areas.[31] An example

| • TABLE 25.2 | Decayed, Missing, and Filled (DMF) Teeth per Child Ages 12–14 Years and Missing Teeth per Child at the End of the Study Term in Four Pioneer Fluoridation Communities[11] | | | | |
|---|---|---|---|---|---|
| Community | Year | Mean DMF Teeth per Child | Percent Difference | Missing Teeth per Child | Percent Difference |
| Grand Rapids (F) | 1944–45 | 9.58 | 55.5 | 0.84 | 65.6 |
| | 1959 | 4.26 | | 0.29 | |
| Evanston (F) | 1946 | 9.03 | 48.4 | 0.19 | 68.4 |
| | 1959 | 4.66 | | 0.06 | |
| Sarnia (non-F) | 1959 | 7.46 | | 0.75 | |
| Brantford (F) | 1959 | 3.23 | 56.7 | 0.22 | 70.7 |
| Kingston[a] (non-F) | 1960 | 12.46 | | 0.92 | |
| Newburgh[a] (F) | 1960 | 3.73 | 70.1 | 0.10 | 89.1 |

[a]Children in Kingston and Newburgh were ages 13 to 14 years.

*Note:* Fluoridated communities are designated by F, nonfluoridated by non-F, after city name.

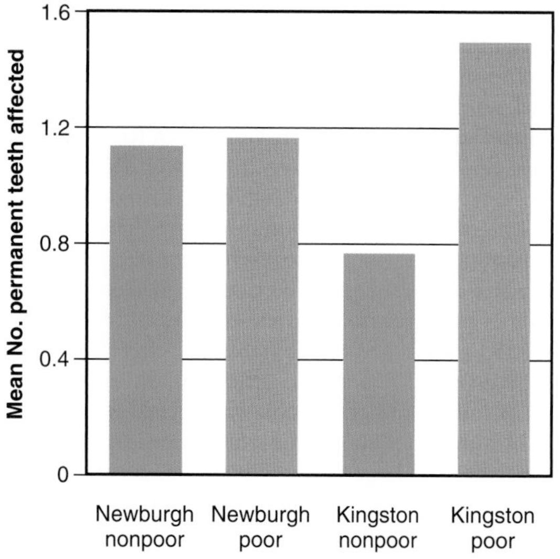

• **Figure 25.3** Caries experience, expressed as covariate adjusted mean decayed, missing, and filled surfaces per child in 7- to 14-year-old children in Newburgh and Kingston, New York, by poverty status ("poor" children were defined as those participating in the school lunch program).[31]

is shown in Figure 25.3, which presents data from the most recent clinical examinations in the Newburgh-Kingston studies in New York. When caries levels found in 7- to 14-year-old poor and non-poor children in the 1995 examinations were compared, the greatest disparity was seen between the poor and nonpoor in nonfluoridated Kingston rather than between poor groups in the two cities. Reducing the disparities in health status between high- and low-SES areas is a United States national health objective for 2020, and fluoridation does its part to help achieve this goal.

Assessments of fluoridation's effectiveness, including its effectiveness in reducing disparities between groups, have come from systematic reviews. The first was carried out by the Centre for Reviews and Dissemination at the University of York in Britain in 2000 (referred to earlier).[95] Systematic reviews place high emphasis on rigorous study design. They have been criticized[118] by the public health community for their overemphasis on randomized clinical trials, which are relatively uncommon in community-based interventions. Similarly, stringent inclusion and exclusion criteria lead to the omission of many reports from consideration.

In the York review, one of the aims was to determine if fluoridation reduced the disparity in caries experience between higher and lower SES groups. Most of the 15 papers selected to examine this question reported data for 5-year-old children. The review found no difference between fluoridated and nonfluoridated areas in the magnitude of the disparities between children of different SES groups when caries *prevalence* was measured. However, a favorable reduction in differences between social groups was seen when caries *severity* was the measure. Data for ages other than 5 years were too limited to permit conclusions. The U.S. Preventive Services Task Force has updated the York systematic review to include studies published between 1999 and 2012. Findings continue to show a decrease in new dental caries of about 15% when community water fluoridation begins.[59]

## Caries Reductions in Children

Studies of the effectiveness of fluoridation in reducing caries experience in children far outnumber studies of its effectiveness in adults. The many fluoridation studies conducted in different parts of the world have varied in quality of design, but their results have still been remarkably uniform.[117] Differences in oral health between fluoridated and nonfluoridated areas are easier to demonstrate when there are relatively few fluoridated areas, because the diffusion effect of fluoride exposure from sources indirectly linked to fluoridated water has less impact. Contemporary evidence supports a benefit for lifetime exposure to fluoridation.[122,126]

Based on a recent systematic review, differences in caries experience between children in fluoridated and nonfluoridated communities are now estimated to be more on the order of 26% to 35%.[72] Fluoridation also increases the proportion of children who are caries free by about 15%.[72] However, how many of fluoride's benefits are due to water fluoridation, rather than to overall fluoride exposure, really cannot be estimated with any precision now for the following reasons:

- The development and almost universal use of fluoridated toothpaste and other dental products containing fluoride, plus the presence of fluoride in food and beverages processed with fluoridated water, means that there are many different fluoride exposures for the average American.
- The mobility of the US population means that most people have had varied exposures to fluoridated water at different times of life. When this is added to the diffusion effect (described earlier), it is clear that there is no way of finding true "unexposed" subjects in the United States.
- History of exposure to fluoridation is difficult to document in research studies. There are no biomarkers for lifetime exposure, and interview data can be unreliable.

## Caries Reductions Across the Lifespan

The caries-inhibitory effects of fluoride are not confined to childhood.[43] Contrary assumptions remain surprisingly common and may stem from beliefs that the primary cariostatic action of fluoride was preeruptive and caries was a disease of childhood. Neither of these beliefs is viewed as true today. Contemporary evidence shows a beneficial effect for young adults.[127] Over a lifetime, there is evidence that fluoridation reduces caries, but the magnitude of the benefit seems to diminish in older age groups.[43]

Root caries is also less prevalent in fluoridated areas than in nonfluoridated areas.[32,111,128] This observation may be important, because with increasing tooth retention in an aging population, the amount of root caries would otherwise be expected to increase and become a greater treatment problem in the future.

Early fluoridation studies reported caries reductions in the primary dentition of about the same range as was found in the permanent dentition.[11,23,132] More recent data show that caries reduction attributable to fluoridation is being maintained.[117] The primary dentition clearly benefits from exposure to fluoridated drinking water.[72]

## Caries Patterns When Fluoridation Ceases

Research on cessation of community water fluoridation is limited. A systematic review of what happens to the caries level in a community after the water supply no longer has optimal fluoride has evaluated 15 studies.[96] The authors highlight the difficulties in assessing the impact of cessation of fluoridation. While eight studies did show clear increases in dental caries after fluoridation was stopped, all 15 studies had methodologic issues that made it difficult to draw conclusions in a pooled manner. Key gaps for further study are a need for an improved understanding of the factors that lead to the decision to stop fluoridation in a community and better investigation of the equity of impact across socioeconomic groups in the community.

The continued decline in caries experience after fluoridation ceases would be expected in communities in which there is regular and frequent exposure to fluoride from toothpaste and other sources, whereas a caries increase would be expected if drinking water were the only fluoride source. These findings emphasize yet again that regular exposure to low-concentration fluoride is what leads to reduced caries experience, not necessarily exposure to any one fluoride vehicle. Water fluoridation is the most efficient way to bring fluoride to a community, but other exposure methods work as well.

## Fluoridation in the Age of Multiple Fluoride Exposure

With caries levels at their lowest ever and fluoride available from a variety of sources, the question arises of whether water fluoridation is still needed. The answer is clearly "yes."[79] Although overall caries experience in the populations of the United States, Canada, Western European nations, Australia, and New Zealand continues to diminish, we have noted that the caries-preventive effects directly attributable to water fluoridation are not as high as they once were.

The pioneering four studies reported caries reductions of 50% to 70% (see Table 25.2), whereas more recent studies of fluoridation's effects produce less clear-cut differences.[117] The prime reason that effects attributable to water fluoridation are reduced while overall caries experience still continues to decline is that an increase has occurred in exposure to fluoride from other sources. The main such source is fluoride toothpaste, but there are also possibly significant amounts of fluoride in processed foods and beverages. The rise in the prevalence of fluorosis (see Chapter 19) also attests to a broad increase in fluoride exposure.

On the other hand, some recent studies of fluoridation's effects in Britain and Australia have yielded results that still show caries experience to be significantly lower in fluoridated communities.[43,104,126] One theory put forward to explain these mixed results is that the clear benefits of water fluoridation tend to be seen more in places where fluoridation is less common, which thus reduces the diffusion effects[65] and emphasizes the impact from water fluoridation. In many studies, the standard method of measuring exposure to fluoridated water has traditionally been ecologic: That is, if you live in a fluoridated community you drink fluoridated water; if you live in a nonfluoridated community you do not. This may have been adequate in earlier days, but in today's world of high mobility, heavy consumption of soft drinks and bottled water, extensive use of water softeners and filtration systems (which can take fluoride from water), and high consumption of processed foods, the ecologic approach to assigning exposure becomes increasingly questionable in research design.

With differences in caries levels between fluoridated and nonfluoridated communities becoming increasingly blurred, the decision to fluoridate a water supply is not always as automatic as it once was. It can be argued that when caries experience is already low, good fluoride exposure comes from other sources, and the economic cost of installing fluoridation is high, so fluoridation is unnecessary. However, there are two good reasons to argue for fluoridation except in the most exceptional circumstances. One is the cost-effectiveness of the measure compared to other methods of caries control, and the second is the social equity benefits of fluoridation. Alone among caries control strategies, fluoridation is a population-based approach that reaches everyone in a community, and as described earlier it has been shown to reduce the strong SES gradient usually seen in the distribution of caries in a community. Caries is still more prevalent and severe in lower SES groups than in higher SES groups in fluoridated communities, but the differences are much less marked than they are in nonfluoridated communities (see Figure 25.3). This factor of social equity alone is a strong argument for fluoridating a community's drinking water. Medicaid costs for dental restorative and extraction procedures have been observed to vary by fluoridation status across comparable communities such that caries-related treatments were more common in counties with low fluoridation coverage.[80]

A recent review[109] of the economic costs and benefits of community water fluoridation demonstrated that there is a favorable return on investment in community water fluoridation interventions and that the cost–benefit ratio is enhanced in communities with larger populations. Little evidence was found for communities with fewer than 1000 people. Another study made use of program cost data from 2013 to demonstrate that $32 per capita in savings for caries averted is attributable to community water fluoridation.[101]

In some parts of the world, water fluoridation is not an easy option, so fluoride is added to salt or milk to accomplish the same population-level objectives of prevention. An excellent summary of these interventions is provided by O'Mullane et al.[102] Briefly, salt fluoridation has enjoyed wide use since the 1950s in Switzerland, where about 85% of domestic salt contains 250 ppm fluoride. Other European countries with varying population exposure include France, Germany, the Czech Republic, and to a lesser extent Austria, Spain, and Slovakia. In the Americas, Mexico, Colombia, Costa Rica, and Uruguay have very good population exposure to fluoridated salt.[94] The concern with salt as a vehicle for fluoride particularly in poor countries, however, is that while we may prevent caries, its effect or role in cardiovascular diseases is a concern.

Milk fluoridation has been shown to have a favorable reduction in dental caries in primary teeth.[144] The approach is used in some parts of the world, including Bulgaria, Russia, Thailand, and Chile. Milk fluoridation takes advantage of the infrastructure that exists for milk production and the fact that many schools provide milk to children to improve nutrition. Many of these children are at elevated risk for dental caries. Levels of fluoride in milk vary depending on other sources of fluoride exposure. Typically, the target range is tailored to provide 0.5 to 0.85 mg fluoride per day for a typical child.[17]

## Dietary Fluoride Supplements

Because the assumption in the 1940s was that the effect of fluoridated water was mainly preeruptive, dietary supplements were intended to mimic the observed action of fluoridated water. Fluoride supplements in the form of tablets, lozenges, drops, liquids, and fluoride-vitamin preparations have been used around the world since the 1940s.

Fluoride supplements have fluoride quantities of 1 mg, 0.5 mg, or 0.25 mg. They were originally made as a 1 mg fluoride pill to be dissolved in a liter of the infant's drinking water, an approach that in time gave way to the simpler once-a-day ingestion of the tablet. Later, chewable tablets and lozenges were manufactured for older children, to be chewed or sucked 1 to 2 minutes before swallowing, the intent here being to obtain both topical and systemic effects. Most tablets contain neutral NaF, although acidulated phosphate fluoride (APF) tablets have been tested. There are also fluoride-vitamin drops for infants, often prescribed by pediatricians.

## Caries Prevention by Fluoride Supplementation

A systematic review[134] of fluoride supplement use to prevent caries in children examined evidence from trials that were at least 2 years in duration. Eleven studies provided sufficient evidence to demonstrate a 24% reduction in caries increment in permanent teeth. The effect of fluoride supplementation on primary teeth was unclear.

## Dosing Schedules

To obtain fluoride supplements in the United States and Canada, a prescription from a dentist or physician is required. The ADA, the American Academy of Pediatric Dentistry (AAPD), and the American Academy of Pediatrics (AAP) maintain the same schedules of recommended doses of fluoride supplements.[115]

As the dosing schedules for fluoride supplements are revised periodically, the trend has been to make them ever more conservative. The current ADA-recommended schedule, based on the age of the child and the concentration of fluoride in the water supply, is shown in Table 25.3. It was updated in 2010 and continues to be reviewed periodically. When the recommended standard for drinking water was changed in 2015, the schedule was reviewed and deemed appropriate in light of the new recommendation of 0.7 ppm fluoride for public water systems. Drawbacks related to fluoride supplement use relate to compliance and cost. Since daily administration is required, compliance will vary from child to child. Cost may be a barrier for some families. Each situation should be evaluated including the water fluoride level tested before a fluoride supplement is prescribed, and efforts to address these challenges should be discussed with parents and caregivers. It can also be questioned whether the emphasis should be on the use of fluoride dentifrice instead of fluoride supplements, although studies are required to determine which approach leads to better caries prevention outcomes.

| • TABLE 25.3 | Recommended Dosage Levels of Supplemental Fluoride as Established by the American Dental Association in 2010 (in mg F/day)[115] |
| --- | --- |

| Age | CONCENTRATION OF FLUORIDE IN WATER (PPM) | | |
| --- | --- | --- | --- |
| | <0.3 | 0.3–0.6 | >0.6 |
| 6 mo to 3 yr | 0.25 | — | — |
| 3–6 yr | 0.50 | 0.25 | — |
| 6–16 yr | 1.00 | 0.50 | — |

## Prenatal Fluoride Supplementation

The question of whether to prescribe fluoride supplements for an expectant woman to increase caries resistance in the offspring has been debated for years. In light of the discussion on dietary fluoride supplements in general and fluoride's predominantly topical mechanism of action in preventing caries, it is not surprising that current views are that any enhanced resistance to caries will be only minor at best. The only prospective randomized trial of prenatal fluoride supplementation found no significant difference in the caries experience of the offspring.[83] Therefore, use of prenatal supplements is not recommended.

## Clinical Guidance on Use of Fluoride Products

The ADA periodically provides clinical practice guidelines. The most recent guideline came out in 2013[142] and is expected to be updated in 2020. The expert panel was convened by the ADA Council on Scientific Affairs and reviewed professionally applied and prescription-strength topical fluoride agents including mouth rinses, gels, foams, pastes, and varnishes.

The panel determined that sufficient evidence supports use of four different options to prevent dental caries in people at risk: 2.26% fluoride varnish; 1.23% APF gel; a prescription-strength, home-use 0.5% fluoride gel or paste; or 0.09% fluoride mouth rinse for individuals 6 years of age or older.[142]

## Fluoride Varnishes

Fluoride varnish is widely accepted as the treatment of choice for preventing caries in high-risk children.[21,90,97] It is especially appropriate for children younger than age 6, due to concerns about fluoride ingestion related to gels and foams.[142] Fluoride varnish is not intended to be as permanent as a fissure sealant (see Chapter 26); rather it is a vehicle for holding fluoride in close contact with the tooth for a period of time. An advantage of varnishes over other methods of professional fluoride application is that varnishes are adhesive and hence should maximize fluoride contact with the tooth surface. Varnishes are a way of using high fluoride concentrations in small amounts of material. Fluoride varnishes have a long history in Europe and Canada and were accepted for use in the United States in 1994 as a cavity liner, but they are used off label in caries prevention. In a systematic review of 22 trials of fluoride varnishes, evidence has clearly established caries reduction for both permanent and primary teeth.[90]

Varnishes must be reapplied at regular intervals to maintain their cariostatic effect, and a dose-response pattern has been demonstrated.[141] Innovative public health collaborative programs in the United States use fluoride varnish to bridge the gap between dental and medical practice. Efforts to bring appropriate use of fluoride varnish into the medical practice include training programs like Smiles for Life[124] and those offered for pediatricians through the AAP[5] and in medical school.[64] In many states, physicians use fluoride varnish to prevent early childhood caries in their at-risk young patients and get reimbursed by the Medicaid program.[78] A recent review[61] found evidence that supports collaborative medical–dental integration that makes use of topical fluoride varnish applications for children. The premise for integrating oral health into primary medical care is based on the fact that a much higher proportion of infants visit a physician's office than visit a dental office (see Chapter 5).

## Fluoride Mouth Rinses

NaF formulations have been tested as a weekly rinse at 0.2% (900 ppm fluoride) and as a daily rinse at 0.05% (230 ppm fluoride). School-based programs have found the weekly regimen to be the most convenient, whereas daily rinsing is most appropriate for individual use. The caries reductions from daily rinsing are only slightly greater than those from weekly rinsing, and the slight differences do not compensate for the greater practicality and lower cost of weekly rinsing in a school-based program. A systematic review of 35 studies demonstrated a preventive fraction of 27% for DMFS increment for interventions of at least 1-year duration.[88] This finding was irrespective of background fluoride exposure from other sources and baseline caries status. For home use, dentists can advise patients to buy fluoride mouthrinse from the drugstore or supermarket. Products come and go; a list of current products with ADA approval can be found on the ADA's website. Fluoride mouthrinses in school-based programs used since the 1970s have come under some scrutiny, with decline of its use in public programs. Box 25.2 provides a discussion.

## Fluoride Gel Applications

Professional fluoride gel-tray applications have long been considered not to be cost-effective for community-based health programs, but use of 1.23% APF gel in a clinical setting or a prescription-strength, home-use 0.5% fluoride gel or paste can be effective for high risk children older than age 6. Although the effectiveness of fluoride varnish compared to fluoride gel is inconclusive, the time savings for application of fluoride varnish make it a reasonable approach for highly susceptible special groups in targeted community programs.[87,89]

## Prophylaxis Pastes Containing Fluoride

Fluoride-containing prophylactic pastes are widely used in dentistry; the reasoning behind their development was that the prophylaxis and the professional fluoride application could be carried out at the same time. However, results from systematic reviews do not demonstrate any benefit attributable to this procedure.[142]

## Estimating Fluoride Intake From Various Formulations

Table 25.4 lists the quantities and concentrations of the fluoride compounds most frequently used in dental practice and those self-applied by individuals. Box 25.3 is a guide to estimating the amounts of fluoride in dental products, and Box 25.4 brings together the information on toxic exposure to fluoride.

## Fluoride Toothpastes

Toothpastes with a fluoride concentration of 1000 to 1500 ppm are proved effective in prevention of dental caries and supported internationally.[45,55,143] Toothpastes without active ingredients, meaning those that contain abrasive and flavoring agents only and thus are intended for oral hygiene and cosmetic benefits, have no anticaries action by themselves. But because toothbrushing is a social norm in high-income countries, a variety of preventive and therapeutic agents (both known and hypothetical) have been added to toothpastes over the years. Early efforts to produce anticariogenic toothpastes included the addition of ammonia, antibiotics, chlorophyll, and various other agents to toothpastes. None of these agents was effective. To date, fluoride is the only nonprescription toothpaste additive that has been shown to prevent caries.

The earliest attempts to add fluoride to toothpaste were unsuccessful because of the incompatible abrasives used in the products, which bound the fluoride and thus made it biologically unavailable. The first successful clinical trials of an fluoride additive used $SnF_2$ with a calcium pyrophosphate abrasive.[99] These positive results were replicated during the 1960s in other American and British studies using the same formulation. Systematic reviews demonstrate caries reductions in children of 24% in studies of at least 1-year duration, and use of fluoride toothpastes in fluoridated

---

### • BOX 25.2    Using Data to Inform Action—Fluoride Mouthrinsing as a Community-Based Preventive Intervention

The Association of State and Territorial Dental Directors (ASTDD) updated the *Best Practice Approach Report: Use of Fluoride in Schools* in 2018.[13] This report noted that the number of states with school-based fluoride mouthrinse programs has dropped from 37 in 2002 to 14 in 2017. The ASTDD report identified recommendations from a 1986 American Public Health Association (APHA) technical report[6] to shift focus and target "mouthrinse programs to at-risk populations in nonfluoridated communities and to primarily focus on dental sealants, reflecting the declining rate of decay on the smooth surfaces of teeth." The APHA report summarized the results of the National Preventive Dentistry Demonstration Program (NPDDP), a large program conducted in 10 US cities in 1976 to 1981 to compare the costs and effectiveness of a series of preventive mechanisms. The NPDDP raised serious doubts about fluoride mouthrinsing as an effective public health procedure.

The NPDDP found that the effectiveness of fluoride mouthrinsing was poor both in overall results[76] and in separate assessments of first-grade children with high and low caries increments.[42] Earlier reviews by the NPDDP researchers had reported serious flaws in the conduct of many earlier studies that did not use concurrent control groups[26] and in some of the economic analyses that led to the assumption of cost-effectiveness.[129] Quite strong criticism was also leveled at the way in which the National Institute of Dental and Craniofacial Research had used its data to promote the use of fluoride mouthrinses in public health programs.[41]

At the same time, the NPDDP itself was criticized on the grounds of faulty design and analysis.[58] The atmosphere of uncertainty was dissipated to some extent at a workshop on the cost-effectiveness of preventive procedures in 1989, where it was concluded that fluoride mouthrinsing is a reasonable procedure to use in high-risk individuals or groups, though of questionable cost-effectiveness as a population-based strategy.[82]

A question for consideration today is this: What should policy makers and program directors do when a large (and expensive) study reports findings that challenge the current practice and conventional wisdom? While systematic reviews to summarize evidence are a relatively newer phenomenon in public health, the number of studies that showed a benefit for a fluoride mouthrinse intervention in 1986 was sufficient to justify such programs in schools. Today, the summary of 35 published studies[88] stands in support of fluoride mouthrinse programs while one study stands in opposition.[6]

A way forward is to recognize the uncertainty and emphasize the importance of the use of data to drive program implementation and evaluation.[28] The costs for proper monitoring of a community program need to be included when planning a preventive intervention. Qualitative and quantitative data should be gathered to ensure smooth implementation and to guide quality improvement over the course of the intervention. Evaluation of the impact of the program serves to inform stakeholders and guide program expansion.

• TABLE 25.4 **Concentration and Quantity of Fluoride in Commonly Used Topical Fluoride Compounds**

| Compound | Concentration (ppm) | Quantity |
|---|---|---|
| **Topically Applied Agents** | | |
| 5% NaF varnish (2.26% F) | 22,600 | 9 mg in 0.4 mL unit dose[a] |
| 1.23% APF gel, foam, or prophylactic paste | 12,300 | 62 mg in 5 g |
| 8% SnF$_2$ solution | 19,363 | 97 mg in 5 mL |
| 2% NaF | 9,050 | 44 mg in 5 mL |
| 38% Silver diamine fluoride (5% F) | 44,800 | 1.3 mg in 0.03 mL (1 drop) |
| **Mouthrinses** | | |
| 0.2% NaF—weekly | 905 | 9 mg in 10 mL[b] |
| 0.05% NaF—daily | 226 | 2 mg in 10 mL |
| 0.1% SnF—daily | 242 | 2 mg in 10 mL |
| APF rinse (0.1% fluoride)—weekly | 1,000 | 10 mg in 10 mL |
| APF rinse (0.022% fluoride)—daily | 200 | 2 mg in 10 mL |
| **Toothpastes** | | |
| 0.76% Na$_2$ FPO$_3$ | 1,000 | 1 mg/g[c] |
| 0.243% NaF | 1,105 | 1.1 mg/g |
| 1.1% NaF | 5,000 | 5.0 mg/g |
| 0.454% SnF$_2$ | 1,100 | 1.1 mg/g |

[a]Amount of material varies by type of topical application.
[b]Amounts of 5 and 10 mL are used in supervised mouthrinsing.
[c]An average load of toothpaste on the brush is about 1 g.
*APF,* Acidulated phosphate fluoride; *F,* fluoride.
*Note:* Some figures are rounded.

areas has demonstrated an additive effect.[86,135] There is some evidence that use of fluoride toothpaste prevents root caries in adults.[62]

In all, more than 90 clinical trials have been conducted with various fluoride compounds as the active ingredient: SnF$_2$, NaF, sodium monofluorophosphate (MFP), and amine fluoride have all been successfully tested.[99] Even more compatible abrasives have been developed and tried: insoluble metaphosphate, sodium trimetaphosphate, hydrated silica gel, calcium carbonate, dicalcium dihydrate, and calcium pyrophosphate are the main ones. New formulations are constantly under investigation and are soon marketed when found effective.

There is some laboratory evidence that toothpastes with NaF are more efficacious than those with MFP, although clinical data on this subject are hard to interpret. Analyses of data available in the early 1990s were split on the issue, with discussion often becoming pedantic. Subsequent clinical trials that gave a slight edge to NaF required very large groups to show statistical significance,[91] and another trial found no difference between NaF and MFP products.[39]

Serious marketing of fluoride toothpastes was underway by the early 1970s, and public acceptance was immediate in virtually all of the high-income nations. By the 1990s, fluoride toothpastes accounted for well over 90% of the toothpaste market in the United States, Canada, and many other countries. Their use in low-income countries, where fluoride toothpastes could potentially fill an important preventive role, is limited by their relatively high cost[63] and poor distribution.

## Quality of the Fluoride Toothpaste Trials

It must be stated at this point that many of the clinical trials for fluoride toothpaste are among the most elegant trials to be found in dentistry—or in all of biomedicine for that matter—to demonstrate the efficacy of a product. All of the essential features of the best clinical trials (see Chapter 12) can be found in many of these studies: randomized groups, double-blind designs, placebo controls, and meticulous procedural protocols. Because the water fluoridation field trials have inherent design limitations as previously discussed, opponents of fluoridation can attack their validity. But if the issue is the efficacy of fluoride exposure, the fluoride toothpaste trials collectively include many studies that meet the gold standard for such trials. Taken together, the toothpaste trials provide the strongest evidence we have that fluoride exposure is efficacious in controlling caries.

## Fluoride Concentrations in Toothpastes

The fluoride toothpastes that first became widely marketed contained about 1000 to 1100 ppm fluoride. When introduced into the oral cavity, fluoride in toothpaste is taken up directly by demineralized enamel,[110,131] although its retention on sound enamel is thought to be of relatively minor importance. It also increases the fluoride concentration in dental plaque fluid,[49] thus leaving a store of fluoride available for remineralization.[84,121] Salivary fluoride levels, normally low in resting saliva, rise 100- or even 1000-fold after toothbrushing with fluoride toothpaste.[49] This level drops over the next few hours. Postbrushing levels of intraoral fluoride are affected by the amount and vigor of water rinsing after brushing[50]; the best advice for adults is to rinse gently after brushing or just spit and not rinse.

Because laboratory studies showed that the uptake of fluoride into demineralized enamel and into plaque was proportional to the concentration of fluoride in the toothpaste, a natural next step was the testing of toothpastes with higher concentrations. Toothpastes with 1500 ppm fluoride have been found slightly more efficacious than the 1000 ppm fluoride products.[143] Clinical trials have also been conducted with toothpastes of 2500 to 5000 ppm fluoride with mixed results. In general, systematic analyses conclude that caries reductions are proportional to the fluoride concentration in the toothpastes.[143] Prescription-strength toothpaste with 5000 ppm fluoride (1.1% NaF) is recommended for high-risk patients based on a systematic review.[142]

At the other end of the spectrum, concerns about the fluorosis risk from the swallowing of toothpaste by children have led to the testing of toothpastes with lower than standard levels of fluoride. Children can swallow between 0.12 and 0.38 mg of toothpaste per brushing.[19] In general, studies of 440 and 550 ppm fluoride products suggest a reduced risk for fluorosis compared to 1000 ppm fluoride toothpastes when used by young children.[143] However, the systematic review of these levels showed that they are not sufficiently different from placebo for preventing caries.[143] While toothpastes containing 400 ppm fluoride have been

---

**• BOX 25.3    How to Estimate the Amount of Fluoride in a Dental Product**

**Basic Information**

$$1 \text{ oz} = 28.4 \text{ g}$$

"Percent" means g or mL per 100 g or mL; e.g., 2% NaF solution means 2 g NaF per 100 mL water

Atomic weights: Na = 23; F = 19, Sn = 119; P = 31; O = 16

Fluoride compounds most often used are NaF, $SnF_2$, $Na_2FPO_3$

**Example 1: How much fluoride is in 10 mL of 0.05% NaF mouthrinse?**

The mouthrinse has 0.05 g of NaF per 100 mL of rinse

= 50 mg of NaF, or 5 mg of NaF per 10 mL

Amount of fluoride = 5 × 19/42 = 2.26 mg

**Example 2: How much fluoride is in a 6.4 oz tube of Colgate MFP toothpaste? (6.4 oz = 181.8 g)**

Colgate with sodium monofluorophosphate (MFP) is 0.76% $Na_2FPO_3$, so it has 0.76 g of MFP per 100 mL of toothpaste

Grams of $Na_2FPO_3$ in a 6.4 oz tube = 0.76 × 181.8/100 = 1.38 g, which is 1380 mg $Na_2FPO_3$

Amount of fluoride in the tube = 1380 × 19/144 = 182.1 mg

**Example 3: How much fluoride is in an 8.2 oz tube of Crest toothpaste? (8.2 oz = 232.9 g)**

Crest contains 0.243% NaF, so it has 0.243 g of NaF per 100 mL of toothpaste

Grams of NaF in an 8.2 oz tube = 0.243 × 232.9/100 = 0.566 g, which is 566 mg NaF

Amount of fluoride in the tube = 566 × 19/42 = 256 mg

---

**• BOX 25.4    Data on Toxic Fluoride Intake Levels in Humans[30,68]**

- Certainly lethal dose (CLD) = 32–64 mg fluoride/kg body weight
- Death is likely in a child who ingests more than 15 mg fluoride/kg body weight
- Probably toxic dose (PTD), defined as the minimum dose that could cause toxic signs and symptoms, including death, and the ingestion of which should trigger immediate intervention and hospitalization = 5 mg fluoride/kg body weight

The 10th and 90th percentiles of weight for children at various ages are as follows:

| Age | Weight |
|-----|--------|
| 1 year | 8–12 kg |
| 2 years | 10–15 kg |
| 3 years | 12–17 kg |
| 4 years | 14–20 kg |
| 6 years | 17–27 kg |
| 8 years | 22–34 kg |

So for a child about 7 years of age, who would weight approximately 20 kg, the PTD would be around 100 mg fluoride.

---

available in Europe, Australia, and New Zealand for years, they have not been tested in clinical trials and are not approved for marketing in the United States and Canada.

The efficacy of fluoride toothpaste is mainly driven by three things: (1) the concentration of available fluoride; (2) the application to the tooth surface and biofilm; and (3) the retention of fluoride after brushing in saliva, plaque fluid, and other tissue reservoirs. However, the tendency to swallow toothpaste can lead to enamel fluorosis in children younger than age 6. Use of less toothpaste and brushing with adult supervision is advocated for this age group and *not* using an ineffective concentration of toothpaste. In 2014, the ADA published guidelines indicating that children under age 3 should be using no more than a smear of toothpaste that is the size of a grain of rice. For children 3 to 6 years old, caregivers should be dispensing no more than a pea-sized amount of fluoride toothpaste.[3]

## Standards for Toothpaste Efficacy

The toothpaste market is a multibillion-dollar industry in the United States, so competition between major manufacturers is keen. Companies incur much research and development expense to secure the ADA's seal of approval for their products; the logo on the package improves marketing and is a guide for consumers as well. Because of the multitude of formulations of fluoride plus abrasive available, the ADA developed guidelines for use in judging applications for its seal of approval for fluoride toothpastes.[1] With newer formulations replacing earlier products and advertising claims being made of superiority over rival products, the ADA Council on Scientific Affairs periodically determines standards such as what evidence would be adequate to substantiate claims of equivalency or superiority of a particular formulation (i.e., fluoride ingredient with compatible abrasives) relative to other formulations. Typically, manufacturer claims need to be backed by rigorous clinical trials in human populations and such trials require the use of the rival product as a positive control. The trials had to be designed to show a 10% difference in caries increment with a power of 80% (see Chapter 13). The ADA's seal of approval goes to particular formulations rather than to products. The list of toothpastes that carry the seal, which can be found on the ADA website, is now quite long and seems to be constantly growing.

## Impact of Fluoride Toothpastes

The impact of fluoride toothpaste use on global caries experience has been profound. Fluoride exposure is accepted as the main reason for the decline of dental caries over recent years, and most authorities believe that fluoride toothpaste has been the most important fluoride vehicle on a global scale.[27] The caries reductions of 15% to 30% achieved in most clinical trials may appear modest compared to those attributed to water fluoridation, but it must be remembered that these were trials of 2 to 3 years' duration, whereas water fluoridation studies usually measured lifetime exposure. Because, as we know, fluoride works most effectively to prevent caries when small amounts are in the oral cavity at all times, there is no reason that regular lifetime use of fluoride toothpaste should not give results that are similar to those of lifetime use of fluoridated water.

Supervised brushing programs using fluoride toothpaste offer an approach for intervention in high-risk groups.[40] Efficacy of fluoride toothpaste appears to be enhanced in supervised settings[86,135] and successful programs have been used in places such as Ireland.[73] However, some investigators find good evidence for supervised programs to be lacking.[44]

## Multiple Fluoride Exposures

The majority of clinical trials of fluoride products test only a single agent. In the modern world, however, exposure to multiple sources of fluoride is the rule rather than the exception. People who live in fluoridated areas brush their teeth with fluoride toothpastes and are periodically given professional fluoride applications by their dentists. Fluoride mouthrinsing is used in public health programs, and some mouthwashes contain fluoride. Then there are dietary supplements, whether used appropriately or not, as well as the poorly quantified fluoride exposures from food and drink. When these are added together, it becomes readily apparent that people in most high-income countries are being exposed to much more fluoride than in the past.

This phenomenon of multiple fluoride exposures can be viewed from several perspectives. In one way it is beneficial because with the several different anticaries actions of fluoride, fuller advantage is being taken of fluoride's potential. On the other hand, the increasing prevalence of fluorosis (see Chapter 19) is almost certain to be a product of these multiple and poorly controlled fluoride exposures. Dentistry's goal, though not an easy one to achieve for either an individual patient or the community, is to maximize the benefits from fluoride exposure while avoiding an unacceptable level of the undesirable side effects.

Multiple fluoride therapies, whether in fluoridated or non-fluoridated areas, are clearly beneficial for patients who are unusually susceptible to caries. For example, excellent results may be attained in preventing caries in patients with salivary disorders such as Sjögren disease or those who have had radiation treatment that can produce dysfunction of the salivary glands and hence loss of salivary caries-protective benefits. Based on a recent systematic review, only a generic recommendation can be made for the use of topical fluoride as the first line of defense in individuals with Sjögren disease due to the lack of sufficient evidence for specific types of fluoride or frequency of use.[149]

Systematic reviews have found caries reductions above those expected from fluoridated water alone among children in studies of fluoride rinse[88] and studies of fluoride toothpaste.[86] In the context of cost-effectiveness, the data on the use of fluoride mouthrinses in fluoridated areas are worth examining in detail; Table 25.5 presents these data for four North American studies. A beneficial effect can be seen in each case, although even in the earlier studies the effects were limited in terms of absolute caries reductions. Cost-effectiveness issues arise given results such as

## • TABLE 25.5 Summarized Results of Studies of Fluoride Mouthrinses in Fluoridated Areas

| Material | Age Groups | Duration | % Reduction | DMFS Reduction | Reference |
|---|---|---|---|---|---|
| 0.1% SnF₂ daily | 8–13 yr | 20 mo | 33.1[a] | 1.00 | Radike et al.[108] |
| | | | 43.3[b] | 1.22 | |
| 0.05% NaF daily | 12 yr | 30 mo | 27.9[a] | 0.72 | Driscoll et al.[46] |
| | | | 49.7[a] | 0.94 | |
| 0.2% NaF weekly | 12 yr | 30 mo | 22.1[a] | 0.57 | Driscoll et al.[46] |
| | | | 55.0[b] | 1.04 | |
| 0.2% NaF weekly | Grades 1–2 | 48 mo | Not given[c] | 0.29 | Bell et al.[18] |
| | Grade 5 | 24 mo | Not given[c] | 0.03 | |

[a]First of two examiners.
[b]Second of two examiners.
[c]Could not be determined from the data provided.
*DMFS*, Decayed, missing, and filled tooth surfaces.

| Age Groups | Duration | F Rinse[a] | F Toothpaste[b] | Rinse + Toothpaste[c] | Placebo | Reference |
|---|---|---|---|---|---|---|
| Approximately 13 yr | 24 mo | 4.81 (13.1%)[d] | 4.44 (17.9%)[d] | 4.12 (22.7%)[d] | 5.61 | Ashley et al.[9] |
| 11 yr | 30 mo | 4.79 (23.4%)[d] | 5.14 (17.8%)[d] | 5.30 (15.2%)[d] | 6.51 | Ringelberg et al.[112] |
| 11–12 yr | 36 mo | 4.72 (24.5%)[d] | 4.60 (26.3%)[d] | 4.76 (26.8%)[d] | 6.25 | Blinkhorn et al.[25] |

• TABLE 25.6  Summarized Results of Studies of Additive Effects of Fluoride Mouthrinsing and Supervised Brushing With Fluoride Toothpastes DMFS Increments

[a]0.05% NaF daily at school.
[b]0.76% Sodium monofluorophosphate except for Ringelberg et al.[112] (0.4% stannous fluoride, unsupervised).
[c]All conducted supervised rinse immediately after brushing.
[d]Percentage reduction compared to placebo control.
DMFS, Decayed, missing, and filled tooth surfaces; F, fluoride.

these: When a new fluoride program is instituted among children who already have some fluoride exposure and low caries experience, is the additional benefit worth the cost?

The last two lines of Table 25.5 showing data from the NPDDP provoked the subsequent criticisms of fluoride mouthrinsing mentioned earlier in this chapter. Table 25.6 gives the results of studies in which supervised brushing with a fluoride toothpaste was combined with supervised daily fluoride mouthrinsing at school, and the results were compared with those for each procedure alone. The results for the combined procedures are, at best, only slightly superior to the use of either alone.

Because caries experience in North American children has generally reached lower levels than those at which the results in Tables 25.5 and 25.6 were produced, it is hard to argue for the cost-effectiveness of fluoride mouthrinsing in fluoridated areas, especially where frequent use of fluoride toothpaste is common, unless there is a way to target the intervention to individuals at high risk for caries. This conclusion was confirmed at the 1989 workshop on cost-effectiveness of preventive programs.[82]

Cost-effectiveness is a less important issue for the private patient than for public health programs, but selection of a preventive regimen for an individual patient should still take into account the likely added benefit of multiple exposures. To illustrate, professional fluoride applications are of dubious additional value to the individual patient in a fluoridated area who brushes daily with fluoride toothpaste and who has little caries problem. However, even in a fluoridated area, more caries-susceptible patients may get reasonable additional benefit from professional fluoride applications or prescribed daily use of fluoride mouthrinses. In these decisions, the clinical judgment should always be guided by sound evidence and can be enhanced by attention to recommendations on fluoride use.[142] The potential benefits of fluoride mouthrinses need to be weighed against the benefits of prescription high-concentration fluoride toothpaste for high caries–risk patients. As we have said already, however, broad exposure to multiple sources of fluoride is the norm in North America today. When introducing a new fluoride program in a community, therefore, a public health administrator must assess whether the program will produce benefits beyond those already being provided by other fluoride exposures. The evidence just cited shows that additional benefits will probably accrue, but the bigger public health question is whether the extra benefits will be worth the cost of the program.

## Nonrestorative Caries Treatment-Arresting Advanced Carious Lesions With Fluoride

In 2018, the ADA Council on Scientific Affairs released the first in a series of clinical practice guidelines for caries management. It presents a viable role for silver diamine fluoride that may optimize patient care in some scenarios.[123]

### Silver Diamine Fluoride

Silver diamine fluoride (SDF) is not new, but around 2014 it re-emerged in the United States as a nonrestorative treatment that is effective for carious lesions.[103,123] The 2018 ADA clinical practice guideline[123] summarizes and highlights the effectiveness of SDF for advanced cavitated coronal and root surface lesions. Application of 38% SDF biannually is shown to be more effective at arresting advanced cavitated lesions on primary teeth than 5% NaF varnish applied once per week for 3 weeks and more effective than a single application of 38% SDF annually. The ADA panel recommends use of 38% SDF biannually to arrest cavitated lesions on primary teeth as a first line of care. The panel was comfortable extrapolating the published research to date to go on and recommend biannual application of 38% SDF for advanced cavitated lesions on permanent teeth as well. Readers should be aware that ongoing research is likely to continue on use of SDF to better outline its comparative effectiveness in a range of settings.

Although the impact of SDF on cavitated lesions in primary teeth is well established, evidence that application of 38% SDF is effective for preventing new smooth surface lesions is building. A systematic review[103] of the beneficial impact of SDF on other teeth (beyond the ones treated with cavitated lesions) yielded only four studies that had data on primary teeth and followed the children at least 12 months. A key finding from a summarization of two studies that met the inclusion criteria was that 38% SDF provides a benefit to the entire primary dentition in children when they were followed at least 24 months. Compared to placebo, the prevented fraction was 77%.[103] More research will clarify these findings.

The formulation that has been approved for use in the United States is 38% SDF, which equates to 44,800 ppm fluoride. Clinical guidelines for treatment of cavitated lesions of coronal surfaces of primary and permanent teeth are for biannual applications of 38% SDF. The application of SDF arrests caries activity and forms a hard, blackened surface at the site. Use of SDF may be desired in situations where traditional restorative options are not favored, such as in uncooperative patients whose parents or caregivers prefer not to undergo use of general anesthesia. The blackened surface that results from the use of SDF may unacceptable to some patients and/or caregivers. Proper informed consent procedures need to be followed when use of SDF is under consideration.

SDF arrests carious lesions and provides a therapeutic result via several complementary mechanisms.[33] First, the silver component has a direct bactericidal effect by affecting sulfhydryl groups and interfering with metabolism. Second, the silver salts that form on the dentin are very resistant to penetration and protect the dentin tubules from exposure, thereby reducing sensitivity. The fluoride component forms fluorapatite to increase the mineral content of the enamel and improve acid resistance.

## Summary

Fluoride is an excellent model for examining preventive strategies in different contexts. However, in this chapter the focus is solely on fluoride in our efforts to prevent dental caries. Essentially, fluoride acts to raise the threshold of protection against injury to enamel from dietomicrobial acids. Injury prevention strategies[67] such as programs aimed to reduce traffic fatalities typically address factors beyond the occupants in the automobile and include efforts to improve the environmental substrate (i.e., the highway) and the factors that intensify the hazard, such as the velocity of the vehicle. It would be shortsighted to only focus on protecting the occupant when prevention of fatal crashes is the objective. Prevention strategies that aim further upstream to interrupt the cascade of factors that lead to the marshalling of the forces that produce the acid should also be deployed. Multiple avenues should be pursued to address biofilm composition[106] and accumulation as well as the role of dietary sugars[98,120] for a more comprehensive approach to prevent dental caries. These aspects are addressed in other chapters of this volume (diet in Chapter 23 and sealants in Chapter 26).

## References

1. ADA. *ADA Seal of Acceptance.* Available from: https://www.ada.org/en/science-research/ada-seal-of-acceptance/how-to-earn-the-ada-seal/general-criteria-for-acceptance; 2011.
2. ADA. *Fluoridation Facts 2018.* Chicago: American Dental Association; 2018.
3. ADA Council on Scientific Affairs. Fluoride toothpaste use for young children. *J Am Dent Assoc.* 2014;145(2):190–191.
4. Allukian M Jr, Carter-Pokras OD, Gooch BF, et al. Science, politics, and communication: the case of community water fluoridation in the US. *Ann Epidemiol.* 2018;28(6):401–410.
5. American Academy of Pediatrics. *Oral Health Education and Training.* Available from: https://www.aap.org/en-us/advocacy-and-policy/aap-health-initiatives/Oral-Health/Pages/Education-and-Training.aspx. Accessed May 22, 2019.
6. APHA Technical Report. Review of the National Preventive Dentistry Demonstration Program. *Am J Public Health.* 1986;76(4):434–447.
7. Arnold FA Jr, Dean HT, Knutson JW. Effect of fluoridated public water supplies on dental caries prevalence: seventh year of Grand Rapids-Muskegon study. *Public Health Rep (1896–1970).* 1953;68(2):141–148.
8. Arnold FA Jr, Likins RC, Russell AL, et al. Fifteenth year of the Grand Rapids fluoridation study. *J Am Dental Assoc.* 1962;65(6):780–785.
9. Ashley FP, Mainwaring PJ, Emslie RD, et al. Clinical testing of a mouthrinse and a dentifrice containing fluoride. A two-year supervised study in school children. *Br Dent J.* 1977;143(10):333–338.
10. Ast DB, Finn SB, McCaffrey I. The Newburgh-Kingston caries fluorine study. I. Dental findings after three years of water fluoridation. *Am J Public Health Nations Health.* 1950;40(6):716–724.
11. Ast DB, Fitzgerald B. Effectiveness of water fluoridation. *J Am Dent Assoc.* 1962;65(5):581–587.
12. Ast DB, Smith DJ, Wachs B, Cantwell KT. The Newburgh-Kingston caries-fluorine study. XIV. Combined clinical and roentgenographic dental findings after ten years of fluoride experience. *J Am Dent Assoc.* 1956;52:314–325.
13. ASTDD. *Directors AoSaTD.* Best Practice Approach Report. Use of fluoride in schools. ASTDD; 2018.
14. Auerbach J. The 3 buckets of prevention. *J Public Health Manage Practice.* 2016;22(3):215–218.
15. Backer Dirks OHB, Kwant GW. The result of 6½ years of artificial drinking water in the Netherlands; the Tiel-Culemborg experiment. *Arch Oral Biol.* 1961;5:284–300.
16. Bailey W. Fluoridation Law. In: *NOHC 2009: National Oral Health Conference*; 2009.
17. Banoczy J, Rugg-Gunn AJ. Clinical Studies. In: Banoczy J, Petersen PE, Rugg-Gunn AJ, eds. *Milk fluoridation for the prevention of dental caries.* Geneva: World Health Organization; 2009.
18. Bell RM, Klein SP, Bohannan HM, Disney JA, Graves RC, Madison R. *Treatment effects in the National Preventive Dentistry Demonstration Program.* Santa Monical, CA: Rand Corporation; 1984.
19. Beltrán ED, Szpunar SM. Fluoride in toothpastes for children: suggestion for change. *Ped Dent.* 1988;10(3):185–188.
20. Beltrán-Aguilar ED, Barker L, Sohn W, Wei L. Water intake by outdoor temperature among children aged 1–10 years: implications for community water fluoridation in the U.S. *Public Health Rep.* 2015;130(4):362–371.
21. Beltrán-Aguilar ED, Goldstein JW, Lockwood SA. Fluoride varnishes: a review of their clinical use, cariostatic mechanism, efficacy and safety. *J Am Dent Assoc.* 2000;131(5):589–596.
22. Blayney JR, Hill IN. Fluorine and dental caries. *J Am Dent Assoc.* 1967;74(Special Issue):233–302.
23. Blayney JR, Hill IN, Wolf W. The Evanston dental caries study. XVI. Reduction in dental caries attack rates in children six to eight years old. *J Am Dent Assoc.* 1956;53(3):327–333.
24. Blayney JR, Tucker WH. The Evanston dental caries study: II. Purpose and mechanism of the study. *J Dent Res.* 1948;27(3):279–286.
25. Blinkhorn AS, Holloway PJ, Davies TGH. Combined effects of a fluoride dentifrice and mouthrinse on the incidence of dental caries. *Community Dent Oral Epidemiol.* 1983;11(1):7–11.
26. Bohannan HM, Graves RC, Disney JA, Stamm JW, Abernathy JB, Bader JD. Effect of secular decline in caries on the evaluation of preventive dentistry demonstrations. *J Public Health Dent.* 1985;45(2):83–89.
27. Bratthall D, Hansel-Petersson G, Sundberg H. Reasons for the caries decline: what do the experts believe? *Eur J Oral Sci.* 1996;104:416–422.
28. Brownson RC, Baker EA, Leet TL, Gillespie KN, True WR. *Evidence-Based Public Health.* 2nd ed. New York: Oxford University Press; 2011.
29. Buchalla W, Attin T, Schulte-Mönting J, Hellwig E. Fluoride uptake, retention, and remineralization efficacy of a highly concentrated fluoride solution on enamel lesions in situ. *J Dent Res.* 2002;81(5):329–333.
30. Burt BA. The changing patterns of systemic fluoride intake. *J Dent Res.* 1992;71:1228–1237.

31. Burt BA. Fluoridation and social equity. *J Public Health Dent.* 2002;62(4):195–200.

32. Burt BA, Eklund SA, Ismail AI. Root caries in an optimally fluoridated and a high-fluoride community. *J Dent Res.* 1986;65(9): 1154–1158.

33. Chibinski AC, Wambier LM, Feltrin J, Loguercio AD, Wambier DS, Reis A. Silver diamine fluoride has efficacy in controlling caries progression in primary teeth: a systematic review and meta-analysis. *Caries Res.* 2017;51(5):527–541.

34. Dawes C. Salivary flow patterns and the health of hard and soft oral tissues. *J Am Dent Assoc.* 2008;139:18S–24S.

35. Dean HT. The investigation of physiological effects by the epidemiological method. In: Moulton FR, ed. *Fluorine and dental health.* Washington DC: American Association for the Advancement of Science; 1942:23–31.

36. Dean HT, Arnold FA Jr, Jay P, et al. Studies on mass control of dental caries through fluoridation of the public water supply. *Public Health Rep.* 1950;65:1403–1408.

37. Dean HT, Arnold Francis A Jr, Elias E. Domestic Water and Dental Caries: V. Additional studies of the relation of fluoride domestic waters to dental caries experience in 4,425 white children, aged 12 to 14 years, of 13 cities in 4 states. *Public Health Rep (1896–1970).* 1942;57(32):1155–1179.

38. Dean HT, Jay P, Arnold FA Jr, et al. Domestic water and dental caries: II. A study of 2,832 white children, aged 12–14 years, of 8 suburban Chicago communities, including Lactobacillus acidophilus studies of 1,761 children. *Public Health Rep (1896–1970).* 1941;56(15):761–792.

39. DePaola PF, Soparkar PM, Triol C, et al. The relative anticaries effectiveness of sodium monofluorophosphate and sodium fluoride as contained in currently available dentifrice formulations. *Am J Dent.* 1993;S7–S12.

40. Dickson-Swift V, Kenny A, Gussy M, et al. Supervised toothbrushing programs in primary schools and early childhood settings: a scoping review. *Community Dent Health.* 2017;34(4):208–225.

41. Disney JA, Bohannan HM, Klein SP, et al. A case study in contesting the conventional wisdom: school-based fluoride mouthrinse programs in the USA. *Community Dent Oral Epidemiol.* 1990;18(1): 46–56.

42. Disney JA, Graves RC, Stamm JW, et al. Comparative effects of a 4-year fluoride mouthrinse program on high and low caries forming grade 1 children. *Community Dent Oral Epidemiol.* 1989;17 (3):139–143.

43. Do L, Ha D, Peres MA, Skinner J, et al. Effectiveness of water fluoridation in the prevention of dental caries across adult age groups. *Community Dent Oral Epidemiol.* 2017;45(3):225–232.

44. dos Santos APP, de Oliveira BH, Nadanovsky P. A systematic review of the effects of supervised toothbrushing on caries incidence in children and adolescents. *Int J Paed Dent.* 2018;28(1):3–11.

45. Dos Santos APP, Nadanovsky P, De Oliveira BH. A systematic review and meta-analysis of the effects of fluoride toothpastes on the prevention of dental caries in the primary dentition of preschool children. *Community Dent Oral Epidemiol.* 2013;41(1): 1–12.

46. Driscoll WS, Swango PA, Horowitz AM. Caries-preventive effects of daily and weekly fluoride mouthrinsing in a fluoridated community: final results after 30 months. *J Am Dent Assoc. (1939).* 1982;105(6):1010–1013.

47. EPA. Drinking Water Regulations. Public Notifications. *Fed Reg.* 1987;52:41534–41550.

48. EPA. *National Primary Drinking Water Regulations; Announcement of the Results of EPA's Review of Existing Drinking Water Standards and Request for Public Comment and/or Information on Related Issues.* Washington, DC: National Archives; January 11, 2017.

49. Duckworth RM. Pharmacokinetics in the oral cavity: fluoride and other active ingredients. *Monographs in Oral Science.* 2013;23: 125–139.

50. Duckworth RM, Knoop D, Stephen KW. Effect of mouthrinsing after toothbrushing with a fluoride dentifrice on human salivary fluoride levels. *Caries Res.* 1991;25(4):287–291.

51. EPA. Interim Primary Drinking Water Regulations. *Fed Reg.* 1980;45(168):57332–57357.

52. EPA. National Primary Drinking Water Regulations. *Fluoride Fed Reg.* 1985;50:20164–20175.

53. EPA. National Primary and Secondary Drinking Water Regulations. Fluoride; Final Rule. *Fed Reg.* 1986;51:11396–11412.

54. Featherstone JDB. Prevention and reversal of dental caries: role of low level fluoride. *Community Dent Oral Epidemiol.* 1999;27(1):31–40.

55. FDI World Dental Federation. *Promoting Dental Health Through Fluoride Toothpaste.* Geneva, 2018.

56. FDI World Dental Federation. Promoting Oral Health Through Fluoride. *Int Dent J.* 2018;68(1):16–17.

57. Fejerskov O. Concepts of dental caries and their consequences for understanding the disease. *Community Dent Oral Epidemiol.* 1997;25(1):5–12.

58. Fleiss JL. A dissenting opinion on the National Preventive Dentistry Demonstration Program. *Am J Public Health.* 1986;76(4):445–447.

59. Community Preventive Services Task Force. Available from: https://www.thecommunityguide.org/sites/default/files/assets/Oral-Health-Caries-Community-Water-Fluoridation_3.pdf.

60. Frieden TR. A framework for public health action: the health impact pyramid. *Am J Public Health.* 2010;100(4):590–595.

61. Gauger TL, Prosser LA, Fontana M, Polverini PJ. Integrative and collaborative care models between pediatric oral health and primary care providers: a scoping review of the literature. *J Public Health Dent.* 2018;78(3):246–256.

62. Gluzman R, Katz RV, Frey BJ, et al. Prevention of root caries: a literature review of primary and secondary preventive agents. *Spec Care Dentistry.* 2013;33(3):133–140.

63. Goldman AS, Yee R, Holmgren CJ, et al. *Global affordability of fluoride toothpaste.* 2008;4:7.

64. Graham E, Negron R, Domoto P, et al. Children's oral health in the medical curriculum: a collaborative intervention at a university-affiliated hospital. *J Dent Ed.* 2003;67(3):338–347.

65. Griffin SO, Gooch BF, Lockwood SA, et al. Quantifying the diffused benefit from water fluoridation in the United States. *Community Dent Oral Epidemiol.* 2001;29(2):120–129.

66. Groeneveld A, Van Eck AAMJ, Backer Dirks O. Fluoride in caries prevention: is the effect pre- or post-eruptive? *J Dent Res.* 1990;69 (Feb Spec Iss):751–755.

67. Haddon W Jr. On the escape of tigers: an ecologic note. *Am J Public Health Nation's Health.* 1970;60(12):2229–2234.

68. Heifetz SB, Horowitz HS. Amounts of fluoride in self administered dental products: safety considerations for children. *Pediatrics.* 1986;77:876–882.

69. Heller KE, Sohn W, Burt BA, Eklund SA. Water consumption in the United States in 1994–96 and implications for water fluoridation policy. *J Public Health Dent.* 1999;59(1):3–11.

70. Hutton WL, Linscott BW, Williams DB. The Brantford fluorine experiment: interim report after five years of water fluoridation. *Can J Public Health/Rev Can Santee Publique.* 1951;42(3):81–87.

71. Hutton WL, Linscott BW, Williams DB. Final report of local studies on water fluoridation in Brantford. *Can J Public Health/Rev Can Santee Publique.* 1956;47(3):89–92.

72. Iheozor-Ejiofor Z, Worthington HV, Walsh T, et al. Water fluoridation for the prevention of dental caries. *Cochrane DB Syst Rev U6.* 2015;(6). CD010856.

73. Irish Oral Health Services Guideline Initiative. Topical fluorides: Evidence-based guidance on the use of topical fluorides for caries prevention in children and adolescents in Ireland. University College Cork. 2008.

74. Ismail AI, Tellez M, Pitts NB, et al. Caries management pathways preserve dental tissues and promote oral health. *Community Dent Oral Epidemiol.* 2013;41(1):e12–e40.

75. Keyes PH. Recent advances in dental caries research. Bacteriology. Bacteriological findings and biological implications. *Int Dent J.* 1962;12(4):443–464.

76. Klein SP, Bohannan HM, Bell RM, et al. The cost and effectiveness of school-based preventive dental care. *Am J Public Health.* 1985; 75(4):382–391.

77. Koo H. Strategies to enhance the biological effects of fluoride on dental biofilms. *Adv Dent Res.* 2008;20(1):17–21.

78. Kranz AM, Preisser JS, Rozier RG. Effects of physician-based preventive oral health services on dental caries. *Pediatrics.* 2015;136(1):107.

79. Kumar JV. Is water fluoridation still necessary? *Adv Dent Res.* 2008;20(1):8–12.

80. Kumar JV, Adekugbe O, Melnik TA. Geographic variation in medicaid claims for dental procedures in New York state: role of fluoridation under contemporary conditions. *Public Health Rep.* 2010;125(5):647–654.

81. Lamont RJ, Koo H, Hajishengallis G. The oral microbiota: dynamic communities and host interactions. *Nat Rev Microbiol.* 2018.

82. Leverett DH. Effectiveness of mouthrinsing with fluoride solutions in preventing coronal and root caries. *J Public Health Dent.* 1989; 49(5):310–316.

83. Leverett DH, Adair SM, Vaughan BW, et al. Randomized clinical trial of the effect of prenatal fluoride supplements in preventing dental caries. *Caries Res.* 1997;31(3):174–179.

84. Li X, Wang J, Joiner A, Chang J. The remineralisation of enamel: a review of the literature. *J Dent.* 2014;42:S12–S20.

85. Margolis HC, Moreno EC, Murphy BJ. Effect of low levels of fluoride in solution on enamel demineralization in vitro. *J Dent Res.* 1986;65(1):23–29.

86. Marinho VC, Higgins JP, Sheiham A, Logan S. Fluoride toothpastes for preventing dental caries in children and adolescents. *Cochrane DB Syst Rev (Online).* 2003;(1).

87. Marinho VC, Higgins JP, Sheiham A, Logan S. One topical fluoride (toothpastes, or mouthrinses, or gels, or varnishes) versus another for preventing dental caries in children and adolescents. *Cochrane DB Syst Rev (Online).* 2004;(1). Available from: https://doi.org/10.1002/14651858.CD002780.pub2.

88. Marinho VCC, Chong LY, Worthington HV, Walsh T. Fluoride mouthrinses for preventing dental caries in children and adolescents. *Cochrane DB Syst Rev.* 2016;2016(7).

89. Marinho VCC, Worthington HV, Walsh T, Chong LY. Fluoride gels for preventing dental caries in children and adolescents. *Cochrane DB Syst Rev.* 2015;2015(6).

90. Marinho VCC, Worthington HV, Walsh T, Clarkson JE. Fluoride varnishes for preventing dental caries in children and adolescents. *Cochrane DB Syst Rev.* 2013;2013(7).

91. Marks RG, Conti AJ, Moorhead JE, et al. Results from a three-year caries clinical trial comparing NaF and SMFP fluoride formulations. *Int Dent J.* 1994;44(3 suppl 1):275–285.

92. Marquis RE, Clock SA, Mota-Meira M. Fluoride and organic weak acids as modulators of microbial physiology. *FEMS Microbiol Rev.* 2003;26(5):493–510.

93. Marshall TA, Levy SM, Broffitt B, et al. Patterns of beverage consumption during the transition stage of infant nutrition. *J Am Dietetic Assoc.* 2003;103(10):1350–1353.

94. Marthaler TM. Salt fluoridation and oral health. *Acta Med Academ.* 2013;42:140–155.

95. McDonagh MS, Kleijnen J, Whiting PF, et al. Systematic review of water fluoridation. *Br Med J.* 2000;321(7265):855–859.

96. McLaren L, Singhal S. Does cessation of community water fluoridation lead to an increase in tooth decay? A systematic review of published studies. *J Epidemiol Community Health.* 2016;70 (9):934–940.

97. Moyer VA. Prevention of dental caries in children from birth through age 5 years: US Preventive Services Task Force recommendation statement. *Pediatrics.* 2014;133(6):1102–1111.

98. Moynihan PJ, Kelly SAM. Effect on caries of restricting sugars intake: systematic review to inform WHO guidelines. *J Dent Res.* 2014;93(1):8–18.

99. Muhler JC, Radike AW, Nebergall WH, Day HG. A comparison between the anticariogenic effects of dentifrices containing stannous fluoride and sodium fluoride. *J Am Dent Assoc. (1939).* 1955;51(5): 556–559.

100. National Research Council. *Fluoride in Drinking Water: A Scientific Review of EPA's Standards.* Washington, DC: The National Academies Press; 2006.

101. O'Connell J, Rockell J, Ouellet J, et al. Costs and savings associated with community water fluoridation in the United States. *Health Affairs.* 2016;35(12):2224–2232.

102. O'Mullane DM, Baez RJ, Jones S, et al. Fluoride and oral health. *Community Dent Health.* 2016;33(2):69–99.

103. Oliveira BH, Rajendra A, Veitz-Keenan A, et al. The effect of silver diamine fluoride in preventing caries in the primary dentition: a systematic review and meta-analysis. *Caries Res.* 2019;53(1):24–32.

104. Parnell C, Whelton H, O'Mullane D. Water fluoridation. *Eur Arch Paediatr Dent.* 2009;10(3):141–148.

105. Petersen PE, Ogawa H. Prevention of dental caries through the use of fluoride - the WHO approach. *Community Dent Health.* 2016;33:66–68.

106. Philip N, Suneja B, Walsh LJ. Ecological approaches to dental caries prevention: paradigm shift or shibboleth? *Caries Res.* 2018;52(1-2): 153–165.

107. Pitts NB, Zero DT, Marsh PD, et al. Dental caries. *Nat Rev Disease Primers.* 2017;3.

108. Radike AW, Gish CW, Peterson JK, et al. Clinical evaluation of stanous fluoride as an anticaries mouthrinse. *J Am Dent Assoc.* 1973;86(2):404–408.

109. Ran T, Chattopadhyay SK. Economic evaluation of community water fluoridation: a community guide systematic review. *Am J Prevent Med.* 2016;50(6):790–796.

110. Reintsema H, Schuthof J, Arends J. An in vivo investigation of the fluoride uptake in partially demineralized human enamel from several different dentifrices. *J Dent Res.* 1985;64(1):19–23.

111. Rihs LB. Da Luz Rosário De Sousa M, et al.. Root caries in areas with and without fluoridated water at the southeast region of São Paulo State, Brazil. *J Appl Oral Sci.* 2008;16(1):70–74.

112. Ringelberg ML, Webster DB, Dixon DO, et al. The caries-preventive effect of amine fluorides and inorganic fluorides in a mouthrinse or dentifrice after 30 months of use. *J Am Dent Assoc. (1939).* 1979;98(2):202–208.

113. Rose G. Sick individuals and sick populations. *Int J Epidemiol.* 1985;14(1):32–38.

114. Rosier BT, Marsh PD, Mira A. Resilience of the oral microbiota in health: mechanisms that prevent dysbiosis. *J Dent Res.* 2018;97(4): 371–380.

115. Rozier RG, Adair S, Graham F, et al. Evidence-based clinical recommendations on the prescription of dietary fluoride supplements for caries prevention: a report of the American Dental Association Council on Scientific Affairs. *J Am Dent Assoc.* 2010;141(12): 1480–1489.

116. Ruff JC, Herndon JB, Horton RA, et al. Developing a caries risk registry to support caries risk assessment and management for children: a quality improvement initiative. *J Public Health Dent.* 2018;78(2):134–143.

117. Rugg-Gunn AJ, Do L. Effectiveness of water fluoridation in caries prevention. *Community Dent Oral Epidemiol.* 2012;40(suppl 2):55–64.

118. Rugg-Gunn AJ, Spencer AJ, Whelton HP, et al. Critique of the review of "Water fluoridation for the prevention of dental caries" published by the Cochrane Collaboration in 2015. *Br Dent J.* 2016;220(7):335–340.

119. Russell AL. Dental fluorosis in Grand Rapids during the seventeenth year of fluoridation. *J Am Dent Assoc.* 1962;65(5): 608–612.

120. Sheiham A, James WPT. Diet and dental caries: the pivotal role of free sugars reemphasized. *J Dent Res.* 2015;94(10):1341–1347.

121. Shellis RP, Duckworth RM. Studies on the cariostatic mechanisms of fluoride. *Int Dent J.* 1994;44(3 suppl 1):263–273.

122. Slade GD, Grider WB, Maas WR, et al. Water fluoridation and dental caries in U.S. children and adolescents. *J Dent Res*. 2018; 97(10):1122–1128.

123. Slayton RL, Urquhart O, Araujo MWB, et al. Evidence-based clinical practice guideline on nonrestorative treatments for carious lesions. *J Am Dent Assoc*. 2018;149(10):837–849. e819.

124. Society of Teachers of Family Medicine. Caries risk assessment, fluoride varnish and counseling—Course 6. Smiles for Life. In: *A National Oral Health Curriculum*; 2017. Available from: http://www.smilesforlifeoralhealth.org/buildcontent.aspx?tut=584& pagekey=64563&cbreceipt=0.

125. Sohn W, Heller KE, Burt BA. Fluid consumption related to climate among children in the United States. *J Public Health Dent*. 2001;61 (2):99–106.

126. Spencer AJ, Do LG, Ha DH. Contemporary evidence on the effectiveness of water fluoridation in the prevention of childhood caries. *Community Dent Oral Epidemiol*. 2018;46(4):407–415.

127. Spencer AJ, Liu P, Armfield JM, et al. Preventive benefit of access to fluoridated water for young adults. *J Public Health Dent*. 2017;77(3): 263–271.

128. Stamm JW, Banting DW, Imrey PB. Adult root caries survey of two similar communities with contrasting natural water fluoride levels. *J Am Dent Assoc. (1939)*. 1990;120(2):143–149.

129. Stamm JW, Bohannan HM, Graves RC, Disney JA. The efficiency of caries prevention with weekly fluoride mouthrinses. *J Dent Ed*. 1984;48(11):617–626.

130. Stoodley P, Sauer K, Davies DG, et al. Biofilms as complex differentiated communities. *Ann Rev Microbiol*. 2002;56: 187–209.

131. Stookey GK, Schemehorn BR, Cheetham BL, et al. In situ fluoride uptake from fluoride dentifrices by carious enamel. *J Dent Res*. 1985;64(6):900–903.

132. Tank G. Storvick CA. Caries experience of children one to six years old in two Oregon communities (Corvallis and Albany). I. Effect of fluoride on caries experience and eruption of teeth. *J Am Dent Assoc. (1939)*. 1964;69(6):749–757.

133. ten Cate JM, Featherstone JDB. Mechanistic aspects of the interactions between fluoride and dental enamel. *Crit Rev Oral Biol Med*. 1991;2(3):283–296.

134. Tubert-Jeannin S, Tramini P, Gerbaud L, et al. Fluoride supplements (tablets, drops, lozenges or chewing gums) for preventing dental caries in children. *Cochrane DB Syst Rev*. 2009;2009(1).

135. Twetman S, Axelsson S, Dahlgren H, et al. Caries-preventive effect of fluoride toothpaste: a systematic review. *Acta Odontol Scan*. 2003;61(6):347–355.

136. US Public Health Service Centers for Disease Control and Prevention. Ten great public health achievements: United States 1900–1999. *Morbid Mortal Weekly Rep*. 1999;48(12):241–243.

137. US Public Health Service Centers for Disease Control and Prevention. Health Impact in 5 Years. Available from: https://www.cdc.gov/policy/hst/hi5/index.html; 2017.

138. US Public Health Service Centers for Disease Control and Prevention. *Fluoridation Statistics*. 2014;Revised July 2016. Available from: https://www.cdc.gov/fluoridation/statistics/2014stats.htm.

139. USDHHS Federal Panel on Community Water Fluoridation. US Public Health Service recommendation for fluoride concentration in drinking water for the prevention of dental caries. *Public Health Rep*. 2015;130(4):318–331.

140. Vogel GL. Oral fluoride reservoirs and the prevention of dental caries. *Monogr Oral Sci*. 2011;22:146–157.

141. Weintraub JA, Ramos-Gomez F, Jue B, et al. Fluoride varnish efficacy in preventing early childhood caries. *J Dent Res*. 2006;85(2): 172–176.

142. Weyant RI, Tracy SL, Anselmo T, et al. Topical fluoride for caries prevention. *J Am Dent Assoc*. 2013;144(11):1279–1291.

143. Wong MCM, Clarkson J, Glenny AM, et al. Cochrane reviews on the benefits/risks of fluoride toothpastes. *J Dent Res*. 2011;90(5): 573–579.

144. Yeung CA, Chong LY, Glenny AM. Fluoridated milk for preventing dental caries. *Cochrane DB Syst Rev*. 2015;2015(9).

145. Zero DT. Adaptations in Dental Plaque. In: Bowen WH, Tabak L, eds. *Cariology for the Nineties*. Rochester, NY: University of Rochester Press; 1993:333–350.

146. Zero DT. Dental caries process. *Dent Clinics North Am*. 1999;43(4): 635–664.

147. Zero DT. Sugars—the arch criminal? *Caries Res*. 2004;38(3):277–285.

148. Zero DT. Dentifrices, mouthwashes, and remineralization/caries arrestment strategies. *BMC Oral Health*. 2006;6(suppl 1):S9.

149. Zero DT, Brennan MT, Daniels TE, et al. Clinical practice guidelines for oral management of Sjögren disease: dental caries prevention. *J Am Dent Assoc*. 2016;147(4):295–305.

150. Zero DT, Raubertas RF, Pedersen AM, et al. Studies of fluoride retention by oral soft tissues after the application of home-use topical fluorides. *J Dent Res*. 1992;71(9):1546–1552.

# 26
# Dental Sealants and Caries Prevention

DARIEN WEATHERSPOON, DDS, MPH

MATT CRESPIN, MPH, RDH

A dental sealant is a professionally applied dental material used to prevent decay in the pits and fissures found on the occlusal surfaces of posterior teeth. Sealants are used as an important means of primary prevention by providing a physical barrier to the impaction of substrate for cariogenic bacteria in the crevices of teeth, thereby preventing caries from developing. They also play a role in secondary prevention, as they can halt the carious process after it has begun and therefore can be used as a form of treatment for early lesions. Different options for sealant materials exist, which will be discussed in this chapter. Sealants are applied to teeth in a liquid form and, depending on the specific material, will set through either a chemical reaction, a polymerization reaction (often referred to as "curing"), or a combination of the chemical and polymerization reactions.[9]

Dental sealant materials are sometimes referred to as *pit-and-fissure sealants*, but they are more commonly referred to as *dental sealants* or simply *sealants*. This chapter discusses the use of sealants in caries prevention, reviews sealant materials, reviews the literature on their efficacy and effectiveness, examines their cost-effectiveness, and provides an evidence-based rationale for to their use at both individual and population levels.

## Historical Development

The idea of physically occluding the pits and fissures of teeth is not new. As long ago as 1923, Hyatt suggested a technique he called "prophylactic odontotomy."[38] Developed in an age of severe and seemingly universal caries, Hyatt's technique involved minimal operative preparation of sound fissures and restoration with amalgam. The idea was not fully accepted even before the days of modern preventive dentistry,[42] but it led to widespread use of "preventive restoration," wherein sound fissures of teeth were prepared and restored on the grounds that without intervention such areas would soon develop decay anyway. For many years, this type of restoration was considered good preventive practice. Although it is not known how many caries lesions this method "prevented." Additionally the use of these preventive restorations resulted in artificially inflating decayed, missing, and filled (DMF) scores.

In the prefluoride era, various chemical agents were placed on tooth surfaces in an effort to prevent caries, but none proved to be successful.[41] Even as fluoride exposure became widespread, interest in a specific preventive agent for pit-and-fissure caries persisted, but it proved difficult to find a material that adhered successfully to enamel in the oral environment. A breakthrough came in 1955 with Buonocore's development of the acid-etch technique.[15] In the late 1960s, the bisphenol A-glycidyl methacrylate or "bis-GMA" formulation (a resin-based sealant that is the reaction product of bisphenol A [BPA] and glycidyl methacrylate with a methyl methacrylate monomer) was developed and proved successful in a feasibility trial.[16] The bis-GMA formulation became the basis of a number of other products that soon came onto the market. The American Dental Association (ADA) issued provisional acceptance of the first bis-GMA material, Nuva-Seal, in 1972[5] and full acceptance in 1976.[6]

Since then, the number and types of accepted sealant materials have grown steadily and will likely continue to grow in the future.[76] Currently, the most widely used sealant materials are resin based, but glass ionomer (cements) sealants are also commonly used, specifically under hydrophilic conditions because they are less moisture sensitive.[47] There is considerable ongoing research comparing the efficacy and effectiveness of different sealant materials in caries prevention and comparing the utility of sealants to other preventive dental materials, such as fluoride varnish.[1,2,20]

## Rationale for Sealants

Dental caries (tooth decay) is a chronic disease that results from the activity of bacterial biofilm on a tooth surface that is exposed to fermentable carbohydrate substrates over time, leading to demineralization and eventually cavitation.[76] It has been recognized for years that the fissured occlusal surfaces of posterior teeth are the tooth surfaces most vulnerable to caries. With the continuing decline in caries prevalence among young children,[22] caries is becoming more commonly a disease of the fissured surfaces, as the rate of interproximal caries development continues to decline faster than the overall rate of caries experience.[12] Occlusal surfaces are also those surfaces least protected by fluorides,[21] so the case for sealant application as an important part of the overall caries management process, complementary to fluoride use, is strong.

Nationally, it has been estimated that approximately 90% of carious lesions are found in the pits and fissures of posterior teeth in school-aged children.[40] By sealing the pits and fissures of occlusal surfaces, carious lesions can either be prevented from the onset or inhibited from further progressing to cavitated lesions.[76]

## Sealant Products and Procedures

The original bis-GMA materials, now referred to as first-generation sealants, polymerized under ultraviolet (UV) light, a procedure that required a bulky UV light source in the oral cavity. Second-generation sealants are chemically polymerized; that is, when they are mixed, the operator has a fixed time to apply the sealant before it hardens. A number of such sealants are currently available. Third-generation sealants are those cured by visible light, which gives the operator the advantage of curing the sealant only when satisfied that it is all correctly in place. That advantage also applied to first-generation UV-cured sealants, but the visible light sources are far more compact and less expensive than the original UV light sources. Some second- and third-generation sealants are colored or opaque to make them more visible at clinical examination.

It should also be noted that in 1996 a research report from Spain concluded that shortly after placement of sealants, bisphenol A and bisphenol A dimethacrylate monomers could be detected in saliva and that these monomers showed estrogen-like activity when tested in in vitro cultures of human breast cell tumors.[52] This effect is of concern, because it theoretically could result in increased tumor cell growth. Some sealant materials are free of these monomers and sealant manufacturers should be consulted to confirm this. To date there is no evidence that the transient amounts of these chemicals in saliva represent an important exposure in humans. In addition, none of the sealants that currently carries the ADA Seal of Acceptance produces detectable levels of bisphenol A.[3,4,76] However, the Spanish finding does point out that any material used in dentistry must be thoroughly evaluated for potential risk and that regardless of how safe it appears to be, practitioners must take care to use any procedure or material only when the patient is likely to benefit from it. In 2016, the *ADA Professional Product Review* published research showing a 6-year-old child is exposed to more BPA from food, drinks, sunscreen, shampoo, body wash, air, and thermal paper (receipt paper) than the amount that is in dental sealants.[4]

Sealant application is a simple though meticulous procedure that requires attention to all details of technique, especially moisture control. Even slight moisture contamination during sealant application and curing will result in failure. When applying a sealant, the operator begins by washing and drying the tooth surface, then etching with acid to demineralize the surface layers of enamel in and around the fissures. The etchant is supplied as either a liquid or a gel; 37% orthophosphoric acid is the most commonly used and recommended agent.[71] Acid etching dissolves out some of the inorganic fraction of the enamel, which subsequently allows "tags" of sealant to penetrate and thus enhances retention. Some of these tags can extend up to 100 μm into enamel, although tags of 15 to 20 μm are more common.[64] After etching, the tooth surface is again washed and dried thoroughly, and the liquid sealant is applied and worked into the fissures and pits. The sealant is then polymerized (by visible light or by self-curing) and trimmed if necessary. Detailed descriptions of the application process are available.[71]

By the early 21st century, the application of sealants as a purely caries-preventive procedure was merging into the popularity of minimally invasive or conservative restoration procedures, many of which also used the acid-etch technique. The trend was stimulated by the caries decline, which meant that practitioners increasingly had to manage small, slowly developing lesions rather than large cavities, and by the rapid developments in composite materials. Dentistry began moving away from placement of amalgams in traditionally prepped Black's preparations with extension for prevention and toward minimum-preparation or minimally invasive restorations, which were far less invasive, lasted longer, and were more aesthetic.[25] The preventive resin and sealed composite restoration,[45] sealed glass ionomer restoration,[36] and even sealed amalgams[45,46] are changing the face of restorative dentistry. Sealants can be used for both prevention on a sound tooth or for the treatment of a noncavitated carious lesion (NCCL) on the pit and fissure surfaces.[76] Clinicians should use the most current evidence-based recommendations available in determining the need for sealants and for proper application technique. The ADA Council on Scientific Affairs published detailed, well developed, evidence-based guidelines in 2008 and 2016.[76] When used for prevention or to treat an NCCL, the technical placement and recommendations are the same. Mechanical preparation of any sort is not recommended.[76]

Sealant materials have continued to evolve and now include "wet bond" sealants that can be applied when moisture is present. Additionally, glass ionomer cements (GIC) are becoming commonly used in cases where moisture control is an issue. The use of GIC has shown to be as effective in reducing caries as a traditional resin-based sealant, but studies show that they are five times more likely to fail.[76] The ability to follow the patient and monitor sealant retention may be a key factor in determining which sealant material is best for each individual patient.[76]

## Sealant Clinical Trial Design

The initial clinical trials for testing the efficacy of sealants necessarily differed from the classical model in several respects:
- The study design was usually a "split-mouth" (or "half-mouth") design, in which the analytic unit was a contralateral pair of teeth, usually first or second molars. Because test and control teeth are in the same mouth, the required number of study participants could be reduced, and controlled for patient factors.
- There was no placebo sealant; the control tooth of each pair in these earlier trials was simply left untreated (a passive control).
- Examiners could not be blinded in a trial with a passive control because they could see the sealant on the test tooth.

Given the overwhelming evidence for the efficacy of sealants, clinical trials testing new sealant products now most commonly apply an accepted sealant as a positive control on the control tooth. As positive controls are used in comparative studies, the examiners should be blind as to which sealant is the test product and which is the positive control. Since differences in efficacy between the test product and the control are expected to be small, the number of participants needed is usually high.

Many current clinical trials involving sealants compare the efficacy or effectiveness of different dental sealant materials in preventing caries or compare sealants to other caries preventive materials, such as fluoride varnish.[1,2] For studies comparing the efficacy/effectiveness of sealants to other caries-preventive agents, a parallel group design is sometimes used rather than a split-mouth study design, where one group of participants receives sealants and another group receives the other caries preventive agent (e.g., fluoride varnish), and the efficacy/effectiveness of the two preventive modalities is compared.[1] Systematic reviews, including meta analyses, are often conducted to provide a comprehensive summary of the current evidence produced from clinical trials that is relevant to answering clinical questions related to sealants.[1]

## Sealant Efficacy and Effectiveness

A large number of well-conducted sealant studies have been carried out, which allows conclusions on their efficacy to be stated with some confidence. The panel at the National Institutes of Health Consensus Conference on dental sealants in 1983, one of the relatively few such conferences held on dental procedures, concluded that sealants were highly efficacious.[50] The panel also noted, however, that practitioners were slow to adopt their use and that insurance carriers were also hesitant about adding sealant application to their list of benefits. The Medicaid programs in all 50 states now cover sealant application, and although precise numbers are unavailable, the number of privately insured groups with sealant coverage continues to grow.

The first clinical sealant studies in the 1960s yielded spectacular results, with caries reductions of 99% reported.[16] These initial studies, however, carefully selected both the patients and the teeth to be sealed. By the end of the 1970s, there was clear evidence from numerous clinical trials in different populations that sealants were highly efficacious when applied correctly.[56] Studies since then using second- and third-generation sealants have almost all yielded results highly favoring their use; reviews of what is now an extensive literature have all reached highly favorable conclusions regarding their efficacy.[2,57,76] Well-controlled clinical trials have shown good results after 5 years[37] and 10 years[57]; and 15-year retrospective reports also showed encouraging results.[66]

In 2004 and 2005, the Centers for Disease Control and Prevention (CDC) sponsored an expert working group to update recommendations for sealant use in school-based sealant programs.[27] As part of this working group, a review of the available evidence on the effectiveness of sealants on sound and carious pit and fissure surfaces occurred. Reviews of three metaanalyses by the group found that sealants are effective in preventing the development of caries on sound pit and fissure surfaces. One of the reviewed metaanalyses (a metaanalysis of 10 studies) found that sealants placed on sound permanent molars in children and adolescents reduced dental caries by 78% at 1 year and 59% at 4 or more years of follow-up.[27] The favorable evidence has led the ADA to strongly support the appropriate use of sealants in general practice.[9]

Evidence for the efficacy of sealant application in private practice, although scanty, also appears favorable. In an observational study in Canada, sealed first permanent molars had a 75% lower incidence of new restorations than originally sound but unsealed molars.[39] The authors acknowledged that use of sealants was more common in caries-free children and in children whose parents had higher levels of education, which could account for some of the lower caries increment, but the differences in caries experience were so large that sealants had to have played a substantial role. It is nevertheless important to be cautious in interpreting outcomes from observational studies in which patients are not randomly assigned to receive or not to receive sealants. As has been pointed out in a study of the use of sealants in a Medicaid program, the children who actually received sealants tended to be at lower risk; that is, they were more likely to have been caries free initially and were more likely to have been classified by the study examiners as not needing sealants.[59] The authors pointed out that this pattern of nonrandom use of sealants in the least caries-prone children could lead to overestimates of sealant effectiveness. Nevertheless, there is ample reason to think that, with appropriate patient selection, sealant application is highly effective in private practice.

Findings from the earlier clinical studies of sealants that have been supported by later research include the following:
- The performance of a sealant is not impacted by side of the mouth or arch placed nor tooth type with the exception of premolars.[53]
- Retention seems better on premolars than on molars. This too is likely to come from better accessibility, plus the fact that in studies in which children have had premolars sealed they were obviously older than children who had only their first molars available for sealing.
- Sealants are better retained when placed in older children. This is thought to be due to the ability to achieve better isolation in more completely erupted teeth and the ability of the older child to cooperate in maintaining a dry field.
- Retention of sealant is synonymous with freedom from caries. An early concern was how the caries status of a tooth could be judged beneath intact sealant, but subsequent clinical research has shown that caries does not progress beneath intact sealant.
- Loss of sealant is greatest in the first 6 months after application. The sealant is probably lost very early in that period, however, because the data suggest that the rapidly lost sealants are those that never properly adhered in the first place. The most likely reason for this kind of failure is moisture contamination. A properly placed sealant will gradually wear down after a period of years, but protection from caries seems to remain, perhaps because of the sealant tags. The quickly lost sealant almost certainly has no tags, so the tooth concerned becomes vulnerable again.

These results demonstrated unequivocally the considerable efficacy of sealants; they also gave hints of the more recent realization that sealants are more difficult to successfully apply and maintain on the very teeth that are most vulnerable, that is, the early erupting molars in caries-prone children. On the other hand, sealants seem to be retained best on teeth that are least caries prone (e.g., bicuspids) and in children with low caries risk.[13] This realization is part of what has led to efforts to target sealant use to the most susceptible groups, individuals, and teeth, an issue discussed later in this chapter.

Later studies of sealant efficacy have led to additional conclusions that have an important bearing on the way sealants are used in clinical practice. These conclusions are discussed in the

**• TABLE 26.1** Summary of Clinical Recommendations on the Use of Pit-and-Fissure Sealants in the Occlusal Surfaces of Primary and Permanent Molars in Children and Adolescents[76]

| Question | Recommendation | Quality of the Evidence | Strength of Recommendation |
|---|---|---|---|
| Should dental sealants, when compared with nonuse of sealants, be used in pits and fissures of occlusal surfaces of primary and permanent molars on teeth deemed to have clinically sound occlusal surfaces or noncavitated carious lesions? | The sealant guideline panel recommends the use of sealants compared with nonuse in permanent molars with both sound occlusal surfaces and noncavitated occlusal carious lesions in children and adolescents. | Moderate | Strong |
| Should dental sealants, when compared with fluoride varnishes, be used in pits and fissures of occlusal surfaces of primary and permanent molars on teeth deemed to have clinically sound occlusal surfaces or noncavitated carious lesions? | The sealant guideline panel suggests the use of sealants compared with fluoride varnishes in permanent molars with both sound occlusal surfaces and noncavitated occlusal carious lesions in children and adolescents. | Low | Conditional |
| Which type of sealant material should be used in pits and fissures of occlusal surfaces of primary and permanent molars on teeth deemed to have clinically sound occlusal surfaces or noncavitated carious lesions? | The panel was unable to determine superiority of one type of sealant over another because of the very low quality of evidence for comparative studies; the panel recommends that any of the materials evaluated (for example, resin-based sealants, resin-modified glass ionomer sealants, glass ionomer cements, and polyacid-modified resin sealants, in no particular order) can be used for application in permanent molars with both sound occlusal surfaces and noncavitated occlusal carious lesions in children and adolescents (conditional recommendation, very low–quality evidence). | Very low | Conditional |

following sections. Table 26.1 summarizes the current clinical recommendations (updated in 2016) on the use of pit-and fissure sealants in the occlusal surfaces of primary and permanent molars in children and adolescents.[76]

## Sealants Can Be Safely Placed Over Incipient Caries

A conclusion of the National Institutes of Health consensus panel in 1983 was that evidence supported the use of sealants to arrest the progress of incipient lesions.[50] Nothing has occurred since then to alter that conclusion.[27,76]

Modern sealants were developed as a primary preventive procedure—that is, to be placed on sound surfaces—but shades of Hyatt's philosophy soon emerged. Given that sealants occluded the fissures, it was logical to question whether caries could progress beneath a sealant. The answer, after a number of studies, is now clear. When a sealant is placed over an incipient carious lesion, meaning a stained fissure in which softness at the base can be detected but in which cavitation has not yet occurred, caries does not progress provided the sealant remains intact. Sealant is retained on carious teeth just as well as on sound teeth,[31] and neither lesion depth nor microbiologic counts progresses under intact sealant.[32] Reviews of these and other studies have concluded that the evidence is strong that caries-active lesions become caries inactive beneath intact sealant.[67] As restorative philosophy continues to evolve toward increasingly conservative cavity preparations, more recent reports confirm that even carious dentin, when isolated under a minimal restoration and sealant, does not progress.[45]

These results provide further assurance that the clinician need not fear the placement of sealant over incipient caries. Indeed, consensus is developing that the placement of sealants over incipient lesions is one of their most effective uses.[76]

The previously mentioned CDC-sponsored expert working group reviewed one metaanalysis (of six studies) to determine the effectiveness of sealants in preventing the progression of noncavitated or incipient caries to cavitation and found that sealants reduced the percentage of noncavitated/incipient lesions that progressed to cavitation by 71% up to 5 years after placement.[27]

## Sealants Are of Uncertain Value on Primary Teeth

Some early research showed poorer retention of sealant on primary tooth enamel, although results were better in some later studies.[55,65] The different enamel structure of primary teeth was thought to be a possible reason, although moisture contamination may also have been greater with younger children. Subsequent laboratory studies have shown that a short etch time is effective for primary enamel,[68] and sealant retention on primary molars in a large Head Start program in Tennessee was equivalent to that on permanent molars.[33] What is not clear, however, is whether the usual caries pattern in primary molars is compatible with optimal sealant effectiveness, despite retentive success. In many children, the occlusal surfaces of primary molars are not highly fissured and thus are not especially caries prone. Further, when caries is a problem in primary molars, the first lesion is often interproximal. Sealants are not effective in these circumstances.

A panel convened by the ADA Council on Scientific Affairs and the American Academy of Pediatric Dentistry in 2016 to update evidence-based guidelines for the use of pit-and-fissure sealants highlighted the need for additional research to assess the effect of sealants in the primary dentition.[76]

## Sealants Are an Important Part of Public Health Programs

With the decline of dental caries among children, especially interproximal caries, sealant programs are becoming more appropriate choices in public caries prevention programs for children. Although many dental public health initiatives are directed toward encouraging the use of sealants in private practice, there is also considerable activity in the development of projects to actually place sealants in public programs. School-based sealant programs operate across the country. These programs operate either in schools, usually with portable equipment, or in community clinics. The CDC reports that school-based sealant programs are a highly effective means of providing sealants to the nearly 7 million children nationwide who do not have them, which could prevent more than 3 million cavities and save up to $300 million in dental treatment costs.[17] The philosophy behind these public sealant programs is to bring this preventive procedure to children who otherwise would be unlikely to receive comprehensive dental care. School-based and school-linked programs are targeted to schools with a high proportion of children from low-income families or schools with a high number of children with untreated dental needs or to areas in which there is a shortage of dentists.[11] For example, Wisconsin has experienced an increase in school-based sealant programs over the past 15 years and seen a decrease in untreated disease in third-grade children as a result. Additionally, disparities have been eliminated and children in these high-risk schools or those where more children participate in free and reduced meal programs have higher incidence of sealed teeth than their more affluent peers.[75] Table 26.2 summarizes updated recommendations for school-based sealant programs.[27]

## Sealant Prevalence

Despite the overwhelming evidence of the efficacy and effectiveness of dental sealants in preventing caries,[2,76] historically the overall prevalence of dental sealants in the United States has been rather low. Data from the 1986 to 1987 national survey of US schoolchildren ages 5 to 17 years indicated that only 7.6% had one or more dental sealants on permanent teeth.[14] By 1991, however, the results from the first part of the third National Health and Nutrition Examination Survey (NHANES III) showed that this proportion had risen to 18.5%.[62] Since the 1990s, there has continued to be an increase in the prevalence of dental sealants. NHANES data on the prevalence of dental sealants on permanent teeth from 1999 to 2004 indicated that 20% of youth ages 6 to 8 years and 40% of youth ages 9 to 11 years had at least one dental sealant, but considerable differences in prevalence were observed based on race/ethnicity and income level.[23] Non-Hispanic black Americans, Mexican Americans, and children or adolescents at the lowest income level had a substantially lower prevalence than non-Hispanic whites and children or adolescents at the highest income level during that time period.[23] Current data show that the overall prevalence of dental sealants continues to increase.[35]

| TABLE 26.2 | Recommendations for School-Based Sealant Programs[27] |
|---|---|
| **Topic** | **Recommendation** |
| Indications for Sealant Placement | Seal sound and noncavitated pit and fissure surfaces of posterior teeth, with first and second permanent molars receiving highest priority. |
| Tooth Surface Assessment | Differentiate cavitated and noncavitated lesions. <br>• Unaided visual assessment is appropriate and adequate. <br>• Dry teeth before assessment with cotton rolls, gauze, or, when available, compressed air. <br>• An explorer may be used to gently confirm cavitations (that is, breaks in the continuity of the surface); do not use a sharp explorer under force. Radiographs are unnecessary solely for sealant placement. <br>• Other diagnostic technologies are not required. |
| Sealant Placement and Evaluation | Clean the tooth surface. <br>• Toothbrush prophylaxis is acceptable. <br>• Additional surface preparation methods, such as air abrasion or enameloplasty, are not recommended. <br>Use a four-handed technique when resources allow. <br>Seal teeth of children even if follow-up cannot be ensured. <br>Evaluate sealant retention within one year. |

Increasing the proportion of children and adolescents who have received a dental sealant on their molar teeth was included as a Healthy People 2020 oral health objective.[34] Healthy People 2020 sets the following goals related to sealant utilization: 1.5% of 3- to 5-year-olds who have received dental sealants on one or more of their primary molar teeth (baseline 1.4% in 1999–2004), 28% of 6- to 9-year-olds who have received dental sealants on one or more of their permanent first molar teeth (baseline 26% in 1999–2004), and 22% of 13- to 15-year-olds who have received dental sealants on one or more of their permanent moral teeth (baseline 20% in 1999–2004).[34]

The most currently available data indicate that all three goals related to sealant utilization have been met and exceed their original targets, with 2011 to 2012 national data indicating that 4.3% of 3- to 5-year-olds have received dental sealants on one or more of their primary molar teeth, and 2013 to 2014 data showed 40.7% of 6- to 9-year-olds and 42.6% of 13- to 15-year-olds have received dental sealants on one or more of their permanent first molar teeth.[35] However, these data continue to show that the prevalence of dental sealants still remains lower in racial/ethnic minorities and those children or adolescents living at or below the federal poverty level as compared to their white and higher-income counterparts.

Disparities in dental sealant prevalence highlights the importance of sealant programs that target vulnerable and underserved groups who are at greater risk for dental caries. Healthy People 2020 also includes a goal to increase the proportion of school-based health centers with an oral health component that includes sealants to 18.8% (baseline 17.1% in 2007–2008). The most recently available data indicate that this goal has been met as well, as 24.4% of school-based health centers in 2010 and 2011 had an oral health component that included sealants.[35]

## Sealant Programs

Research has shown that licensed dental hygienists can apply sealant just as successfully as dentists can.[44] This is an important finding in public health, as the cost effectiveness of sealant programs virtually depends on deployment of the most appropriate provider type.[2] It is unfortunate that regulations in some states do not permit dental hygienists and assistants to apply sealants, a provision that is hard to defend as being in the public's interest. The on-site presence of a dentist will obviously add to the cost of a public program without necessarily improving its outcome. Several public health sealant programs have managed to deal with these problems and have subsequently flourished. Restrictive dental practice regulations limit the expansion of school-based programs across the country.[70]

In 2000, Wisconsin allowed dental hygienists to place sealants in schools without the prior authorization and supervision of a dentist and in 2006 allowed dental hygienists to bill Medicaid directly for these services. After 2006, funding for school-based programs increased through greater investments from the state budget, and private foundations and sealant programs now cover more than 75% of the high-risk schools statewide. Allowing dental hygienists the opportunity to provide high-risk children with direct access to sealant and get reimbursed for the service is one method to promote school-based sealant programs. The American Dental Hygienists' Association reports that 42 states allow dental hygienists direct access and 19 reimburse them directly through Medicaid.[10]

In addition to sealant programs geographically targeting schools in more deprived communities, most public sealant programs also treat only children at specific stages of dental development (i.e., soon after eruption of the first and second molars). In the United States, where children begin school at age 6, grades 1 to 2 are the best times for sealing first molars, and grades 6 to 7 for sealing second molars.[43] Sealing of bicuspids and primary teeth is not usually a part of public programs because far fewer bicuspids decay than do molars[7,24] and a primary molar that is sound in grade 1 will probably stay that way. A good body of experience in the operation of programs with sealant teams has now accumulated, and excellent guides to the development and operation of public sealant programs are available.[19,60]

## Sealants and Fluorides

We referred earlier in this chapter to the prospect of using sealants and fluoride together to reduce caries levels lower than could even have been imagined only a few decades ago. Sealant placement is an obvious adjunct to water fluoridation; a comprehensive 1989 review found that sealants were more effective in fluoridated areas than in nonfluoridated areas, although the difference was slight.[73] Sealants also have been tested in combination with fluoride mouth-rinsing. In a New York study, after 2 years the 84 children in grades 2 to 3 with sealants had an increment of only 0.03 decayed, missing, and filled surfaces (DMFS), compared with an increment of 0.47 DMFS in the control group. In the 84 children in the sealant-rinse group, there were only three new decayed or filled surfaces over the 2 years, two of them occlusal, whereas in the 51 controls, there were 24 new decayed or filled surfaces, 15 of them occlusal.[58] In

another study that used a sequential cross-sectional comparison group, a 23% decline in occlusal caries over a 4-year period in 14- to 17-year-olds was attributed to the addition of sealant placement to an ongoing school-based fluoride program.[61]

These data suggest that nearly complete prevention of caries at levels that require invasive restorations is indeed theoretically possible, but its achievement might be costly. As we saw with topical fluoride application, there comes a point at which the underlying risk of caries in some individuals is so low that additional fluoride exposure is not warranted. The same is likely to be true for sealant placement. In those individuals (and teeth, in the case of sealants) in whom the risk of occlusal caries is very low, the cost of placing and maintaining sealants may outweigh the potential benefit that sealants can be expected to provide. This is the biggest question a public health administrator has to deal with when considering sealant programs: Can we afford it, and is the benefit from sealants worth the cost?

## Cost-Effectiveness of Sealants

Questions about the cost-effectiveness of sealants were a central issue at the inception of their use in public programs. An early economic assessment of the cost-effectiveness of sealants as part of public health programs was not encouraging.[26] However, in this economic review, dentists, rather than other dental professionals (such as dental hygienists), applied the sealants, and retention of the first-generation sealant was not high.

*Cost-effectiveness* can be defined as the net cost per gained health outcome.[30] It differs from *cost–benefit*, which is the ratio of an activity's cost to the monetary benefit it produces, although it is conceptually similar to *efficiency*, which is the return on effort expended.[72] A *cost-effective program* is virtually synonymous with an *efficient program*.

The issue of cost-effectiveness arises in public dental programs when a dental director, whose objective is to reduce the caries experience in a population by a specified amount over a specified time, considers the use of a variety of different preventive programs to meet that objective. The director weighs the costs of each program against the anticipated benefit. In a fluoridated community where people routinely use fluoride toothpaste, have high utilization of dental services, and have very low caries levels, it might be a rational alternative to decide not to introduce an additional preventive program (i.e., a sealant program). Considering cost-effectiveness has moved dentistry away from an attitude of "the more prevention the better" to careful selection of preventive programs. Cost-effectiveness is also a central consideration when targeting preventive programs to the most susceptible groups and individuals rather than applying them to the population at large.

When determining the expense of sealants, consideration must be given to what the alternative prevention or treatment options are. For example, compared to community water fluoridation and other types of self-applied fluorides, sealants are a relatively expensive alternative, as they require application by a dental professional. However, the average fee for sealant application by dentists in private practice is less than half of the fee for a one-surface restoration. The ADA's 2018 survey of fees charged by general practitioners found that the mean fee for sealant application was $56.77 per tooth compared to a mean fee of $145.77 for placement of a one-surface amalgam in a posterior permanent tooth and $189.73 for a one-surface composite resin restoration on a posterior tooth.[8] In public programs, such as school-based sealant programs, sealant application has been shown to be even less expensive than in private practice settings.[29,30] A Community Guide systematic economic review of school sealant programs, discussed in more detail later in this chapter, found the median, one-time cost per tooth sealed to be $11.64.[30] The ability to provide sealants at a lower cost in public programs is attributable in part to the economies of scale that are possible through treating large numbers of children in settings such as schools and through the extensive use of nondentist personnel, such as dental hygienists, as allowable by state practice acts.[29,30]

In addition to cost or expense, effectiveness must also be considered when deciding whether the use of sealants in population-based prevention programs is cost-effective. Favorable cost-effectiveness data indicate that sealant use in public health programs is cost-effective under the right conditions.[29,30] However, research exploring the cost-effectiveness of sealants must consider several factors. For example, sealant programs will be more cost-effective in nonfluoridated areas as compared to fluoridated areas, because children living in nonfluoridated regions will have a higher burden of caries and will, therefore, also have a greater number of occlusal surfaces susceptible to caries that can potentially be prevented with sealants.[48] Although the majority of communities in the United States are now served by fluoridated water, and the availability of fluoride products is rather ubiquitous, data still demonstrate the cost-effectiveness of sealant programs that target those children at high risk for dental caries, such as those who attend schools in low socioeconomic neighborhoods, and that apply sealants to teeth at greatest risk for developing decay.[30,49]

A 2017 updated Community Guide systematic economic review of school-based sealant programs (SSPs) reviewed the following economic outcomes: (1) SSP resource costs, (2) economic benefit of sealants, (3) cost-effectiveness of SSPs, and (4) costs and benefits of sealants delivered to Medicaid-enrolled children.[30] Related to SSP costs, five studies were reviewed that reported the number of sealed teeth, and the median cost per sealed tooth was found to be $11.64 (range: $8.34–$52.13), which is substantially lower than the $56.77 sealant per tooth fee reported in the ADA's 2018 survey of fees.[8] The median per-child cost of 12 SSPs (that had complete cost information) was found to be $76.09 (range: $33.36–163.16). SSP costs included: labor, equipment, supplies, travel, and other related costs.

This economic review calculated economic benefit based on averted treatment costs attributable to placing sealants. Treatment costs and productivity losses were used to estimate the averted treatment costs in the reviewed studies. The median annual economic benefit (annual averted cost per tooth) for studies reviewed was $6.29.[30] One study stratified economic benefit by the children's caries risk and found that the economic benefit of sealants increased as the caries risk of the teeth increased.[74] In this study, the reduction in receipt of restorations and averted treatment costs over 5 years were 53.3%, 62.6%, and 70.7% and $10.04, $34.61, and $53.04, respectively, for low-, medium-, and high-risk teeth.

The economic review compared data on median SSP cost and benefit per tooth and found that the SSP benefit exceeded cost 2 years after sealant placement and saved $11.73 per sealed tooth over 4 years.[30] Four studies were reviewed that modeled the cost-effectiveness of SSPs sealing first molars.[30] Each of the four studies used caries or caries-free children as the health outcome to determine cost-effectiveness. Two of the four studies calculated cost-effectiveness ratios for SSPs, which were determined to be $13.13 and $1.63 per averted decayed tooth surface in the respective studies, while the other two studies found that SSPs saved

societal resources because of improved dental outcomes. Finally, studies reviewed using Medicaid claims data found the delivery of sealants to children enrolled in Medicaid to be cost saving to society.

Issues of cost-effectiveness arise in private practice too, although the issues are sometimes different from those related to public programs.[7] Private practitioners are likely challenged as to whether they should seal or restore a deeply fissured molar. Private practitioners must consider the susceptibility of the pits and fissures of teeth and the unique anatomy that individuals may have when considering the cost-effectiveness of sealants. Additionally, a patient's individual caries risk and the extent to which other preventive modalities are being used must be considered when determining cost-effectiveness of sealants in a practice. Lastly, evidence-based guidelines related to sealant use should be followed.[27] Risk-based sealing has been shown to be cost-effective and improve clinical outcomes.[49]

## Public and Professional Attitudes Toward Sealants

Even though the trend of widespread use of sealants in modern dental practice developed slowly, it has been consistent. Steady growth in the numbers of dentists using sealants was evident through the 1980s, and by the early 1990s several states reported that more than 90% of general dentists were using sealants.[63] A survey conducted among Florida dentists in 2013 found that nearly all (98%) of the dentist participants reported that they use dental sealants as a routine preventive measure in their clinical practices, indicating that dental sealant use has become a mainstay of the modern dental practice.[28] Lack of dental insurance coverage was previously cited as a major factor in the slow initial acceptance of sealants,[63] but all state Medicaid programs currently reimburse for sealant placement on permanent teeth,[18] and several private insurers also cover their placement.

While the use of dental sealants has become ubiquitous in dental practice, overall knowledge regarding the evidence-based use of sealants among dentists has been found to be low.[28] A large-scale survey of US dentists' practices related to sealants indicated that many dentists have not adopted evidence-based, clinical recommendations for sealant use.[69] This 2011 survey of 2400 randomly selected US general dentists and pediatric dentists was conducted to understand their practices regarding the 2010 ADA recommendation to seal noncavitated carious lesions in children and young adults. The survey found that in the absence of radiographic evidence of caries, only 37% of general dentists and 42% of pediatric dentists surveyed indicated that they would follow evidence-based recommendations to seal noncavitated carious lesions in molar teeth. Additionally, less than 40% of the dentists surveyed indicated that they sealed noncavitated carious lesions.

A qualitative study was conducted with a small convenience sample of private-practice dentists to better understand and assess barriers to the use of evidence-based clinical recommendations for sealant use in the treatment of noncavitated carious lesions. The study found that personal clinical experience was the determining factor regarding whether dentists followed evidence-based clinical recommendations.[51] Other barriers to adherence to evidence-based guidelines for sealant use that have been reported include concerns of sealing in decay, being unaware of sealant clinical practice guidelines, and mistrust of evidence-based recommendations.[28,51,54] In summary, although the adoption of sealants as a part of overall preventive dental practice has greatly increased over time, studies indicate that dentists do not always adhere to evidence-based clinical guidelines regarding their use. These findings indicate the need for further implementation research and associated strategies to increase dentists' adherence to clinical guidelines for sealant use that go beyond the simple dissemination of evidence-based information.

As with any other tool in the dental armamentarium, sealants must be used appropriately, in a way that is (1) compatible with the properties of the material, (2) consistent with the nature of the condition that they are meant to prevent or treat, and (3) acceptable in terms of cost to the provider and patient. New sealant materials will continue to expand, and the standards for sealant use will undoubtedly continue to progress. At the same time, optimal use of sealants is also likely to remain somewhat different in public programs than in private practice. In public programs, sealants continue to be highly effective in reducing the burden of caries in high-risk children (such as low socioeconomic status and minority children).[27] This is because the children are selected based on untreated disease and limited access to routine dental care, and large numbers of high-risk children can be treated with sealants.

On the other hand, for patients who have access to regular care in private practice, the trend toward a more selective, individual approach to sealant use continues. Here the decision to treat is made on the basis of the expected risk for the individual child and tooth surface, with the knowledge that sealants are part of a conservative approach to restorative care. The role of sealants and the related restorative materials in improving the oral health of the public is substantial. The challenge for dental practitioners is to be alert and accepting of the inevitable evolution of the evidence-based recommendations for the most appropriate use of these materials, with timely implementation into their practices.

* This manuscript was prepared by Dr. Weatherspoon in his personal capacity. The opinions expressed in this chapter are the author's own and do not reflect the view of the National Institute of Dental and Craniofacial Research, the National Institutes of Health, the Department of Health and Human Services, or the United States government.

# References

1. Ahovuo-Saloranta A, Forss H, Hiiri A, et al. Pit and fissure sealants versus fluoride varnishes for preventing dental decay in the permanent teeth of children and adolescents. *Cochrane DB Syst Rev.* 2016;(1): Cd003067.

2. Ahovuo-Saloranta A, Forss H, Walsh T, et al. Pit and fissure sealants for preventing dental decay in permanent teeth. *Cochrane DB Syst Rev.* 2017;(1):Cd001830.

3. American Dental Association. ADA Council on Scientific Affairs position statement: estrogenic effects of bisphenol A lacking in dental sealants. *J Gt Houst Dent Soc.* 1998;70(2):11.

4. American Dental Association. BPA in Dental Sealants Safe. *Research Shows a Child's Exposure From BPA Mostly From Food, Drinks*; 2016. Available from: https://www.ada.org/en/publications/ada-news/2016-archive/august/bpa-in-dental-sealants-safe.

5. American Dental Association Council on Dental Materials and Devices. Nuva-Seal pit and fissure sealant classified as provisionally acceptable. Council on Dental Materials and Devices. *J Am Dent Assoc.* 1972;84(5):1109.

6. American Dental Association Council on Dental Materials and Devices. Pit and fissure sealants. Council on Dental Materials and Devices. *J Am Dent Assoc.* 1976;93(1):134.

7. American Dental Association Council on Dental Research. Cost-effectiveness of sealants in private practice and standards for use in prepaid dental care. Council on Dental Research. *J Am Dent Assoc.* 1985;110(1):103–107.

8. American Dental Association Health Policy Insitute. *Survey of Dental Fees.* 2018. Available from: https://success.ada.org/en/practice-management/finances/survey-of-dental-fees.

9. American Dental Association Oral Health Topics. *Oral Health Topics: Dental Sealants.* 2016. Available from: https://www.ada.org/en/member-center/oral-health-topics/dental-sealants.

10. American Dental Hygienists' Association Direct Access. Available from: http://www.adha.org/direct-access. Accessed February 24, 2019.

11. Association of State and Territorial Dental Directors. *School-Based and School-Linked Public Health Dental Sealant Programs in the United States, 1992–93.* Columbus, OH: ASTDD; 1997.

12. Bohannan HM. Caries distribution and the case for sealants. *J Public Health Dent.* 1983;43(3):200–204.

13. Bravo M, Osorio E, Garcia-Anllo I, et al. The influence of dft index on sealant success: a 48-month survival analysis. *J Dent Res.* 1996;75(2): 768–774.

14. Brunelle JA. Prevalence of dental sealants in U.S. schoolchildren [abstract]. *J Dent Res.* 1989;68:183.

15. Buonocore MG. A simple method of increasing the adhesion of acrylic filling materials to enamel surfaces. *J Dent Res.* 1955;34(6): 849–853.

16. Buonocore MG. Caries prevention in pits and fissures sealed with an adhesive resin polymerized by ultraviolet light: a two-year study of a single adhesive application. *J Am Dent Assoc.* 1971;82(5):1090–1093.

17. Centers for Disease Control and Prevention. Available from: https://www.cdc.gov/oralhealth/dental_sealant_program/index.htm.

18. Chi DL, Singh J. Reimbursement rates and policies for primary molar pit-and-fissure sealants across state Medicaid programs. *J Am Dent Assoc.* 2013;144(11):1272–1278.

19. Children's Dental Health Project (2017). *School-Based Dental Sealant Programs: Recommendations.* Available from: https://www.cdhp.org/resources/334-school-based-dental-sealant-programs-recommendations.

20. Deery C. Fissure seal or fluoride varnish? *Evid Based Dent.* 2016; 17(3):77–78.

21. Dirks OB. The benefits of water fluoridation. *Caries Res.* 1974; 8(0):2–15.

22. Dye BA, Mitnik GL, Iafolla TJ, et al. Trends in dental caries in children and adolescents according to poverty status in the United States from 1999 through 2004 and from 2011 through 2014. *J Am Dent Assoc.* 2017;148(8):550–565.e557.

23. Dye BA, Tan S, Smith V, et al. Trends in oral health status: United States, 1988–1994 and 1999–2004. *Vital Health Stat.* 2007;11 (248):1–92.

24. Eklund SA, Ismail AI. Time of development of occlusal and proximal lesions: implications for fissure sealants. *J Public Health Dent.* 1986;46(2):114–121.

25. Elderton RJ. Restorations without conventional cavity preparations. *Int Dent J.* 1988;38(2):112–118.

26. Foch CB. *The Costs, Effects, and Benefits of Preventive Dental Care: A Literature Review. Rand Report No. N-1732-RWJF.* Santa Monica, CA: Rand; 1981.

27. Gooch BF, Griffin SO, Gray SK, et al. Preventing dental caries through school-based sealant programs: updated recommendations and reviews of evidence. *J Am Dent Assoc.* 2009;140(11):1356–1365.

28. Govindaiah S, Bhoopathi V. Dentists' levels of evidence-based clinical knowledge and attitudes about using pit-and-fissure sealants. *J Am Dent Assoc.* 2014;145(8):849–855.

29. Griffin SO, Jones K, Naavaal S, et al. Estimating the cost of school sealant programs with minimal data. *J Public Health Dent.* 2018; 78(1):17–24.

30. Griffin SO, Naavaal S, Scherrer C, et al. Evaluation of school-based dental sealant programs: an updated community guide systematic economic review. *Am J Prev Med.* 2017;52(3):407–415.

31. Handelman SL, Leverett DH, Espeland M, Curzon J. Retention of sealants over carious and sound tooth surfaces. *Community Dent Oral Epidemiol.* 1987;15(1):1–5.

32. Handelman SL, Leverett DH, Espeland M, Curzon J. Clinical radiographic evaluation of sealed carious and sound tooth surfaces. *J Am Dent Assoc.* 1986;113(5):751–754.

33. Hardison JR, Collier DR, Sprouse LW, et al. Retention of pit and fissure sealant on the primary molars of 3- and 4-year-old children after 1 year. *J Am Dent Assoc.* 1987;114(5):613–615.

34. Healthy People 2020. *Oral Health Objectives.* Available from: https://www.healthypeople.gov/2020/topics-objectives/topic/oral-health/objectives.

35. Healthy People 2020 Data Search. Available from: https://www.healthypeople.gov/2020/data-search/.

36. Henry RJ, Jerrell RG. The glass ionomer rest-a-seal. *ASDC J Dent Child.* 1989;56(4):283–287.

37. Horowitz HS, Heifetz SB, Poulsen S. Retention and effectiveness of a single application of an adhesive sealant in preventing occlusal caries: final report after five years of a study in Kalispell, Montana. *J Am Dent Assoc.* 1977;95(6):1133–1139.

38. Hyatt T. Prophylactic odontotomy. *Dent Cosmos.* 1923;65:234–241.

39. Ismail AI. Gagnon P. A longitudinal evaluation of fissure sealants applied in dental practices. *J Dent Res.* 1955;74(9):1583–1590.

40. Kaste LM, Selwitz RH, Oldakowski RJ, et al. Coronal caries in the primary and permanent dentition of children and adolescents 1–17 years of age: United States, 1988–1991. *J Dent Res.* 1996;75:631–641. Spec No.

41. Klein H, Knutson J. Studies on dental caries. Effect of ammoniacal silver nitrate on caries in the first permanent molars. *J Am Dent Assoc.* 1942;29:1420–1426.

42. Klein H, Palmer C. Therapeutic odontotomy and preventive dentistry. *J Am Dent Assoc.* 1940;27:1054–1055.

43. Kuthy RA, Ashton JJ. Eruption pattern of permanent molars: implications for school-based dental sealant programs. *J Public Health Dent.* 1989;49(1):7–14.

44. Leske GS, Pollard S, Cons N. The effectiveness of dental hygienist teams in applying a pit and fissure sealant. *J Prev Dent.* 1976; 3(2):33–36.

45. Mertz-Fairhurst EJ, Adair SM, Sams DR, et al. Cariostatic and ultra-conservative sealed restorations: nine-year results among children and adults. *ASDC J Dent Child.* 1995;62(2):97–107.

46. Mertz-Fairhurst EJ, Call-Smith KM, Shuster GS, et al. Clinical performance of sealed composite restorations placed over caries compared with sealed and unsealed amalgam restorations. *J Am Dent Assoc.* 1987;115(5):689–694.

47. Mickenautsch S, Yengopal V. Caries-preventive effect of glass ionomer and resin-based fissure sealants on permanent teeth: an update of systematic review evidence. *BMC Res Notes.* 2011;4:22.

48. Morgan MV, Crowley SJ, Wright C. Economic evaluation of a pit and fissure dental sealant and fluoride mouthrinsing program in two nonfluoridated regions of Victoria, Australia. *J Public Health Dent.* 1998;58(1):19–27.

49. Naaman R, El-Housseiny AA, Alamoudi N. The use of pit and fissure sealants—a literature review. *Dent J (Basel).* 2017;5(4).

50. National Institutes of Health. National Institutes of Health consensus development conference statement. Dental sealants in the prevention of tooth decay. *J Dent Educ.* 1984;48(2 suppl):126–131.

51. O'Donnell JA, Modesto A, Oakley M, et al. Sealants and dental caries: insight into dentists' behaviors regarding implementation of clinical practice recommendations. *J Am Dent Assoc.* 2013;144(4):e24–e30.

52. Olea N, Pulgar R, Perez P, et al. Estrogenicity of resin-based composites and sealants used in dentistry. *Environ Health Perspect.* 1996;104(3):298–305.

53. Papageorgiou SN, Dimitraki D, Kotsanos N, et al. Performance of pit and fissure sealants according to tooth characteristics: a systematic review and meta-analysis. *J Dent.* 2017;66:8–17.

54. Polk DE, Weyant RJ, Shah NH, et al. Barriers to sealant guideline implementation within a multi-site managed care dental practice. *BMC Oral Health.* 2018;18(1):17.

55. Ripa LW. Sealant retention on primary teeth: a critique of clinical and laboratory studies. *J Pedod.* 1979;3(4):275–290.

56. Ripa LW. Occlusal sealants: rationale and review of clinical trials. *Int Dent.* 1980;30(2):127–139.

57. Ripa LW. Sealants revisted: an update of the effectiveness of pit-and-fissure sealants. *Caries Res.* 1993;27(suppl 1):77–82.

58. Ripa LW, Leske GS, Forte F. The combined use of pit and fissure sealants and fluoride mouthrinsing in second and third grade children: final clinical results after two years. *Pediatr Dent.* 1987;9(2):118–120.

59. Robison VA, Rozier RG, Weintraub JA, et al. The relationship between clinical tooth status and receipt of sealants among child Medicaid recipients. *J Dent Res.* 1997;76(12):1862–1868.

60. Seal America. *Seal America: The Prevention Invention, Third Edition.* 2016. Available from: https://www.mchoralhealth.org/seal/.

61. Selwitz RH, Nowjack-Raymer R, Driscoll WS, Li SH. Evaluation after 4 years of the combined use of fluoride and dental sealants. *Community Dent Oral Epidemiol.* 1995;23(1):30–35.

62. Selwitz RH, Winn DM, Kingman A, et al. The prevalence of dental sealants in the US population: findings from NHANES III, 1988–1991. *J Dent Res.* 1996;75:652–660.

63. Siegal MD, Garcia AI, Kandray DP, et al. The use of dental sealants by Ohio dentists. *J Public Health Dent.* 1996;56(1):12–21.

64. Silverstone LM. State of the art on sealant research and priorities for further research. *J Dent Educ.* 1984;48(suppl 2):107–118.

65. Simonsen RJ. Fissure sealants in primary molars: retention of colored sealants with variable etch times, at twelve months. *ASDC J Dent Child.* 1979;46(5):382–384.

66. Simonsen RJ. Retention and effectiveness of dental sealant after 15 years. *J Am Dent Assoc.* 1991;122(10):34–42.

67. Swift EJ Jr. The effect of sealants on dental caries: a review. *J Am Dent Assoc.* 1988;116(6):700–704.

68. Tandon S, Kumari R, Udupa S. The effect of etch-time on the bond strength of a sealant and on the etch-pattern in primary and permanent enamel: an evaluation. *ASDC J Dent Child.* 1989;56(3): 186–190.

69. Tellez M, Gray SL, Gray S. Lim, et al. Sealants and dental caries: dentists' perspectives on evidence-based recommendations. *J Am Dent Assoc.* 2011;142(9):1033–1040.

70. The Pew Charitable Trusts. *When Regulation Block Access to Oral Health Care, Children at Risk Suffer. School Dental Sealant Program Dilemma.* 2018. https://www.pewtrusts.org/en/research-and-analysis/issue-briefs/2018/08/when-regulations-block-access-to-oral-health-care-children-at-risk-suffer.

71. Waggoner WF, Siegal M. Pit and fissure sealant application: updating the technique. *J Am Dent Assoc.* 1996;127(3):351–361. quiz 391–352.

72. Warner KE. Issues in cost effectiveness in health care. *J Public Health Dent.* 1989;49:272–278.

73. Weintraub JA. The effectiveness of pit and fissure sealants. *J Public Health Dent.* 1989;49:317–330.

74. Weintraub JA, Stearns SC, Rozier RG, Huang CC. Treatment outcomes and costs of dental sealants among children enrolled in Medicaid. *Am J Public Health.* 2001;91(11):1877–1881.

75. Wisconsin Department of Health Services. Healthy Smiles/Healthy Growth. In: *Wisconsin's Third Grade Children*: 2013. https://www.dhs.wisconsin.gov/publications/p0/p00589.pdf.

76. Wright JT, Crall JJ, Fontana M, et al. Evidence-based clinical practice guideline for the use of pit-and-fissure sealants: a report of the American Dental Association and the American Academy of Pediatric Dentistry. *J Am Dent Assoc.* 2016;147(8):672–682. e612.

# 27

# Plaque Control and Promotion of Periodontal Health

VLADIMIR W. SPOLSKY, DMD, MPH

## CHAPTER OUTLINE

## Introduction

Chronic diseases are a growing burden on all people across the world pervading all socioeconomic classes.[73] The World Health Organization (WHO) estimates that the major chronic diseases currently account for about 40% of this burden and will increase to 60% by 2020 in developing countries.[96,97] Periodontal disease is one of the two major oral diseases contributing to the global burden of chronic diseases.[73,74]

In the United States the prevalence of periodontal disease is high (see Chapter 15). NHANES III (1988–1999) was the last national survey to record the prevalence of gingivitis, with more than half of US adults having gingival bleeding.[3] The 2009 to 2010 NHANES data showed the prevalence of periodontitis was 47.2% with anywhere from 6.7% to 11.2% having severe periodontitis.[26] Later years of NHANES survey data (2009–2014) showed an improvement in periodontal health in adults 30 years of age and older, with 42.2% having periodontitis and 7.8% having severe periodontitis.[27]

The etiology of this burden of chronic oral disease is dental plaque. Supragingival plaque is responsible for reversible gingivitis, and if nothing is done it may become subgingival plaque, contributing to irreversible periodontitis.[21]

## Nature of Plaque

Dental plaque was first observed by van Leeuwenhoek in the 17th century and was associated with the common dental diseases. The proposed hypothesis at that time was that dental infections were caused by an overgrowth of all of the microorganisms in dental plaque.[54] Controversy over the hypothesis took place over a century.[54] This hypothesis was labeled the nonspecific plaque hypothesis (NSPH) and was predicated on the quantity of plaque that determined the pathogenicity without considering the virulence of the various microorganisms.[79]

As culturing techniques and microscopy improved in the 1970s, it became possible to identify specific microorganisms in plaque. Experiments with the antibiotic kanamycin, for example, showed that removing streptococcus reduced dental caries formation. In 1976, Loesche proposed the specific plaque hypothesis (SPH), which stated that dental caries was an infectious disease due to mutans streptococci.[55] When anaerobic hoods were developed, it was possible to cultivate strict anaerobic species that were proposed as specific periopathogens and extending the SPH. Numerous potent periopathogens were isolated such as Gram-negative anaerobic rods (*Prevotella melaninogenica*) and cultured. They included protozoa, spirochetes, streptococci, and actinomyces. In addition, Gram-negative anaerobic rods (*Prevotella melaninogenica* and *Campylobacter*) and facultative anaerobes, Gram-negative rods (*Capnocytophaga*, *Eikenella*, and *Actinobacillus*) were also cultivated. Collectively all of this led to the idea that many different species could initiate periodontal disease.[79] These findings led Socransky to investigate and characterize bacterial clusters that were associated with periodontal disease. He found that the red complex microorganisms were strongly associated with periodontal disease and that they can be detected in low numbers in healthy sites.[85] *Porphyromonas gingivalis*, *Treponema denticola*, and *Tannerella forsythia* are the microorganisms that make up the red cluster.[41]

The next evolution in plaque hypotheses came when Marsh proposed the ecological plaque hypothesis (EPH). The EPH states that "disease is the result of an imbalance in the total microflora due to ecological stress, resulting in an enrichment of some 'oral pathogens' or disease-related microorganisms." He attributed the changes in microbial composition to changes in the environment such as redox potential, the presence of nutrients, and pH. More simply, the composition of plaque depends on the environment.[60]

The most recent discussion of plaque hypotheses is derived from the EPH and is called the keystone pathogen hypothesis (KPH). The KPH posits that certain low-abundance microbes that are relatively disproportionate to the overall abundance can cause inflammatory disease by increasing the quantity of the normal microbes and changing its composition. The host-immune system is critical to the KPH.[79] One other aspect of this environmental picture is that there are differences in susceptibility for oral diseases that can be attributed to genetic factors. Genetic factors play an important role in health and disease.[92] Genetic predispositions are believed to contribute as much 50% to periodontitis.[64] See Chapter 15 for more on periodontal disease etiology.

## Approaches to Plaque Control

The study by Löe showed that cessation of oral hygiene can cause gingivitis.[54] Lang found that removal of plaque every second day could prevent gingivitis, but removal every third or fourth day did not prevent gingivitis.[48] These studies firmly established the evidence base that gingivitis could be prevented by removal of supragingival plaque.

Formation of plaque is a natural ongoing process on the tooth surface. Dental plaque is a "diverse microbial community found on the tooth surface embedded in a matrix of polymers of bacterial and salivary enzymes."[61] Shortly after a tooth surface is cleaned, a salivary pellicle made up of mucoproteins covers the tooth. The plaque is the result of the interaction between the initial microbial colonizers and the acquired enamel pellicle. Secondary colonizers attach to the early colonizers in a definite pattern of succession. This process starts within 6 to 8 hours after a tooth surface is cleaned. After 7 to 14 days a more complex or mature microflora develops. Plaque protects the tooth physically and chemically. Physically it protects the tooth from exogenous microorganisms and chemically by serving as a reservoir for calcium, phosphorus, and fluoride.[61]

Since plaque has both positive and negative properties, disturbing this balance or homeostasis will result in a disease more severe than any microorganisms entering the mouth. This concept is called the ecologic plaque hypothesis (EPH) and is the basis for believing that controlling early plaque is better than complete plaque eradication.[60]

The goal is to keep plaque supragingivally where mechanical and chemical means can control it. Once plaque becomes established subgingivally, it requires removal by a professional and more intense mechanical removal by the individual. Hence the goal of primary prevention is to keep supragingival plaque from accumulating.

There are several approaches that work for removing or controlling the buildup of plaque, yet there are others that lack an evidence basis. For example, rinsing with water may loosen food particles, but it does not remove the tenacious plaque. Although finger or brush massaging of the gums is alleged to increase blood circulation of the gingiva, there is no body of evidence to support this practice. It may loosen food particles after toothbrushing. Neither does chewing fibrous foods, which may clean the incisal one-third of the tooth but not the middle or gingival thirds.[52,78] Chewing gum for plaque removal is also without merit,[63,65] but it does simulate salivary flow with its strong buffering effect. Sugarless gum and gum containing xylitol would be the gum of choice. Although the benefits of sound nutrition and diet are important to the resistance of the host and immune system, current evidence does not support their role in preventing periodontal disease.[4,87]

There are essentially three approaches to controlling plaque. They are physical or mechanical removal of plaque by the individual, removal by the dental professional, and chemotherapeutic control of plaque.

## Mechanical Removal of Plaque by the Individual

The most fundamental care that we can provide our patients is to teach them how to take care of their mouths. Toothbrushing is the most common method for cleaning the plaque from the tooth. Questions then arise about methods of brushing, frequency, type of brush, and comparison of powerbrushes.

### Manual Toothbrushing

In theory, brushing the teeth once per day should work in persons with healthy gingiva, but very few people are capable of removing the plaque sufficiently to maintain a healthy gingiva.

In Western society, brushing the teeth twice a day with a fluoridated toothpaste is more common.[25] Although fluoride is probably more beneficial in preventing decalcification, fluoride has a modest effect on bacterial enzymes. Brushing twice a day has been shown to improve gingival heath.[5] In a 30-year prospective study that provided regular dental care, Axelsson and colleagues showed that brushing with a fluoride toothpaste more than once per day and using interproximal cleaning aides was effective in plaque removal.[9] Suomi found less gingivitis, plaque, and calculus in a prison population that brushed twice or more daily.[86] The American Dental Association (ADA) recommends brushing twice a day, and this frequency of brushing is substantiated by research.[83]

### Methods of Brushing

Methods of brushing may be classified by the brushing motion with specific techniques of brushing falling into one or more classifications: vertical (Leonard), horizontal, roll technique, vibratory (Charters, Stillman, Bass) technique, circular (Fones), physiologic (Smith), sulcular (Bass), and scrub-brush methods. Many comparisons of brushing methods have been done. Bergenholtz compared four methods (Bass, roll, circular scrub, horizontal scrub) and found that the Bass method was more effective in removing plaque on lingual aspects. There was some consensus that the horizontal scrub was more effective in preschool children.[46] The multitude of brushing methods reflects the fact that no one method is superior to another.

Based on our current understanding about the formation of plaque, the method that offers the best approach to removing plaque from the dentogingival margin is the Bass technique, which was first described in 1954. Also, with this technique the toothbrush can remove plaque subgingivally by as much as 1 mm.[19]

### Type of Toothbrush

Numerous designs of toothbrush heads have been developed. These designs include flat, rippled, dome, bi-level, and v-shaped heads. Brush handles also vary, with some handles being at an angle relative to the brush head. Additional variables include the bristle material (nylon), length and diameter of the filaments, the rounded and polished ends of the filaments, arrangement of the filaments into tufts, and the arrangement of the tufts relative to each other. Soft nylon brushes with small brush heads are recommended because they can clean beneath the gingival margin when used with the sulcus brushing method (e.g., Bass) and minimize pressure on the gingival tissues.[20]

### Power Toothbrushes

Electric or powerbrushes were introduced in the 1960s when they became available as an alternative to manual toothbrushing. In general, powerbrushes were able to remove more plaque during a comparable period than a manual brush.[19] Powerbrushes are grouped by the action of their brush heads: rotational oscillation, side-to-side, counter oscillation (adjacent tufts rotate in opposite directions), circular, and ultrasonic (brush head vibrates at ultrasonic frequency). All of the powerbrushes were at least as effective as manual brushes in reducing plaque and gingivitis. Of all of the powerbushes, the rotational oscillation and side-to-side brushes had the largest number of clinical trials and study populations.

Systematic reviews conducted by the Cochrane Collaboration concluded that only the rotational oscillation is better than a manual toothbrush at removing plaque and in reducing gingivitis and is unlikely to cause injury to the gums.[20] The rotational oscillation powerbrush was superior to the side-to-side powerbrush.[98] Several other attributes of the powerbrushes make it desirable. The wider handle and small brush head make it highly desirable for individuals with dexterity problems. Additionally, some of the brushes have timers that assist the individual in brushing at least 2 minutes. This is helpful, as many individuals spend only 40 to 60 seconds brushing.[17] For individuals with gingival recession, the powerbrush placed less pressure on the gingiva (100 g less) than a manual brush.[91]

### Tongue Cleaning

Any discussion about brushing the teeth would be incomplete without mentioning brushing or scraping the tongue. The dorsum of the tongue harbor numerous microorganisms and desquamated epithelial cells with easy access to nutrients in the saliva. One study identified commensal organism on the tongue that have been associated with pneumonia in frail elderly adults.[6] The tongue also plays an important role in the production of oral malodor.[90] Hence, from a practical point of view, individuals may benefit from routine scraping of the tongue. Scraping removed more sulfur compounds from the tongue than brushing.[72]

### Pulsating Irrigation

Studies of powered pulsating irrigation devices have shown that in addition to removing food particles and bacteria, they don't appear to reduce plaque but do reduce gingivitis.[16,32] This lack of correlation between plaque and gingivitis may be explained by a change in the composition of the microorganisms in the plaque, even though the plaque's mass does not appear to change. The remaining plaque is less toxic and irritating to the gingiva.[18]

### Interproximal Cleaning

In spite of the fact that the majority of time spent on bushing is to remove plaque from the teeth, 40% of the tooth surfaces are never cleaned by brushing. Of all of the tooth surfaces, the interproximal tooth surface has the most inflammation.[54] Cleaning beneath the contact is the target area most vulnerable to periodontitis.

The use of floss with brushing has been highly praised by health educators in oral hygiene programs in reducing plaque and gingivitis more than brushing alone,[53] in spite of the fact that only 31% of adults floss daily.[31] There are no differences in waxed and unwaxed nylon floss, except that floss made of Gore-Tex does not fray easily and is especially useful in tight interproximal contact areas.[12,13] Flossing requires considerable digital skill. There are conflicting reviews on the benefits of brushing and flossing. One systematic review concluded that there was no additional benefit to flossing with brushing.[11] However, another review concluded that there was a statistically significant benefit to flossing with brushing compared to brushing alone.[82] The sequence of flossing and brushing is also important. Flossing followed by brushing significantly reduced plaque compared to brushing and then

flossing.[62] Although the evidence for flossing and brushing is weak, Drisko concluded that until reviews are published to contradict the use of floss for interproximal plaque control, it does have limited support in the literature.[25]

Alternatives to flossing include triangular shaped wooden cleaners and interproximal brushes. The key to selecting an appropriate interdental aid is determined by the size of the embrasure space. Triangular shaped wooden sticks made of compressible wood are included with interdental brushes of various diameters. In a systemic review, it was concluded not surprisingly that using interdental brushes as an adjunct to toothbrushing removes more interproximal plaque than brushing alone.[59] They also showed a positive effect on removing more plaque than wood sticks and dental floss.[13,45] Marchesan and colleagues found a higher percentage of interproximal sites with Clinical Attachment Loss (CAL) of 3 mm or greater and Probing Depth (PD) greater than 4 mm in participants who did not use interproximal cleaning aids compared to regular interproximal users.[59]

In addition to removing supragingival plaque interproximally, the interdental brush removed subgingival plaque to a depth of 2.5 mm below the gingival margin.[93] One of the supposed advantages of the interdental brushes over flossing is that it can be carried by the individual and used throughout the day. Although floss is also portable, it is not used as readily in public. Recently, "soft-picks" made of flexible latex rubber have become available that permit access to tight embrasures and under pontics and orthodontic wires.

### Individual Motivation

The success of any oral hygiene regimen ultimately depends on the motivation of the individual. For individuals who are willing to change their oral hygiene practices, it must fit into their lifestyle and not be burdensome. A study in British schoolchildren illustrates this issue. Children who reported frequent toothbrushing also reported frequent personal hygiene habits such as the use of deodorant and washing of their hands after using the bathroom.[57] Hence, oral hygiene fit into these children's daily health behavior.

Although knowledge is always thought to precede action, that may not always be the case. In a North Carolina study, there was a poor correlation between understanding the process of periodontal disease and maintaining periodontal health.[10] In a study of supervised toothbrushing in school children, gingivitis was reduced, but the improvement disappeared when supervision was ended.[50,51] Serious doubts have been raised about the effects of one-on-one chairside instruction. In general, dentists have less than enthusiastic belief that oral health education has positive benefits. Several studies of brushing and flossing have shown a 50% rate of compliance.[70] This is comparable to reported adherence in long-term medical regimens.[81] The compliance model that many have followed in oral health education, however, may be flawed in light of our current contemporary lifestyle. Compliance by definition focuses on the provider and not on the patient. In this model, the communication is a one-way authoritarian message directed at the patient, with no more than 50% responding.[94] (See Chapter 21.)

A more contemporary concept is adherence, which is a more proactive behavior resulting in a positive lifestyle initiated by the patient and not dictated by the doctor.[42] Preventive activities are critical in a chronic disease such as periodontal disease, where the patient must initiate and maintain a high level of oral hygiene in conjunction with professional care for successful periodontal maintenance.[76] The concept of self-care, or having the patient involved in the process, is predicated on pretesting the patient's self-skills, realizing that not everyone is ready to change self-care habits, and believing that communication is critical. In this instance, the communication is praise and feedback by the dentist encouraging the patient to set a goal of plaque removal. This model comes close to the concept of adherence.[70] Conceptually, another model of behavioral change in periodontal patients is based on goal setting, planning, and self-monitoring.[69]

Finally, one operational model of encouraging behavioral change in controlling plaque is having the patient demonstrate his/her skill within their own mouth, followed by instruction by the health provider while the patient uses a hand mirror. Probably the most important step in this model is having the patient demonstrate within the mouth the instruction just given. The health provider can give any suggested technique adjustments within his/her mouth and to give encouragement. The use of a disclosing solution at this time is an excellent educational and motivational aide. The patient can see the plaque and understand the goal of thorough plaque removal.

## Mechanical Calculus Removal by the Dental Professional

Once the supragingival plaque becomes established in the gingival sulcus and becomes mineralized, it can only be removed by a dental professional. Subgingival plaque creates the environment for periodontitis. One of the first controlled trials to demonstrate the benefits of subgingival calculus removal in conjunction with daily oral hygiene was conducted by Lövdal and colleagues.[56] Factory workers in Olso were given a thorough removal of their supra- and subgingival calculus every 6 months and in more severe conditions as often as every 3 months. They received instruction in oral hygiene and the use of toothpicks. After 5 years (n = 808), those who started the study with good oral hygiene showed a 60% decreased incidence of gingivitis. The factory workers who started with poor oral hygiene showed a 30% decreased incidence of gingivitis. These differences illustrate the importance of self-care and the limitations of professional cleaning. In the controlled oral hygiene study by Suomi et al., the treatment group received oral hygiene instruction and professional prophylaxis every 3 to 4 months.[86] The matched control group continued their routine dental care. After 3 years (n = 652), the treatment group had less plaque and gingivitis and only 0.01 mm of attachment loss (AL) per year (none radiographically) compared to the control group that experienced 0.33 mm AL per year and radiographic loss of 0.19 mm of bone loss.[88] Axelsson had similar results in a 6-year study.[8]

The common thread that goes through all of these studies is that oral hygiene instruction was given prior to the study and reinforced at every prophylaxis appointment. A commentary in the American Academy of Periodontology centennial issue succinctly summarizes the practice of frequent prophylaxis as periodontitis is preventable.[8]

## Chemotherapeutic Methods of Controlling Plaque

Considering that toothbrushing only removes anywhere from 40% to 60% of supragingival plaque and that many individuals brush for less than a minute, the idea of a mouthrinse as an adjunct to toothbrushing to remove more plaque is appealing. Culturally, like toothpaste, mouthrinse or mouthwash use is simple and widely accepted. Mouthrinses have been developed for many different oral conditions, such as halitosis, xerostomia, dental caries, anticalculus, topical pain relief, and gingivitis. Our focus will be on supragingival plaque control.

Some of the most common antimicrobial mouthrinses are chlorhexidine, phenolic compounds, halogens (iodine and sodium hypochlorite), oxygenating agents, and quaternary ammonium compounds (cetylpyridinium chloride).[68] All of them have broad spectrum activity except for cetylpyridinium chloride (CPC) that is only effective against Gram-positive microorganisms.

Chlorhexidine (CHX, 0.12%; pH 5.5) has been researched the most of all of the rinses listed and is considered the "gold standard" of mouthrinses. Based on two studies of 6-month durations, its efficacy in plaque reduction was 48% to 61% and in gingivitis reduction 27% to 67%.[29] The active site of the molecule is cationic and binds to the negatively charged tooth surface. CHX is time dependent and requires a two-step process to be effective. First, it attaches to the teeth and oral tissues and second, it remains in the mouth for up to 12 hours.[15] This property is called substantivity. Fifty percent of a single rinse of CHX may bind to the oral tissues within 15 seconds.[66] Chlorhexidine rinses require a prescription in the United States because the the Food and Drug Administration (FDA) wants professional supervision of its use. The only side effects of CHX are that it stains the teeth (easily removable by rubber cup polishing) and interferes temporarily with taste. It is also available in a nonalcoholic formulation. Several studies have demonstrated that the nonalcoholic formulation is comparable in efficacy to the alcohol-based CHX.[28,49]

The best example of a phenolic mouthrinse is a rinse that contains essential oils (eucalyptol, thymol, methyl salicylate) dissolved in alcohol ranging from 21.6% to 26.9%, pH 4.3. It is currently available in a water base. Its efficacy against plaque reduction (19%–35%) and gingivitis reduction (15%–37%) is more modest than CHX.[29] Compared to CHX, an essential oil rinse has about 60% of the antigingivitis and dental plaque effect.[25]

Cetylpyridinium chloride (CPC, pH 5.5–6.5) represents the quaternary ammonium compounds. The alcohol content is between 14% to 18%. Based on limited studies, its efficacy on plaque reduction and gingivitis reduction is 14% and 24%, respectively.[29] CPC is absorbed into the teeth and oral tissues but does not last long because of low substantivity.

The halogens are the least researched of the antimicrobial mouthrinses, but they will become more important in the future because they are inexpensive, readily available, and effective. Sodium hypochlorite (NaOCl) has been used safely in dentistry primarily in endodontics for many years and has proven to be effective against microorganisms, funguses, and viruses. Unlike CHX, which is time sensitive to be effective, NaOCl acts by direct contact. It lacks the substantivity of CHX. It is clear and has neutralizing and deodorizing properties. In a 3-week study, participants who used 15 cc of 0.05% NaOCl twice daily experienced a 48% reduction in supragingival plaque.[23] Galvin and colleagues performed a 3-month study using a 0.25% solution of NaOCl with participants rinsing twice weekly and experienced a 58% reduction in supragingival plaque.[37] Slots recommends a 0.2% to 0.3% NaOCl solution for supragingival rinsing. The same concentration has been used with positive results in lavaging periodontal pockets prior to scaling and root planing.[84]

There is less evidence to support the antiplaque properties of povidone iodine (10% sol. 1% iodine) as a mouthrinse and its effect on supragingival plaque.[2] Povidone iodine (PVI) is reported to kill periodontopathic bacteria in vitro within 15 to 30 seconds, which would make it valuable in periodontal therapy.[84] Like

NaOCl, PVI kills by direct contact and is effective again *S. mutans*. In addition to its antimicrobial properties, it has a mild anesthetic effect. DenBesten and Berkowitz used it as a topical application on the teeth of high caries–risk children and found that it reduced mutans streptococci and lactobacilli for up to 3 months.[24] Berkowitz and colleagues were also able to decrease mutans streptococci for up to 3 months in high caries-risk children.[14] It may be used topically to remove supragingival plaque, as a subgingival lavage, or as a coolant in conjunction with an ultrasonic scaler.[77,80] The only objection to using iodine is its strong metallic taste when used as a rinse. It is less objectionable when applied topically for a minute and wiped or rinsed with water. The only precaution is that it not be used in persons with hyperthyroidism.

## Toothpaste

Since toothpastes are used more frequently than mouthrinses, manufacturers have made progress in incorporating antimicrobial entities into their products. In addition to cleaning the tooth surface with a mild abrasive, the two most common antimicrobial ingredients are stabilized stannous fluoride and triclosan/copolymer. The commercial products containing both these ingredients have received the ADA Seal of Acceptance. Although the FDA placed a ban on many over-the-counter products containing triclosan due to concerns about the effects of triclosan on the environment and promotion of bacterial resistance, the FDA excluded toothpastes from this ban because the health benefits outweighed the risks.[33-35]

Davies reviewed 16 clinical trials, each lasting at least 6 months, in which adults brushed with triclosan/copolymer and fluoride toothpastes. The triclosan/copolymer (pH 7.5) averaged a 30% decrease in supragingival plaque compared with the fluoride toothpaste.[22] It was also found to be effective in decreasing plaque and gingivitis in unsupervised studies.[40] In the United States, new formulations in toothpaste technology may replace triclosan because of FDA requirements.

Another systematic review, comparing a stannous fluoride toothpaste with a sodium fluoride toothpaste, concluded that the stannous fluoride toothpaste reduced gingivitis compared to the sodium toothpaste. The magnitude of the differences in gingivitis and plaque were difficult to determine because of the heterogeneity of the studies.[71] Also, the stannous fluoride toothpaste was less effective than the triclosan/copolymer toothpaste as an antiplaque and antigingivitis agent.[38]

In addition to adding antimicrobial agents to toothpastes, anticalculus and neutralizing agents were developed for incorporation into toothpaste.[44,89] Fleisch found that pyrophosphates prevented calcification by interfering with the conversion of amorphous calcium phosphate to hydroxyapatite.[30] When this was coupled with the observation that low calculus formers had higher concentrations of pyrophosphates than high calculus formers, the background was set for commercial development of anticalculus toothpaste.[58] Pyrophosphates in concentrations of 3.35% to 5% inhibited supragingival calculus formation when used with fluorides. It is important to point out that the remineralization of enamel and fluoride in demineralized enamel does not interfere with the crystal-inhibiting power of the pyrophosphate.[1] A review of the many agents that enhance pyrophosphates, such as copolymers, zinc citrate, and triclosan, appeared in *Advances in Dental Research*.[1]

One manufacturer of toothpastes has added sodium bicarbonate with the hope of neutralizing the acidity in plaque. It was also combined with a 1.3% pyrophosphate to formulate toothpaste. One of the more promising agents to be added to toothpastes is arginine. Although it is being developed as an anticaries agent, it will indirectly influence the gingival tissues by altering the pH of the plaque and causing less irritation to the gingiva. Originally discovered in saliva, bacteria in the plaque can metabolize arginine to ammonia, which neutralizes acid, thus raising the plaque pH.[47] When 1.5% arginine is combined with fluoride in a toothpaste, it has a greater anticaries effect than a fluoride toothpaste.[95] Currently, arginine is available in the United States as a desensitizing agent, but it is not available as a toothpaste with fluoride.

## Community Programs for Controlling Periodontal Disease

In the United States, 7.8% of the population have severe periodontitis and are high-risk periodontal patients.[27] Even with intensive periodontal therapy such as scaling and root planing supplemented with antimicrobial agents, many of these susceptible individuals will lose their teeth and become edentulous. Plaque control and removal of calculus is critical for the high-risk population. However, even with dental care this may be insufficient.

A cornerstone of public health programs has always been dental health education to improve oral hygiene and dental health. Although evaluating their effectiveness is difficult to determine, several Scandinavian countries have demonstrated successful public health programs.[39,43]

Frandsen proposed a total population approach.[36,75] In the overall strategy, manpower includes educating dentists about prevention, greater utilization of dental hygienists, midlevel providers, and nondental professionals such as school teachers. Interprofessional education opens the door to working with physicians, nurses, pharmacists, and allied health workers. All of these individuals can be instrumental in advancing the prevention message to the population. This will be a good opportunity to employ the principles of combining interprofessional education and health literacy.[7]

Taking the health education message to the broader audience might benefit from partnering with commercial advertisers who have experience in getting messages to the population. This is an opportunity to show that dental infections place a burden on the immune system and are risk factors in individuals with diabetes, cigarette smokers, smokeless tobacco users, and individuals with systemic diseases. The critical issue with this approach is twofold: educating all of the providers about the periodontal disease message and having providers who internalize the message and integrate it into every encounter they have with patients. Whatever public oral hygiene programs are launched, their impact might be greater on populations with little exposure to the middle class values targeted by advertisers. Perhaps targeting of the population below the poverty level by advertisers might be fruitful. Whatever programs are developed, they will need to be accepted by the target population and periodically monitored for effectiveness and maintained with a broad base of resources.

## Acknowledgment

The author is indebted to Ernest Newbrun, DMD, PhD, for his constructive and critical comments. Additional thanks are extended to Raul Garcia, DMD, CAGS, MMsc, and David Cappelli, DMD, MPH, PhD.

# References

1. Adams D. Calculus-inhibition agents: a review of recent clinical trials. *Adv Dent Res.* 1995;9(4):410–418.
2. Addy M. Oral hygiene products: potential for harm to oral and systemic health? *Periodontol 2000.* 2008;48:54–65.
3. Albadar JM, Rams TE. Global epidemiology of periodontal diseases: an overview. *Periodontol 2000.* 2002;29:7–10.
4. Alfano MC. Controversies, perspectives and clinical implications of nutrition in periodontal disease. *Dent Clin North Am.* 1976;20(3):519–548.
5. Ariaudo AA, Arnim SS, Greene JC, Löe H. In our opinion: how frequently must patients carry out effective oral hygiene procedures in order to maintain gingival health? *J Periodontol.* 1971;42(5):309–313.
6. Asakawa M, Takeshita T, Furuta M, et al. Tongue microbiota and oral health status in community-dwelling elderly adults. *mSphere.* 2018;3(4). e00332-18. https://doi.org/10.1128/mSphere.00332-18.
7. Atchison KA, Rozier RG, Weintraub JA. Integrating oral health, primary care, and health literacy: considerations for health professional practice, education and policy. In: *Roundtable on Health Literacy of the National Academies of Sciences, Engineering and Medicine;* 2017. Available from: http://nationalacademies.org/hmd/~/media/Files/Activity%20Files/PublicHealth/HealthLiteracy/Commissioned%20Papers%20-Updated%202017/Atchison%20K%20et%20al%20 2017%20Integrating%20oral%20health%20primary%20care%20 and%20health%20literacy.pdf. Accessed May 23, 2019.
8. Axelsson PA. Commentary: periodontitis is preventable. *J Periodontol.* 2014;85(10):1303–1307.
9. Axelsson P, Nyström B, Lindhe J. The long-term effect of a plaque control program on tooth mortality, caries and periodontal disease in adults. Results after 30 years of maintenance. *J Clin Periodontol.* 2004;31(9):749–757.
10. Bader JD, Rozier RG, McFall WT Jr, et al. Association of dental health knowledge with periodontal conditions among regular patients. *Community Dent Oral Epidemiol.* 1990;18(1):32–36.
11. Berchier CE, Slot DE, Haps S, Van der Weijden GA. The efficacy of dental floss in addition to a toothbrush on plaque and parameters of gingival inflammation: a systematic review. *Int Dent Hyg.* 2008; 6(4):265–279.
12. Bergenholtz A, Brithon J. Plaque removal by dental floss or toothpicks. An intra-individual comparative study. *J Clin Periodontol.* 1980;7(6):516–524.
13. Bergenholtz A, Olsson A. Efficacy of plaque-removal using interdental brushes and waxed dental floss. *Scand J Dent Res.* 1984; 92(3):198–203.
14. Berkowitz RJ, Koo H, McDermott MP, et al. Adjunctive chemotherapeutic suppression of mutans streptococci in the setting of severe early childhood caries: an exploratory study. *J Public Health Dent.* 2009;69(3):163–167.
15. Bonesvoll P, Lökken P, Rölla G, et al. Retention of chlorhexidine in the human oral cavity after mouth rinses. *Arch Oral Biol.* 1974; 19(3):209–212.
16. Brownstein CN, Briggs SD, Schweitzer KL, et al. Irrigation with chlorhexidine to resolve naturally occurring gingivitis. A methodologic study. *J Clin Periodontol.* 1990;17(8):588–593.
17. Cancro LP, Fischman SL. The expected effect on oral health of dentl plaque control through mechanical removal. *Periodontol 2000.* 1995;8:6–74.
18. Chancio S. Chemical agents: plaque control, calculus reduction and treatment of dentinal hypersensitivity. *Periodontol 2000.* 1995;8:75–86.
19. Claydon NC. Current concepts in toothbrushing and interdental cleaning. *Periodontol 2000.* 2008;48:10–22.
20. Danser MM, Timmerman MF, IJzerman Y, et al. Evaluation of the incidence of gingival abrasion as a result of toothbrushing. *J Clin Periodontol.* 1998;25(9):701–706.
21. Darveau RP. Periodontitis: a polymicrobial disruption of host homeostasis. *Nat Rev Microbiol.* 2010;8(7):481–490.
22. Davies RM, Ellwood RP, Davies GM. The effectiveness of a toothpaste containing triclosan and polyvinyl-methylethermaleic acid copolymer in improving plaque control and gingiva health. *J Clin Periodontol.* 2004;31(12):1029–1033.
23. De Nardo R, Chiappe V, Gómez M, Romanelli H, Slots J. Effects of 0.05% sodium hypochlorite oral rinse on supragingival biofilm and gingival inflammation. *Int Dent J.* 2012;62(4):208–212.
24. DenBesten P, Berkowitz R. Early childhood caries: an overview with reference to our experience in California. *J Calif Dent Assoc.* 2003; 31(2):139–143.
25. Drisko CL. Periodontal self-care: evidence-based support. *Periodontol 2000.* 2013;62(1):243–255.
26. Eke PI, Dye BA, Wei L, Thornton-Evans GO, Genco RJ. Prevalence of periodontitis in adults in the United States: 2009 and 2010. *J Dent Res.* 2012;91(10):914–920.
27. Eke PI, Thornton-Evans GO, Wei L, et al. Periodontitis in US adults: National Health and Nutrition Examination Survey 2009–2014. *J Am Dent Assoc.* 2018;149(7):576–588.e6.
28. Eldridge KR, Finnie SF, Stephens JA, et al. Efficacy of an alcohol-free chlorhexidine mouthrinse as an antimicrobial agent. *J Prosthet Dent.* 1998;80(6):685–690.
29. Fine DH. Chemical agents to prevent and regulate plaque development. *Periodontol 2000.* 1995;8(1):87–107.
30. Fleisch H, Russell RG, Bisaz S, et al. The influence of pyrophosphate on the transformation of amorphous to crystalline calcium phosphate. *Calcif Tissue Res.* 1968;2(2):49–59.
31. Fleming EB, Nguyen D, Afful J, et al. Prevalence of daily flossing among adults by selected risk factors for periodontal disease—United States, 2009–2014. *J Periodontol.* 2018;89(8):933–939.
32. Flemmig TF, Newman MG, Doherty FM, et al. Supragingival irrigation with 0.6% chlorhexidine in naturally occurring gingivitis: I. 6 months clinical observations. *J Periodontol.* 1990;61:112–117.
33. Food and Drug Administration. Drug approval package. Total toothpaste. *NDA: 20231.* July 11, 1997. Available from: https://www.accessdata.fda.gov/drugsatfda_docs/nda/97//020231_total_toc.cfm.
34. Food and Drug Administration. Safety and effectiveness of health care antiseptics; topical antimicrobial drug products for over-the counter human use. *Fed Reg 2017-27317,* Dec. 20, 2017. Available from: https://www.federalregister.gov/documents/2017/12/20/2017-27317/safety-and-effectiveness-of-health-care-antiseptics-topical-antimicrobial-drug-products-for.
35. Food and Drug Administration. *5 Things to Know about Triclosan.* Dec. 19, 2017. Available from: https://www.fda.gov/ForConsumers/ConsumerUpdates/ucm205999.htm.
36. Frandsen A, ed. *Public health aspects of periodontal disease. Proceedings of a workshop held in Copenhagen, Denmark, Dec. 3–5, 1982.* Chicago, IL: Quintessence; 1984:241–242.
37. Galván M, Gonzalez S, Cohen CL, et al. Periodontal effects of 0.25% sodium hypochlorite twice-weekly oral rinse. A pilot study. *J Periodont Res.* 2014;49(6):696–702.
38. Gunsolley JC. A meta-analysis of six-month studies of antiplaque and antigingivitis agents. *J Am Dent Assoc.* 2006;137(12):1649–1657.
39. Hamp SE, Lindhe J, Fornell J, et al. Effect of a field program based on systematic plaque control on caries and gingivitis in schoolchildren after 3 years. *Community Dent Oral Epidemiol.* 1978;6(1):17–23.
40. Hioe KP, van der Weijden GA. The effectiveness of self-performed mechanical plaque control with triclosan containing toothpastes. *Int J Dent Hyg.* 2005;3(4):192–204.
41. Holt SC, Ebersole JL. *Porphyromonas gingivalis, Treponema denticola,* and *Tannerella forsythia:* the "red complex," a prototype polybacterial pathogenic consortium in periodontitis. *Periodontol 2000.* 2005; 38:72–122.
42. Horne R, Weinman J, Barber N, et al. Concordance, adherence and compliance in medicine taking. In: *Report for the National Coordinating Centre for NHS Service Delivery and Organisation R & D (NCCSDO):* December 2005. Available from: https://www.aph.gov.au/DocumentStore.ashx?id=defbfbc9-5206-42c1-8093-3d408ebbe09f.

43. Hugoson A, Koch G. Thirty year trends in the prevalence and distribution of dental caries in Swedish adults (1973–2003). *Swed Dent J.* 2008;32(2):57–67.

44. Jackson D. The efficacy of 2 percent sodium ricinoleate in toothpaste to reduce gingival inflammation. *Br Dent J.* 1962;112:487–493.

45. Kiger RD, Nylund K, Feller RP. A comparison of proximal plaque removal using floss and interdental brushes. *J Clin Periodontol.* 1991;18(9):681–684.

46. Kimmelman BB, Tassman GC. Research in designs of children's toothbrushes. *J Dent Child.* 1960;27(1):60–64.

47. Kleinberg I, Kanapka J, Chatterjee R, et al. Metabolism of nitrogen by oral mixed bacteria. In: Kleinberg I, Ellison SA, Mandel ID, eds. *Proceedings, Saliva and Dental Caries. Microbiology Abstracts.* New York, NY: Information Retrieval Ltd; 1979:357–377.

48. Lang NP, Cumming BR, Löe H. Toothbrushing frequency as it relates to plaque development and gingival health. *J Periodontol.* 1973;44(7):396–405.

49. Leyes Borrajo JL, Garcia Varela L, Lopez Castro G, et al. Efficacy of chlorhexidine mouthrinses with and without alcohol: a clinical study. *J Periodontol.* 2002;73(3):317–321.

50. Lindhe J, Koch G. The effect of supervised oral hygiene on the gingival of children. Progression and inhibition of gingivitis. *J Periodontal Res.* 1966;1(4):260–267.

51. Lindhe J, Koch G. The effect of supervised oral hygiene on the gingivae of children. *J Periodontal Res.* 1967;2(3):215–220.

52. Lindhe J, Wicén PO. The effects on the gingivae of chewing fibrous foods. *J Periodontal Res.* 1969;4(3):193–200.

53. Lobene RR, Soparkar PM, Newman MB. Use of dental floss. Effect on plaque and gingivitis. *Clin Prev Dent.* 1982;4(1):5–8.

54. Löe H, Theilade E, Jensen SB. Experimental gingivitis in man. *J Periodontol.* 1965;36:177–187.

55. Loesche WJ. Chemotherapy of dental plaque infections. *Oral Sci Rev.* 1976;9:65–107.

56. Lövdal A, Arno A, Schei O, et al. Combined effect of subgingival scaling and controlled oral hygiene on the incidence of gingivitis. *Acta Odontol Scand.* 1961;19:537–555.

57. Macgregor ID, Balding JW. Toothbrushing frequency and personal hygiene in 14-year-old English schoolchildren. *Br Dent J.* 1987;162(4):141–144.

58. Mallatt ME, Beiswanger BB, Stookey GK, et al. Influence of soluble pyrophosphate on calculus formation in adults. *J Dent Res.* 1985;64(9):1159–1162.

59. Marchesan JT, Morelli T, Moss K, et al. Interdental cleaning is associated with decreased oral disease prevalence. *J Dent Res.* 2018;97(7):773–778.

60. Marsh PD. Microbial ecology of dental plaque and its significance in health and disease. *Adv Dent Res.* 1994;8(2):263–271.

61. Marsh PD, Bradshaw DJ. Dental plaque as a biofilm. *J Ind Microbiol.* 1995;15(3):169–175.

62. Mazhari F, Boskabady M, Moeintaghavi A, et al. The effect of toothbrushing and flossing sequence on interdental plaque reduction and fluoride retention: a randomized controlled clinical trial. *J Periodontol.* 2018;89(7):824–832.

63. McCall CM Jr, Szmyd L, Hartman BO, et al. A method for selecting an oral hygiene technic for use in space cabin simulator flights. *J Periodontol.* 1964;35(2):160–165.

64. Michalowicz BS, Diehl SR, Gunsolley JC, et al. Evidence of a substantial genetic basis for risk of adult periodontitis. *J Periodontol.* 2000;71(11):1699–1707.

65. Moller IJ, Poulsen S. Effect of sorbitol-containing chewing gum on the occurrence of dental caries, plaque, and gingivitis. *Tandlaegebladet.* 1974;(1):1–11.

66. Moran JM. Home-use oral hygiene products: mouthrinses. *Periodontol 2000.* 2008;48(1):42–53.

67. Deleted in Review.

68. Newbrun E. Chemical and mechanical removal of plaque. *Compend Contin Educ Dent.* 1985;(Suppl 6):S110–S116.

69. Newton JT, Asimakopoulou K. Behavioral models for periodontal health and disease. *Periodontol 2000.* 2018;78(1):201–211.

70. Nikias MK, Budner NS, Glassman MB, et al. Planning and delivery of dental health care. Compliance with preventive oral home care regimens. In: Holloway PJ, Lennon MA, eds. Oral disease prevention: its implications and applications. Proceedings of the eighth international conference on oral biology, Tokyo, Japan. *J Dent Res.* 1980;59(Spec Issue D, Part II):2216–2225.

71. Paraskevas S, van der Weijden GA. A review of the effects of stannous fluoride on gingivitis. *J Clin Periodontol.* 2006;33(1):1–13.

72. Pedrazzi V, Sato S, de Mattos Mda G, et al. Tongue-cleaning methods: a comparative clinical trial employing a toothbrush and a tongue scraper. *J Periodontol.* 2004;75(7):1009–1012.

73. Petersen PE, Baehni PC. Periodontal health and global public health. *Periodontol 2000.* 2012;60:7–14.

74. Petersen PE, Bourgeois D, Ogawa H, et al. The global burden of oral diseases and risks to oral health. *Bull World Health Organ.* 2005;83:661–669.

75. Pilot T. Implementation of preventive periodontal programmes at the community level. In: Frandsen A, ed. *Public Health Aspects of Periodontal Disease. Proceedings of a Workshop Held in Copenhagen, Denmark, December 3–5.* Chicago, IL: Quintessence; 1984:181–196.

76. Pratt L. The significance of the family in medication. *J Comp Family Studies.* 1973;4(1):13–35.

77. Rams TE, Slots J. Local delivery of antimicrobial agents in the periodontal pocket. *Periodontol 2000.* 1996;10:139–159.

78. Reece JA, Swallow JN. Carrots and dental health. *Br Dent J.* 1970;128(11):535–539.

79. Rosier BT, De Jager M, Zaura E, et al. Historical and contemporary hypotheses on the development of oral diseases: are we there yet? *Front Cell Infect Microbiol.* 2014;4:92.

80. Rosling BG, Slots J, Christersson LA, et al. Topical antimicrobial therapy and diagnosis of subgingival bacteria in the management of inflammatory periodontal disease. *J Clin Periodontol.* 1986;13(10):975–981.

81. Sackett DL, Snow JC. The magnitude of compliance and non-compliance. In: Haynes RB, Sackett DL, Taylor DW, eds. *Compliance in Health Care.* Baltimore, MD: John Hopkins University Press; 1979:11–22.

82. Sambunjak D, Nickerson JW, Poklepovic T, et al. Flossing for the management of periodontal diseases and dental caries in adults. *Cochrane DB Syst Rev.* 2011;7(12):CD008829.

83. Sheiham A. Section 6: Prevention and control of periodontal disease. Position report and review of literature. In: *International Conference on Research in the Biology of Periodontal Disease.* Chicago, IL: University of Illinois College of Dentistry; 1977:309–376.

84. Slots J. Selection of antimicrobial agents in periodontal therapy. *J Periodontal Res.* 2002;37(5):389–398.

85. Socransky SS, Haffajee AD, Cugini MA, et al. Microbial complexes in subgingival plaque. *J Clin Periodontol.* 1998;25(2):134–144.

86. Suomi JD. Periodontal disease and oral hygiene in an institutionalized population: report of an epidemiological study. *J Periodontol.* 1969;40(1):5–10.

87. Suomi JD. Prevention and control of periodontal disease. *J Am Dent Assoc.* 1971;83(6):1271–1287.

88. Suomi JD, Greene JC, Vermillion JR, et al. The effect of controlled oral hygiene procedures on the progression of periodontal disease in adults: results after third and final year. *J Periodontol.* 1971;42(3):152–160.

89. Suomi JD, Horowitz HS, Barbano JP, et al. A clinical trial of a calculus-inhibitory toothpaste. *J Periodontol.* 1974;45(3):139–145.

90. Tonzetich J. Production and origin of oral malodor: a review of mechanisms and methods of analysis. *J Periodontol.* 1977;48(1):13–20.

91. Van der Weijden GA, Timmerman MF, Reijerse E, et al. Toothbrushing force in relation to plaque removal. *J Clin Periodontol.* 1996;23(8):724–729.

92. Vieira AR, Albandar JM. Role of genetic factors in the pathogenesis of aggressive periodontitis. *Periodontol 2000*. 2014;65(1):92–106.

93. Waerhaug J. The interdental brush and its place in operative and crown and bridge dentistry. *J Oral Rehabil*. 1976;3(2):107–113.

94. Weinstein P, Getz T, Milgrom P. Oral self-care: a promising alternative behavior model. *J Am Dent Assoc*. 1983;107(1):67–70.

95. Wolff MS, Schenkel AB. The anticaries efficacy of a 1.5% arginine and fluoride toothpaste. *Adv Dent Res*. 2018;29(1):93–97.

96. World Health Organization. *Oral Health Surveys Basic Methods*. 4th ed. Geneva, Switzerland: World Health Organization; 1997.

97. World Health Organization. *Preventing Chronic Disease—A Vital Investment*. Geneva, Switzerland: World Health Organization; 2005.

98. Yaacob M, Worthington HV, Deacon SA, et al. Powered versus manual toothbrushing for oral health. *Cochrane DB Syst Rev*. 2014;(6): CD002281.

# 28

# Tobacco Control and Oral Health

SCOTT L. TOMAR, DMD, MPH, DRPH

BENJAMIN W. CHAFFEE, DDS, MPH, PhD

## CHAPTER OUTLINE

## Introduction

Tobacco use is a major risk factor for diseases affecting nearly every organ in the human body, and it is the leading preventable cause of premature mortality in the United States and worldwide.[66] On average, cigarette smokers die 10 years earlier than nonsmokers,[38] and there are more than 480,000 deaths each year—about one in five deaths—directly attributable to tobacco use in the United States.[38] Worldwide, tobacco use causes nearly 6 million deaths per year, and current trends show that tobacco use will cause more than 8 million deaths annually by 2030.[72] As staggering as the death toll is due to tobacco use, for every person who dies because of smoking, at least 30 people live with a serious smoking-related illness.[65] More than 50 years after the U.S. Surgeon General declared that there was sufficient evidence to conclude that smoking caused cancer in humans,[60] each day more than 3200 people younger than 18 years of age smoke their first cigarette.[66]

The history of tobacco use began in the Americas, where indigenous peoples in Central and South America started cultivating tobacco for social and sacred purposes about 5000 years ago.[62] Tobacco was introduced to Europeans in 1492, when tobacco leaves were offered to Christopher Columbus in the West Indies as a token of friendship. The explorers brought tobacco back to Europe, where its use rapidly grew. Although tobacco was a major cash crop in the Americas throughout the colonial period and early American history (and fueled the slave trade), the modern history of tobacco use really began 1880 with the invention of the Bonsack cigarette machine.[7] The mechanization of cigarette manufacturing increased production from four cigarettes per minute to 200 per minute, dramatically revolutionizing the industry and largely enabling the global epidemic of tobacco use. The subsequent fortunes amassed by cigarette companies provided them with the political and economic power to massively promote tobacco use and addiction and to avoid meaningful regulation for more than a century. Large transnational corporations dominate today's tobacco industry, with net sales of the world's seven largest tobacco companies exceeding $150 billion annually.[53] Looking at the tobacco epidemic through the classic epidemiologic perspective of agent, host, and vector, tobacco is the causative agent for death and disease, humans are the hosts who experience those adverse health effects, but tobacco manufacturers are the vectors propagating the epidemic.

## Tobacco Products

**Cigarettes** remain the most common form of tobacco used in the United States. Mass-produced and consisting of processed tobacco and additives in a paper wrapper, cigarettes are designed for rapid delivery of nicotine to the brain. Although nicotine is the addictive chemical in tobacco, cigarettes deliver thousands of other compounds, including toxins and dozens of human carcinogens.[63] Irrefutable evidence causally links cigarette smoking to death and serious illness affecting virtually all organs of the body.[66] In addition to cancer and pulmonary and cardiovascular diseases among smokers, exposure to secondhand smoke leads to approximately 50,000 child and adult deaths per year.[65] Cigarette smoking costs US society more than $300 billion annually in healthcare expenditures and lost productivity.[66,73]

Changing social attitudes and effective tobacco control have led to a steady decline in the prevalence of smoking in the United States, from 42% among adults in 1965 to 15% in 2017[9,71]—ongoing progress rightly considered one of 10 great public health achievements of the 20th century.[8] Despite this meaningful success, disparities in smoking remain, particularly among groups who are harder to reach with tobacco control policies. Smoking prevalence remains persistently higher in rural areas, low-income populations, and among some racial/ethnic and gender minorities.[36]

**Cigars, pipes, and other combustible tobacco** products are used less often than cigarettes but in aggregate account for a substantial portion the of US tobacco market. Large cigars can contain as much tobacco as a pack of cigarettes and deliver enough nicotine to establish dependence.[29] Little cigars and cigarillos resemble cigarettes in appearance and health risks, yet because they are nominally marketed as cigars, these products often evade flavor restrictions and cigarette excise taxes, thus increasing appeal to youth and low-income populations.[52]

**Smokeless tobacco (ST)** includes a range of noncombustible tobacco products placed in the oral cavity: most prominently in the United States, chewing tobacco and oral moist snuff. ST use is much higher among men than women in the United States, with the prevalence of use notably elevated among young adults, rural dwellers, and lower socioeconomic groups.[31] While cigarette smoking has declined among US adolescents, youth use of ST has remained largely unchanged for more than a decade.[1]

In the mid-2010s, the multinational cigarette makers Altria and Reynolds America purchased the major American ST manufacturers, followed by a dramatic increase in ST marketing expenditures.[20] New marketing campaigns aimed to reposition ST as more attractive to mainstream cigarette smokers.[16] Around that time, ST products modeled after Swedish snus—a lower carcinogen, drier, high-nicotine form of oral snuff—were introduced in the United States.[28] However, snus sold in the United States does not necessarily contain lower carcinogen levels than conventional ST.[54]

**Hookah**, also known as waterpipe, shisha, narghile, or goza, involves inhaling tobacco smoke that has passed through water. Hookah has been used for centuries in parts of South Asia and the Middle East. More recently, hookah use substantially increased in popularity in other parts of the world, especially among adolescent and young adults,[46] often under the perception that hookah use is associated with few health risks.[49] However, hookah smoking exposes individuals to levels of nicotine, smoke, and carbon monoxide comparable to or exceeding those resulting from cigarette smoking.[18]

**Electronic cigarettes** are part of a heterogeneous class of battery-powered electronic nicotine delivery systems commonly referred to as vapor pens, e-hookah, or e-cigarettes. E-cigarettes heat a liquid mixture, typically consisting of propylene glycol or glycerin, nicotine, flavorings, and other additives, and deliver a nicotine-containing aerosol ("vapor") to the user.[24] As e-cigarettes do not burn tobacco, users are exposed to significantly lower levels of carcinogens and other toxins than found in cigarette smoke. Thus, the products have been marketed heavily as less harmful than smoking.[17,24] E-cigarette awareness and use expanded rapidly after 2010, and by 2014, e-cigarettes surpassed conventional cigarettes as the tobacco product used most commonly among high school students.[35]

Despite lower carcinogen levels than found in tobacco smoke, e-cigarette aerosol is not free of potentially dangerous chemicals,[25] and no data exist regarding the health implications of long-term use. Concerns have been raised regarding potential effects on pulmonary[12] and cardiovascular[6] health and that e-cigarette experimentation among youth may presage future cigarette smoking.[50] Limited evidence supports e-cigarette efficacy for smoking cessation,[27] yet some public health agencies, notably in the United Kingdom, have embraced e-cigarettes as an alternative to combustible tobacco.[42] US public health agencies have been more cautious, leaving clinicians and public health practitioners to evaluate new evidence as it accumulates.

## Prevalence of Tobacco Use

Although cigarette smoking remains the leading preventable cause of premature death in the United States, the prevalence of this behavior among adults is now at its lowest point since the federal government began tracking it in 1965 (Figure 28.1). In the mid-1960s, more than one-half of men and more than one-third of women in this country were smokers. In 2018, 15.6% of men and 12.1% of women were current smokers.[44] Similarly, the prevalence of smoking among high school seniors—a period that typically marks the transition from adolescence to adulthood—is at the lowest level since monitoring began in 1975[39] (Figure 28.2).

ST use in the United States has long been most prevalent among adolescent and young adult males.[57] The prevalence of past-30-day use of ST among male high school seniors was declining for more than decade, from a high of 23.6% in 1995 to 11.0% in 2006.[39] The prevalence of ST use then increased for several years, reaching 15.8% in 2009, during the period in which Reynolds American and Altria largely took over the ST market and invested in new products and promotions.[57] The prevalence of past-30-day ST use has since been gradually declining and was estimated at 9.9% in 2017, not much lower than the prevalence of smoking (10.6%).[39] In 2017, about 4% of adult males in the United States reported current ST use.[69] The emerging pattern of ST use in recent years is one of dual use: Nearly 40% of male high school students and 15% of adult males who used ST daily were also current smokers.[57]

Hookah smoking has been widespread in the Middle East and South Asia for centuries but gained popularity in the United States in the early 2000s.[46] As with most tobacco products, the increase of hookah smoking in this country occurred mostly among

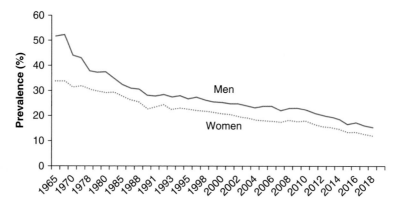

• **Figure 28.1** Prevalence of current* cigarette smoking among adults. United States, 1965–2018. (*Smoked ≥100 cigarettes lifetime and now smoke every day or some days)

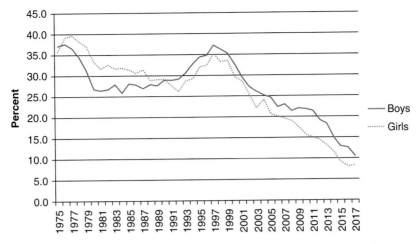

• **Figure 28.2** Prevalence of cigarette smoking* among high school seniors, 1975–2017. (*Smoked on ≥1 of the 30 days preceding the survey)

adolescents and young adults. The prevalence of hookah smoking among US high school students peaked at about 9% in 2014 and has been declining since then, and it was estimated at 3.3% in 2017.[69] Similarly, the prevalence of past-30-day hookah smoking among college students peaked in 2013 at about 10% but has since declined to less than 3% in 2018.[3] Hookah smoking remains relatively rare among US adults, with current prevalence of hookah smoking estimated at less than 1% in 2017.[69]

Use of e-cigarettes is currently the most prevalent form of tobacco use among young people in the United States.[70] In 2017, an estimated 12% of US high school students used e-cigarettes in the preceding 30 days, down from the peak of 16% reported in 2015.[70] In 2017, fewer than 3% of US adults used e-cigarettes.[69]

## Adverse Effects on Oral Health

All tobacco products carry their own documented or probable adverse oral health effects. Cigarette smoking has been well established as a major preventable risk factor for cancer of the oral cavity and pharynx and is responsible for the majority of those neoplasms.[32,64] More than 60 confirmed carcinogens have been identified in cigarette smoke in addition to thousands of other chemical compounds, many of which are toxic. Other combusted tobacco products, such as cigars, produce smoke that generally contains the same carcinogenic agents as cigarettes and, consequently, also have been identified as risk factors for head and neck cancer.[43,48] Although some of those carcinogens are produced by burning tobacco, very high levels of a class of carcinogens known as tobacco-specific N-nitrosamines (TSNA) are present in smokeless tobacco products. The typical pattern of ST use involves keeping the product in the oral cavity throughout the day and leaves the user exposed to high levels of TSNA. Comprehensive reviews conducted by the International Agency for Research on Cancer and the U.S. Department of Health and Human Services have concluded that use of smokeless tobacco is a cause of oral cancer.[33,61] Smokeless tobacco use also increases the risk for lesions on oral mucosa.[26,59,61]

There is consistent and compelling epidemiologic and laboratory evidence that smoking is a major cause of chronic periodontitis.[64] By one estimate, approximately one-half of chronic periodontitis cases among US adults is attributable to cigarette smoking.[58] The probable mechanisms of disease etiology likely include alterations in periodontal microbiota, impairment of various local immune functions, and interference with periodontal healing mechanisms.[64] Although there are far fewer studies on the periodontal health effects of other combusted tobacco products, there is some evidence that cigar or hookah smoking is associated with periodontitis.[2,41,45] Oral surgical procedures have higher rates of complications and poorer wound healing among smokers than among nonsmokers.[56,51,37] Rapidly accumulating evidence is consistent in suggesting that smoking increases the risk for failure of dental implants.[30,11,55] Although only a few studies reported an association between smokeless tobacco use and periodontitis,[5,22] its use is strongly associated with localized gingival recession.[61]

## Reducing Tobacco Use

Effective tobacco control requires a comprehensive approach that combines educational, clinical, regulatory, economic, and social strategies.[10] Dentists and dental hygienists can play a critical role within a comprehensive tobacco control strategy, including advocacy on the political front, community education, and counseling individual patients.

## Comprehensive Tobacco Control

There is widespread consensus among public health experts that the most effective approach to reducing tobacco use—and its resulting devastating health effects—is comprehensive tobacco control. The goals of comprehensive tobacco control efforts are to prevent initiation of tobacco use by young people, to promote quitting, to eliminate exposure to secondhand tobacco smoke, and to identify and eliminate tobacco-related disparities among population groups.[10] The elements of a comprehensive tobacco control approach include state and community interventions, mass-reach health communication interventions, cessation interventions, surveillance and evaluation, and development of infrastructure, administration, and management to support these initiatives.

State and community interventions include evidence-based policies and programs that are effective in reducing tobacco use initiation and promoting cessation. One of the earliest and most effective tobacco control policies is to raise the unit price of tobacco products through excise taxes.[15,34,71] This policy is based on consistent evidence that, like many consumer products, tobacco use follows a basic principle of economics: Consumption of tobacco products declines as the cost of those products increase. Increasing tobacco prices leads to lower rates of initiation, increases quit rates, reduces consumption among those who continue to use tobacco, increases worker productivity (due to better health), and reduces healthcare costs.[34,15]

Smoke-free policies are public-sector regulations and private-sector rules that prohibit smoking in indoor spaces and designated public areas.[13] State and local ordinances establish smoke-free standards for all or some indoor workplaces, indoor spaces, and outdoor public places. Private-sector smoke-free policies may ban all tobacco use on private property or restrict smoking to designated outdoor locations. There is strong evidence that smoke-free policies are effective in reducing exposure to secondhand smoke, reducing the prevalence of tobacco use, increasing the number of tobacco users who quit, reducing the initiation of tobacco use among young people, and reducing tobacco-related morbidity and mortality, including acute cardiovascular events.[13,23] In addition, economic evidence indicates that smoke-free policies can reduce healthcare costs substantially and do not have an adverse economic impact on businesses, including bars and restaurants.[13]

There is strong evidence that mass-reach health communication interventions, such as the national "Truth" campaign that began in 2000,[19] can be powerful tools for preventing the initiation of tobacco use, promoting and facilitating cessation, and shaping social norms related to tobacco use.[14] Through vehicles such as television, radio, and social media, these widespread health communications interventions and tobacco countermarketing campaigns can make meaningful changes in population-level awareness, knowledge, attitudes, and behaviors.[10]

Promoting cessation is a core component of comprehensive tobacco control. Population-wide cessation efforts—including policy, systems, or environmental changes—are the most efficient and effective at reaching many people.[10] Comprehensive tobacco control cessation activities focus on promoting health systems change that support individual behavior change, expanding insurance coverage and use of effective evidence-based cessation treatments, and supporting the capacity of quitlines.

Comprehensive tobacco control programs need to have accountability and demonstrate effectiveness. These programs need timely data that can be used for program improvement and decision-making. Therefore, a surveillance and evaluation system that can monitor and document key short-term, intermediate, and long-term outcomes within populations is a critical infrastructure component of any comprehensive tobacco control program.[10]

Finally, comprehensive tobacco control programs require considerable funding to implement.[10] Therefore these programs must have a fully functioning infrastructure in place to achieve the capacity to implement effective interventions. That infrastructure includes appropriate leadership, staffing, and financial support to be able to operate an effective comprehensive tobacco control program.

## Tobacco Regulation

In 1996, the U.S. Food and Drug Administration (FDA) attempted to regulate cigarettes and smokeless tobacco under the Federal Food, Drug, and Cosmetic Act, under the premise that nicotine is an active drug that tobacco products are intended to deliver.[40] However, the U.S. Supreme Court ruled in 2000 that the FDA was not authorized to regulate tobacco. Later, in 2009, the Family Smoking Prevention and Tobacco Control Act explicitly granted the FDA regulatory authority over tobacco products, including their marketing, warning labels, and nicotine content.[4] Actions under the Tobacco Control Act include banning characterizing flavors in cigarettes and new funding for public information campaigns and research. The FDA officially asserted its authority to regulate all forms of tobacco products in 2016 but 1 year later announced that it would delay any regulatory process for e-cigarettes until 2022.[67]

Some of the most impactful and innovative tobacco regulation occurs at the state and local levels. State excises taxes and comprehensive smoke-free air laws that ban smoking in public areas and workplaces are two of the most powerful policy tools for reducing smoking prevalence.[10,13] Recently, local jurisdictions have considered measures to ban menthol and other flavors in all tobacco products to reduce appeal to youth and to extend existing smoking restrictions to the use of e-cigarettes and other tobacco.

## What Dental Professionals Can Do

Oral healthcare professionals have a potentially major role to play in educating patients about the hazards of tobacco use and in helping patients to quit.[68] *Treating Tobacco Use and Dependence*, a clinical practice guideline issued by the U.S. Public Health Service, provides recommendations for clinicians on evidence-based, effective steps that dentists, dental hygienists, and other healthcare providers can use to treat tobacco use and dependence.[21] The 10 key recommendations from those guidelines are summarized in Box 28.1.

Leading health authorities recommend that all clinicians provide "The 5 As" for all of their patients who use tobacco products (Table 28.1): **ask** about patients' tobacco use at every visit; **advise** all tobacco users to quit; **assess** every tobacco users' readiness to quit; **assist** tobacco users with a quit plan; and **arrange** follow-up visits for those trying to quit.[21]

While oral health professionals are encouraged to provide active, evidence-based counseling and assistance for their patients who are willing to try quitting tobacco use, there are brief alternative approaches that bring in the expertise of professional behavioral interventionists. Some of these alternatives include the Ask, Advise, and Refer model, in which healthcare providers **ask** their patients about their use of tobacco products, **advise** current users to quit, and **refer** interested patients to a counselor or a telephone quitline.[47] Many state health departments operate free tobacco quitlines, and the U.S. Department of Health and Human Services provides a national toll-free number (1-800-QUITNOW) that will route callers to the appropriate service in their area.

Dentists and dental hygienists do not necessarily need to be behavioral counselors if they are not comfortable in that role, but they do have a professional obligation to help treat tobacco addiction by enhancing patients' motivation to quit and connecting them with appropriate support. Tobacco cessation resources should be available in every dental office, and helping patients to become tobacco-free needs to be a primary step in any dental treatment plan. After all, tobacco use is a serious matter—in fact, it is a matter of life and death.

## BOX 28.1   Ten Key Recommendations from Treating Tobacco Use and Dependence: 2008 Update[21]

1. Tobacco dependence is a chronic disease that often requires repeated intervention and multiple attempts to quit. Effective treatments exist, however, that can significantly increase rates of long-term abstinence.
2. It is essential that clinicians and healthcare delivery systems consistently identify and document tobacco use status and treat every tobacco user seen in a healthcare setting.
3. Tobacco dependence treatments are effective across a broad range of populations. Clinicians should encourage every patient willing to make a quit attempt to use the counseling treatments and medications recommended in this Guideline.
4. Brief tobacco dependence treatment is effective. Clinicians should offer every patient who uses tobacco at least the brief treatments shown to be effective in this Guideline.
5. Individual, group, and telephone counseling are effective, and their effectiveness increases with treatment intensity. Two components of counseling are especially effective, and clinicians should use these when counseling patients making a quit attempt:
   - Practical counseling (problem-solving/skills training)
   - Social support delivered as part of treatment
6. Numerous effective medications are available for tobacco dependence, and clinicians should encourage their use by all patients attempting to quit smoking—except when medically contraindicated or with specific populations for which there is insufficient evidence of effectiveness (i.e., pregnant women, smokeless tobacco users, light smokers, and adolescents).
   - Seven first-line medications (5 nicotine and 2 non-nicotine) reliably increase long-term smoking abstinence rates:
     - Bupropion SR
     - Nicotine gum
     - Nicotine inhaler
     - Nicotine lozenge
     - Nicotine nasal spray
     - Nicotine patch
     - Varenicline
   - Clinicians also should consider the use of certain combinations of medications identified as effective in this Guideline.
7. Counseling and medication are effective when used by themselves for treating tobacco dependence. The combination of counseling and medication, however, is more effective than either alone. Thus, clinicians should encourage all individuals making a quit attempt to use both counseling and medication.
8. Telephone quitline counseling is effective with diverse populations and has broad reach. Therefore, both clinicians and healthcare delivery systems should ensure patient access to quitlines and promote quitline use.
9. If a tobacco user currently is unwilling to make a quit attempt, clinicians should use the motivational treatments shown in this Guideline to be effective in increasing future quit attempts.
10. Tobacco dependence treatments are both clinically effective and highly cost-effective relative to interventions for other clinical disorders. Providing coverage for these treatments increases quit rates. Insurers and purchasers should ensure that all insurance plans include the counseling and medication identified as effective in this Guideline as covered benefits.

## TABLE 28.1   The 5 As Model for Treating Tobacco Use and Dependence[21]

| | |
|---|---|
| **As**k about tobacco use. | Identify and document tobacco use status for every patient at every visit. |
| **Ad**vise to quit. | In a clear, strong, and personalized manner, urge every tobacco user to quit. |
| **As**sess willingness to make a quit attempt. | Is the tobacco user willing to make a quit attempt at this time? |
| **As**sist in quit attempt. | For the patient willing to make a quit attempt, offer medication and provide or refer for counseling or additional treatment to help the patient quit. For patients unwilling to quit at the time, provide interventions designed to increase future quit attempts. |
| **Ar**range follow-up. | For the patient willing to make a quit attempt, arrange for follow-up contacts, beginning within the first week after the quit date. For patients unwilling to make a quit attempt at the time, address tobacco dependence and willingness to quit at next clinic visit. |

From Fiore MC, Jaén CR, Baker TB, et al. *Treating Tobacco Use and Dependence: 2008 Update. Clinical Practice Guideline.* Rockville, MD: U.S. Department of Health and Human Services. Public Health Service; 2008. Available from: www.ahrq.gov/professionals/clinicians-providers/guidelines-recommendations/tobacco/index.html.

## References

1. Agaku IT, Vardavas CI, Ayo-Yusuf OA, et al. Temporal trends in smokeless tobacco use among US middle and high school students, 2000–2011. *JAMA.* 2013;309(19):1992–1994.
2. Albandar JM, Streckfus CF, Adesanya MR, et al. Cigar, pipe, and cigarette smoking as risk factors for periodontal disease and tooth loss. *J Periodontol.* 2000;71(12):1874–1881.
3. American College Health Association. *National College Health Assessment Reference Group Data Report, Spring 2018.* Silver Spring, MD: American College Health Association; 2018. Available from: http://www.acha.org.
4. Ashley DL, Backinger CL. The Food and Drug Administration's regulation of tobacco: the Center for Tobacco Products' Office of Science. *Am J Prev Med.* 2012;43(5 suppl 3):S255–S263.
5. Beck JD, Koch GG, Offenbacher S. Incidence of attachment loss over 3 years in older adults–new and progressing lesions. *Community Dent Oral Epidemiol.* 1995;23(5):291–296.
6. Benowitz NL, Fraiman JB. Cardiovascular effects of electronic cigarettes. *Nat Rev Cardiol.* 2017;14(8):447–456.
7. Brandt AM. *The Cigarette Century: The Rise, Fall, and Deadly Persistence of the Product the Defined America.* New York, NY: Basic Books; 2007.
8. Centers for Disease Control and Prevention. Ten great public health achievements–United States, 1900–1999. *Morb Mortal Wkly Rep.* 1999;48(12):241–243.
9. Centers for Disease Control and Prevention. *Trends in current cigarette smoking among high school students and adults, United States, 1965–2014.* Available from: http://www.cdc.gov/tobacco/data_statistics/tables/trends/cig_smoking/index.htm. Last updated March 30, 2016.
10. Centers for Disease Control and Prevention. *Best practices for comprehensive tobacco control programs—2014.* Atlanta, GA: National Center for Chronic Disease Prevention and Health Promotion, Office on Smoking and Health; 2014.

11. Chrcanovic BR, Albrektsson T, Wennerberg A. Smoking and dental implants: a systematic review and meta-analysis. *J Dent.* 2015;43(5):487–498.

12. Chun LF, Moazed F, Calfee CS, et al. Pulmonary toxicity of e-cigarettes. *Am J Physiol Lung Cell Mol Physiol.* 2017;313(2): L193–L206.

13. Community Preventive Services Task Force. Guide to Community Preventive Services. Tobacco Use and Secondhand Smoke Exposure: Smoke-Free Policies. Available from: https://www. thecommunityguide.org/findings/tobacco-use-and-secondhand-smoke-exposure-smoke-free-policies. Last updated August 21, 2018.

14. Community Preventive Services Task Force. Guide to Community Preventive Services. Tobacco Use and Secondhand Smoke Exposure: Mass-Reach Health Communication Interventions. Available from: https://www.thecommunityguide.org/findings/tobacco-use-and-secondhand-smoke-exposure-mass-reach-health-communication-interventions. Last updated: August 21, 2018.

15. Contreary KA, Chattopadhyay SK, Hopkins DP, et al. Community Preventive Services Task Force. Economic impact of tobacco price increases through taxation: a community guide systematic review. *Am J Prev Med.* 2015;49(5):800–808.

16. Curry LE, Pederson LL, Stryker JE. The changing marketing of smokeless tobacco in magazine advertisements. *Nicotine Tob Res.* 2011;13(7):540–547.

17. de Andrade M, Hastings G, Angus K. Promotion of electronic cigarettes: tobacco marketing reinvented? *Br Med J.* 2013;347:f7473.

18. Eissenberg T, Shihadeh A. Waterpipe tobacco and cigarette smoking. Direct comparison of toxicant exposure *Am J Prev Med.* 2009; 37(6):518–523.

19. Farrelly MC, Nonnemaker J, Davis KC, Hussin A. The influence of the national truth campaign on smoking initiation. *Am J Prev Med.* 2009;36(5):379–384.

20. Federal Trade Commission. Federal Trade Commission smokeless tobacco report for. Washington, DC: Federal Trade Commission; 2015:2017. www.ftc.gov/system/files/documents/reports/federal-trade-commission-cigarette-report-2015-federal-trade-commission-smokeless-tobacco-report/2015_smokeless_tobacco_report.pdf.

21. Fiore MC, Jaén CR, Baker TB, et al. Treating Tobacco Use and Dependence: 2008 Update. Clinical Practice Guideline. Rockville, MD: US Department of Health and Human Services. In: *Public Health Service*. 2008. www.ahrq.gov/professionals/clinicians-providers/guidelines-recommendations/tobacco/index.html.

22. Fisher MA, Taylor GW, Tilashalski KR. Smokeless tobacco and severe active periodontal disease, NHANES III. *J Dent Res.* 2005;84(8):705–710.

23. Frazer K, Callinan JE, McHugh J, et al. Legislative smoking bans for reducing harms from secondhand smoke exposure, smoking prevalence and tobacco consumption. *Cochrane DB Syst Rev.* 2016;(2). CD005992.

24. Glasser AM, Collins L, Pearson JL, et al. Overview of electronic nicotine delivery systems: a systematic review. *Am J Prev Med.* 2017; 52(2):e33–e66.

25. Goniewicz ML, Knysak J, Gawron M, et al. Levels of selected carcinogens and toxicants in vapour from electronic cigarettes. *Tob Control.* 2014;23(2):133–139.

26. Greer RO Jr. Oral manifestations of smokeless tobacco use. *Otolaryngol Clin North Am.* 2011;44(1):31–56.

27. Hartmann-Boyce J, McRobbie H, Bullen C, et al. Electronic cigarettes for smoking cessation. *Cochrane DB Syst Rev.* 2016;(9):Cd010216.

28. Hatsukami DK, Ebbert JO, Feuer RM, Stepanov I, Hecht SS. Changing smokeless tobacco products new tobacco-delivery systems. *Am J Prev Med.* 2007;33(6 suppl):S368–S378.

29. Henningfield JE, Fant RV, Radzius A, et al. Nicotine concentration, smoke ph and whole tobacco aqueous ph of some cigar brands and types popular in the United States. *Nicotine Tob Res.* 1999;1(2):163–168.

30. Hinode D, Tanabe S, Yokoyama M, et al. Influence of smoking on osseointegrated implant failure: a meta-analysis. *Clin Oral Implants Res.* 2006;17(4):473–478.

31. Howard-Pitney B, Winkleby MA. Chewing tobacco: who uses and who quits? Findings from NHANES III, 1988–1994. National Health and Nutrition Examination Survey III. *Am J Public Health.* 2002;92(2):250–256.

32. International Agency for Research on Cancer. IARC Monographs on the Evaluation of Carcinogenic Risks to Humans. In: *Volume. Tobacco Smoke and Involuntary Smoking.* Lyon, France: International Agency for Research on Cancer; 2004:83.

33. International Agency for Research on Cancer. IARC Monographs on the Evaluation of Carcinogenic Risks to Humans. In: *Volume. Smokeless Tobacco and Some Tobacco-Specific N-Nitrosamines.* Lyon, France: International Agency for Research on Cancer; 2007:89.

34. International Agency for Research on Cancer. *IARC Handbooks of Cancer Prevention: Tobacco Control Volume 14. Effectiveness of Price and Tax Policies for Control of Tobacco.* Lyon, France: International Agency for Research on Cancer; 2011.

35. Jamal A, Gentzke A, Hu SS, et al. Tobacco use among middle and high school students—United States, 2011–2016. *Morb Mortal Wkly Rep.* 2017;66(23):597–603.

36. Jamal A, King BA, Neff LJ, et al. Current cigarette smoking among adults—United States, 2016. *Morb Mortal Wkly Rep.* 2018; 67(2):53–59.

37. Javed F, Al-Rasheed A, Almas K, et al. Effect of cigarette smoking on the clinical outcomes of periodontal surgical procedures. *Am J Med Sci.* 2012;343(1):78–84.

38. Jha P, Ramasundarahettige C, Landsman V, et al. 21st century hazards of smoking and benefits of cessation in the United States. *N Engl J Med.* 2013;368:341–350.

39. Johnston LD, Miech RA, O'Malley PM, et al. *Demographic Subgroup Trends Among Adolescents in the Use of Various Licit and Illicit Drugs.* 1975–2017 (Monitoring the Future Occasional Paper No. 90), Ann Arbor, MI: Institute for Social Research, University of Michigan; 2018. Available from: http://www.monitoringthefuture.org/pubs/occpapers/mtf-occ90.pdf.

40. Kessler DA, Witt AM, Barnett PS, et al. The Food and Drug Administration's regulation of tobacco products. *N Engl J Med.* 1996; 335(13):988–994.

41. Krall EA, Garvey AJ, Garcia RI. Alveolar bone loss and tooth loss in male cigar and pipe smokers. *J Am Dent Assoc.* 1999;130(1):57–64.

42. McNeill A, Brose L, Calder R, et al. *E-Cigarettes: An Evidence Update.* London, England: Public Health England; 2015.

43. Munshi T, Heckman CJ, Darlow S. Association between tobacco waterpipe smoking and head and neck conditions: a systematic review. *J Am Dent Assoc.* 2015;146(10):760–766.

44. National Center for Health Statistics. *Early Release of Selected Estimates Based on Data From January–June 2018 National Health Interview Survey.* Atlanta, GA: National Center for Health Statistics; December 2018. Available from: http://www.cdc.gov/nchs/nhis/releases/released2018 12.htm#TechNotes.

45. Ramôa CP, Eissenberg T, Sahingur SE. Increasing popularity of waterpipe tobacco smoking and electronic cigarette use: implications for oral healthcare. *J Periodontal Res.* 2017;52(5):813–823.

46. Salloum RG, Thrasher JF, Kates FR, Maziak W. Water pipe tobacco smoking in the United States: findings from the National Adult Tobacco Survey. *Prev Med.* 2015;71:88–93.

47. Schroeder SA. What to do with a patient who smokes. *JAMA.* 27; 294(4):482–487.

48. Shanks TG, Burns DM. Disease consequences of cigar smoking. In: National Cancer Institute. *Tobacco Control Monograph 9: Cigars: Health Effects and Trends.* Bethesda, MD: US Department of Health and Human Services, National Institutes of Health, National Cancer Institute; 1998.

49. Smith-Simone S, Maziak W, Ward KD, et al. Waterpipe tobacco smoking: knowledge, attitudes, beliefs, and behavior in two U.S. samples. *Nicotine Tob Res.* 2008;10(2):393–398.

50. Soneji S, Barrington-Trimis JL, Wills TA, et al. Association between initial use of e-cigarettes and subsequent cigarette smoking among

adolescents and young adults: a systematic review and meta-analysis. *JAMA Pediatr.* 2017;171(8):788–797.
51. Sørensen LT. Wound healing and infection in surgery: the pathophysiological impact of smoking, smoking cessation, and nicotine replacement therapy. A systematic review. *Ann Surg.* 2012;255(6):1069–1079.
52. Star Tribune. *A Cigarette in All But Its Name.* Minneapolis, MN: Star Tribune; 2011. Available from: http://www.startribune.com/editorial-a-cigarette-in-all-but-its-name/116625028/.
53. Statistica. *Tobacco Industry—Statistics & Facts.* New York, NY: Statistica, Inc.; 2018. Available from: https://www.statista.com/topics/1593/tobacco/.
54. Stepanov I, Biener L, Yershova K, et al. Monitoring tobacco-specific N-nitrosamines and nicotine in novel smokeless tobacco products: findings from round II of the new product watch. *Nicotine Tob Res.* 2014;16(8):1070–1078.
55. Strietzel FP, Reichart PA, Kale A, Kulkarni M, Wegner B, Küchler I. Smoking interferes with the prognosis of dental implant treatment: a systematic review and meta-analysis. *J Clin Periodontol.* 2007;34(6):523–544.
56. Tarakji B, Saleh LA, Umair A, et al. Systemic review of dry socket: aetiology, treatment, and prevention. *J Clin Diagn Res.* 2015;9(4). ZE10-3.
57. Tomar SL, Alpert HR, Connolly GN. Patterns of dual use of cigarettes and smokeless tobacco among US males: findings from national surveys. *Tob Control.* 2010;19(2):104–109.
58. Tomar SL, Asma S. Smoking-attributable periodontitis in the United States: findings from NHANES III. *J Periodontol.* 2000;71(5):743–751.
59. Tomar SL, Winn DM, Swango GA, et al. Oral mucosal smokeless tobacco lesions among adolescents in the United States. *J Dent Res.* 1997;76(6):1277–1286.
60. US Department of Health, Education, and Welfare. *Smoking and Health: Report of the Advisory Committee to the Surgeon General of the Public Health Service.* PHS Publication No. 1103. Washington, DC: US Department of Health, Education, and Welfare; 1964.
61. US Department of Health and Human Services. *The Health Consequences of Using Smokeless Tobacco: A Report of the Advisory Committee to the Surgeon General.* DHHS Publication No. (NIH) 86-2874. Washington, DC: US Department of Health and Human Services; 1986.
62. US Department of Health and Human Services. *Smoking and Health in the Americas.* DHHS Publication No. (CDC) 92-8419. Atlanta, GA: US Department of Health and Human Services; 1992.
63. US Department of Health and Human Services. *Risks Associated with Smoking Cigarettes With Low Machine-Measured Yields of Tar and Nicotine.* Bethesda, MD: US Department of Health and Human Services; 2001.
64. US Department of Health and Human Services. *The Health Consequences of Smoking: A Report of the Surgeon General.* Atlanta, GA: US Department of Health and Human Services; 2004.
65. US Department of Health and Human Services. *The Health Consequences of Involuntary Exposure to Tobacco Smoke: A Report of the Surgeon General.* Atlanta, GA: US Department of Health and Human Services; 2006.
66. US Department of Health and Human Services. *The Health Consequences of Smoking—50 Years of Progress: A Report of the Surgeon General.* Atlanta, GA: US Department of Health and Human Services; 2014.
67. US Food and Drug Administration. *FDA News Release: FDA Announces Comprehensive Regulatory Plan to Shift Trajectory of Tobacco-Related Disease, Death.* July 28, 2017. Available from: http://www.fda.gov/newsevents/newsroom/pressannouncements/ucm568923.htm.
68. Walsh MM, Ellison JA. Treatment of tobacco use and dependence: the role of the dental professional. *J Dent Educ.* 2005;69(5):521–537.
69. Wang TW, Asman K, Gentzke AS, et al. Tobacco product use among adults—United States, 2017. *Morb Mortal Wkly Rep.* 2018;67:1225–1232.
70. Wang TW, Gentzke A, Sharapova S, et al. Tobacco product use among middle and high school students—United States, 2011–2017. *Morb Mortal Wkly Rep.* 2018;67:629–633.
71. Wilson LM, Avila Tang E, Chander G, et al. Impact of tobacco control interventions on smoking initiation, cessation, and prevalence: a systematic review. *J Environ Public Health.* 2012;2012:1–36.
72. World Health Organization. *WHO Report on the Global Tobacco Epidemic.* Geneva, Switzerland: World Health Organization; 2011.
73. Xu X, Bishop EE, Kennedy SM, et al. Annual healthcare spending attributable to cigarette smoking: an update. *Am J Prev Med.* 2015;48(3):326–333.

# Index

Note: Page numbers followed by *f* indicate figures, *t* indicate tables, and *b* indicate boxes.